Rheumatic Diseases in the Arab World

Khalid A. Alnaqbi • Ghaydaa Aldabie
Editors

Rheumatic Diseases in the Arab World

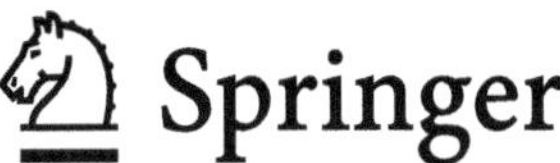

Editors
Khalid A. Alnaqbi
Rheumatology Division
Sheikh Tahnoon bin Mohammed Medical City and Tawam Hospital, SEHA / PureHealth
Al Ain, UAE

College of Medicine
RAK Medical and Health Sciences University
Ras Al Khaimah, UAE

College of Medicine and Health Sciences
UAE University
Al Ain, UAE

Ghaydaa Aldabie
Rheumatology Unit
Farwaniya Hospital
Kuwait City, Kuwait

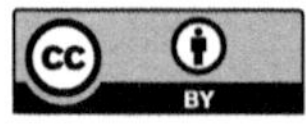

ISBN 978-981-92-0966-8 ISBN 978-981-92-0967-5 (eBook)
https://doi.org/10.1007/978-981-92-0967-5

This Springer imprint is published by the registered company Springer Nature Singapore Pte Ltd.
The registered company address is: 152 Beach Road, #21-01/04 Gateway East, Singapore 189721, Singapore

Foreword

Diseases desperate grown
By desperate appliance are relieved,
Or not at all. —Shakespeare

Shakespeare reminds us that serious diseases need to be taken seriously. That is certainly the case for rheumatic diseases which impose enormous cost in terms of disability and healthcare expenditures, and in terms of symptomatic burden of disease. There is an unmet need to globally address the challenges presented by rheumatic diseases. *Rheumatic Diseases in the Arab World* represents an important step toward addressing that challenge, as it includes 22 countries with a population of over 480 million individuals. This is the first publication to comprehensively address rheumatic diseases in these regions. The book has included a multidisciplinary range of authors who include not only healthcare professionals but also patients.

Respond to every call that excites your spirit. —Rumi

Building a team which incorporates adult and pediatric rheumatologists, nurses, and pharmacists—as well as patients—is a monumental challenge. It could only have been accomplished by the vision and commitment of the lead editors, Prof. Khalid A. Alnaqbi and Dr. Ghaydaa Aldabie. Clearly, the authors felt a call which excited their spirits. To assemble this many professionals from this many countries presented an enormous challenge for the authors. The fact that this has come to successful fruition is testimony to their dedication to the goal of team-building. This clearly will be of major significance for the diagnosis and management of rheumatic diseases in these nations, but also for educators and health policy planners, who now will have country-specific metrics to utilize. Ultimately, it will be the patients with rheumatic diseases who are the major beneficiaries of this comprehensive textbook.

Robert D. Inman, MD, FRCPC, FACP, FRCP Edin
Co-Director Schroeder Arthritis Institute,
Deputy Physician in Chief Research
University Health Network
Professor of Medicine and Immunology
University of Toronto
Toronto, Canada

Preface

It is my great pleasure to introduce *Rheumatic Diseases in the Arab World*, the first comprehensive book dedicated to understanding rheumatic diseases across the Arab region. The Arab world consists of 22 countries across Western Asia, North Africa, and the Horn of Africa, with a combined population of approximately 480 million in 2024. Although culturally and linguistically diverse, the Arab world is united by Arabic as a common language. The region is known for its rich historical heritage as the cradle of numerous ancient civilizations and the birthplace of major world religions.

To date, no comprehensive work has been published that discusses the care of patients with rheumatic diseases in each Arab country in detail. Since completing my graduate and postgraduate training in Toronto, Canada, in December 2012, I have dreamed of leading a project that would engage rheumatologists across the Arab world. This aspiration eventually led to the conception of the present book in 2020.

This landmark reference examines the state of rheumatic diseases across the Arab countries and is authored by a diverse group of nearly 100 expert contributors, including rheumatologists, nurses, pharmacists, and patients predominantly from the Arab region. It is organized around two overarching themes: country-specific chapters and special topics.

The former meticulously examine each Arab nation's healthcare system, rheumatology services for both pediatric and adult patients, and highlight epidemiological and clinical characteristics of rheumatic diseases, clinical research, specialization in rheumatology, and suggestions for service enhancement. Unfortunately, we could not find rheumatologists from Somalia, Djibouti, and the Union of Comoros; however, we were able to write a summary of the available information.

The latter explore key themes shaping rheumatology throughout the region, including the role of the Arab League of Associations for Rheumatology (ArLAR), pediatric rheumatology in the Arab world, the impact of war and conflict on patient care, patient perspectives on living with rheumatic diseases, and future directions for strengthening rheumatology systems across the region.

Designed to serve a broad audience—including rheumatologists, pharmacists, professionals from nonprofit organizations, regulators, epidemiologists, and individuals from the pharmaceutical industry—this book provides a comprehensive resource for understanding rheumatic diseases in the Arab world. It may also serve as a useful reference for graduate and postgraduate education, particularly in addressing clinical questions relevant to patients across the Arab region.

The journey of bringing this book to completion has been both exciting and demanding, requiring many evenings, weekends, and annual leave devoted to reviewing chapters and coordinating with contributors from across the region. Throughout this process, chapters were carefully revised and updated to ensure that the information presented reflects the most current knowledge available. Despite the challenges, the experience has been immensely rewarding and has offered valuable lessons in collaboration, communication, and scholarly editing.

I wish to acknowledge the dedicated authors who generously contributed their time, expertise, and commitment to this project. I am particularly grateful to Dr. Ghaydaa Aldabie, Rheumatology Consultant at Al Farwaniya Hospital (Kuwait) and co-editor of this book, whose invaluable support throughout this project has left me deeply indebted. I also extend my sincere thanks to Dr. Vanessa Shaar and Karine Noufaily, Project Managers at InfoMed, for their administrative assistance during this journey.

In memory of my late mother Mariam, sister Fatima, brother Ali, and uncle Mohammed. Their unwavering belief in me continues to inspire me, and I remain forever indebted. I express profound appreciation to my father, Abdalla, for his continuous love and support throughout my life.

To my beloved wife, Tamador, and our children—Mahra, Mayed, Bader, and Fatima—your enduring love and support have been my greatest blessings.

I wish to extend my heartfelt gratitude to the individuals who have profoundly influenced my medical journey. I am especially grateful to my mentor, Prof. Robert D. Inman (Co-Director of the Spondylitis Program at the University Health Network and Professor of Medicine and Immunology at the University of Toronto), whose guidance and support have been invaluable throughout my career.

During my graduate and postgraduate training in Toronto, I had the privilege of learning from many outstanding rheumatology professors, including Prof. Murray Urowitz and Prof. Dafna Gladman, whose contributions to rheumatology continue to inspire generations of physicians. I am also indebted to Dr. Heather McDonald-Blumer, Dr. Arthur A.M. Bookman, Dr. Carl Laskin, and Dr. Zareen Ahmed for their mentorship and support.

I also wish to acknowledge the late Prof. Earl Dunn (Family Medicine, University of Toronto), who welcomed me warmly and supported me throughout my decade-long journey in Toronto.

Finally, I extend my sincere appreciation to the patients in the Arab world whose resilience and support are truly commendable.

We hope you find this book as fulfilling to read as it was for the authors to write.

Al Ain, Abu Dhabi, UAE Khalid A. Alnaqbi

Contents

About the Editors

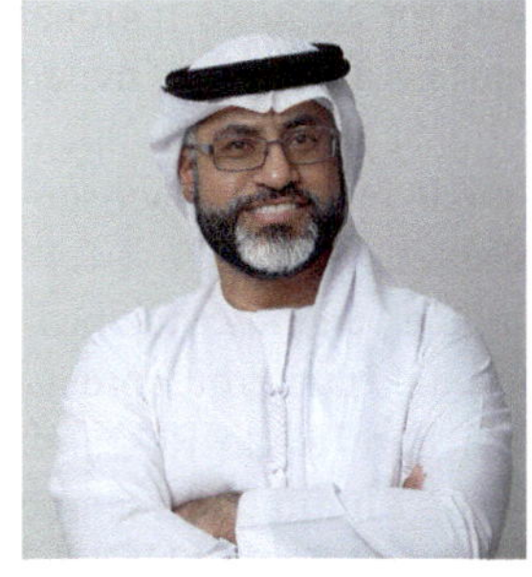

Khalid A. Alnaqbi MBBS, MSc, CCD, FRCPC, FACP, FACR is a Consultant Rheumatologist and Chief of Rheumatology at Sheikh Tahnoon bin Mohammed Medical City and Tawam Hospital in Al Ain, United Arab Emirates (UAE). He holds academic appointments as Adjunct Professor at RAK Medical and Health Sciences University and Adjunct Associate Professor at the College of Medicine and Health Sciences, UAE University. He holds triple board certification from the Royal College of Physicians and Surgeons of Canada in Internal Medicine, Rheumatology, and the Clinician Investigator Program. He completed advanced subspecialty training in Spondyloarthritis at the University of Toronto, Canada, and holds a Master of Science from the Institute of Medical Science at the same institution, alongside a certificate in the Patient Safety and Quality Improvement Program.

Beyond his clinical practice, Prof. Alnaqbi serves as Physician Lead of the Rheumatology and Immunology Committee at the SEHA Medical Council. He previously led the Rheumatology Clinical Care Programs Certification (CCPC) at Al Ain Hospital (2018–2020), overseeing accreditation of programs in Spondyloarthritis, Systemic Lupus Erythematosus, Rheumatoid Arthritis, and Juvenile Idiopathic Arthritis—all of which received accreditation via Joint Commission International.

He has served as Chairman of the Emirati Board of Pediatric and Adult Rheumatology Fellowship Programs at the National Institute of Health Specialties (NIHS), where he played a central role in advancing rheumatology graduate medical education in the UAE. He additionally serves as Vice Chair of the Rheumatology Committee at the Arab Board of Health Specializations.

He is an active member of several leading international professional organizations, including the American College of Rheumatology (as International Advisor), the Assessment of Spondyloarthritis International Society (ASAS), the Group for Research and Assessment of Psoriasis and Psoriatic Arthritis (GRAPPA), and the Outcome Measures in Rheumatology (OMERACT) Working Groups for Systemic Lupus Erythematosus and Psoriatic Arthritis. He has been elected as the European, Middle Eastern, and African (EMEA) Regional Representative of the International Society for Clinical Densitometry (ISCD).

He serves as a peer reviewer for multiple regional and international journals and is a regular invited speaker at national and international conferences spanning rheumatology, internal medicine, pharmacoeconomics, and health technology assessment.

His contributions to rheumatology and internal medicine have been recognized through numerous prestigious distinctions, including the PureHealth Research Excellence Award (2025), the Lifetime Research Achievement Award at Al Ain Research Day (2025), the Annual Outstanding Research Faculty Award (2024), First Prize for Clinical Research at the Middle East Rheumatology Conference (2022), and the Cleveland Clinic Young Clinician Runner-up Award (2015), among others.

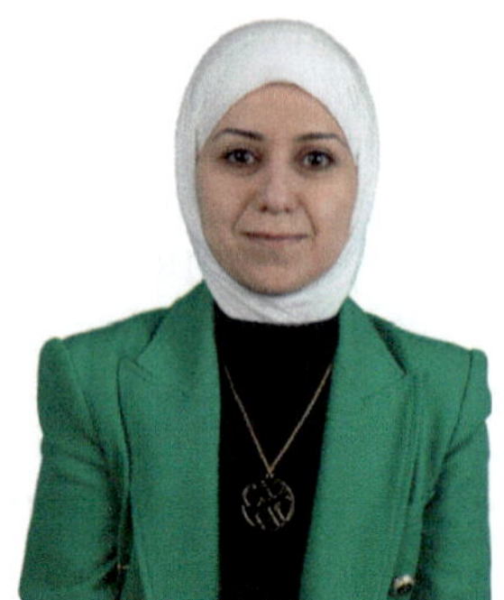

Ghaydaa Aldabie BMBCh, KBIM, MRCP, SEAP is a Consultant in the Rheumatology and Internal Medicine Department at Farwaniya Hospital in Kuwait. She obtained her Bachelor of Medicine and Bachelor of Surgery from the Faculty of Medicine, Kuwait University, in 2008, and subsequently completed her internal medicine residency training in Kuwait, acquiring broad and substantive clinical experience.

She holds Membership of the Royal College of Physicians (MRCP) and undertook advanced subspecialty training through two consecutive fellowship programs at the University of Toronto, Canada: the first in adult rheumatology and the second focused on the clinical management of systemic lupus erythematosus and psoriatic arthritis.

In 2021, she successfully completed the subspecialty examination of the Royal College of Physicians and Surgeons of Canada, attaining recognition as a Subspecialist Affiliate—a distinction that reflects her sustained commitment to the highest standards of subspecialty care in rheumatology.

She currently serves as Program Director of the Kuwait Adult Rheumatology Fellowship Program, a role in which she shapes the next generation of rheumatology specialists in the region.

Contributors

Algeria

Prof. Chafika Haouichat Professor of Rheumatology, Head of Rheumatology Department, Djillali Bounaama University Hospital, Algiers, Algeria

Faculty of Medicine Saad Dahlab, Blida, Algeria

Dr. Chafia Makhloufi-Dahou Department of Rheumatology, Mohamed Lamine Debaghine University Hospital, BD Said Touati, Bab El Oued, Algiers, Algeria

Faculty of Medicine, Algiers, Algeria

Dr. Malik Djennane Department of Rheumatology, CHU Tizi Ouzou, University of Medicine Mouloud Mammeri, Tizi-Ouzou, Algeria

Prof. Manal El Rakawi Professor of Rheumatology, Rheumatology Department, Djillali Bounaama University Hospital, Douera, Algiers, Algeria

Faculty of Medicine Saad Dahlab, Blida, Algeria

Bahrain

Prof. Sahar Saad Consultant Rheumatologist, Head of Rheumatology Division, King Hamad University Hospital, Busaiteen, Bahrain

Professor, Assiut Medical School, Assiut, Egypt

Dr. Redha Ali Consultant Rheumatologist, Department of Rheumatology, Salmaniya Medical Complex, Manama, Bahrain

Dr. Saadeya Abdulkarim Consultant Rheumatologist, Department of Rheumatology, Salmaniya Medical Complex, Manama, Bahrain

Egypt

Dr. Lobna A. Maged Associate Professor, Rheumatology and Clinical Immunology, Cairo University, Cairo, Egypt

Prof. Kamal El-Garf Professor, Rheumatology and Clinical Immunology, Cairo University, Cairo, Egypt

Prof. Mervat Eissa Professor of Rheumatology and Clinical Immunology, Cairo University, Cairo, Egypt

Dr. Walaa Abdelrahman Associate Professor, Rheumatology Department, Faculty of Medicine, Cairo University, Cairo, Egypt

Prof. Bassel El Zorkany Professor, Rheumatology and Clinical Immunology, Cairo University, Cairo, Egypt

Iraq

Prof. Ziad Shafeeq Al-Rawi Professor, College of Medicine, University of Baghdad, Baghdad, Iraq

Prof. Sami Salman Professor, College of Medicine, University of Baghdad, Baghdad, Iraq

Prof. Nizar Abdulateef Jassim Professor, College of Medicine, University of Baghdad, Baghdad, Iraq

Dr. Asal Adnan Assistant Professor, College of Medicine, University of Baghdad, Baghdad, Iraq

Jordan

Prof. Khaldoon Alawneh Professor, Rheumatology Program Director, King Abdullah University Hospital, Department of Medicine, Jordan University of Science and Technology, Irbid, Jordan

Dr. Basel Masri Consultant Rheumatologist, Department of Internal Medicine, Jordan Hospital, Amman, Jordan

Dr. Raed Alzyoud Consultant Pediatrician, Head of Immunology, Allergy and Rheumatology, Queen Rania Children's Hospital, Amman, Jordan

Dr. Wafa Madanat Consultant Rheumatologist, Private Clinic, Amman, Jordan

Kuwait

Dr. Ahmed Thuweni Alenizi Consultant Rheumatologist, Al-Jahra Hospital, Ministry of Health, Al Jahra, Kuwait

Dr. Eman Haji Hasan Consultant Rheumatologist, Rheumatic Disease Unit, Amiri Hospital, Ministry of Health, Kuwait City, Kuwait

Dr. Muna Almutairi Consultant Pediatric Rheumatologist, Rheumatic Disease Unit, Al-Adan Hospital, Ministry of Health, Hadiya, Kuwait

Prof. Adel Alawadhi Professor of Rheumatology, Department of Medicine, College of Medicine, Kuwait University, Kuwait City, Kuwait

Lebanon

Dr. Georges El Hasbani Division of Rheumatology, Department of Medicine, Mayo Clinic, Rochester, NY, USA

Dr. Kamel Mroue Consultant and Head of Rheumatology Division, Department of Internal Medicine, Al Zahra University Medical Center, Beirut, Lebanon

Prof. Imad Uthman Professor, Department of Internal Medicine, American University of Beirut Medical Center, Beirut, Lebanon

Libya

Prof. Khaled Elmuntaser Consultant in Internal Medicine and Rheumatology, Kadisia Clinic, Tripoli, Libya

Prof. Soad Hashad Consultant Pediatric Rheumatologist and Professor, University of Tripoli, Tripoli, Libya

Mauritania

Dr. Mohamed K. Ahmed Ghassem Assistant Professor, Department of Internal Medicine, National Hospital Centre (CHN), Nouakchott, Mauritania

Dr. Saleck Ahmed Vall Specialist in Rheumatology, Cheikh Zayed Hospital (HCZ), Nouakchott, Mauritania

Dr. Noura Biha Assistant Professor, Department of Internal Medicine, Military Hospital, Nouakchott, Mauritania

Prof. Sidi El Wafi Baba Professor, Faculty of Medicine, University Al Aasriya, Nouakchott, Mauritania

Morocco

Dr. Ihsane Hmamouchi Vice Dean, Assistant Professor, Epidemiologist, and Rheumatologist, Faculty of Medicine, Health Sciences Research Center (CReSS), International University of Rabat (UIR), Rabat, Morocco

Rheumatology Unit, Temara Hospital Center, Temara, Morocco

Prof. Bouchra Amine Professor of Rheumatology, Faculty of Medicine and Pharmacy of Rabat, Rabat, Morocco

Department of Rheumatology A, El Ayachi Hospital, Ibn Sina University Hospital Salé, Morocco

Dr. Ibtissam Bentaleb Specialist Rheumatologist, Private Practice of Rheumatology, Salé, Morocco

Dr. Abir Souissi Specialist Rheumatologist, Rheumatology Unit, Mohammed VI Hospital Center, Al Hoceima, Morocco

Dr. Salma Zemrani Assistant Professor, Department of Rheumatology A, El Ayachi Hospital, Ibn Sina University Hospital, Salé, Morocco

Prof. Rachid Bahiri Professor of Rheumatology, Faculty of Medicine and Pharmacy of Rabat, Rabat, Morocco

Head of Department of Rheumatology, El Ayachi Hospital, Ibn Sina University Hospital, Salé, Morocco

Oman

Dr. Nasra K. Al Adhoubi Senior Consultant Rheumatologist, Rheumatology Unit, Royal Hospital, Muscat, Oman

Dr. Zakariya Alismaeili Consultant Rheumatologist, Rheumatology Unit, Nizwa Hospital Nizwa, Oman,

Dr. Maha Ali Consultant Rheumatologist, Rheumatology Unit, Al Nahdha Hospital Muscat, Oman,

Palestine

Dr. Sima Abu Al-Saoud Consultant Pediatric Rheumatologist and Assistant Professor of Pediatrics, Department of Pediatrics, Division of Pediatric Rheumatology, Al-Quds University, Faculty of Medicine, Makassed Hospital, Jerusalem, Palestine

Prof. Nezam Altorok Professor, Division of Rheumatology, Department of Internal Medicine, University of Toledo, Toledo, OH, USA

Dr. Muaath Itmaizeh Department of Internal Medicine, Division of Rheumatology, Makassed Hospital, Faculty of Medicine, Al-Quds University, Jerusalem, Palestine

Qatar

Dr. Omar Alsaed Consultant Rheumatologist, Division of Rheumatology, Department of Medicine, Hamad Medical Corporation, Doha, Qatar

Dr. Mohamed Hammoudeh Senior Rheumatologist Consultant, Division of Rheumatology, Department of Medicine, Hamad Medical Corporation, Doha, Qatar

Dr. Samar Al Emadi Senior Rheumatology Consultant, Division of Rheumatology, Department of Medicine, Hamad Medical Corporation, Doha, Qatar

Associate Professor, Weill Cornell Medicine – Qatar, Doha, Qatar

Saudi Arabia

Dr. Fahdah Al Okaily Consultant and Head of Rheumatology Division, Prince Sultan Military Medical City, Riyadh, Saudi Arabia

Prof. Sami Bahlas Professor, King Abdulaziz University Hospital, Jeddah, Saudi Arabia

Dr. Ibrahim Al-Homood Consultant Rheumatologist, King Fahad Medical City, Riyadh, Saudi Arabia

Adjunct Associate Professor, AlFaisal University, Riyadh, Saudi Arabia

Chairman of Postgraduate and Scholarship Department, Riyadh, Saudi Arabia

Somalia, Djibouti, and the Union of Comoros

Dr. Shamma Al Nokhatha Consultant Rheumatologist, Rheumatology Division, Sheikh Tahnoon Medical City, SEHA/PureHealth, Al Ain, UAE

Prof. Khalid A. Alnaqbi Consultant and Chief of Rheumatology, Sheikh Tahnoon Medical City and Tawam Hospital, SEHA/PureHealth, Al Ain, UAE

Adjunct Professor, RAK Medical and Health Sciences University, Ras Al Khaimah, UAE

Adjunct Associate Professor, College of Medicine and Health Sciences, UAE University, Al Ain, UAE

Sudan

Dr. Ziryab Imad Taha Mahmoud Associate Professor, Department of Internal Medicine, University of Bahri, Khartoum, Sudan

Consultant Physician and Rheumatologist, Merowe Medical City, Merowe, Sudan

Dr. Elnour Mohamed Elageb Senior Consultant Physician and Rheumatologist, Military Teaching Hospital, Omdurman, Sudan

Dr. Wafaa Hassan Ahmed Albashir Consultant Physician and Rheumatologist, Friendship Teaching Hospital, Omdurman and Aliaa Specialist Hospital, Omdurman, Sudan

Sudanese Association of Rheumatology, Khartoum, Sudan

Al Rehab Medical Centre in Cairo, Cairo, Egypt

Syria

Prof. Salwa Al Cheikh Professor of Medicine and Rheumatology, Faculty of Medicine, Damascus University, Damascus, Syria

Dr. Mohammad Said Al Sawaf Senior Consultant Rheumatologist, Syrian Association for Rheumatology, Damascus, Syria

Dr. Mohammed Alaswad Medical Centre Hospital, Hama, Syria

Dr. Layla Kazkaz Honorary President of the Syrian Association for Rheumatology, Damascus, Syria

Tunisia

Dr. Hiba Boussaa Assistant Professor in Rheumatology, Faculty of Medicine of Tunis, University of Tunis El Manar, Tunis,Tunisia

Department of Rheumatology, Mongi Slim University Hospital, Tunis, Tunisia

Dr. Hanene Lassoued Ferjani Associate Professor of Rheumatology, Department of Rheumatology, Mohamed Kassab Institute of Orthopedics, La Manouba, Tunisia

Faculty of Medicine of Tunis, University of Tunis El Manar, Tunis, Tunisia

Dr. Saoussen Miladi Assistant Professor in Rheumatology, Faculty of Medicine of Tunis, University of Tunis El Manar, Tunis, Tunisia

Department of Rheumatology, Mongi Slim University Hospital, Tunis, Tunisia

Dr. Nejla El Amri University of Sousse, Faculty of Medicine of Sousse, Department of Rheumatology, Farhat Hached University Hospital, Sousse, Tunisia

Prof. Kawther Ben Abdelghani Professor of Rheumatology, Faculty of Medicine of Tunis, University of Tunis El Manar, Tunis, Tunisia

Department of Rheumatology, Mongi Slim University Hospital, Tunis, Tunisia

Dr. Elyes Bouajina University of Sousse, Faculty of Medicine of Sousse, Department of Rheumatology, Farhat Hached University Hospital, Sousse, Tunisia

The United Arab Emirates (UAE)

Dr. Suad Hannawi Consultant Rheumatologist, Alkuwait Hospital, Emirates Health Services, Dubai, UAE

Dr. Amna Almheiri Research and Innovation, Rheumatology Division, Sheikh Shakhbout Medical City, PureHealth, Abu Dhabi, UAE

Dr. Mohamed Almarzooqi Sheikh Khalifa Medical City, SEHA/PureHealth, Abu Dhabi, UAE

Prof. Khalid A. Alnaqbi Consultant and Chief of Rheumatology, Sheikh Tahnoon Medical City and Tawam Hospital, SEHA/PureHealth, Al Ain, UAE

Adjunct Professor, RAK Medical and Health Sciences University, Ras Al Khaimah, UAE

Adjunct Associate Professor, College of Medicine and Health Sciences, UAE University, Al Ain, UAE

Yemen

Dr. Arwa Aljohi Consultant in Rheumatology and Rehabilitation, Alsheikh Othman Polyclinic, Aden, Yemen

Dr. Nabil Al-Ashmory Rheumatology and Rehabilitation, University of 21 September, Sanaa, Yemen

Dr. Thekra Alabsi Internal Medicine and Rheumatology, Kuwait University Hospital, Sanaa University, Sanaa, Yemen

Dr. Abdulrahman Jamel Rheumatology and Rehabilitation at Taiz University, Taiz, Yemen

Arab League of Associations for Rheumatology (ArLAR)

Dr. Fatemah Abutiban Consultant Rheumatologist, Jaber AlAhmed Hospital, Department of Medicine, Ministry of Health, Kuwait City, State of Kuwait

Dr. Hebah AlHajeri Consultant in Internal Medicine and Rheumatology, Mubarak Al Kabeer Hospital, Department of Medicine, Ministry of Health, Kuwait City, State of Kuwait

Dr. Amjad Alkadi Consultant in Internal Medicine and Rheumatology, Al-Sabah Hospital, Department of Medicine, Ministry of Health, Kuwait City, State of Kuwait

Dr. Fatemah Baroun Consultant in Internal Medicine and Rheumatology, Jaber AlAhmed Hospital, Department of Medicine, Ministry of Health, Kuwait City, State of Kuwait

Rheumatology Research in the Arab World

Dr. Hadeel Zaghloul Research Associate, Weill Cornell Medicine-Qatar, Doha, Qatar

Hubaib Haider Medical Student, Weill Cornell Medicine-Qatar, Doha, Qatar

Prof. Thurayya Arayssi Professor of Medicine and Vice Dean for Academic and Curricular Affairs, Weill Cornell Medicine-Qatar, Doha, Qatar

Accreditation of Rheumatology Programs in the Arab World

Nafaja Alhasni Patient Clinical Navigator, Sheikh Tahnoon Medical City, SEHA/PureHealth, Al Ain, UAE

Hodan Hussein Jama Registered Nurse, Sheikh Tahnoon Medical City, SEHA/PureHealth, Al Ain, UAE

Prof. Khalid A. Alnaqbi Consultant and Chief of Rheumatology Division, Sheikh Tahnoon Medical City, SEHA/PureHealth, Al Ain, UAE

Rheumatology Leader of Clinical Care Programs Certification (CCPC) for Rheumatology Programs at Al Ain Hospital (2018–2020), Adjunct Professor, RAK Medical and Health Sciences University, Ras Al Khaimah, UAE

College of Medicine and Health Sciences, UAE University, Al Ain, UAE

Pediatric Rheumatology in the Arab World

Prof. Soad Hashad Consultant Pediatric Rheumatologist and Professor, University of Tripoli, Tripoli, Libya

Prof. Djohra Hadef Pediatric Rheumatologist and Professor, Batna 2 University, Batna, Algeria

Dr. Buthaina Al Adba Senior Attending Physician and Pediatric Rheumatologist, Sidra Medicine, Doha, Qatar

Pharmacoeconomics of Rheumatic Diseases in the Arab World

Dr. Nicole Gebran Clinical Pharmacy Service Lead, Pharmacy Department, Dubai Health, Dubai, UAE

Clinical Pharmacy Residency Program Director, Mohammed Bin Rashid University of Medicine and Health Sciences, Dubai, UAE

Dr. Lamia AlHajri Assistant Professor (Pharmacy) and Dean of Academic Operations, Higher Colleges of Technology, Dubai, UAE

Dr. Abdulrazaq S. Al-Jazairi Clinical Pharmacy Consultant and Deputy Executive Director, Research and Innovation, King Faisal Specialist Hospital and Research Center, Riyadh, Saudi Arabia

Dr. Solaiman Alhawas Medication Use Safety and Policy Consultant, Saudi Pharmacovigilance Group, Saudi Pharmaceutical Society, Riyadh, Riyadh, Saudi Arabia

Perspectives of Arab Patients on Rheumatic Diseases

Dr. Shaimaa Alasfour Public Authority of Food and Nutrition (PAFN), Kuwait Lupus Group, Kuwait City, Kuwait

Nida Abul Kuwait Lupus Group, Kuwait City, Kuwait

Prof. Khalid A. Alnaqbi Consultant and Chief of Rheumatology Division, Sheikh Tahnoon Medical City, SEHA/PureHealth, Al Ain, UAE

Adjunct Professor, RAK Medical and Health Sciences University, Ras Al Khaimah, UAE

College of Medicine and Health Sciences, UAE University, Al Ain, UAE

Complementary and Alternative Medicine Use in Rheumatic Diseases

Dr. Noria Ghulam Nabi Specialist Internal Medicine, Department of Internal Medicine, Sheikh Tahnoon Medical City, SEHA/PureHealth, Al Ain, UAE

Dr. Hazem Taifour Postgraduate Year 4 Resident, Department of Medicine, Rochester Regional Health/Unity Hospital, Rochester, NY, USA

Prof. Khalid A. Alnaqbi Consultant and Chief of Rheumatology Division, Sheikh Tahnoon Medical City, SEHA/PureHealth, Al Ain, UAE

Adjunct Professor, RAK Medical and Health Sciences University, Ras Al Khaimah, UAE

College of Medicine and Health Sciences, UAE University, Al Ain, UAE

Dr. Yossra Suliman Assistant Professor of Rheumatology, Assiut University, Assiut, Egypt

Specialist Rheumatologist, Mediclinic—Al Ain Hospital, Abu Dhabi, UAE

War, Conflict, and Rheumatic Diseases in the Arab World

Prof. Sami Salman Professor, College of Medicine, University of Baghdad, Baghdad, Iraq

Dr. Sima Abu Al-Saoud Consultant Pediatric Rheumatologist and Assistant Professor of Pediatrics, Department of Pediatrics, Division of Pediatric Rheumatology, Al-Quds University, Faculty of Medicine, Makassed Hospital, Jerusalem, Palestine

Dr. Arwa Aljohi Consultant in Rheumatology and Rehabilitation, Alsheikh Othman Polyclinic, Aden, Yemen

Dr. Ziryab Imad Taha Mahmoud Consultant Physician and Rheumatologist, Merowe Medical City, Merowe, Sudan

Associate Professor, Department of Internal Medicine, University of Bahri, Khartoum, Sudan

Prof. Khalid A. Alnaqbi Consultant and Chief of Rheumatology, Sheikh Tahnoon bin Mohammed Medical City and Tawam Hospital, SEHA/PureHealth, Al Ain, UAE

Adjunct Professor, College of Medicine, RAK Medical and Health Sciences University, Ras Al Khaimah, UAE

Adjunct Associate Professor, College of Medicine and Health Sciences, UAE University, Al Ain, UAE

Dr. Mira Merashli Consultant and Associate Professor of Clinical Medicine, Department of Internal Medicine, Division of Rheumatology, American University of Beirut, Beirut, Lebanon

COVID-19 Crisis and Rheumatology Care in the Arab World

Dr. Nelly Ziadé Consultant and Head of Rheumatology Department, Saint-Joseph University and Hotel-Dieu de France Hospital, Beirut, Lebanon

Prof. Wafa Hamdi Professor of Rheumatology and Head of Rheumatology Department, Kassab Institute, Tunis, Tunisia

Faculty of Medicine of Tunis, University of Tunis El Manar, Tunis, Tunisia

Dr. Martin Lee Consultant Rheumatologist, Northumbria Healthcare Trust, North Shields, UK

Dr. Krystel Aouad Assistant Professor of Rheumatology, Saint George Hospital University Medical Center, Saint George University of Beirut, Beirut, Lebanon

Prof. Manal El Rakawi Professor of Rheumatology, Rheumatology Department, Djillali Bounaama University Hospital, Douera, Algiers, Algeria

Faculty of Medicine Saad Dahlab, Blida, Algeria

Future Directions of Rheumatology Care in the Arab World

Prof. Khalid A. Alnaqbi Consultant and Chief of Rheumatology, Sheikh Tahnoon bin Mohammed Medical City and Tawam Hospital, SEHA/PureHealth, Al Ain, UAE

Adjunct Professor, College of Medicine, RAK Medical and Health Sciences University, Ras Al Khaimah, UAE

Adjunct Associate Professor, College of Medicine and Health Sciences, UAE University, Al Ain, UAE

Chapter 1
Rheumatic Diseases in Algeria

Chafika Haouichat, Chafia Makhloufi-Dahou, Malik Djennane, and Manal El Rakawi

Abstract Algeria is the largest country in Africa, the Arab world, and the Mediterranean basin.

The Algerian health system is ranked fourth in Africa, behind Nigeria, Tunisia, and South Africa.

Although the burden of rheumatic diseases has been well documented globally and widely presented at scientific events, data from Algeria remain limited. This limits the visibility of national progress in rheumatology care, service development, and rheumatologist training.

This chapter aims to provide a comprehensive overview of the healthcare system, with a specific focus on rheumatology practice. It will explore various rheumatic diseases, including rheumatoid arthritis, spondyloarthritis, juvenile idiopathic arthritis, and osteoarthritis, through a review of several Algerian publications and local data presented at scientific events. Throughout this chapter, we will present a detailed report on the progress and stages involved in the diagnosis and therapeutic management of rheumatic diseases. Ultimately, the

C. Haouichat (✉)
Rheumatology Department, Djillali Bounaama University Hospital, Algiers, Algeria

Faculty of Medicine Saad Dahlab, Blida, Algeria
e-mail: chaouichat@yahoo.fr

C. Makhloufi-Dahou
Department of Rheumatology, Mohamed Lamine Debaghine University Hospital, Algiers, Algeria

Faculty of Medicine, Algiers, Algeria
e-mail: makhloufi-dahou@hotmail.com

M. Djennane
Department of Rheumatology CHU Tizi Ouzou, University of Medicine Mouloud Mammeri Tizi-Ouzou, Tizi-Ouzou, Algeria
e-mail: Malik.djennane@hotmail.com

M. El Rakawi
Rheumatology Department, Douera Hospital, Faculty of Medicine Saad Dahlab, Blida, Algeria
e-mail: m.elrakawi@gmail.com

K. A. Alnaqbi, G. Aldabie (eds.), *Rheumatic Diseases in the Arab World*,
https://doi.org/10.1007/978-981-92-0967-5_1

authors propose a strategic action plan to improve the management of rheumatic diseases in Algeria in the coming years.

Keywords Algeria · North africa · Algerian healthcare system · Rheumatic diseases · Rheumatology services · Rheumatology workforce · Non-communicable diseases · Rheumatology training · Biologic therapy · Biosimilars

1.1 Introduction

Algeria is the biggest country in Africa, the Arab world, and the Mediterranean basin because of its surface of 2.381.741 km2. With a coast of 1200 km, the country shares more than 6385 km of land borders with Tunisia to the Northeast, Morocco to the Northwest, Libya to the East, Niger to the Southeast, and Mali to the Southwest, in addition to Mauritania and Western Sahara to the West [1].

The relief of Algeria is made up of the Tell in the North, the high plateaus and the Saharan Atlas in the center, the Sahara in the South, and the highest peak in the country (Tahat) is located at an altitude of 3003 meters at the North of Tamanrasset [1, 2]. Algeria has a humid Mediterranean environment in the North and an arid Saharan climate in the South. Approximately, 91% of Algeria's population lives along the Mediterranean coast on 12% of its land mass.

Algiers is the capital and largest city of Algeria. Algeria is administratively divided into 58 wilayas, which are subdivided into daïras and municipalities [3].

The largest cities in Algeria are: Algiers; Oran, the largest city in the West, which houses the second-largest port in the country; Constantine, or a city "with suspension bridges"; Annaba, a booming industrial city; and Bejaia, which has a giant Mediterranean port. The other big cities of Algeria are Sétif, Batna, Blida, Djelfa, Sidi Bel Abbès, and Biskra [3, 4].

The history of the country, its geography, and its demography explain the disparity in the characteristics of the different Wilayas. These differ in their areas, several Daïras, and population.

As of January 1, 2022, Algeria's population was estimated at 45,137,119 people, predominantly concentrated in the North [5]. The overall population density is 20 people per square kilometer. By 2024, males accounted for 50.7% and females 49.3% of the population, with a median age of 29.1 years [6].

1.2 Health Sectors at the National Level

The Algerian health system is ranked fourth in Africa behind Nigeria, Tunisia, and South Africa by the Bloomberg Healthiest Country Index in 2019 [7]. In Algeria, healthcare is provided by two types of care: public and private. Health care is free in hospitals, and public structures are run by the State.

The 2020 Ministry of Health report outlines Algeria's health sector as follows:

- A total of 15 University Hospital Centers (CHU), with 13,125 beds.
- One University Hospital Establishment (EHU), with 1029 beds.
- A total of 79 Specialized Hospital Establishments (EHS), with 12,843 beds across various specialties (see Tables 1.1 and 1.2).
- Nine Hospitals with Specific Management (EH), including five general and four ophthalmology hospitals, totaling 1316 beds.
- A total of 210 Public Hospital Establishments (EPH), with 39,522 beds.
- A total of 273 Local Public Health Establishments (EPSP), featuring 1748 polyclinics (390 with integrated maternity, totaling 2849 maternity beds), 13 rural and maternities with 151 beds, and 6160 treatment rooms. The polyclinics also have 4607 emergency beds and 170 hemodialysis beds.

In the private sector, a significant portion of healthcare is provided by diverse facilities, detailed in Table 1.3: 46 medical clinics, 299 medical and surgical clinics, 62

Table 1.1 Breakdown of public healthcare establishments by type of structure

Establishment	Number	Percentage (%)
CHU	15	2.56
EHU	1	0.17
EHS	79	13.46
EPH	210	35.78
EH	9	1.53
EPSP	273	46.5
Total	587	100.0

CHU University Hospital Centers, *EHU* University Hospital Establishment, *EHS* Specialized Hospital Establishments, *EPH* Public Hospital Establishments, *EH* Hospitals with Specific Management, *EPSP* Local Public Health Establishments

Table 1.2 Distribution of specialties

Specialty	Number
Mothers and children	33
Psychiatry	21
Functional rehabilitation	7
Ophthalmology	3
Heart surgeries	4
Cancer centers	10
Plastic surgery	1
Neurosurgery	2
Infectiology	1
Ortho-traumatology	1
Medical and surgical emergency	1
Nephrology	1
Pediatrics	1
Organ and tissue transplantation	1
Musculoskeletal system	1

Table 1.3 Distribution of private practices

Private practices	Number
Specialists	11,591
General practitioners	8848
Dental surgeons	8266
Pharmacies	10,985
Group practices	1074

diagnostic clinics, 176 hemodialysis centers, 1074 group practices, 11,591 specialists' offices, 8848 general practitioners' practices, 8266 dental surgeries, and 10,985 pharmacies.

1.3 Health Services in Rheumatology in Algeria

1.3.1 The Number of Rheumatologists

At the national level, nine hospital–university rheumatology departments (five departments in Algiers, one in Tizi-Ouzou, one in Oran, one in Constantine, and one in Annaba) provide residents' training.

There are 81 residents in rheumatology specialization programs, predominantly female. The faculty comprises 43 hospital–university teachers, including professors, lecturers, and assistant teachers. In public health establishments, there are two rheumatology departments (Blida and Ain Turk), which treat patients with rheumatic and osteoarticular pathologies but do not offer resident training.

At the national level, the number of public health specialists is 112. According to the 2020 report from the Ministry of Health, there are 229 rheumatologists in Algeria's private sector. This includes 197 working in private practices and 32 in private clinics. This number has seen an increase over the last decade. Additionally, there are 24 newly graduated rheumatologists from the classes of 2021 and 2022, and 7 who have retired. In total, there are approximately 415 rheumatologists in Algeria.

1.3.2 Number of Certified Rheumatology Nurses

In Algeria, there are currently no nurses specifically trained for rheumatology departments, particularly in areas like biotherapies and their administration methods or side effects. However, continuing medical training sessions are regularly organized across various hospital–university structures. These sessions are dedicated to paramedics and cover topics such as therapeutic education, biological management, and more.

1.3.3 Accredited Centers of Excellence in Rheumatology

In Algeria, there are no accredited centers of excellence in rheumatology. Nevertheless, six university–hospital centers are equipped with the necessary technical platforms and equipment to fulfill the training objectives outlined in the rheumatology resident's handbook. These departments are generally well-equipped, featuring bone densitometers, ultrasound machines, capillaroscopes, microscopes, and other essential tools. There are nine primary training centers: five located in the center of Algiers, one center in Tizi-Ouzou, two in the east of the country (Constantine and Annaba), and one in the west of Algeria (Oran).

1.3.4 Pediatric Rheumatology

There are few centers specializing in pediatric rheumatology. In Algeria, six university–hospital rheumatology departments collaborate with pediatricians to manage Juvenile Idiopathic Arthritis (JIA), highlighting the crucial role of rheumatologist–pediatrician collaboration. An example of this collaborative effort is the study conducted by the African League of Associations for Rheumatology during the COVID-19 pandemic. This study, which included Algeria, focused on identifying changes in rheumatology practice and patient behavior amidst the pandemic [8]. A national JIA management guide in Algeria has been developed in French.

According to published data, there are ten pediatric rheumatology reference centers in Africa, including one in Algeria, with ten beds caring for nearly 100 children on an outpatient basis [9].

1.3.5 Evolution of Hospital–University Training Centers

The evolution of hospital–university training centers in rheumatology is illustrated in Fig. 1.1, showing their establishment and growth over the past decades.

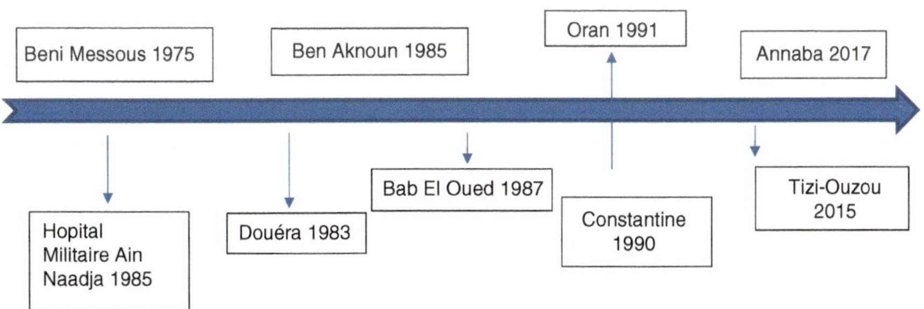

Fig. 1.1 Timeline showing the establishment of hospital–university training centers in rheumatology in Algeria

1.3.6 *Official Societies of Rheumatology*

In Algeria, the key official rheumatology societies include the Algerian Society of Rheumatology (SAR), the Algerian Anti-Rheumatic League, and the Association of Private Algerian Rheumatologists, Furthermore, there are various patient associations for chronic inflammatory rheumatism, such as Anaya.

1.4 Overview of Rheumatic Diseases in Algeria

The impact of rheumatic diseases in Algeria, and broadly across Africa, is likely more severe than in other regions, both in terms of morbidity and mortality. This is particularly due to patients frequently presenting at more advanced stages of the disease [10]. In the following section, we will discuss some specific rheumatic diseases.

1.4.1 *Rheumatoid Arthritis*

The first series of patients with rheumatoid arthritis (RA) was identified at the end of the 1970s, primarily in university hospital rheumatology centers located in major urban areas. Since then, the number of identified cases has increased, a trend likely influenced by the country's growing population, the establishment of free healthcare post-independence, and the expansion of rheumatology departments across various regions. These developments have given the opportunity for patients to receive treatment of rheumatic and autoimmune diseases.

1.4.1.1 Prevalence and Risk Factors

Data on the prevalence of RA in Algeria are scarce. However, a local study conducted by Slimani et al. in the urban commune of Barika, which has a population of 52,504 residents, reported a relatively low RA prevalence of 0.13% [11]. Dahou-Makhlouf et al. conducted a study in the Bab el Oued district of Algiers to examine RA's prevalence and management strategies. The study involved 157,991 individuals who were covered by health insurance. Out of the participants, 244 were diagnosed with RA, with 89.34% of them being female. The researchers estimated the prevalence of RA to be 0.15% [12].

In a case-control study conducted by Acheli et al., the genetic association between HLA class II alleles and RA in Algerian patients was investigated. The study included 159 unrelated patients with RA, and HLA class II typing was performed using a molecular biology method known as Polymerase Chain

Reaction–Sequence-Specific Primers (PCR-SSP). The frequencies of HLA-DRβ1*0405 and HLA-DRB1* SE+ alleles were significantly higher in RA patients compared to the control group. This indicates the role of HLA-DRB1*SE+ alleles as a marker for susceptibility to RA, although they do not seem to influence the clinical expression of the disease. Additionally, these alleles are associated with the production of Anti-Citrullinated Protein Antibodies [13].

Louahchi S et al. investigated the association of Interleukin 23R (IL-23R), Interleukin 17A (IL-17A), and Interleukin 17F (IL-17F) gene single-nucleotide polymorphisms (SNPs) with RA susceptibility in the Algerian population. Three hundred forty-three patients with RA and 323 healthy subjects were genotyped for IL-23R (rs11209026, rs1343151, and rs10489629), IL-17F (rs763780 and rs2397084), and IL-17A (rs2275913) variants by TaqMan technology. The study emphasizes the lack of association of IL-23R and IL-17 polymorphisms with RA susceptibility in the Algerian population. However, the data showed the relationship between IL-23R and IL-17A polymorphisms and the production of the different rheumatoid factor (RF) isotypes in RA patients [14].

In a study performed in Algeria in 2013 by Slimani and colleagues, the characteristics of RA were investigated. A total of 249 patients, consisting of 213 women and 36 men, participated in the study. Among them, ten patients (4%) had a juvenile onset of the disease. The average age of the participants was 50.1 ± 14.5 years, and the average duration of RA was 8.4 ± 7.8 years. In terms of comorbidities, 18.9% of patients had arterial hypertension, and 5.2% had diabetes mellitus. The mean Disease Activity Score 28 (DAS28) at the beginning of the study was 4.3 (95% CI 4.1–4.5), with 14.0% of patients achieving remission (DAS28 ≤2.6). The mean Health Assessment Questionnaire score, which measures functional disability, was 0.81 ± 0.82. RF was found to be positive in 78.5% of cases, and when measured, anticitrullinated protein/peptide antibodies (anti-CCP) were positive in 69.0% of cases. The study showed that RA in Algeria was more prevalent in women and had a higher occurrence of seronegative oligoarticular forms [15].

In a 2020 study led by Ouali et al., involving 281 RA patients, it was found that 86% of the patients were female. The study revealed that patients with positive anti-CCP antibodies (97.7%) had high disease activity ($p < 0.0001$), a longer duration of the disease ($p = 0.016$), and more structural damage ($p < 0.0001$). This indicates a strong correlation between positive anti-CCP antibodies and the development of RA in Algerian patients, suggesting that anti-CCP could be a useful predictor of disease severity [16]. These results are consistent with those from a previous study by Acheli and colleagues [17].

Dahou et al. conducted a multicenter cross-sectional prospective study aiming to determine the prevalence of periodontitis and its relationship with RA severity, treatment, and patient characteristics. The study showed that the frequency of periodontitis was 37.3% (51.1% related to the *Porphyromonas gingivalis*) among the 204 patients with RA. The tooth loss frequency was 31.4%. However, there was no significant difference between the subjects with periodontitis and patients without periodontitis in terms of RA severity or treatment [18].

1.4.1.2 Demographics, Presentation, and Care

In Algeria, the presentation of RA exhibits variability. The majority of affected patients experience the onset of RA at an average age of 48 years, predominantly in females. Interestingly, this population has a low occurrence of subcutaneous nodules and extra-articular manifestations. Generally, the disease tends to be mild, with less severe radiographic changes observed [13]. However, it is worth mentioning that fatigue, a prevalent symptom of RA, substantially impacts RA patients' quality of life [19]. Moreover, osteoporosis and vertebral fractures have been reported in women with RA in various studies [20, 21]. In addition, ocular involvement and cervical spine damage have been investigated in other studies [21, 22].

The majority of RA patients are prescribed low doses of corticosteroids [23]. Disease modifying anti-rheumatic drugs (DMARDs)-based treatments are widely used in Algeria. Methotrexate is the most commonly used conventional DMARD for its efficacy and tolerability. The biological therapies available since 2009 are accessible according to their availability to patients at the level of hospital structures. They are provided free of charge due to the free care policy in Algeria.

1.4.2 Spondyloarthritis

The first description of spondyloarthritis (SpA) in North Africa came from a series of 78 cases of reactive arthritis (ReA) during the Algerian War [24]. The wide distribution of HLA-B27 explains the prevalence and severity of SpA in Algeria [25].

1.4.2.1 Genetic Characteristics

In their study, Amron et al. examined the influence of MHC class I chain-linked A (MICA)—129met (methionine) polymorphisms in MICA molecules on SpA susceptibility. They conducted their research on a cohort of 129 SpA patients and 76 healthy controls. The results showed a significant correlation between the MICA-129 met/met genotype and juvenile SpA, regardless of the presence of HLA-B27 [26]. Many SNPs have been explored in the Algerian population to assess genetic risk factors associated with ankylosing spondylitis (AS) [27–30]. The JAK-STAT pathway and gene-to-gene interactions were also assessed in Algerian and Han Chinese SpA cohorts. The findings confirmed the correlation between genes in the IL-23 signaling pathway and the development of AS. Specifically, the association was observed with the variant rs3212227 in the 3′ untranslated region (3'UTR) of interleukin (IL)-12β [28; 29].

1.4.2.2 Demographics, Presentation, and Care

Algerian rheumatologists use the Assessment of SpondyloArthritis International Society (ASAS) Classification Criteria to diagnose nonradiographic axial SpA (nr-axSpA); as in other regions, their use for diagnostic purposes remains a significant challenge. Physicians diagnosing nr-axSpA often encounter the pressure of establishing and confirming an early diagnosis based only on magnetic resonance imaging (MRI) imaging. This can contribute to a slightly longer delay in diagnosing nonradiographic disease than other forms of SpA as a small proportion of patients have positive HLA-B27 [31].

In North Africa and the Middle East (MENA), disease measures used for the diagnosis and monitoring of patients with SpA include the various physical components of the disease, such as morning stiffness, lumbar flexion (Schober's test), thoracic expansion, lateral flexion of the spine, occiput-wall distance, and tragus-wall distance. Regional experts from MENA region reported that conventional scoring methods are routinely used for patient visits, including the Bath Ankylosing Spondylitis Disease Activity Index (BASDAI), Bath Ankylosing Spondylitis Functional Index, Bath Ankylosing Spondylitis Metrology Index, and Visual Analog Scale for assessing spinal pain and Ankylosing Spondylitis Quality of Life questionnaire (ASQoL) to measure health-related quality of life [32].

Information is limited on the prevalence and clinical features of nr-axSpA in patients with inflammatory back pain (IBP) in African countries. A global study conducted in 19 countries across Latin America, Europe, Asia, and Africa estimated the prevalence of nr-axSpA in patients with IBP. Out of the 2517 patients with chronic low back pain identified in the study, 974 (38.70%) met the criteria for IBP. Among the IBP patients, 29.10% fulfilled the criteria for nr-axSpA and 53.72% met the criteria for AS. The prevalence of nr-axSpA varied significantly across regions ($p < 0.05$), with the highest prevalence observed in Asia (36.46%) and the lowest in Africa (16.02%) [33].

In another study involving 206 African patients with IBP, the prevalence of nr-axSpA was comparable between patients from North West Africa (Morocco and Algeria) and South Africa. Northwest Africa had a higher proportion of male patients, and both regions experienced delays in diagnosis compared to the global average. Additionally, increased disease activity levels (Ankylosing Spondylitis Disease Activity Score and BASDAI scores) were found in both regions, suggesting suboptimal disease control [34].

In Maghreb countries, hip involvement in SpA, particularly AS, is frequent and often severe. Local studies have reported prevalence of hip involvement ranging from 30% to over 75% in patients with ankylosing spondylitis (AS) [35]. The same study also reported a substantial diagnostic delay, with the average time from symptom onset to diagnosis of AS being 5.68 ±5.54 years, especially prolonged in HLA-B27–negative patients. One of the key contributors to this delay is the limited awareness and understanding of axial SpA among nonrheumatologists [36].

Despite their widespread availability, access to MRI facilities in Algerian hospitals is restricted to selected patients. This limitation can be attributed to long waiting lists in some hospitals, causing delays in diagnosis. Additionally, general practitioners, orthopedic specialists, and even radiologists may face challenges in identifying sacroiliac alterations, further contributing to the delay in diagnosing these cases [32].

Algeria has a public health system where most people can access conventional disease modifying anti-rheumatic drugs (DMARDs). However, patient access to biological therapies is limited, as they are only available free of charge in public hospitals. Other measures are necessary before initiating treatment with a TNF inhibitor. Latent tuberculosis (TB) is a problem in the African region, with positive TB tests occurring in 20–25% of patients [37]. Rheumatologists use the most recent recommendations of the Assessment of SpondyloArthritis International Society (ASAS) and the European Alliance of Associations for Rheumatology to manage SpA [38]. There are several challenges in the management of SpA in Algeria. For example, the consistent availability of biologics is often affected by the country's economic situation. Furthermore, convincing some patients to adhere to their medication regimen can be difficult. This reluctance may be attributed to the chronic nature of the disease and concerns, particularly among young patients, about the long-term implications of treatment. Additionally, the method of administering treatments can contribute to patient hesitancy.

1.4.3 Juvenile Idiopathic Arthritis (JIA)

JIA is the most common chronic heterogeneous rheumatological disorder that presents in patients under the age of 16 and, in some cases, can lead to severe impairment and disability. It constitutes various subtypes with clinical manifestations, genetic markers, and pathogenesis.

Aiche et al. adapted and validated the Algerian Arabic version of the Juvenile Arthritis Multidimensional Assessment Report (JAMAR) in 70 children with JIA who mainly presented with oligoarticular forms (35.7%), polyarticular forms with negative rheumatoid factor (21.4%), polyarticular seronegative forms (2%), and systemic forms (10%). The results obtained for the parent version of the JAMAR are very similar to those obtained for the child version [39].

1.4.4 Systemic Sclerosis

Tahiti et al. assessed the profile of *systemic sclerosis* (SSc)-related autoantibodies and their clinical characteristics in 150 Algerian patients. One hundred thirty-five (90.0%) patients were positive for SSc-related autoantibodies [40].

In a study by Lahcene et al., the average age of 183 SSc patients was 40.4 ± 13.3 years, with an average disease duration of 6.8 ± 7.5 years. Among the cases, 81% had a localized cutaneous form, while 19% had a diffuse form [41]. Esophageal motility disorders of 183 SSc patients were observed in 81% of cases, with 62% also showing lower esophageal sphincter hypotonia. Esophageal symptoms and esophagitis were reported in 59% and 37% of patients, respectively. Interestingly, motor disturbances were found in 64% of asymptomatic patients [42].

In a case-control study conducted by Mellal et al., the genetic association of IL-17A, IL-17F, IL-21, IL-23R, and STAT3 genes with SSc susceptibility and their impact on clinical and immunological phenotypes were investigated. The study included 136 SSc patients and 317 healthy controls from the Algerian population. The findings revealed that IL-17F and IL-21 genes were linked to an increased susceptibility to SSc. Additionally, IL-17A, IL-17F, IL-21, and IL-23R genes were found to influence clinical characteristics and immunological factors, suggesting the involvement of Th17 cells in the development of SSc [43].

1.4.5 Reactive Arthritis (ReA)/Undifferentiated Arthritis (UA)

A study conducted by Kuipers et al. aimed to investigate the potential involvement of *Chlamydia trachomatis* in patients with reactive arthritis or undifferentiated arthritis (UA) in North Africa. The study included 8 cases of posturethritic arthritis, 2 cases of postenteritic arthritis, 23 cases of undifferentiated arthritis (UA), 13 cases of osteoarthritis (OA), and 12 cases of RA in Algeria, Morocco, and Tunisia. Polymerase chain reaction (PCR) was used to analyze synovial specimens in this population. The findings revealed a low prevalence of Chlamydia trachomatis PCR-positive synovial samples in North African ReA/UA patients. The study also highlighted the importance of standardizing PCR testing procedures, as better concordance among the three testing laboratories could have improved the accuracy of the results [44].

1.4.6 Osteoarthritis (OA)

OA is a prevalent condition worldwide. In an epidemiological study conducted in a semiurban locality of Algiers, the prevalence of radioclinical OA of the knee was estimated at 21%, while OA of the hands was found to be 31.7% in the general population. Age, body mass index, and type 2 diabetes were risk factors linked to the occurrence of OA [45].

A cross-sectional study conducted by Slimani et al. aimed to estimate the overall prevalence of symptomatic OA among rheumatology outpatients in Northern

Algeria and the prevalence based on the specific joint sites affected. The study included adult outpatients (age >18 years) attending secondary and tertiary rheumatology clinics, and only patients with a confirmed diagnosis were consecutively enrolled. Of the 500 patients included in the study, 389 were females, and 111 were males, with a median age of 56 [range 15–88] years. The findings revealed a high frequency of OA among the rheumatology outpatient clinics in Algeria, with an overall prevalence of approximately 50%. Interestingly, the study also highlighted that hip OA was relatively uncommon compared to knee and spine OA, with a hip-to-knee OA ratio of 1:27. OA was identified as the most prevalent rheumatic condition, with the knee, spine, hip, and hand joints being the most commonly affected sites [46]. The prevalence of comorbidities of Algerian patients with OA of the knees and hands was studied by Haouichat et al. in a multicenter study carried out on 289 patients [47].

1.5 Screening Programs for Rheumatic Diseases in Algeria

The screening program for rheumatic diseases in Algeria is primarily driven by our rheumatology societies. Through various events and scientific congresses, they issue directives and recommendations aimed at raising awareness among rheumatologists, as well as other specialists (internists, gastroenterologists, dermatologists, and pulmonologists), and general practitioners regarding the importance of early-stage screening for rheumatic diseases and optimizing their management. Similarly, continuing education programs are frequently carried out in the various health structures intended mainly for general practitioners who are often on the front line in the care of patients.

Within the framework of inflammatory rheumatic diseases such as RA and AS, the Algerian Society of Rheumatology recommends promptly referring patients presenting with recent onset arthralgia or arthritis of the hands and feet for RA, and inflammatory low back pain, buttock pain, heel pain, and arthritis of the lower limbs for AS, to a specialist. This recommendation particularly applies if the inflammatory assessment and immunological assessment (including RF and anti-CCP antibodies for RA and HLA-B27 typing for AS) are positive. Additionally, it is advised to request specific X-rays at the onset of symptoms, focusing on the hands and feet to identify signs suggestive of RA, and to consider the utility of musculoskeletal ultrasound in detecting early forms. In patients with suspected AS, MRI of the sacroiliac and spinal joints can be utilized for early diagnosis. The patients are then referred to the rheumatologist to initiate treatment with close follow-up for the disease and potential associated medical conditions.

For patients with suspected OA, training programs exist to emphasize the interest of referring patients to the hospital in case of diagnostic doubt, with a view to a local procedure, and to direct patients requiring a preventive or curative orthopedic procedure.

1.6 Diagnostic Resources for Rheumatic Diseases in Algeria

Most healthcare facilities in the country are equipped with biochemistry laboratories, enabling them to conduct standard screening assessments at no cost. Prebiological tests, such as QuantiFERON tests, are accessible upon special orders and are conducted free of charge by specialized hospital centers and private laboratories.

Genetic tests such as HLA-B27 (for SpA) and HLA-B51 (for Behcet disease) have restricted access because they are carried out by a few specialized hospital laboratories, depending on the availability of reagents. Some private laboratories subcontract with foreign partners.

1.6.1 Imaging of Rheumatic Diseases in Algeria

Most public health centers in Algeria are equipped with standard imaging units that offer free access to patients. However, the availability of scanners and MRI machines is limited underscoring the need for an increase in the number of MRI machines. Capillaroscopy is now widely available in the majority of rheumatology and internal medicine departments.

Unfortunately, some imaging services provided in the private sector are either not reimbursed or are under-reimbursed by Social Security. For several years, ultrasounds dedicated to the musculoskeletal system have been available in all hospital rheumatology departments and all imaging centers.

In Algeria, two imaging centers have the positron emission tomography scanner; the first is private, opened in December 2016, and another public, recently inaugurated in April 2021 in a hospital center in Algiers.

The vast majority of radiologists practice in the private sector. This has led to significant pressure on hospital imaging centers due to a consistent shortage of radiologists.

1.7 Management of Rheumatic Diseases in Algeria

The facilities that provide immunomodulatory treatment are distributed on the national territory; they are divided into four regions: the central region (83 facilities), the West region (43 facilities), the Eastern region (49 facilities), and the Southern region (28 facilities).

Accessibility to multidisciplinary specialties, especially rehabilitation and orthopedic surgery, is facilitated according to established guidelines or protocols. These specialties are generally available in the university–hospital centers, and the private sector also has clinics and offices of orthopedic surgery and rehabilitation. There are no formal rheumatology nursing programs available.

1.8 Education and Research

There is currently no formal training program with a diploma specifically tailored for physicians interested in specializing in rheumatology, nor are there any formal programs for rheumatology nursing in Algeria. However, numerous theses have been conducted, primarily focusing on inflammatory rheumatic diseases, osteoarthritis, and bone diseases.

1.9 Cost of Rheumatic Diseases Care

The cost of care for rheumatic diseases is significant, as shown in Table 1.4 (unpublished data from the Ministry of Health). To regulate these costs, policies have been implemented that encourage the use of biosimilars as a more affordable alternative to original biological drugs. For example, the original version of infliximab (TNF inhibitor) was replaced by its biosimilar version in 2019.

Table 1.4 Cost of treatment of immune-mediated rheumatic diseases for 2022 in Algeria

Product	Dosage	Cost/year
Adalimumab injection	40 mg	2,581,683,234 DA
Etanercept injection	50 mg	1,076,919,160 DA
Anakinra injection	100 mg	316,045,306 DA
Infliximab injection	100 mg	618,707,206 DA
Rituximab injection	500 mg	1,502,824,640 DA
Methotrexate pill	2.5 mg	2,936,942 DA
Methotrexate injection	20 mg	533,934,800 DA
Mycofenolate mofetil pill	500 mg	138,206,718 DA

DA Algerian Dinar

1.10 Future Directions for Rheumatology Workforce and Service Development

The available human resources for managing rheumatic diseases remain insufficient, not adequately meeting current and future demands, especially with the increase in life expectancy [48, 49]. This underscores the urgent need to optimize the workforce responsible for treating patients with rheumatic diseases and compel national authorities to implement action plans to strengthen the workforce in rheumatology.

Algeria requires additional accredited training programs to develop and establish specialization in rheumatology, followed by training programs in subspecialties. This initiative will significantly address the demand for rheumatologists and facilitate the establishment of specialized clinics for rheumatic diseases.

While the policy of providing free care governs patient treatment, there is still a need to establish medical tourism in Algeria.

1.11 Future Directions for Rheumatic Disease Management in Algeria

Rheumatic diseases should be recognized as a public health problem in Algeria. Appropriate treatments and care represent a significant challenge for all those involved in caring for patients with rheumatic diseases. The problem posed by rheumatic diseases will continue to increase in the coming years, not only due to demographic changes with the rise of life expectancy but also because of changes in lifestyle.

Rheumatic diseases were not given due consideration in the development of the national strategy "National multi-sector strategic plan for the integrated fight against the risk factors of non-communicable diseases 2015–2019," unlike cancer, diabetes mellitus, cardiovascular diseases, and respiratory tract diseases [49]. They are also not part of the World Health Organization (WHO) Global Action Plan 2013–2020 for preventing and controlling noncommunicable diseases [50].

The national strategy must prioritize and facilitate coordination among various stakeholders. This strategy against rheumatic diseases will contribute to enhancing our health system and improving the quality of life in Algeria. It should complement the national strategy for preventing noncommunicable diseases established by the Ministry of Health. Therefore, the primary objective of the action plan must be to reduce risk factors and establish a comprehensive and appropriate management strategy, necessitating a multisectoral and intersectoral approach. Additionally, disease-specific strategies should be developed.

To achieve this objective, the authors propose three strategic fields of action: prevention and early detection, support and care, and research and training.

1.11.1 Prevention and Early Detection

1.11.1.1 Disease Prevention

Disease prevention controls the risk factors that promote the onset of diseases mainly determined by modifiable factors, apart from unmodifiable risk factors such as age, sex, and genetic factors. It considers the domains of primary and secondary prevention and the domain of treatment and care (tertiary prevention).

Raising awareness among the population about rheumatic diseases, their risk factors, and effective prevention strategies is crucial. This can be achieved by providing comprehensive and tailored information accessible to all. The focus should be on general modifiable risk factors, which can be categorized into three strategic axes:

Axis 1: Promotion of sufficient, varied, and balanced healthy food.
Axis 2: Promotion of physical activity and the practice of sports.
Axis 3: Tobacco control.

Algeria demonstrated its commitment to combating tobacco use by ratifying and implementing the WHO Framework Convention for Tobacco Control in June 2006 [51].

1.11.1.2 Early Detection by

- Promoting the early detection of rheumatic diseases and identification of the risk of chronicity.
- Conducting awareness campaigns about risk factors for developing rheumatic diseases with primary care medical personnel (general practitioners) and specialists.
- Developing diagnostic algorithms and recommendations for physicians, generalists, and specialists supporting disease screening.

1.11.2 Support and Care

Support and care are essential when rheumatic diseases have already become symptomatic, aiming to mitigate consequences, prevent sequelae, and avoid recurrences. The following measures are necessary to ensure that patients receive high-quality care:

- Establishing early diagnosis in more individuals suffering from rheumatic diseases.
- Promoting clinical examination methods, imaging, and laboratory examinations during the diagnostic stage to utilize resources efficiently.
- Ensuring that patients with rheumatic diseases receive high-quality treatment and care tailored to their specific needs throughout their illness.
- Educating healthcare professionals in all fields and specialties about the different manifestations of rheumatic diseases and training them to identify patients earlier.
- Facilitating collaboration between healthcare professionals in diagnosing these diseases.
- Guaranteeing patients easy access to a comprehensive range of services, including information, training, advice, and support throughout their illness.

1.11.3 Research and Training

1.11.3.1 Research

- Promoting and supporting high-quality scientific research and development efforts to combat rheumatic diseases.
- Establishing and maintaining registries on diseases and their treatments, including biotherapy registries, and encouraging participation in these registries through providing more information, incentives, and simplified participation processes.
- Ensuring the sharing of research findings among healthcare professionals.

1.11.3.2 Training by

- Providing continuing educational programs for healthcare professionals involved in the care of rheumatic patients.
- Organizing scientific congresses.

Supporting materials of the plan, such as funding and human resource development, are complementary axes that reinforce the three strategic fields of action. Funding aims to ensure sustainable and equitable financing for health action plans in Algeria, while human resource development aims to optimize and strengthen the workforce for combating rheumatic diseases.

1.12 Conclusion

In Algeria, the care of patients with rheumatic diseases is expanding, and the number of specialists is increasing gradually. One of the strengths of the healthcare system is the provision of free access and full coverage by the state for expensive drugs such as biologics and injectable antirheumatic treatments.

Numerous epidemiological studies in Algeria pertaining to clinical, genetic, and risk factors of rheumatic diseases have been published. The availability of biological DMARDs will probably increase with the introduction of biosimilars, decreasing the risk of intermittent supply and reducing the cost of the treatment.

An essential action plan for improving the management of rheumatic diseases involves increasing the number of trained rheumatology physicians and enhancing screening, diagnosis, and treatment options.

Conflict of Interest The authors declare that there is no conflict of interest.

References

1. Julien C. Histoire de l'Afrique du nord. Paris: Editions Payot et Rivages; 2015.
2. Algérie géographie physique. n.d. In: Larousse. [cited 2025 Sept 17]. Available from: https://www.larousse.fr/encyclopedie/divers/Alg%C3%A9rie_g%C3%A9ographie_physique/185613.
3. Wikipedia. Algeria [Internet]. San Francisco: Wikimedia Foundation; [cited 2026 May 11]. Available from: https://en.wikipedia.org/wiki/Algeria.
4. Loi no 19–12 du 11 décembre 2019, relative à l'organisation territoriale du pays. (2019, December 18). Journal officiel algérien. 2019 Dec 18;(2019–078):12 et suivantes. [cited 2025 Sept 17]. Available from: https://www.joradp.dz/.
5. Office National des Statistiques ONS. [Internet]. [cited 2025 Sept 17]. Available from: https://www.ons.dz/.
6. Central Intelligence Agency. Algeria – The World Factbook [Internet]. 2025 Sept 2 [cited 2025 Sept 17]. Available from: https://www.cia.gov/the-world-factbook/countries/algeria/.
7. Le système de santé algérien classé 4e en Afrique. TSA [Internet]. 2019 Feb 27 [cited 2025 Sept 17]. Available from: https://www.tsa-algerie.com/le-systeme-de-sante-algerien-classe-4e-en-afrique/.
8. Akintayo RO, Adelowo OO, Akintayo AA, et al. COVID-19 and rheumatology practice in Africa: significant changes to services from the shockwave of a pandemic. Ann Rheum Dis 2020;annrheumdis-2020.
9. Migowa AN, Hadef D, Hamdi W, Mwizerwa O, Ngandeu M, Taha Y, Ayodele F, et al. Pediatric rheumatology in Africa: thriving amidst challenges. Pediatr Rheumatol Online J. 2021;19(1):69. https://doi.org/10.1186/s12969-021-00557-7. PMID: 33962643; PMCID: PMC8103667.
10. Mody GM. Rheumatology in Africa – challenges and opportunities. Arthritis Res Ther. 2017;19(1):49.
11. Slimani S, Ladjouze-Rezig A. Prevalence of rheumatoid arthritis in an urban population of Algeria: a prospective study. Rheumatology (Oxford). 2014;53(3):571–3.

12. Makhloufi-Dahou C, et al. Prévalence et modalités de prise en charge de la polyarthrite rhumatoïde dans la circonscription de Bab El Oued. Rev Algerienne Immunol Immunopathol. 2022; ISSN: 1112-8739.
13. Acheli D, et al. Étude de l'association entre les allèles HLA classe II et la polyarthrite rhumatoïde chez des patients algériens. [dissertation]. Blida: University of Blida; 2022. Available from: http://di.univ-blida.dz:8080/jspui/handle/123456789/5711 [cited 2025 Sept 17].
14. Louahchi S, et al. Association study of single nucleotide polymorphisms of IL23R and IL17 in rheumatoid arthritis in the Algerian population. Acta Reumatol Port. 2016;41:151–7.
15. Slimani S, Abbas A, Ben Ammar A, Kebaili D, Ali el H, Rahal F, et al. Characteristics of rheumatoid arthritis in Algeria: a multicenter study. Rheumatol Int. 2014;34(9):1235–9. https://doi.org/10.1007/s00296-014-2981-7.
16. Ouali S, Zemri K, Sellam F, Harir N, Benaissa Z, Hebri ST, et al. Is there an association between anti-citrullinated peptide antibodies and the severity of rheumatoid arthritis parameters in Algerian patients? J Drug Deliv Ther. 2020;10(4):52–8.
17. Acheli D, Salah S, Ouardi W, Benidir M, lken A, Metatla S, et al. Les anticorps anti-protéines citrullinées et la polyarthrite rhumatoïde: quelles sont les caractéristiques de la PR avec ACPA chez les patients algériens. Rev Rhum. 2012;79(Suppl 1):A98.
18. Dahou C, Mechid F, Salah S, et al. [abstract THU0089] Rheumatoid arthritis and periodontal disease in Algerian people. Ann Rheum Dis. 2016;75(Suppl 2):1491.
19. Rupp I, Boshuizen HC, Jacobi CE, Dinant HJ, van den Bos GA. Impact of fatigue on health-related quality of life in rheumatoid arthritis. Arthritis Rheum. 2004;51(4):578–85. https://doi.org/10.1002/art.20539.
20. Djennane M, et al. Identification des fractures vertébrales des patientes atteintes de polyarthrite rhumatoïde à l'aide de la densité minérale osseuse et du Trabecular bone score (TBS). Rev Rhum. 2018;85S:A173-A335.
21. Djennane M, et al. Prévalence des fractures vertébrales au cours de la Polyarthrite rhumatoïde. Rev Rhum. 2017;84S:A159–334.
22. Bahaz N, Mechid F, Dahou-Makhlouf C. Anticorps anti-protéines citrullinées et atteinte du rachis cervical au cours de la polyarthrite rhumatoïde. Rev Rhum. 2021;88:A121–237.
23. Slimani S, Abbas A, Ben Ammar A, Kebaili D, Ali EH, Rahal F, et al. Characteristics of rheumatoid arthritis in Algeria: a multicenter study. Rheumatol Int. 2014 Sep;34(9):1235–9.
24. Pernod J, Bruneaux J. The Fiessinger-Leroy-Reiter syndrome in Algeria. A propose of 78 cases. Bull Mem Soc Med Hop Paris. 1960 Mar 4–11; 76:351–356.
25. Djoudi H. Etude du système HLA dans la population applications en rhumatologie. Thèse de doctorat en sciences médicales 1985.
26. Amroun H, Djoudi H, Busson M, Allat R, El Sherbini SM, Sloma I, et al. Early-onset ankylosing spondylitis is associated with a functional MICA polymorphism. Hum Immunol. 2005 Oct;66(10):1057–61.
27. Dahmani CA, Benzaoui A, Amroun H, Mecabih F, Sediki FZ, Zemani-Fodil F, et al. Association of the HLA-B27 antigen and the CTLA4 gene CT60/rs3087243 polymorphism with ankylosing spondylitis in Algerian population: a case-control study. Int J Immunogenet. 2018;45(3):109–17.
28. Saadi A, Dang J, Shan S, Ladjouze-Rezig A, Lefkir-Tafiani S, Gong Y, Liu Q, Benhassine T. Ankylosing spondylitis: analysis of gene-gene interactions between IL-12β, JAK2, and STAT3 in Han Chinese and Algerian cohorts. Cent Eur J Immunol. 2019;44(1):65–74.
29. Khan MA, Kushner I, Braun WE, Zachary AA, Steinberg AG. HLA-B27 homozygosity in ankylosing spondylitis: relationship to risk and severity. Tissue Antigens. 1978;11:434–8.
30. Dahmani CA, Benzaoui A, Amroun H, Zemani-Fodil F, Petit-Teixeira E, Boudjema A. Association study of copy number variants in CCL3L1, FCGR3A and FCGR3B genes with risk of ankylosing spondylitis in a West Algerian population. Int J Immunogenet. 2019 Dec;46(6):437–43.
31. Al Attia HM, Sherif AM, Hossain MM, et al. The demographic and clinical spectrum of Arab versus Asian patients with ankylosing spondylitis in the UAE. Rheumatol Int. 1998;17:193–9.

32. Hammoudeh M, et al. Challenges of diagnosis and management of axial spondyloarthritis in North Africa and the Middle East: an expert consensus. Int Med Res. 2016;44(2):216–30.
33. Burgos-Varga R, Wei JC, Rahman MU, Akkoc N, Haq SA, Hammoudeh M, et al. The prevalence and clinical characteristics of nonradiographic axial spondyloarthritis among patients with inflammatory back pain in rheumatology practices: a multinational, multicenter study. Arthritis Res Ther. 2016;18(1):132. https://doi.org/10.1186/s13075-016-1027-9.
34. Shirazy K, Hajjaj-Hassouni N, Hammond C, Jones H, Rezig AL, Pedersen R, et al. The prevalence of non-radiographic axial spondyloarthritis among patients with inflammatory back pain from northwest and South Africa: data from a noninterventional, cross-sectional study. Rheumatol Ther. 2018;5:437–45.
35. Haouichat C, et al. Particularités de l'atteinte de la hanche au cours des Spondyloarthropathies [abstract]. Rev Rhum. 2005;72:958–1159. https://doi.org/10.1016/j.rhum.2005.10.003. Available from: https://www.sciencedirect.com/science/article/pii/S1169833005003200.
36. Hammoudeh M, Al Rayes H, Alawadhi A, Gado K, Shirazy K, Deodhar A. Clinical assessment and management of Spondyloarthritides in the Middle East: a multinational investigation. Int J Rheumatol. 2015;2015:178750.
37. Kizza FN, List J, Nkwata AK, Okwera A, Ezeamama AE, Whalen CC, et al. Prevalence of latent tuberculosis infection and associated risk factors in an urban African setting. BMC Infect Dis. 2015;15:165.
38. Ramiro S, Nikiphorou E, Sepriano A, Ortolan A, Webers C, Baraliakos X, et al. ASAS-EULAR recommendations for the management of axial spondyloarthritis: 2022 update. Ann Rheum Dis. 2023;82:19–34. https://doi.org/10.1136/ard-2022-223296.
39. Aiche MF, Djoudi H, Al-Mayouf S, Consolaro A, Bovis F, Ruperto N, Paediatric Rheumatology International Trials Organisation (PRINTO). The Algerian Arabic version of the Juvenile Arthritis Multidimensional Assessment Report (JAMAR). Rheumatol Int. 2018;38(Suppl 1):27–33. https://doi.org/10.1007/s00296-018-3937-0.
40. Tahiat A, Allam I, Abdessemed A, Mellal Y, Nebbab R, Ladjouze-Rezig A, Djidjik R. Autoantibody profile in a cohort of Algerian patients with systemic sclerosis. Ann Biol Clin (Paris). 2020;78(2):126–33. https://doi.org/10.1684/abc.2020.1532.
41. Lahcene M, Oumnia N, Matougui N, Boudjella M, Tebaibia A, Touchene B. Esophageal involvement in scleroderma: clinical, endoscopic, and manometric features. ISRN Rheumatol. 2011;2011:325826. https://doi.org/10.5402/2011/325826.
42. Lahcene M, Oumnia N, Matougui N, Boudjella M, Tebaibia A, Touchene B. Esophageal dysmotility in scleroderma: a prospective study of 183 cases. Gastroenterol Clin Biol. 2009;33(6–7):466–9. https://doi.org/10.1016/j.gcb.2009.01.014.
43. Mellal Y, Allam I, Tahiat A, Abessemed A, Nebbab R, Ladjouze A, et al. Th17 pathway genes polymorphisms in Algerian patients with systemic sclerosis. Acta Rheumatol Port. 2018;43:269–78.
44. Kuipers JG, Sibilia J, Bas S, Gaston H, Granfors K, Vischer TL, Hajjaj-Hassouni N, Ladjouze-Rezig A, Sellami S, Wollenhaupt J, Zeidler H, Schumacher HR, Dougados M. Reactive and undifferentiated arthritis in North Africa: use of PCR for detection of Chlamydia trachomatis. Clin Rheumatol. 2009;28:11–6.
45. Haouichat C, Lekhal F, Mellal S, Aiche MF, Djoudi EH. Prévalence de l'arthrose des genoux et des mains chez les Femmes de la localité de Douéra (Alger). Rev Rhum. 2013;80S:A119–352.
46. Slimani S, Bencharif I, Haddouche A, Bendjenna D, Kebaili D, Khaled T, et al. The Algerian study of osteoarthritis. A shallow frequency of hip osteoarthritis. Press Med. 2017;
47. Haouichat C, et al. Prevalence of comorbidities in Algerian patients with knee and/or hand osteoarthritis attending outpatient clinics: a multicenter study [Abstract]. Rev Rhum Ed Fr. 2014;81(Suppl 1):A388–400.
48. Office National des Statistiques (Algérie). 5e Recensement Général de la Population et de l'Habitat (RGPH) 2008. Algeria: Office National des Statistiques; 2008.
49. Ministère de la Santé, de la Population et de la Réforme Hospitalière (Algérie). Plan stratégique national multisectoriel de lutte intégrée contre les facteurs de risque des

maladies non transmissibles 2015-2019 [Internet]. Algeria: Ministère de la Santé; 2015 [cited 2026 May 9]. Available from: https://www.iccp-portal.org/resources/plan-strategique-national-multisectoriel-de-lutte-integree-contre-les-facteurs-de-risque.
50. World Health Organization (WHO). Global Action Plan for the Prevention and control of non-communicable Diseases 2013-2020. [cited 2025 Sep 17]. Available from: https://www.who.int/publications/i/item/9789241506236.
51. Ministère de la Santé, de la Population et de la Réforme Hospitalière (Algérie). Stratégie nationale d'aide au sevrage tabagique Algérie 2017–2019 [Internet]. Algeria: Ministère de la Santé; 2017 [cited 2025 Sep 17]. Available from: https://extranet.who.int/ncdccs/Data/DZA_D1bib_Tabac%20strategie%20Algerie.pdf.

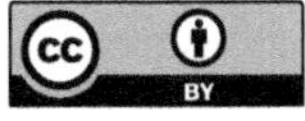

Chapter 2
Rheumatic Diseases in the Kingdom of Bahrain

Sahar Saad, Redha Ali, and Saadeya Abdulkarim

Abstract The Kingdom of Bahrain is the smallest member of the Gulf Cooperation Council countries. Its healthcare system began in 1960. Bahrain adopted the Universal Declaration of Alma-Ata in 1978 and the Astana Declaration in 2018, aiming for universal health coverage. The nation prioritizes public health, ensuring disease prevention and treatment by establishing various hospitals and a comprehensive network of health centers throughout the country. The implementation of an Electronic Medical Record system and the connectivity between the two main hospitals and health centers have significantly improved healthcare services and the referral system to the three major tertiary hospitals.

Until 1989, rheumatology cases in Bahrain were managed by orthopedic surgeons. The first dedicated rheumatology clinic was established in January 1990 at Salmaniya Medical Complex (SMC) and was overseen by a single rheumatology consultant. Since then, rheumatology practice in Bahrain has seen significant advancements in the services provided. Today, the rheumatology unit at SMC boasts six consultants, along with residents and chief residents.

In 2011, a second rheumatology division was inaugurated at King Hamad University Hospital. Since its inception, this division has made notable strides, by expanding its services and introducing specialized clinics for the early detection of arthritis, osteoporosis, spondyloarthritis, and lupus.

Being teaching institutions, both healthcare facilities host undergraduate students from Arabian Gulf University and Royal College of Surgeons in Ireland medical schools for their rheumatology rotations. These students gain experience at the rheumatology divisions of these major tertiary hospitals.

In this chapter, we delve deeper into the evolution and current state of rheumatology practice in Bahrain.

S. Saad (✉)
Rheumatology Division, King Hamad University Hospital, Busaiteen, Kingdom of Bahrain
e-mail: sahar.saad@rms.bh; saharsaad68@gmail.com

R. Ali · S. Abdulkarim
Department of Rheumatology, Salmaniya Medical Complex, Manama, Kingdom of Bahrain
e-mail: redha231@yahoo.com; drsnaji@gmail.com

K. A. Alnaqbi, G. Aldabie (eds.), *Rheumatic Diseases in the Arab World*,
https://doi.org/10.1007/978-981-92-0967-5_2

Keywords Bahrain · Rheumatic diseases · Rheumatology services · Rheumatology workforce · Arthritis · Rheumatoid arthritis · Spondyloarthritis · Osteoporosis · Pediatric rheumatology · Biologic therapy · Healthcare system · Rheumatology training · Patient education

2.1 Country Demographics

The Kingdom of Bahrain, comprised of 33 islands in the Arabian Gulf, is the smallest country in the Arab League of Nations, spanning an area of 661 km^2 (255.21 square miles) [1]. To the west, across the Gulf of Bahrain, lies its neighboring country, Saudi Arabia, connected by the 25-km (15-mile) King Fahd Causeway. To the east of the Gulf of Bahrain is the Qatar peninsula.

According to a 2024 statistical report published by the Government of Bahrain, the country's total population was estimated at 1,588,670. Bahrainis represented 47.8% of the population, while expatriates comprised the remaining 52.2% [2]. The overall sex ratio was 1.5 males per female. Approximately 18.1% of the population were aged 0–14 years, 77.7% were between 15 and 64 years, and 4.3% were aged 65 years and above. Figure 2.1 illustrates the age distribution of the population [3].

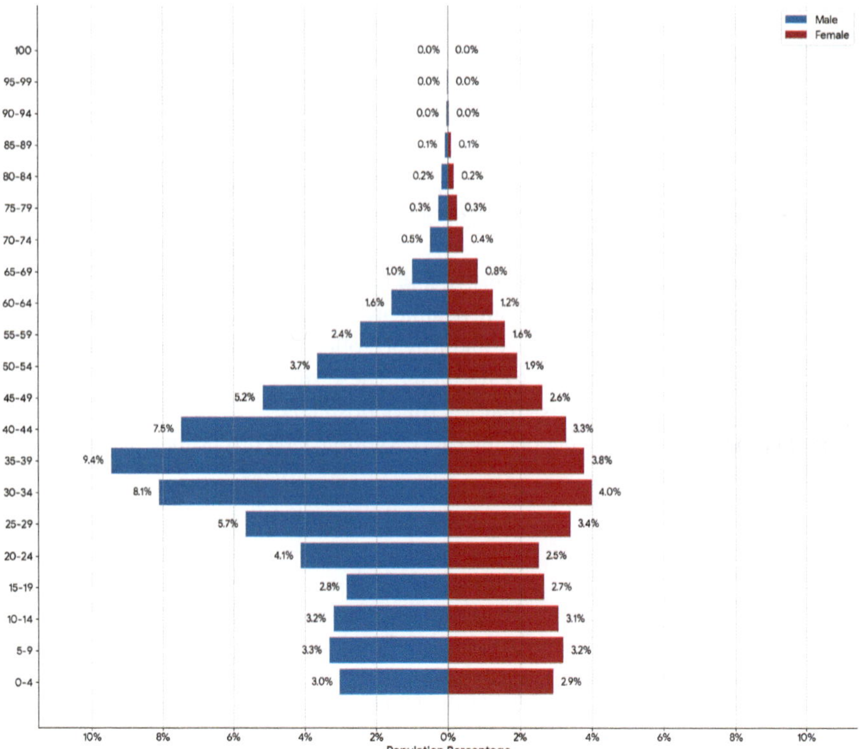

Fig. 2.1 Population pyramid of the Kingdom of Bahrain, 2024. (© 2024 by PopulationPyramid.net [3], Adapted and made available under a Creative Commons license CC BY 3.0 IGO (http://creativecommons.org/licenses/by/3.0/igo/))

The population grew by about 0.82% compared to 2023. Life expectancy in Bahrain in 2024 was 82.7 years for females and 78.1 years for males [4].

As of 2023, most of the population (89.9%) resided in urban areas, reflecting rapid growth and urban development. Bahrain accounts for approximately 0.02% of the world's total population [4].

Administratively, the Kingdom is divided into four governorates: the Capital (Manama), Al Muharraq, Northern, and Southern. The overall population density is 2002.16 people per square kilometer [2]. Bahrain has nine major cities: Manama (the most populous), Al Muharraq, Al Riffa, Dar Kulayb, Madinat Hamad, Madinat Isa, Sitrah, Jidhafs, and Al Hidd.

2.2 Bahrain Healthcare Sectors

Bahrain established its universal healthcare system in 1960 [5]. The American Mission Hospital, the country's first hospital, began as a modest dispensary in 1893. It transitioned into a clinic and, after the construction of a proper facility, was formally inaugurated as the Mason Memorial Hospital on 26 January 1903. The hospital retained this name until 1962 [6–8].

Bahrain has a modern, technologically advanced, and comprehensive healthcare system. Overseen by the Ministry of Health (MOH), this system encompasses a vast network of hospitals, clinics, and specialized centers. These facilities offer free services to nationals and are available to expatriates for a nominal fee. Healthcare in government hospitals is categorized into three levels: primary, secondary, and tertiary. The primary healthcare acts as the initial point of contact for individuals and is founded on a robust system that includes health centers spread throughout the country. This primary care is delivered by qualified family physicians, community health nurses, health promotion specialists, and social workers. They provide a range of curative and preventive services and refer patients to secondary and tertiary care when necessary.

In 1957, the Salmaniya Medical Complex (SMC) in the Manama governorate became the first public tertiary hospital in the Kingdom of Bahrain. The SMC is a multispecialty healthcare facility that offers emergency, secondary, and tertiary care to all citizens and residents of Bahrain [9]. Following the SMC, the Bahrain Defence Force Royal Medical Services Hospital was established in 1968, and the King Hamad University Hospital (KHUH) was founded in 2010 [10, 11].

Currently, there are 831 public and private healthcare facilities throughout the country, including 21 hospitals, 301 centers, and 96 clinics. Accordingly, the National Health Regulatory Authority was formed as a separate body in 2009 and is responsible for regulating and inspecting public and private facilities, licensing medicines, conducting examinations for and licensing medical personnel, and handling complaints [12].

The Supreme Council for Health, founded in 2012, is responsible for strategic planning. Over the longer term, it aims to restructure hospital administration to make each public hospital in Bahrain autonomous and give patients more choices.

Private hospitals are also present throughout the country. Healthcare expenditure accounted for 4.5% of Bahrain's gross domestic product [13].

There are two medical universities in Bahrain: the Arabian Gulf University and the Royal College of Surgeons of Ireland—Medical University of Bahrain. Both offer medicine and nursing programs to the Kingdom's population. Additionally, the College of Health and Science at the University of Bahrain provides programs in scientific disciplines, including nursing, pharmacy, and laboratory studies [14, 15].

2.3 Rheumatology Health Services in the Kingdom of Bahrain

Currently, Bahrain boasts a total of 17 rheumatologists. In the public sector, the primary rheumatology divisions are situated at SMC, Bahrain Defense Force Hospital-Royal Medical Service (BDF-RMS), and the most recently established one at King Hamad University Hospital (KHUH), inaugurated in September 2011. Specifically, SMC has six consultants and two specialists, KHUH has one consultant, and Bahrain Defense Force Hospital has one consultant and one specialist. Additionally, there are six consultants operating in the private sector.

Bahrain continues to advance in the field of rheumatology through the "Visiting Professor Program" organized by the MOH. This program periodically invites esteemed rheumatology professors to share insights on complex cases and deliver lectures to postgraduate fellows.

There are currently no certified rheumatology nurses, nurse practitioners, or physician assistants in Bahrain. However, there are nurses who work closely with rheumatologists.

2.3.1 Rheumatology Health Services in Salmaniya Medical Complex (SMC)

2.3.1.1 Evolution of Rheumatology Services in SMC

Before December 1989, orthopedic surgeons and general physicians handled all cases involving joint issues. The first dedicated rheumatology clinic was established at SMC in January 1990. This clinic was led by a single adult consultant rheumatologist, assisted by a junior and senior medical resident, and offered two clinics weekly. Notably, this rheumatologist was also tasked with overseeing patients with HIV/AIDS and sickle cell disease. This dual responsibility hindered the growth and advancement of rheumatology services, as the focus was not solely on rheumatological cases.

By 2005, two Bahraini infectious disease consultants were appointed at SMC to manage infectious diseases, including HIV. This shift allowed the rheumatology team to devote more attention to their specialty, although they continued to care for sickle cell patients.

As of April 2026, SMC hosts 12 outpatient clinics each week. The department is staffed by six consultants, including two chiefs, in addition to one pediatric rheumatology consultant. Another consultant pediatric rheumatologist previously affiliated with SMC has since retired from the institution and transitioned to private-sector practice.

Patients are referred to the SMC Rheumatology Clinic from various sources, including local health centers, SMC's Accident and Emergency Department, other subspecialties such as orthopedics and nephrology, private hospitals or clinics, and through self-referral.

A clear referral pathway exists between local health centers and SMC, allowing urgent cases to be referred and seen within a few days. Currently, there are a few established screening programs for selected rheumatologic diseases.

While specific statistics are unavailable, the primary rheumatological conditions treated at SMC include rheumatoid arthritis (RA), spondyloarthritis (SpA), psoriatic arthritis, systemic lupus erythematosus (SLE), gout, various vasculitis conditions (especially Behçet disease, polyangiitis with granulomatosis, and Takayasu disease), scleroderma, myositis, fibromyalgia, and osteoarthritis.

2.3.2 *Rheumatology Health Services in King Hamad University Hospital (KHUH)*

2.3.2.1 Evolution of Rheumatology Services in KHUH

KHUH, located in the Muharraq Governorate and spanning an area of 64,000 m^2, was established by Royal Decree No. 31 of 2010 and is affiliated with the Bahrain Defense Force. Both public and private services are available to all citizens and residents of the Kingdom.

The hospital is state-of-the-art, housing 410 beds, 9 operating rooms, and 9 wards. It has two intensive care units: one for adults with 26 beds and a neonatal unit comprising 34 nurseries. Additionally, there is an emergency department, a suite for admitted patients with a total of 54 beds, a day-case ward, and units for physiotherapy, hydrotherapy, and hyperbaric therapy. Every facility is equipped with the latest medical devices and technologies.

In its early stages, the hospital adopted the I-Seha Electronic Medical Record system, similar to the one used at SMC. Later on, the Healthcare Operation and Patient Environment (HOPE) system was introduced. Tailored to meet the needs of all specialties, HOPE demonstrated considerable success in clinical practice. Its implementation provided KHUH staff with enhanced adaptability, gradually phasing out paper use within the hospital. HOPE was later replaced by the ALCARE electronic health information system

KHUH delivers high-quality healthcare across a variety of departments, including but not limited to general surgery, orthopedics, ophthalmology, and internal medicine. These departments are staffed by 80 physicians, ranging from senior house officers to consultants. The internal medicine department is particularly diverse, encompassing subspecialties such as neurology, infectious diseases, endocrinology, pulmonology, nephrology, cardiology, hyperbaric medicine, psychiatry, gastroenterology, and rheumatology.

The rheumatology department at KHUH features a consultant, a registrar (who was promoted to senior registrar in 2022), and a nurse. This department is dedicated to providing optimal patient care through a collaborative clinical approach, aligning with the hospital's overarching mission. Figure 2.2 depicts important events in the development of rheumatology services at KHUH.

Upon the hospital's establishment, a dedicated day-care ward for rheumatology cases was introduced. This ward primarily facilitates parenteral injections for patients, including subcutaneous medications such as methotrexate, biologic disease-modifying antirheumatic drugs (DMARDs), osteoporosis drugs, and intravenous (IV) medications such as pulse steroid therapy, intravenous immunoglobulin, IV biologics, and IV osteoporosis drugs (e.g., zoledronic acid). The goal of this setup was to closely monitor patients, ensuring adherence to their treatment plans, thus optimizing outcomes. The day ward also serves as a platform to better understand patient responses to treatments, allowing for the prompt reporting of any drug side effects.

The approach prioritizes outpatient treatment: only critical rheumatology cases are admitted as inpatients. This system not only facilitates easier access to treatments but also strengthens the bond between healthcare providers and arthritis patients. The concept proved fruitful, with patients showing good adherence to their injection appointments. The need for this day ward originated from patients who previously received intramuscular methotrexate injections at health centers via intramuscular means.

Referrals are conveniently managed through the ALCARE system during patient consultations. The day ward team ensures each patient is contacted to schedule an appointment fitting their availability for the necessary treatments and injections.

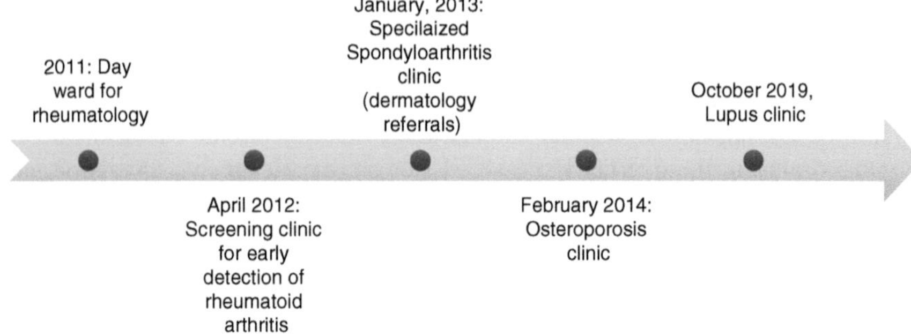

Fig. 2.2 Development of KHUH services over the years

Following the success of the day ward, a screening clinic was initiated in April 2012 for the early detection of RA. This clinic handles referrals from the five health centers within the KHUH catchment area, based on specific criteria:

- Joint pain primarily in the hands and feet.
- Temporary relief with nonsteroidal anti-inflammatory drugs (NSAIDs).
- Persistent symptoms for at least 6 weeks.
- Elevated levels of erythrocyte sedimentation rate, C-reactive protein, or both.

These criteria were designed after a thorough audit of the health centers in the catchment area. Initial visits revealed that many patients consulted their family physicians with a variety of health issues, typically in appointments lasting 5–10 min. Through sustained collaboration with these health centers, the hospital aims to improve patient outcomes by diligently following these criteria, ensuring no arthritis cases go undetected. Upon receiving a referral based on early detection criteria for RA, the KHUH clinic thoroughly reviews the patient's medical history and conducts both a clinical examination and any necessary investigative tests. If RA is confirmed, patients continue with follow-up appointments at the clinic. If not, they are discharged. However, for inconclusive results, patients undergo additional follow-ups and tests until a clear diagnosis is reached.

In January 2013, the rheumatology department introduced a specialized Spondyloarthritis (SpA) Clinic, held monthly. Initially, it relied on internal referrals, predominantly from dermatology, to assess potential cases of psoriatic arthritis in patients with psoriasis. Later, the gastroenterology clinic referred patients with inflammatory bowel conditions such as Crohn's disease and ulcerative colitis who reported joint pain. Over the past 4 years, the service expanded to accept referrals from the orthopedic department for chronic low back pain, specifically those showing symptoms of inflammatory back pain in certain age groups. The clinic's primary objective was early diagnosis and management of spondyloarthritis. However, due to manpower constraints and limited consultation time, outcomes such as metrology and patient-reported outcome measures (PROMs) have not been recorded.

In February 2014, following the inclusion of orthopedic referrals from the SpA clinic, the osteoporosis clinic was established under the umbrella of the rheumatology specialty. Although referrals were welcomed from all hospital departments, including the Bahrain Oncology Center and various specialties, the majority came from the orthopedic department. The clinic screens for osteoporosis based on medical history, laboratory test results, the Fracture Risk Assessment tool, and the dual-energy X-ray absorptiometry scan. Recognizing the varied treatments osteoporosis requires, the hospital pharmacy stocks most of the necessary medications. The osteoporosis clinic convenes once a month.

Furthermore, in October 2019, the Lupus clinic was launched in response to a growing number of rheumatic cases. Designed for the close monitoring of complex lupus cases, the clinic has seen a significant increase in patients over the past 2 years, particularly during the COVID-19 pandemic. This surge resulted in longer waiting lists [16, 17]. Tables 2.1 and 2.2 detail rheumatology visits (including external referrals) and appointments over the past 5 years, ending in September 2025

Table 2.1 Number of rheumatology visits at KHUH from 2016 to September 2025 (includes external referrals)

Year	Number of rheumatology visits	% increase between years
2016	3063	–
2017	3923	28.07%
2018	5758	46.77%
2019	6740	17.05%
2020	7873	16.81%
2021	7445	−5.43%*
2022	2564	−6.55%*
2023	7817	204.87%
2024	8364	6.99%
2025	8865	5.98%

*Negative values indicate reduced rheumatology clinic visits compared with the previous year during the COVID-19 pandemic

Table 2.2 Number of new rheumatology clinic patients at KHUH from 2016 to September 2025

Year	Number of new patients
2016	205
2017	237
2018	271
2019	255
2020	276
2021	323
2022	300
2023	1140
2024	1162
2025	1103
Grand total	5272

(unpublished data from KHUH). A growing trend in the number of RA patients was observed in Bahrain, a notable observation given Bahrain's relatively small population. In addition, there was a marked increase in arthritis cases during the COVID-19 pandemic, with many of these patients later diagnosed with RA post-COVID infection. Various studies have documented a rise in antibodies such as anticardiolipin, anti-β2-glycoprotein I, anticitrullinated protein, and antinuclear antibodies following SARS-CoV-2 infection [18–21].

The breakdown of cases diagnosed at KHUH from 2016 to September 2025 has been summarized in Table 2.3 (unpublished data).

2.3.3 Accredited Rheumatology Centers in Bahrain

Currently, there are no accredited rheumatology centers in Bahrain.

Table 2.3 Rheumatic diseases at KHUH from 2016 to September 2025

Diagnosis	Number of patients
Low back pain	8971
Vitamin D deficiency	7121
Generalized osteoarthritis	6772
Knee osteoarthritis	1965
Osteoporosis	1800
Rheumatoid arthritis	1430
Psoriasis	1204
Trigger finger	919
Plantar fascial fibromatosis	679
Carpal tunnel syndrome	648
Gout	509
Systemic lupus erythematosus	495
Sciatica	443
Spondylosis	426
Adhesive capsulitis of shoulder	422
Cervicalgia	377
Dorsalgia	257
Lateral epicondylitis	235
Psoriatic arthropathy	191
Sicca syndrome [Sjogren]	156
Fibromyalgia	150
Axial spondyloarthritis (ankylosing spondylitis and nonradiographic axial spondyloarthritis)	135
Achilles tendinitis	131
Age-related osteoporosis with current pathological fracture	121
Hallux valgus (acquired)	106
Vasculitis	81
Episcleritis	56
Trochanteric bursitis	52
Medial epicondylitis	51
Systemic sclerosis	41
Olecranon bursitis	36
Behçet disease	22
Erythema nodosum	20
Juvenile arthritis	15
Primary Raynaud's syndrome	13
Other dermatomyositis	11
Other vitamin B12 deficiency anemias	11
Sarcoidosis	9
Progressive systemic sclerosis	8
Polymyositis	6

(continued)

Table 2.3 (continued)

Diagnosis	Number of patients
Granulomatosis with polyangiitis (formerly Wegener's granulomatosis)	5
Microscopic polyangiitis	3
Other overlap syndromes	3
Adult onset still's disease	3
Aortic arch syndrome (Takayasu)	3
Relapsing polychondritis	2

2.3.4 Diagnosis of Rheumatology Patients in Bahrain

SMC offers most modern serological and radiological services, including tests for various rheumatic diseases, HLA genetic markers (HLA-B27 and HLA-B51), and imaging techniques such as CT, MRI, and musculoskeletal ultrasound (MSUS).

The laboratory at KHUH is equipped to diagnose a variety of rheumatic diseases, including tests for rheumatoid arthritis, SLE, other connective tissue disorders, and vasculitis. Furthermore, the hospital's Pathology Department offers a range of laboratory services, from routine tests to advanced diagnostics for autoimmune connective tissue diseases. The hospital's radiology department is equipped with advanced imaging facilities required for diagnosing and monitoring different rheumatic diseases. The imaging modalities include X-rays, musculoskeletal ultrasound, computed tomography, magnetic resonance imaging, positron emission tomography scan (available in Bahrain only at KHUH), and bone scan. There is a musculoskeletal radiologist.

2.3.5 Management of Rheumatology Patients in Bahrain

At SMC, a wide range of NSAIDs and disease-modifying antirheumatic drugs (DMARDs), including conventional synthetic DMARDs, targeted synthetic DMARDs, and biological DMARDs, are available. The day-care unit, which opened in February 2010, was the only unit providing intravenous Infliximab (Remicade). Over time, various other TNF inhibitors and interleukin inhibitors were introduced.

Rheumatic disease management at KHUH hospital adheres to the guidelines and regulations set by the Pharmaceutical Services. Most arthritis medications, including NSAIDs and all conventional synthetic DMARDs, are provided free of charge to public patients. Moreover, the majority of biological DMARDs and other necessary medications for autoimmune rheumatic diseases are available. Biosimilars use started with the introduction of infliximab biosimilar, Remsima. The hospital's private pharmacy stocks all required rheumatology medications, and it offers biologic DMARDs for non-Bahrainis through insurance or as out-of-pocket expenses. Additionally, anti-osteoporosis medications are available such as oral bisphosphonates, subcutaneous teriparatide, subcutaneous denosumab, and intravenous zoledronic acid. Romosozumab and abaloparatide are unavailable.

2.3.6 *Accessibility to Multidisciplinary Specialties*

SMC's orthopedic surgery department conducts a wide range of major procedures for rheumatology patients, including joint replacement, arthroscopy, carpal tunnel release, and spinal stenosis decompression. Additionally, physiotherapy and occupational therapy at SMC play crucial roles in rehabilitating rheumatology patients.

Rehabilitation for rheumatic patients is tailored to their specific needs. Services, including physiotherapy and orthopedic surgery, are available for those with additional comorbidities or cases of arthritis with systemic involvement necessitating a multidisciplinary approach. The rheumatologist oversees all referrals to the physiotherapy and electrophysiology units, as well as other specialties, with all referrals documented in the ALCARE system.

Regarding pediatric rheumatology at KHUH, cases are reviewed by an adult rheumatologist, and all cases under the age of 14 are transferred to SMC for further investigation. There is a shortage in the Kingdom of Bahrain as only three pediatric rheumatology consultants are available: one at SMC and one at BDF-RMS. A chief resident and a consultant recently retired from SMC, further contributing to the shortage.

Additionally, for unique and complex cases that are rarely seen in Bahrain's clinical practice, the hospital arranges overseas rheumatology treatment. Decisions for such transfers are made by the hospital's overseas treatment committee.

2.4 Bahrain Rheumatology Society

Bahrain Rheumatology Society was established in December 2021.

2.5 Patient Support Groups

In Bahrain, there is no arthritis patient support group related to rheumatic disease.

2.6 Education in Rheumatology in Bahrain

2.6.1 *Continuous Medical Education*

In March 2013, KHUH hosted its inaugural rheumatology conference, featuring distinguished speakers from Gulf Cooperation Council (GCC) countries such as the UAE, Qatar, and Egypt. The target audience consisted of family physicians, general practitioners, and rheumatology fellows.

To further the Kingdom of Bahrain's commitment to medical education, KHUH established the Education and Proficiency Centre. This center encompasses the Scientific Research Department and the Healthcare Academy, both designed to offer healthcare professionals resources to continue their professional development.

Established in 2013, the Healthcare Academy is dedicated to providing top-tier continuing education and training for healthcare professionals and undergraduate students. Its educators, having a mix of advanced qualifications and practical clinical experience, offer a range of programs from certificate courses and workshops to formal academic programs. Importantly, the Higher Education Council of the Kingdom of Bahrain recognizes the Healthcare Academy as a governmental institution. This recognition grants it the authority to design and deliver programs, certify degrees and qualifications, and issue certificates in compliance with the law and its internal governance.

2.6.2 *Rheumatology Fellowship Training Programs*

Currently, there are no rheumatology fellowship programs in Bahrain. Specialty applications primarily funnel through the Saudi Medical Board or the Arab Medical Board. At KHUH, Senior House Officers (SHO) have the option to apply for training programs via the Saudi Medical Board. Conversely, at SMC, they can choose between the Saudi Medical Board and the Arab Medical Board, while at BDFRMS, the pathway is exclusively through the Saudi Medical Board. Once SHOs have successfully completed the internal medicine residency program, they become eligible to apply for the rheumatology fellowship program abroad. This pivotal step allows them to progress to the role of rheumatology registrars. With dedication to consistent practice and research, these registrars can elevate to senior registrar positions, eventually culminating in the esteemed role of rheumatology consultants. Notably, at SMC, two candidates have recently concluded their postgraduate training, two are actively undergoing training, and three more are poised to embark on their training journey.

2.6.3 Rheumatology Nurses/Nurse Practitioner/ Physician Assistant

Currently, there are no certified rheumatology nurse, nurse practitioner, or physician assistant specialized in rheumatology.

2.6.4 Patient Education and Awareness

Since the establishment of the Rheumatology Department at KHUH in September 2011, enhancing patient and public awareness about common rheumatic diseases has been a paramount priority. The primary focus lies on RA, SLE, osteoporosis, and osteoarthritis.

To further this goal, the department has developed patient information booklets in both English and Arabic. These booklets detail the services available to patients with rheumatic diseases, aiding in understanding the nature of arthritis and its management. They also offer booklets about various biological therapies, providing comprehensive details about these drugs, including recommended administration and dosage.

To solidify their commitment to raising awareness, every October, KHUH celebrates World Arthritis Day, further emphasizing the importance of understanding rheumatology. Furthermore, every February, Arab Arthritis Day is celebrated through various educational activities. Other awareness days that are recognized in Bahrain include World Arthritis Day, Rheumatoid Arthritis Awareness Day, SLE Awareness Day, and the awareness month of Osteoporosis.

In Bahrain, one of the major health concerns is obesity, a known risk factor for certain types of arthritis. Addressing this, the 2018 “Obesity does not suits me” campaign aimed to heighten awareness about the connection between obesity and health conditions, particularly arthritis. Feedback indicates the campaign’s success, with numerous individuals reporting positive lifestyle changes as a result.

Further emphasizing the importance of international collaboration, rheumatology in Bahrain is represented in the Arab Adults Arthritis Awareness Group, launched in 2019 [22]. Spanning 18 countries, this group actively engages in webinars and patient discussions, even offering support from allied professionals such as psychologists, physiotherapists, and nutritionists. Notably, they effectively addressed global challenges in rheumatology services during the COVID-19 pandemic [23–25].

Moreover, one rheumatologist serves as a board member of the Bahrain Health Mate Society, which focuses on educating the public about a healthy lifestyle to reduce comorbidities. This mission is realized in partnership with dieticians, family physicians, physiotherapists, and psychologists, all united in supporting arthritis patients. The group fervently works to promote a healthy lifestyle among the general public, leveraging campaigns, virtual interactions, lectures, and articles in both Arabic and English local newspapers.

2.6.5 *Screening Programs for Rheumatic Diseases*

Currently, there are no national screening programs for rheumatic diseases in Bahrain.

2.7 Rheumatology Research in Bahrain

Much of the collaborative research with rheumatologists outside Bahrain is initiated on a personal basis. For example, some rheumatologists at SMC have published over 20 articles in local and regional medical journals, with the majority being epidemiological studies and case reports.

The Scientific Research Department at KHUH plays a pivotal role in overseeing all research protocols and supporting the advancement of the healthcare system. Upholding research ethics is paramount to ensure the safety and well-being of our patients. Consequently, research approvals are exclusively granted by the research department based on a project's viability within the healthcare system. Moreover, this department aids physicians throughout various stages of the research cycle, offering assistance ranging from guidance on research projects, review and editing, statistical analysis, and refining the final manuscript.

The department at KHUH has facilitated the publication of numerous rheumatology research studies. Many of these are collaborative efforts, not only with GCC countries but also with other national and international partners. Initiated by rheumatologists at KHUH, these collaborations include notable initiatives such as the creation of an educational video for RA self-assessment. This was subsequently followed by qualitative studies evaluating the video's reception. The AUTO-DAS study explored patients' perceptions of RA and their abilities to self-assess disease activity after viewing educational videos. In addition, KHUH was part of a multicenter regional study that evaluated the concordance between physician and patient assessments of RA disease activity [26, 27].

In Bahrain, collaboration in the field of rheumatology has extended beyond national borders. Notably, one rheumatologist partnered with the Pediatric Rheumatology International Trial Organization (PRINTO) to translate essential information about rheumatic diseases and medications into Arabic. This valuable resource is available on the PRINTO website [28]. Thanks to the efforts of multiple nations, PRINTO has translations in various languages. Specifically for the Arab world, these translations aim to equip parents of children and adolescents with rheumatic diseases with comprehensive knowledge about the diseases and their treatments.

2.8 Future Directions and Recommendations for Rheumatology Care in Bahrain

The prevalence of RA in the Kingdom could be influenced by several factors, such as genetics, lifestyle habits such as smoking, obesity, and consanguinity. There is great potential in mitigating these numbers through enhanced awareness campaigns, strategic screening programs, and the expansion of rheumatology services in Bahrain.

SMC has ambitious plans to expand its day-case unit from 2 beds to 10 beds. Meanwhile, KHUH is keen on enhancing its rheumatology department by leveraging the hospital's resources. A notable initiative is the collaboration with the Healthcare Academy to launch a specialized rheumatology training program for nurses. This move is anticipated to strengthen the nursing workforce in rheumatology and potentially support research endeavors in the field.

Given its population size, the Kingdom of Bahrain faces a notable shortage of pediatric and adult rheumatologists. There is a pressing need to boost the number of rheumatologists in the public sector. Taking a cue from many advanced nations, the objective is to establish a ratio of one consultant rheumatologist for every 80,000 residents in Bahrain. This strategic move can enhance the care of patients with rheumatic diseases by:

1. Reducing wait times at rheumatology clinics.
2. Ensuring patients, especially outpatients with rheumatic diseases, receive ample consultation time.
3. Advocating for certifications in musculoskeletal ultrasound (MSUS)—a tool gaining traction in rheumatology clinics for its role in diagnosis, management, and follow-up in patients with rheumatic diseases [29–31].
4. Paving the way for specialized subspecialty clinics.
5. Championing research to tailor care for Bahrain's patient population.

Achieving these improvements necessitates:

1. Transparent communication between rheumatologists and high-level administrative stakeholders to gauge and address the gap between rheumatology care demands and the current supply of rheumatologists.
2. Introducing medical students, interns, and internal medicine residents to rheumatology earlier in their training.
3. Motivating Senior House Officers (SHOs) to specialize in rheumatology.

Bahrain's healthcare system has seen numerous advancements in rheumatology, with several research studies still ongoing. With the growing rheumatology case load in the Kingdom of Bahrain, the focus has shifted more toward providing immediate care rather than conducting research. This underscores the need for increasing the number of specialized physicians in rheumatology.

2.9 Conclusion

Rheumatology services in Bahrain have undergone significant transformations, consistently aiming to deliver top-notch care to patients. A key remaining challenge is the disparity between the expanding rheumatology services and the healthcare workforce available to support them.

Conflict of Interest The Authors declare that there is no conflict of interest.

References

1. Musaiger AO. The state of nutrition in Bahrain. Nutr Health. 2000 Jan;14(1):63–74.
2. Bahrain National Portal [Internet]. Kingdom of Bahrain; [cited 2025 Oct 13]. Available from: https://bahrain.bh/wps/portal/en/!ut/p/z1/rZJLc4IwFIX_ChuXTBKRh0tb28Ha1icq2TghJJCKASFip7%2D%2D0GkXtRXsTLPITDLnJvd-5wAMNgBLUoqIKJFKklRnH1tbNDKh69xC6D5Ph9CauI7dtW-MiYXA-rsALT0IZ6vRYD65HyLYQwBfUw8vrA-Fsq18BDHCh6p1KlakY-IHMtkx2IAnSo9JUzLSdkFGY7r-uAhLnRFSKnCVEsVBTaSZo0YGcUFVoRIYaF9ExZ0X9bEZFCHzHoP0w4IZOu4ap9whCuuMgppsWItTilt2z%2D%2DcwzrqdGdfBaBDgZlYPjR9MjdpO8XI44EFFK5WKvSqwqXGR_Fdcn6CElrBIFMlHKIqf2FROOBe0ah9_b-AsDWPYIqjj0jYjbpyxYuxXEO2LgicI1qVgJ-DJNN9XCV_80WO3DXNl0yXM_5XKBZMg23veLnjj40czKbO7uXNa8jgpo3fJsDCk/.
3. PopulationPyramid.net. Bahrain — 2024 Population Pyramid [Internet]. 2024 [cited 2025 Oct 13]. Available from: https://www.populationpyramid.net/bahrain/2024/.
4. CIA. Bahrain. The World Factbook [Internet]. [cited 2025 Oct 13]. Available from: https://www.cia.gov/the-world-factbook/countries/bahrain/.
5. Clarke A. Through the changing scenes of life 1983–1993. Bahrain: The American Mission Hospital Society; 1993. ISBN 1-898357-00-5.
6. Mason AD, Barny FJ. History of the Arabian Mission. New York: Board of Foreign Missions, Reformed Church of America; 1926. p. 117.
7. Scudder LR 3rd. The Arabian Mission's story: in search of Abraham's other son. 1st ed. Grand Rapids (MI): Wm. B. Eerdmans Publishing Co.; 1998. p. 168. ISBN: 0802846165. Available from: https://archive.org/download/arabianmissionit00fagg/arabianmissionit00fagg.pdf [cited 2025 Oct 13].
8. Salmaniya Medical Complex [Internet]. [cited 2025 Oct 13]. Available from: https://www.moh.gov.bh/HealthInstitution/SalmaniyaMedicalComplex?lang=en.
9. Bahrain Defence Force Royal Medical Services [Internet]. [cited 2025 Oct 13]. Available from: https://rms.bh/en/.

10. King Hamad University Hospital [Internet]. [cited 2025 Oct 13]. Available from: https://www.khuh.org.bh/en.
11. National Health Regulatory Authority [Internet]. [cited 2025 Oct 13]. Available from: https://www.nhra.bh/.
12. Supreme Council of Health [Internet]. [cited 2025 Oct 13]. Available from: https://www.sch.org.bh/.
13. Arabian Gulf University [Internet]. [cited 2025 Oct 13]. Available from: https://www.agu.edu.bh/en.
14. Royal College of Surgeons in Ireland Medical University of Bahrain [Internet]. [cited 2025 Oct 13]. Available from: https://www.rcsi.com/Bahrain.
15. Gheita TA, Salem MN, Eesa NN, Khalil NM, Gamal NM, Noor RA, Moshrif AH, Shereef RE, Ismail F, Noshy N, Fawzy RM. Rheumatologists' practice during the coronavirus disease 2019 (COVID-19) pandemic: a survey in Egypt. Rheumatol Int. 2020;40(10):1599–611.
16. Chan A, Suarez A, Kitchen J, Bradlow A. Teleclinics in rheumatology introduced during the first lockdown phase of the COVID-19 pandemic of 2020. Future Healthc J. 2021;8(1):e27.
17. Slouma M, Mhemli T, Abbes M, Triki W, Dhahri R, Metoui L, et al. Rheumatoid arthritis occurring after coronavirus disease 2019 (COVID-19) infection: case based review. Egypt Rheumatol. 2022;44(3):275–8.
18. Tripathy A, Swain N, Gupta B. The COVID-19 pandemic: an increased risk of rheumatoid arthritis. Future Virol. 2021;16(6):431–42.
19. Derksen VF, Kissel T, Lamers-Karnebeek FB, Van Der Bijl AE, Venhuizen AC, Huizinga TW, et al. Onset of rheumatoid arthritis after COVID-19: coincidence or connected? Ann Rheum Dis. 2021;80(8):1096–8.
20. Vlachoyiannopoulos PG, Magira E, Alexopoulos H, Jahaj E, Theophilopoulou K, Kotanidou A, et al. Autoantibodies related to systemic autoimmune rheumatic diseases in severely ill patients with COVID-19. Ann Rheum Dis. 2020;79:1661–3.
21. Borghi MO, Beltagy A, Garrafa E, Curreli D, Cecchini G, Bodio C, et al. Anti-phospholipid antibodies in COVID-19 are different from those detectable in the anti-phospholipid syndrome. Front Immunol. 2020;11:584241.
22. Arab Adult Arthritis Awareness Group [Internet]. [cited 2025 Oct 13]. Available from: https://www.arabrheumatology.org/aaaa-group.
23. Ziade N, Hmamouchi I, El Kibbi L, Daou M, Abdulateef N, Abutiban F, et al. Telehealth in rheumatology: the 2021 Arab league of rheumatology best practice guidelines. Rheumatol Int. 2022;42(3):379–90. https://doi.org/10.1007/s00296-021-05078-w.
24. Lewandowski LB. Tackling global challenges in pediatric rheumatology. Curr Opin Rheumatol. 2020;32(5):414–20.
25. Ziadé N, Saad S, Al Mashaleh M, El Kibbi L, Elzorkany B, Badsha H, et al. Perceptions of patients with rheumatoid arthritis about self-assessment of disease activity after watching an educational video: a qualitative pilot study from the AUTO-DAS in middle eastern Arab countries project. Rheumatol Int. 2021;41(4):733–40.
26. Ziade N, Arayssi T, Elzorkany B, Daher A, Karam GA, Jbara MA, et al. Development of an educational video for self-assessment of patients with rheumatoid arthritis: steps, challenges, and responses. Mediterr J Rheumatol. 2021;32(1):66–73. https://doi.org/10.31138/mjr.32.1.66.
27. Ziade N, Abi Karam G, Daher A, Abu Jbara M, Aiko A, Alam E, et al. Development and implementation of an educational video that instructs patients with rheumatoid arthritis for self-assessment of disease activity: methodology of the AUTO-DAS in Middle Eastern Arab countries study. Eur Med J, EULAR highlight special edition, July 2018.
28. Paediatric Rheumatology INternational Trials Organisation (PRINTO) [Internet]. [cited 2025 Oct 13]. Available from: https://www.printo.it/.
29. Lautwein A, Ostendorf B, Vordenbäumen S, Liedmann A, Brinks R, Giulini M, et al. Musculoskeletal ultrasound as a screening-tool for rheumatoid arthritis: results of the "Rheuma-Truck" screening and awareness initiative. Adv Rheumatol 2022;62.

30. Rezaei H, Torp-Pedersen S, af Klint E, Backheden M, Kisten Y, Györi N, et al. Diagnostic utility of musculoskeletal ultrasound in patients with suspected arthritis – a probabilistic approach. Arthritis Res Ther. 2014;16(5):448. https://doi.org/10.1186/s13075-014-0448-6.
31. Mandl P, Baranauskaite A, Damjanov N, Hojnik M, Kurucz R, Nagy O, Nemec P, Niedermayer D, Perić P, Petranova T, Pille A. Musculoskeletal ultrasonography in routine rheumatology practice: data from Central and Eastern European countries. Rheumatol Int. 2016;36(6):845–54.

Chapter 3
Rheumatic Diseases in Egypt

Lobna A. Maged, Kamal El-Garf, Mervat Eissa,
Walaa Abdelrahman, and Bassel El Zorkany

Abstract Egypt is one of the oldest civilizations in the world and the most populous Arab country, with an estimated population of 103 million people in 2022. Despite a free healthcare services policy, the healthcare system in Egypt faces some challenges, including a low level of government health expenditure (4–5% of gross domestic product, GDP) with a resultant high out-of-pocket expenditure (57.2% of total health expenditure). Although there are no formal screening programs for rheumatic diseases in Egypt, the estimated burden of rheumatic diseases was 0.04% of the total disease burden in Egypt in 2014. The laboratory and radiological investigations necessary for diagnosing rheumatic diseases, as well as the facilities required for their proper management, pose minor obstacles. Economic and financial constraints, however, present a significant challenge to ensuring equity in provided services. There are ongoing attempts to improve insurance coverage to face such challenges. With around 1200 rheumatologists and some rheumatology associations, including the Egyptian Society of Rheumatic Diseases, Egypt has an active pivotal role in research and managing rheumatic diseases in the Arab world.

Keywords Egypt · Rheumatic diseases · Prevalence · Health care system · Rheumatology workforce · Arab world

3.1 Historical Background

Egypt is one of the oldest civilizations in the world and has historically contributed significantly to the development of medicine and science. Besides its unparalleled architectural achievements, medical practice in ancient Egypt was highly

L. A. Maged (✉) · K. El-Garf · M. Eissa · B. El Zorkany
Rheumatology and Clinical Immunology, Cairo University, Cairo, Egypt
e-mail: lobnamaged@kasralainy.edu.eg; kamalelgarf@kasralainy.edu.eg;
mervateissa@kasralainy.edu.eg; basselelzorkany@kasralainy.edu.eg

W. Abdelrahman
Rheumatology Department, Faculty of Medicine, Cairo University, Cairo, Egypt
e-mail: walaaabdelrahman@kasralainy.edu.eg

K. A. Alnaqbi, G. Aldabie (eds.), *Rheumatic Diseases in the Arab World*,
https://doi.org/10.1007/978-981-92-0967-5_3

advanced, serving as a guiding influence for centuries in Greek and Roman civilizations [1].

Ancient Egyptians were as equally renowned for pharmacy as they were for medicine. Historical records show they were familiar with drug preparation from plants and herbs such as cumin, caraway, aloe, safflower, pomegranates, castor, and linseed oil. Other drugs were made of mineral substances such as copper salts, plain salt, and lead. Eggs, liver, hair, milk, animal horns and fat, honey, and wax were also used in drug preparation [2].

Ancient Egyptians experienced a wide range of diseases similar to those present today, as demonstrated by the analysis of mummies, which serves as a valuable resource for understanding ancient diseases. Rheumatic and musculoskeletal diseases (RMDs), including gout and osteoarthritis (OA), were among the spectrum of known and treated diseases at that time [3].

Forensic and radiological studies conducted on the well-preserved bodies of the royal mummies from the eighteenth to early twentieth Dynasties (1492–1153 BC) at the Egyptian Museum in Cairo have proposed the diagnosis of ankylosing spondylitis in at least three pharaohs of the 18th and 19th Dynasties: Amenhotep II, Ramesses II, and his son Merenptah [4]. However, the presumed antiquity of this diagnosis was later questioned when further computed tomography (CT) reassessment revealed no evidence of sacroiliac joint erosions or fusion, nor facet joint fusion. Instead, the CT findings in Ramesses II and his son Merenptah were more consistent with those seen in modern populations affected by Diffuse Idiopathic Skeletal Hyperostosis (DISH) [5].

3.2 Demographics

Egypt is a large country with approximately 1 million square kilometers. However, the majority of its land is desert; hence, most inhabitants are concentrated around the Nile Valley. As a result, 98% of Egyptians live on just 3% of the territory [6].

Egypt has an estimated population of approximately 118.4 million in 2025. The country has a relatively young demographic structure, with about 32% of the population aged 0–14 years and approximately 63% in the working-age group (15–64 years). Older adults aged 65 years and above account for roughly 5% of the population [7].

3.3 Health Care Sectors

The healthcare system in Egypt consists of three main sectors [8, 9]:

1. The governmental sector comprises the Ministry of Health and Population facilities (MOHP), the Ministry of Higher Education facilities (university facilities and teaching hospitals), and healthcare services affiliated with the Ministries of Defense and Interior.

2. The semi-governmental sector includes Health Insurance Organizations (HIOs) and Curative Care Organizations (CCOs).
3. The private sector encompasses private hospitals, clinics, non-governmental organizations (NGOs), and facilities affiliated with social or religious organizations, such as mosques and churches.

Government health expenditure in Egypt remains relatively low. Public spending accounts for roughly 30–32% of total health expenditure, while total health spending represents about 4–5% of gross domestic product (GDP). Although total health expenditure per capita reached about US$141 in 2023, limited public financing contributes to a high reliance on out-of-pocket payments, which accounted for approximately 57.2% of total health expenditure. This heavy dependence on direct household payments negatively limits the availability of safe and high-quality care [10]. As a result, private providers play a major role in healthcare delivery. Out-of-pocket payments constitute the largest source of health financing in Egypt, accounting for roughly two-thirds of total health expenditure. A substantial proportion of this spending is directed toward private providers, particularly private clinics and hospitals [8]. According to recent statistics, private sector facilities accounted for about 63.3% of all hospitals and 29.3% of hospital beds in Egypt in 2021 [11].

Historically, Egypt introduced free healthcare services following the 1952 revolution to improve public access. However, budget shortages led to declining service quality. From the late 1980s, health sector policies increasingly encouraged privatization and reduced government spending. In 1997, the Health Sector Reform Program was launched to improve equity, efficiency, quality, and sustainability in healthcare services. As part of this reform, the Family Health Model was introduced to expand primary healthcare services for underserved populations, including rural residents and women without regular employment [12].

High out-of-pocket payments expose many households to catastrophic health expenditures [8]. More than 20% of Egyptians experience catastrophic health spending, a proportion higher than in several other lower-middle-income countries such as India or Bangladesh [13, 14]. Despite the relatively low cost of services in public health facilities, patients are often required to purchase consumables for diagnostic tests and treatments when these are unavailable in public facilities [12].

Physical access to health facilities is a significant obstacle in Egypt, particularly in rural areas like Upper Egypt. Factors such as distance, limited transportation options, restricted hours of services, and limited healthcare offerings at public facilities contribute to these challenges. Additionally, commuting, waiting times, physician-patient interactions, and time allocated to each patient further hinder the provision of satisfactory medical services [12].

The limited number of physicians in public clinics makes it very difficult for physicians to follow and manage patients on a proper paper or electronic filing system. The availability and feasibility of reaching patients' medical records wherever and whenever needed are vital issues to enhancing healthcare, which is still deficient in Egypt [15]. A significant challenge is the variability of work environments and operating systems in most hospitals belonging to the Ministry of Health (MOH).

The shortage of computers and electronic resources in some hospitals and the weakness in computer skills and the English language for most administrative and staff assistants are other obstacles [16]. However, a recent positive outcome emphasized the readiness of health stakeholders to adopt an e-health system in Egypt [17].

As users and international partners reported, private health facilities differ from public health services in several ways. While they tend to be more expensive, private facilities provide a wide range of services and good quality of care. They prioritize equity by minimizing waiting times for consultations and ensuring easy access to healthcare facilities. Private facilities also aim to provide more reliable services by utilizing appropriate equipment, although there may be variations in quality [12].

3.4 Rheumatology Health Services

Despite gradual improvement, physician density in Egypt remains relatively low, reaching 11.8 physicians per 10,000 population in 2021, compared with 4.9 per 10,000 in 2003, according to WHO data [18]. The emigration of Egyptian physicians due to low income and challenging working conditions has become an increasing concern, contributing to workforce shortages in several medical specialties. It is estimated that approximately 1200 rheumatologists practice in Egypt, and they are unevenly distributed across cities, governorates, and regions [19].

In addition to workforce distribution challenges, rheumatology services still face structural limitations, as there are currently no formally accredited rheumatology centers of excellence and no well-established dedicated rheumatology nurses, despite sporadic attempts to establish them.

3.4.1 Pediatric Rheumatology Centers in Egypt

1. The pediatric rheumatology department at Cairo University (Abu El-Reesh Hospital) has an inpatient, outpatient, and daycare unit (for infusions). This department receives thousands of patients seeking medical advice from all over the country. The average number of patients per year is around 17,630 (pre-COVID data).
2. Pediatric Allergy, Immunology, and Rheumatology unit (PAIR unit) at Ain Shams University has an outpatient clinic, inpatient unit, transfusion center, and an immunology lab for basic rheumatological investigations.
3. The pediatric rheumatology unit at Minia University includes an outpatient clinic and a small inpatient unit (4 beds supported with monitors and infusion pumps).
4. Pediatric Allergy, Immunology, and Rheumatology unit, Assiut University: An outpatient clinic (2 days a week) and an inpatient unit with eight beds.

5. Pediatric Rheumatology Department, Alexandria University.
6. At Tanta and Banha Universities, pediatric rheumatology care is provided by adult rheumatologists.

3.5 Rheumatology Associations in Egypt

In Egypt, there are several rheumatology associations. The Egyptian Society of Rheumatic Diseases (ESRd), established in 1977, is the largest and currently includes 1442 members, of whom 991 are females (68.7%), as of 2024. ESRd has two major activities. Firstly, it organizes an annual national congress that has been running for nearly 50 years, with attendees from across Egypt and many Arab countries. Secondly, ESRd publishes a well-recognized quarterly journal called The Egyptian Rheumatologist, which has been published by Elsevier for nearly five decades. The journal is indexed in Scopus and the Web of Science Core Collection and is currently ranked Q3 [20].

Other rheumatology associations include the Egyptian Society of Rheumatology (ESR), the Egyptian Society of Rheumatology and Rehabilitation (EGYRAR), the Egyptian Society for Clinical Immunology and Rheumatology (EGYSIR), and Upper Egypt Rheumatology, Rehabilitation, and Immunology Society (UERRIS). These societies were established partially based on geography (e.g., ESR is locally based in Alexandria, and UERRIS is based in Minia, the large city in Upper Egypt).

3.6 Overview of the Prevalence of Rheumatic Diseases Among Egyptians

Nationwide studies estimating the overall prevalence of RMDs in Egypt remain limited. Data obtained from the MOH estimated that musculoskeletal (MSK) disorders and connective tissue disease accounted for approximately 0.04% of the total disease burden in 2014 [12]. Table 3.1 shows the prevalence studies of some RMDs in Egypt.

As a part of the WHO—International League of Associations for Rheumatology (WHO-ILAR), Community Oriented Program for Screening of Rheumatic Diseases (COPCORD), a cross-sectional study including 3988 subjects in a rural area in Upper Egypt (2013 females and 1975 males) estimated that the prevalence rate of RMDs was 16.22%; prevalence was higher in females (10.4% vs. 5.8% for males), and patients with RMDs were older (46.89 ± 15.25 years) than healthy individuals (29.56 ± 18.95 years) [21]. The most frequently identified RMDs were OA (8.5%), soft tissue rheumatism (6.57%), spinal disorders (6.47%), fibromyalgia (0.60%), rheumatoid arthritis (RA) (0.30%), spondyloarthropathy (SpA) (0.15%), gout (0.6%), pseudogout (0.08%), systemic lupus erythematosus (SLE) (0.5%), juvenile

Table 3.1 The prevalence of some rheumatic diseases in Egypt

Study	Number of participants	Setting	Year	Disease	Prevalence	Female/Male
Rashed et al. [21]	3988	Upper Egypt	2020	OA, soft tissue rheumatism, spinal disorders, fibromyalgia, RA, SpA, gout, pseudogout, SLE, JIA, MCTD	OA (8.5%), soft tissue rheumatism (6.57%), spinal disorders (6.47%), fibromyalgia (0.60%), RA (0.30%), SpA (0.15%), gout (0.6%), pseudogout (0.08%), SLE (0.5%), JIA (0.03), MCTD (0.03%)	F (10.4%) M (5.8%)
Abdel-Tawab et al. [22]	5120	Upper Egypt	2004	OA	8.1%	F (53.2%) M (50.8%)
Abdel-Wahab [23]	4625	Upper Egypt	1991	RA	0.2%	F (0.35%) M (0.1%)
Gheita et al. [24]	3661	Nationwide	2017–2018	Adult SLE	6.1/100,000	F (11.3/100,000), M (1.2/100,000)
Easa et al. [25]	404	Nationwide	2018	Childhood SLE	1/100,000	F (1.8/100,000) M (0.24/100,000)
Gheita et al. [26]	1526	Nationwide	2017	BD	3.6/100,000	M:F (2.6:1)
Assad-Khalil [27]		Delta	1997	BD	7.6/100,000	M:F (5.4:1)
El-Soud et al. [28]	132	Delta	2009–2010	JIA	3.43/100,000	F (4.33/100,000) M (2.58/100,000)
Selim et al. [29]	581	Upper Egypt	2009	Postmenopausal osteoporosis	47.8%	–
Fuda et al. [30]	2000	Kalubia	2012	Juvenile fibromyalgia	1.25%	F (72%) M (28%)

Abbreviations: *BD* Behcet Disease, *F* Female, *JIA* Juvenile Idiopathic Arthritis, *M* Male, *MCTD* Mixed Connective Tissue Disease, *OA* Osteoarthritis, *RA* Rheumatoid Arthritis, *SLE* Systemic Lupus Erythematosus, *SpA* Spondyloarthropathy idiopathic arthritis (JIA) (0.03), and mixed connective tissue disease (MCTD) (0.03%).

Many studies have attempted to estimate the prevalence of RMDs in Egypt. OA was the most common RMD encountered in Egypt, constituting more than half of patients with RMD in the Minia governorate, according to the COPCORD study [21]. OA was the most common morbidity among the elderly population, with a reported incidence as high as 73.5% in one study in the Fayoum governorate [31].

In the COPCORD study, the prevalence of RA in the Minia governorate was found to be 0.3% [28]. The COMORA study revealed that Egyptian RA patients were younger, had more active disease, and experienced more significant disability compared to non-Egyptians from 16 other countries. A possible reason for this difference is Egyptian patients' lower use of biological disease-modifying anti-rheumatic drugs (DMARDs). Additionally, Egyptian RA patients had the highest prevalence of Hepatitis C (HCV), while non-Egyptians had lower rates of depression, hypertension, smoking, and dyslipidemia [32, 33].

In a nationwide study including 3661 adults from 15 governorates, the overall estimated prevalence of adult SLE patients in Egypt was 6.1/100,000 population (1.2/100,000 males and 11.3/100,000 females). The median age at disease onset was 25 years (4–75 years); the highest age at onset was in the South, whereas the lowest was observed in Cairo ($p < 0.0001$) [24].

A study conducted at Cairo University Hospital (a large tertiary center that receives referrals from all over Egypt) showed that the 5- and 10-year survival rates for 770 patients with SLE were 97.4% and 96.3%, respectively, while the rates for patients with nephritis were 96% and 92%, respectively [34]. In the other two centers' experience, the mortality rate among 771 patients diagnosed with SLE was 4.4%. The main reasons for death among SLE patients were infectious (35.3%), cardiopulmonary causes (26.5%), renal involvement (14.7%), and neuropsychiatric manifestations (5.9%) [35]. Additionally, mortality was associated with higher disease activity, damage scores, and the use of more aggressive immunosuppressives in both studies [34, 35].

In a nationwide multicenter study on childhood SLE patients, the estimated prevalence was 1/100,000 population (0.24/100000 males and 1.8/100000 females) [36]. Compared to adult-onset SLE disease, juvenile patients had more severe disease with a higher prevalence of nephritis and seizures [25].

In another multicenter study involving 630 patients, of which 264 were males (41.9%), with ages ranging from 9 months to 74 years, the following associations with vasculitides were observed: HCV infection in 151 patients (24%), Behcet disease (BD) in 148 patients (23.5%), immunoglobulin A vasculitis (IgAV) in 101 patients (16%), vasculitis associated with SLE in 93 patients (14.8%), Takayasu arteritis in 33 patients (5.2%), and Kawasaki disease (KD) in 22 patients (3.5%). Mortality was recorded in 36 patients (5.7%), with 27 deaths being vasculitis-related. Frequencies of KD, IgAV, and HCV-associated vasculitis were higher among patients from Lower Egypt ($p = 0.009$), while BD and ANCA-associated vasculitis were more common among patients from Upper Egypt [37].

In a different multicenter study, BD (76%), HCV-associated vasculitis (13.9%), and granulomatosis with polyangiitis (3.9%) were the most frequently encountered vasculitides. However, lower mortality (1.3%) was noted [38].

In a nationwide study on BD that included 1526 patients, the mean age of onset was 29.37 ± 8.6 years; 91 were juvenile onset (JoBD). The male-to-female ratio was 2.6:1. The overall estimated prevalence of BD in Egypt was 3.6/100,000. However, the rate could be underestimated, as many patients are seen in the private sector. The highest prevalence per 100,000 was observed in Alexandria (15.27) and Cairo (8.72) [26]. An earlier single-center study in Alexandria reported a prevalence of 7.6/100,000 in the population and a male-to-female ratio of 5.4:1 [27].

Recent nationwide studies estimating the prevalence of SpA still need to be improved. In the international ASAS-COMOSPA study, including 224 Egyptians, the bamboo spine was seen in 25% instead of 7% in the global cohort of about 4000 patients. This could be attributed to the infrequent use of biologics [39].

The prevalence of JIA was 3.43/100,000 in a study performed in the Sharkia governorate [28] and 3.3/100,000 in another study conducted in Alexandria [40]. In another cohort from Cairo, the male-to-female ratio was 1:1.09, whereas the mean age of disease onset was 6.257 ± 3.41 years [41].

The prevalence of osteoporosis in Egypt is 28.4% in women and 21.9% in men [42]. In rural areas of Upper Egypt, the prevalence of osteoporosis in postmenopausal women is even higher, reaching up to 47.8% [29, 43].

Studies reporting the incidence of primary fibromyalgia are rare, yet it is a prevalent disease in practice. The prevalence of fibromyalgia among students in the Qalubia governorate was 1.25% [30].

3.7 Risk Factors of Rheumatic Diseases

3.7.1 Consanguinity

The rate of consanguineous marriage is considered high in Egypt (35.3%), especially among first cousins (86%) [44]. Consanguinity was investigated as a risk factor for developing autoinflammatory disorders such as Familial Mediterranean fever (FMF) [45]; however, the data on its impact on autoimmune disorders is scarce. In a study investigating genotypic mutations in Egyptian children with FMF, it was found that 22.1% of patients had a positive family history, while kinship was detected in 37.9% of cases [45].

3.7.2 Infections

Infections are considered one of the most critical environmental factors that may induce the initiation or exacerbation of autoimmune diseases with several postulated mechanisms, including molecular mimicry, epitope spreading, and bystander activation. One of the suggested mechanisms is the constant activation of the immune system in persistent infections [46]. This mechanism is fundamental in HCV, a virus that can evade the immune system, resulting in chronic infection in 80% of infected patients [47].

Patients with chronic HCV infection may present with different rheumatic manifestations, including arthralgia, myalgia, arthritis, vasculitis, sicca symptoms, mixed cryoglobulinemia, and fibromyalgia, in addition to proposed associations with autoimmune diseases such as SLE and Sjogren syndrome [48].

Egypt had the highest worldwide prevalence of HCV infection, with an estimated prevalence of 14.7% in 2008 [49] and 7% in 2015 [50]. In collaboration with the World Health Organization (WHO), the MOH launched a successful program that screened and treated HCV, aiming for complete elimination [51].

Hepatitis B virus (HBV), which is of moderate endemicity in Egypt (2–8%) [52, 53], has been associated with a variety of extrahepatic manifestations, including membranoproliferative glomerulonephritis, cutaneous vasculitis, essential mixed cryoglobulinemia, and polyarteritis nodosa [54], as well as with several RMDs such as RA, polymyositis, and polymyalgia rheumatica. After the national immunization program in 1992, its prevalence dropped in 2015 to 1.4% [53], and later in the HCV campaign, patients treated for HCV received immunization for HBV [51].

3.7.3 Air Pollution and Smoking

Air pollution is another public health problem in Egypt. It was estimated that around 19,200 people died prematurely in 2017, and over 3 billion days were lived with illness in Egypt in 2017 due to air pollution alone in Cairo governorate. Open burning (including the burning of agricultural waste), secondary particulates (sulfates, nitrates, chlorides), and motor vehicles were found to be the major determinants of air pollution in Egypt [55]. Another significant issue is the deterioration of ground and surface water due to the discharge of insufficiently treated, heavily polluted industrial and domestic wastewater into its waterways [56].

Air pollution generally and specific pollutants such as silica were linked to systemic autoimmune disorders, including connective tissue diseases (particularly RA), JIA, ANCA-associated vasculitis, and inflammatory bowel diseases [57–60]. Polluted drinking water was an important predisposing factor to SLE, particularly renal involvement [61]. Silicosis is Egypt's most common occupational lung disease, with an estimated prevalence of 18.5–45.8% among workers exposed to free crystalline silica dust. An Egyptian study showed that the values of C-reactive protein, rheumatoid factor, C3, IgA, IgG, and IgM were significantly higher in the exposed group with silicosis than in the sensitive group without silicosis and in healthy unexposed control subjects [62].

Smoking, which was estimated to have a prevalence of 22% in the Egyptian population in 2010, poses a significant public health challenge. It has been identified as a contributing factor to high seropositivity of RA patients in the post-hoc analysis of the COMORA study [33]. Passive smoking was found to contribute to higher disease activity [63] and parenchymal lung involvement [64] in Egyptian RA patients. In the ASAS-COMOSPA, 17% of Egyptian patients were smokers [39]. It was also linked to higher disease activity, inflammatory markers, functional disability, and radiological progression [65, 66]. Smoking was associated with higher Psoriasis Area and Severity Index (PASI) scores in a large tertiary center study. However, it was not identified as a risk factor for the development of psoriatic arthritis [67].

3.7.4 Diet and Obesity

Obesity is often a result of poor dietary habits and low physical activity. Egypt ranks 18th globally for its high prevalence of obesity, according to the WHO [68].

In Egyptian adults, obesity has been shown to induce chronic inflammation by triggering the release of inflammatory adipokines, such as interleukin-6 (IL-6) and leptin. This has been observed in conditions like OA, where higher serum leptin levels have been associated with knee pain, cartilage degeneration, and functional impairment [69, 70].

Obese individuals with RA in Egypt have higher levels of inflammatory markers, increased disease activity, and a greater likelihood of experiencing deformities and extra-articular manifestations [71].

Poor dietary habits in patients with SLE have been associated with poorer disease control [72]. Similarly, obesity has been linked to increased organ damage in SLE, particularly lupus nephritis [71].

3.8 Screening Programs for Rheumatic Diseases in Egypt

In Egypt, although there is an adequate number of rheumatologists, accessing specialized rheumatologic assessment remains a challenge, especially in rural areas and Upper Egypt. In addition to other healthcare-related issues, this creates obstacles to receiving proper rheumatology care [73]. The absence of centralized hospitals or healthcare systems and patient registries in Egypt makes it challenging to implement screening programs and accurately estimate the incidence and prevalence of rheumatologic diseases. This can lead to a skewed representation with higher prevalence reported in urban areas. Furthermore, there is a need to enhance public knowledge about the rheumatology specialty, as many patients with RMDs seek care from healthcare professionals other than rheumatologists, such as general practitioners, orthopedic specialists, and neurologists [74].

The increased burden of RMDs in the African region is due to a series of unmet needs, including limited disease awareness, sociocultural beliefs, delays in diagnosis and initiation of treatment, lack of country-specific treatment guidelines, and difficulties accessing treatment. These constraints accounted for the scarcity of data and limitations in epidemiological studies about the prevalence of rheumatologic disorders in developing countries [75].

The rheumatology community in Africa, including Egypt, faces a significant challenge in changing the perception among both healthcare professionals and the public that little can be done for those with RMDs [76]. However, by adopting a screening strategy similar to the "100 million Seha campaign," there is potential for a remarkable advancement in the field of rheumatology in Egypt and, subsequently, the entire African continent [77].

Models used in the UK and Europe, such as training specialized nurses and enhancing their role in caring for RMD patients, can address some of these difficulties [78]. Another model from Kenya was proposed to develop a teaching program for MSK care skills directed at all health professionals, including front-line medical officers in rural health centers [76].

The collaboration with international academic institutions is also recommended to establish effective approaches for prevention, diagnosis, and affordable interventions that are applicable in low-resource settings. This collaboration will also contribute to the training of more rheumatologists. Adequate support should be provided to these trained professionals to enhance rheumatology services and enhance the knowledge and skills of medical students, physicians, and other healthcare providers.

Raising public awareness about RMDs and the rheumatology specialty and patient work groups should be assembled for the cause, and young physicians should be inspired to consider joining this challenging and rewarding field [73].

3.9 Diagnosis of Rheumatic Diseases in Egypt

3.9.1 Laboratory Services

Most routine laboratory tests do not pose a significant obstacle to healthcare providers in Egypt because of the abundant availability. However, the lack of standardized pricing may still mean a challenge for the financially constrained, especially if not covered by public or private medical insurance.

Most university hospitals and public facilities offer genetic testing either for free or at a low cost. The national health insurance organization, which covers elementary school students, provides a refund for investigations as well as treatment and rehabilitation services. However, the coverage of genetic tests by the public sector is limited, and services for low-income citizens are frequently provided through donations from NGOs or charities. Genetic services offered by the private sector are covered mainly by out-of-pocket payments or reimbursed by private health insurance companies. A huge step toward standardization, improvement, and coverage of healthcare services is expected after the establishment of the new health insurance system in Egypt in 2018, which aimed at maintaining health records for all patients with coverage of most of the service costs, even in the private sector [79].

However, such limitations may not pose a significant obstacle to the diagnosis of some rheumatic diseases. For example, in axial SpA, the diagnostic utility of genetic testing may be lower in the Middle East compared with Western populations because of the lower prevalence of HLA-B27. Reviewing HLA-B27 status in the Middle East region, including Egypt, reveals significantly lower prevalence rates in normal populations in Arab countries (ranging from 0.3% to 6.8%) than rates reported in the United States and Europe (ranging from 6% to 25%) [80].

3.9.2 *Imaging Services*

Egypt has a well-established radiology residency training. In addition, there is a local formal sub-specialization training program with a particular orientation toward interventional radiology and women's imaging [81]. The radiology workforce in Egypt has expanded substantially, increasing from about 600 radiologists in the mid-1990s to approximately 1250 radiologists by 2012 [82]. This number is expected to continue increasing over time.

MSK ultrasound (MSUS) has gained much attention in the rheumatology community over the past few years. In addition to being a simple bedside tool, MSUS has many advantages, including safety and non-invasiveness, relatively low cost compared to MRI or CT, and the ability to detect inflammation and structural damage. As of 2022, approximately 100 rheumatologists in Egypt are trained in MSUS, including at least 10 EULAR-certified MSUS trainers [83].

Nuclear medicine has also been gaining tremendous attention due to its important role in the diagnosis, risk stratification, and management of most non-communicable diseases, including RMDs. In 2015, Egypt had 58 nuclear medicine centers with 65 gamma cameras, including SPECT/CT and PET/CT systems, and an estimated 105 physicians, 95 technologists, 32 medical physicists, and 12 radiopharmacists/radiochemists [84].

Egypt's technical medical equipment market is supplied mainly by imports. Very few ultrasound scanners are produced by a single Egyptian company, El Gomhoureya, wholly owned by the government and distributed by a minority of companies in different countries. Accordingly, private sector stakeholders are restricted to choosing from the limited governmental offers for the choice/price of medical devices or to personally import the needed equipment according to the customs laws [85].

3.10 Management of Rheumatic Diseases in Egypt

Over the past years, despite significant advances in managing RMDs, particularly in the era of biological therapy, conventional synthetic DMARDs remain the cornerstone and initial treatment across RMDs in Egypt; RA is a representative example, where nationwide data show methotrexate as the most widely used agent and biologic therapy received by only a minority of patients [86]. Pressing economic constraints represent a chief hurdle in managing RMDs for patients of low socio-economic status in low- and middle-income countries, where low income and socio-economic deprivation are consistently associated with delayed access to care, treatment non-adherence, and poorer disease outcomes [87]. Reimbursement of biological therapy by health insurance or third-party payers remains a critical challenge in Egypt, where out-of-pocket payments constitute the principal source of health financing, although the state funds a substantial share of the expenditure on expensive medications such as biologics through public mechanisms [88].

Furthermore, the current pharmaceutical pricing system in Egypt does not permit price adjustments to account for inflation, which makes it challenging for Egyptian pharmaceutical companies to operate under a pricing system controlled by the MOH. This has resulted in the need for innovative pricing strategies to ensure affordability and accessibility of medication for the public. Recognizing this, the MOH is actively exploring alternative pricing and reimbursement methods, particularly for innovative drugs like biologics [89].

The biologics market in the Middle East and Africa (MEA) has expanded substantially in recent years. Between 2015 and 2019, the regional biologics market reached approximately USD 4.1 billion, growing at an annual rate of about 14.5% [90, 91]. Within the region, Saudi Arabia represents the largest biologics market in the region, with sales exceeding USD 1.8 billion, followed by the United Arab Emirates, Egypt, and Algeria, each with biologics sales of approximately USD 450 million [90, 91]. Notably, the biologics market in Egypt has shown particularly rapid expansion, with annual growth rates approaching 20% during the same period [90].

Biosimilars have emerged as an important development within the biologics landscape. Despite the increasing availability of these products, biosimilar adoption in the MEA region remains at a relatively early stage, creating opportunities for future market expansion. In 2019, biosimilar sales in Egypt were estimated at approximately USD 6 million [90]. To encourage biosimilar uptake, the Central Administration of Pharmaceutical Affairs in Egypt introduced a pricing policy whereby the first five biosimilars are priced at 35% below the originator product, while subsequent biosimilars are priced at 40% below the originator [90].

3.11 Research and Education

As previously mentioned, at least 1200 physicians specialize in rheumatology in Egypt [19]. After completing 5 years in the Faculty of Medicine and two internships, a medical graduate can specialize in rheumatology directly by applying to the rheumatology residency program in academic hospitals. There are mainly two routes to becoming a specialist in rheumatology in Egypt. The first is applying for a master's degree (MSc) in one of 18 governmental universities; the physician can apply for a medical doctorate (MD) to be a consultant in rheumatology. The second route is applying for an Egyptian fellowship program (5 years) in rheumatology [92].

Research in rheumatology is mainly conducted in universities and national research centers. To obtain a complete degree of MSc and MD, a candidate should complete a training program, pass a written and clinical examination, and submit a thesis. A paper from the thesis must be published in a ranked international journal indexed in Scopus or Web of Science to have a full MSc or MD degree. For the academic promotion of staff members in rheumatology departments in universities and national research centers, five to eight papers must be published in the rheumatology field before attaining associate professor and professor degrees.

According to the SCImago Journal & Country Rank database, Egypt ranks third in the Middle East in rheumatology research productivity, with 1861 publications indexed between 1996 and 2024 that have accumulated 22,942 citations (excluding self-citation), corresponding to an H-index of 66 [93].

There are several rheumatology peer-reviewed journals in addition to The Egyptian Rheumatologist, the official journal of the ESRd hosted and produced by Elsevier. The Egyptian Rheumatology and Rehabilitation Journal is the official journal of the Egyptian Rheumatology and Rehabilitation Society and is published by Springer Open. Finally, the most recent is The Egyptian Journal of Rheumatology and Clinical Immunology, Journal of the Egyptian Society for Clinical Immunology and Rheumatology (EGYSIR) [94].

Many scientific conferences are held annually; the largest is the annual meeting of the Egyptian Society of Rheumatic Diseases, with about 1500 members of ESRd every year.

3.12 Financing and Access to Rheumatic Disease Treatment

The MOH ensures that at least 50% of Egyptians do. Coverage has been extended to different groups of beneficiaries under other legislation. This includes government employees, pensioners, widows, beneficiary family members, school students, women-headed households, and farmers. The private sector must also ensure all employees have access to private and national health insurance companies. Egyptian citizens not covered by health insurance are eligible for treatment at the state's expense [95].

The MOH is the leading purchaser of DMARDs and biologic agents for covered patients. Other purchasers, namely the Ministry of Higher Education and the Health Military Services, continue funding tertiary/university hospitals and military health services through budget allocations. Private health insurance schemes also continue purchasing services from contracted private providers. Availability of expensive biologics was a challenge in Egypt, as Egypt is a lower-middle-income country according to the World Bank country classification 2019, with limited public expenditure on health, as previously mentioned [96].

The Egyptian MOH published the first Egyptian guidelines for the registration of biologics in Egypt in 2015. Detailed protocols for managing different RMDs (RA, SpA, PsA, and JIA) were released to guide all sectors providing government health insurance. Biologic therapy was introduced in these protocols; tumor necrosis factor inhibitors (TNFi) were first introduced, followed by IL-6 inhibitors, B-cell depleting agents, and Janus kinase (JAK) inhibitors, as well as biosimilars. More biosimilars are expected to be introduced.

More recent data show a rising percentage of patients currently on biologics, which is expected to reach 80–88% after 2017 with the introduction of biological DMARDs by health insurance and MOH. This change is noted in patients included from Egypt in several global Assessment of SpondyloArthritis international Society (ASAS) studies [97–99].

3.13 Opportunities and Specific Challenges

Egypt is a well-known tourist destination and an emerging destination for medical tourism. Egypt attracts around 50,000 medical tourists yearly, mainly from Libya, the Gulf area, and Yemen. Major medical centers attracting international patients are located in Cairo, Marsa Alam, Alexandria, the Northwest Coast, Sharm El-Sheikh, and Hurghada [100].

The growing healthcare infrastructure and large patient population also provide opportunities to further advance rheumatology care and research in Egypt. Expanding specialized rheumatology services, strengthening multidisciplinary care, and increasing participation in international research collaborations may help improve disease outcomes and regional scientific contributions.

Thermal or health tourism involves traveling to locations that offer natural therapeutic resources such as mineral waters, mud, or spa treatments that may help manage certain diseases through therapies such as balneotherapy [101, 102]. Such therapeutic environments may also create opportunities for clinical research and participation in international collaborative studies in rheumatology.

The New Valley Governorate has 752 curative sites, including 564 in the Dakhla Oases and 188 in the Kharga Oases. These sites represent approximately 56% of Egypt's total therapeutic locations. They offer treatments such as sand burial therapy and sulfur water baths, which are traditionally believed to provide benefits for conditions including skin diseases (such as scabies, eczema, acne, and psoriasis), gout, obesity, metabolic disorders, and disorders affecting the locomotor system, nerves, joints, and bones. Despite this potential, the development of medical and curative tourism remains underutilized and requires further investment and infrastructure development to maximize its health and economic benefits [102].

3.14 The Future of Rheumatic Disease Care in Egypt

Universal health coverage (UHC) is defined as all people having access to quality health services without the financial hardship of paying for care. UHC is a strategic vision for Egypt's health sector, and the Sustainable Development Strategy (SDS

2030) health pillar has incorporated the objective of UHC into the overall vision for Egypt's development for 2030. Egypt Vision 2030 aims to achieve the aspirations of Egyptians for a dignified and decent life. Extending health insurance coverage geographically and demographically and increasing the level of service will hopefully make expensive drugs more readily available to all rheumatic disease patients. Such a significant health sector leads to profound institutional, functional, and regulatory changes, creating several technical, legal, and institutional challenges, all requiring substantial technical expertise and process management. The government will roll out the new system in six phases over 15 years [103].

Formal rheumatology nursing programs, availability of fellowship training accredited programs in certain diseases, and official subspecialty clinics incorporating patient-reported outcomes are planned in the future with the participation of academic departments in different Egyptian universities.

3.15 Conclusion

Egypt, known for its ancient civilization and large population, faces challenges within its healthcare system. Despite offering free healthcare services, the country struggles with low government health expenditures and high out-of-pocket expenses. While there are no formal screening programs for RMDs, they still contribute to the overall disease burden. Although there are some obstacles in terms of diagnostic investigations and facilities, economic constraints remain a significant barrier to equitable healthcare services. Nonetheless, Egypt actively contributes to research and the management of RMDs in the Arab world, with a substantial number of specialized physicians and active rheumatology associations, such as the ESRd. Ongoing efforts to improve insurance coverage demonstrate a commitment to addressing these challenges.

Conflict of Interest The authors declare they have no conflicts of interest.

References

1. Mark JJ. Egyptian medicine [Internet]. World History Encyclopedia. 2017; [cited 2026 Mar 14]. Available from: https://www.worldhistory.org/Egyptian_Medicine/.
2. Aboelsoud NH. Herbal medicine in ancient Egypt. J Med Plants Res. 2010;4(2):082–6.
3. Saleem SN, Hawass Z. Ankylosing spondylitis or diffuse idiopathic skeletal hypertosis (DISH) in Royal Egyptian mummies of 18th–20th Dynasties? CT and archaeology studies. Arthritis Rheumatol. 2014.
4. Rogers J, Watt I, Dieppe P. Arthritis in Saxon and mediaeval skeletons. Br Med J (Clin Red Ed). 1981;283(6307):1668–70.
5. Chhem RK, Schmit P, Fauré C. Did Ramesses II really have ankylosing spondylitis? A reappraisal. Can Assoc Radiol J. 2004 Oct;55(4):211–7.
6. Fouberg EH, Murphy AB, de Blij. Human geography: people, place, and culture. Wiley; 2009.
7. United Nations Population Fund (UNFPA). Egypt population data [Internet]. New York: UNFPA; [cited 2026 Mar 14]. Available from: https://www.unfpa.org/data/world-population/EG

8. Fasseeh A, ElEzbawy B, Adly W, ElShahawy R, George M, Abaza S, et al. Healthcare financing in Egypt: a systematic literature review. J Egypt Public Health Assoc. 2022;97:1. https://doi.org/10.1186/s42506-021-00089-8.
9. Radwan G, Adawy A. The Egyptian health map: a guide for evidence-based decision-making. East Mediterr Health J. 2019;25(5):350–61. [Internet]. [cited 2026 Mar 14]. Available from: https://www.emro.who.int/emhj-volume-25-2019/volume-25-issue-5/the-egyptian-health-map-a-guide-for-evidence-based-decisionmaking.html.
10. World Health Organization. Global Health Expenditure Database: Country profile [Internet]. Geneva: World Health Organization; [cited 2026 Mar 14]. Available from: https://apps.who.int/nha/database/country_profile/Index/en.
11. Central Agency for Public Mobilization and Statistics (CAPMAS). Egypt in Figures 2025: Health statistics. Cairo: CAPMAS; 2025.
12. Japan International Cooperation Agency (JICA). Health sector cooperation planning survey in the Arab Republic of Egypt: final report [internet]. Tokyo: JICA; 2017 Mar [cited 2026 Mar 14]. Available from: https://openjicareport.jica.go.jp/pdf/12285300.pdf.
13. Rashad A. The catastrophic economic consequences of illness and their effect on poverty estimates in Egypt, Jordan, and Palestine. Econ Res Forum. 2014.
14. Van Doorslaer E, O'Donnell O, Rannan-Eliya RP, Somanathan A, Adhikari SR, Garg CC, et al. Catastrophic payments for health care payments in Asia. Health Econ. 2007;16(11):1159–84.
15. Mohamed H. A model for computerization and implementation of electronic health records in primary health care in Egypt. J Commun Manage. 2020;3:1017.
16. Mursi MF, Salama MA, Galal SE. Towards a secure E-health system for public healthcare sector in Egypt using HL7. MEJ Mansoura Eng J. 2021;46(2):11–22.
17. Badran MF. eHealth in Egypt: the demand-side perspective of implementing. Telecommun Policy. 2019;43(6):576–94.
18. World Health Organization. Density of physicians (per 10 000 population) [Internet]. Geneva: WHO; [cited 2026 Mar 14]. Available from: https://data.who.int/indicators/i/CCCEBB2/217795A.
19. Ziade N, Hmamouchi I, Haouichat C, Baron F, Al Mayouf S, Abdulateef N, et al. The rheumatology workforce in the Arab countries: current status, challenges, opportunities, and future needs from an ArLAR cross-sectional survey. Rheumatol Int. 2023 Dec;43(12):2281–92. https://doi.org/10.1007/s00296-023-05427-x.
20. The Egyptian Rheumatologist [Internet]. Amsterdam: Elsevier; [cited 2026 Mar 14]. Available from: https://www.sciencedirect.com/journal/the-egyptian-rheumatologist.
21. Rashad S, Abda E, Selim Z, Hussein S, Metwally T, Fouad H. Prevalence of rheumatic musculoskeletal disorders in a rural area of Upper Egypt: WHO-ILAR COPCORD based community study. Ann Rheum Dis. 2020;79:1904–5. Abstract AB1227.
22. Abdel-Tawab RR, Abdel-Nasser AM, Darmawan J, et al. The prevalence of rheumatic diseases in rural Egypt: COPCORD-Egypt: abstract proceedings book, 11th APLAR Congress, Jeju, Korea. 2004.
23. Abdel-Wahab J. Some epidemiological aspects of various rheumatic diseases in Egyptian population of El-Minia Governorate. Doctoral thesis, Minia University, Egypt. 1991.
24. Gheita TA, Noor RA, Abualfadl E, et al. Adult systemic lupus erythematosus in Egypt: the nation-wide spectrum of 3661 patients and world-wide standpoint. Lupus. 2021;30(9):1526–35.
25. El Hadidi KT, Medhat BM, Abdel Baki NM, et al. Characteristics of systemic lupus erythematosus in a sample of the Egyptian population: a retrospective cohort of 1109 patients from a single center. Lupus. 2018;27(6):1030–8.
26. Gheita TA, El-Latif EA, El-Gazzar II, et al. Behçet's disease in Egypt: a multicenter nationwide study on 1526 adult patients and review of the literature. Clin Rheumatol. 2019;38(9):2565–75.
27. Assaad-Khalil SH, Kamel FA, Ismail EA. Starting a regional registry for patients with Behçet's disease in North West Nile Delta region in Egypt. In: Hamza M, editor. Behçet's disease. Tunis: Pub Adhoua; 1997.

28. El-Soud A, Amany M, El-Najjar AR, et al. Prevalence of juvenile idiopathic arthritis in Sharkia governorate, Egypt: epidemiological study. Rheumatol Int. 2013;33(9):2315–22.
29. Selim MA, Mahran DG, Khalil SA, et al. Prevalence and risk factors of osteoporosis in post-menopausal rural women in Upper Egypt using ultrasound densitometry.
30. Fuda A, Soliman YA, Hashaad NE, et al. The prevalence of fibromyalgia among school children in Kalubia. Egypt Rheumatol Rehabil. 2014;41(3):135–8.
31. El-Sherbiny NA, Younis A, Masoud M. A comprehensive assessment of the physical, nutritional, and psychological health status of the elderly populace in the Fayoum Governorate (Egypt). Arch Gerontol Geriatr. 2016;66:119–26.
32. Dougados M, Soubrier M, Antunez A, et al. Prevalence of comorbidities in rheumatoid arthritis and evaluation of their monitoring: results of an international, cross-sectional study (COMORA). Ann Rheum Dis. 2014;73(1):62–8.
33. El-Zorkany B, Mokbel A, Gamal SM, Mousa M, Youssef M, Hmamouchi I. Comparison of comorbidities of the Egyptian rheumatoid arthritis patients to the global cohort of the COMORA study: a post-hoc analysis. Clin Rheumatol. 2016;35(5):1153–9. https://doi.org/10.1007/s10067-015-3142-4.
34. Mahmoud GA, Shahin AA, Zayed HS, et al. Clinical and immunological pattern and outcome of Egyptian systemic lupus erythematosus patients: a single center experience. Lupus. 2018;27(9):1562–9.
35. Moghazy A, Ibrahim AM. Mortality in a cohort of Egyptian systemic lupus erythematosus patients: retrospective two-center study. Egypt Rheumatol Rehabil. 2021;48(1):1–9.
36. Eesa NN, Abdel Nabi H, Owaidy RE, et al. Systemic lupus erythematosus children in Egypt: homeland spectrum amid the global situation. Lupus. 2021;30(13):2135–43.
37. Shahin AA, Zayed HS, Elrefai RM, et al. The distribution and outcome of vasculitic syndromes among Egyptians: a multi-centre study including 630 patients. Egypt Rheumatol. 2018;40(4):243–348.
38. Attia DHS, Abdel Noor RA, Salah S. Shedding light on vasculitis in Egypt: a multicenter retrospective cohort study of characteristics, management, and outcome. Clin Rheumatol. 2019;38(6):1675–84.
39. Moltó A, Etcheto A, Van Der Heijde D, et al. Prevalence of comorbidities and evaluation of their screening in spondyloarthritis: results of the international cross-sectional ASAS-COMOSPA study. Ann Rheum Dis. 2016;75(6):1016–23.
40. Tayel MY, Tayel KY. Prevalence of juvenile chronic arthritis in school children aged 10 to 15 years in Alexandria. J Egypt Public Health Assoc. 1999;74(5–6):529–46.
41. Salah S, Hamshary A, Lotfy H, Rahman HA. Juvenile idiopathic arthritis, the Egyptian experience. J Med Sci (Pakistan). 2009;9(2):98–102.
42. Taha M. Prevalence of osteoporosis in Middle East systemic literature review, 10th ECOO. 2011.
43. Mahran DG, Hussein M, Farouk O. Bone mineral density among reproductive age women in rural upper Egypt. J Public Health. 2012;20(4):453–60.
44. Shawky RM, El-Awady MY, Elsayed SM, Hamadan GE. Consanguineous matings among Egyptian population. Egypt J Med Hum Genet. 2011;12(2):157–63.
45. Talaat HS, Sheba MF, Mohammed RH, Gomaa MA, El Rifaei N, Ibrahim MF. Genotype mutations in Egyptian children with familial Mediterranean fever: clinical profile, and response to colchicine. Mediterr J Rheumatol. 2020;31(2):206.
46. Anaya JM, Shoenfeld Y, Rojas-Villarraga A, Levy RA, Cervera R, editors. Autoimmunity: from bench to bedside [Internet]. Bogota (Colombia): El Rosario University Press; 2013. [cited 2026 Mar 16]. Available at: https://www.ncbi.nlm.nih.gov/books/NBK459447/
47. Kwon YC, Ray RB, Ray R. Hepatitis C virus infection: establishment of chronicity and liver disease progression. EXCLI J. 2014;13:977.
48. Palazzi C, D'Amico E, D'Angelo S, Gilio M, Olivieri I. Rheumatic manifestations of hepatitis C virus chronic infection: indications for a correct diagnosis. World J Gastroenterol. 2016;22(4):1405–10.

49. El-Zanaty F, Way A. Egypt demographic and health survey 2008. Int Fam Plan Perspect. 2009;29:158–66.
50. El-Zanaty F, Ministry of Health and Population [Egypt], El-Zanaty and associates [Egypt], ICF International. Egypt health issues survey 2015. Cairo, Rockville: Ministry of Health and Population, ICF International; 2015.
51. Omran D, Alboraie M, Zayed RA, Wifi MN, Naguib M, Eltabbakh M, et al. Towards hepatitis C virus elimination: Egyptian experience, achievements and limitations. World J Gastroenterol. 2022;24(38):4330.
52. Emara MH. Occult hepatitis B: the Egyptian situation. Trop Gastroenterol. 2012;33(4):242–50.
53. Elbahrawy A, Alaboudy A, El Moghazy W, Elwassief A, Alashker A, Abdallah AM. Occult hepatitis B virus infection in Egypt. World J Hepatol. 2015;7(12):1671.
54. Maya R, Gershwin ME, Shoenfeld Y. Hepatitis B virus (HBV) and autoimmune disease. Clin Rev Allergy Immunol. 2008;34(1):85–102.
55. Cost of environmental degradation: air and water pollution [Internet]. Washington (DC): World Bank; 2019 [cited 2026 Mar 15]. Available from: https://openknowledge.worldbank.org/entities/publication/0f982bee-6368-5895-a501-75f8dabfefcf.
56. Abdel-Satar AM, Ali MH, Goher ME. Indices of water quality and metal pollution of Nile River, Egypt. Egypt J Aquat Res. 2017;43(1):21–9.
57. Sun G, Hazlewood G, Bernatsky S, Kaplan GG, Eksteen B, Barnabe C. Association between air pollution and the development of rheumatic disease: a systematic review. Int J Rheumatol. 2016;2016:5356307.
58. Adami G, Pontalti M, Cattani G, Rossini M, Viapiana O, Orsolini G, et al. Association between long-term exposure to air pollution and immune-mediated diseases: a population-based cohort study. RMD Open. 2022;8(1):e002055.
59. Blanco-Pérez JJ, Arnalich-Montiel V, Salgado-Barreira Á, Alvarez-Moure MA, Caldera-Díaz AC, et al. Prevalence and clinical impact of systemic autoimmune rheumatic disease in patients with silicosis. Arch Bronconeumol (English Edition). 2021;57(9):571–6.
60. Farhat SC, Silva CA, Orione MA, Campos LM, Sallum AM, Braga AL. Air pollution in autoimmune rheumatic diseases: a review. Autoimmun Rev. 2011;11(1):14–21.
61. Chen J, Qu W, Sun L, Chen J, Kong W, Wang F, Pan W, et al. The relationship of polluted air and drinking water sources with the prevalence of systemic lupus erythematosus: a provincial population-based study. Sci Rep. 2021;11(1):18591.
62. Kalliny MS, Bassyouni MI. Immune response due to silica exposure in Egyptian phosphate mines. J Health Care Poor Underserved. 2011;22(5):91–109.
63. Hammam N, Gheita TA. Impact of secondhand smoking on disease activity in women with rheumatoid arthritis. Clin Rheumatol. 2017;36(11):2415–20.
64. Elemary AM, Elshawaf WM, Motawea SM, Raafat HA, Metawie SA. Predictors of airway and parenchymal lung abnormalities in patients with rheumatoid arthritis. Egypt Rheumatol. 2021;43(2):125–30.
65. Farouk HM, Abdel-Rahman MA, Hassan RM. Relationship between smoking, clinical, inflammatory, and radiographic parameters in patients with ankylosing spondylitis. Egypt Rheumatol Rehabil. 2021;48(1):1–10.
66. Gaber W, Hassen AS, Abouleyoun II, Nawito ZO. Impact of smoking on disease outcome in ankylosing spondylitis patients. Egypt Rheumatol. 2015;37(4):185–9.
67. El-Garf A, Teleb DA, Said ER, Eissa M. Psoriatic arthritis among Egyptian patients with psoriasis attending the dermatology clinic: prevalence, comorbidities, and clinical predictors. Reumatologia. 2021;59(6):394–401. https://doi.org/10.5114/reum.2021.112238.
68. Aboulghate M, Elaghoury A, Elebrashy I, Elkafrawy N, Elshishiney G, Abul-Magd E, et al. The burden of obesity in Egypt. Front Public Health. 2021;9:718978. https://doi.org/10.3389/fpubh.2021.718978.
69. El-Mikkawy DM, EL-Sadek MA, EL-Badawy MA, Samaha D. Circulating level of interleukin-6 in relation to body mass indices and lipid profile in Egyptian adults with overweight and obesity. Egypt Rheumatol Rehabil. 2020;47(1):1–7.

70. Hussein NA, Sharara G. Correlation between serum leptin, cytokines, cartilage degradation and functional impact in obese knee osteoarthritis patients. Egypt Rheumatol Rehabil. 2016;38(2):117–22.
71. Rizk A, Gheita TA, Nassef S, Abdallah A. The impact of obesity in systemic lupus erythematosus on disease parameters, quality of life, functional capacity and the risk of atherosclerosis. Int J Rheum Dis. 2012;15(3):261–7.
72. Behiry ME, Salem MR, Alnaggar AR. Assessment of nutritional status and disease activity level in Systemic Lupus Erythematosus patients at a tertiary care hospital. Revista Colombiana de Reumatología. 2019;26(2):97–104.
73. Mody GM. Rheumatology in Africa—challenges and opportunities. Arthritis Res Ther. 2017;19(1):1–3.
74. Almoallim H, Al Saleh J, Badsha H, Ahmed HM, Habjoka S, Menassa JA, et al. A review of the prevalence and unmet needs in the management of rheumatoid arthritis in Africa and the Middle East. Rheumatol Ther. 2021;8(1):1–16.
75. Usenbo A, Kramer V, Young T, Musekiwa A. Prevalence of arthritis in Africa: a systematic review and meta-analysis. PLoS One. 2015;10:e0133858.
76. Tikly M, McGill P. The challenge of practicing rheumatology in Africa. Nat Rev Rheumatol. 2016;12(11):630–1.
77. World Health Organization. Global Health expenditure database: country profile—Egypt [internet]. Geneva: World Health Organization; 2018–2019 [cited 2026 Mar 15]. Available from: https://open.who.int/2018-19/country/EGY.
78. Backhouse MR, Ndosi M, Oliver S. Developing a rheumatology team to meet a growing need in Africa: let's not forget to feed the cow. Afr J Rheumatol. 2016;4:39–41.
79. Khalifa AY, Jabbour JY, Mataria A, Bakr M, Farid M, Mathauer I. Purchasing health services under the Egypt's new Universal Health Insurance law: What are the implications for universal health coverage? Int J Health Plann Manage. 2022;37(2):619–31. https://doi.org/10.1002/hpm.3354.
80. Khan MA. HLA-B27 and its subtypes in world populations. Curr Opin Rheumatol. 1995;7:263–9.
81. Haddad MC, Loutfi SI, Tamraz JC, Al-Kutoubi AO. The status of radiology in the Arab world. First world report. J Med Liban. 2007;55(02):94–8.
82. Iyawe EP, Idowu BM, Omoleye OJ. Radiology subspecialisation in Africa: a review of the current status. SA J Radiol. 2021;25(1):1–7.
83. Fotouh AA, Hamdy M, Ali F, Mohamed EF, Allam A, Hassan WA, et al; Egyptian College of Rheumatology (ECR) Musculoskeletal Ultrasound Study Group. The emerging era of interventional imaging in rheumatology: an overview during the coronavirus disease-2019 (COVID-19) Pandemic. Open Access Rheumatol. 2022; 14:43–56.
84. Paez D, Becic T, Bhonsle U, Jalilian AR, Nuñez-Miller R, Osso JA Jr. Current status of nuclear medicine practice in the Middle East. Semin Nucl Med. 2016;46: WB Saunders, Philadelphia:265.
85. International Trade Administration (U.S. Department of Commerce). Egypt: medical equipment and supplies [Internet]. Washington (DC): International Trade Administration; 2025 Nov 21 [cited 2026 Mar 15]. Available from: https://www.trade.gov/country-commercial-guides/egypt-medical-equipment-supplies.
86. Gheita TA, Raafat HA, El-Bakry SA, Elsaman A, El-Saadany HM, Hammam N, et al; Egyptian College of Rheumatology (ECR) Rheumatoid Arthritis Study Group. Rheumatoid arthritis study of the Egyptian College of Rheumatology (ECR): nationwide presentation and worldwide stance. Rheumatol Int. 2023;43(4):667–76. https://doi.org/10.1007/s00296-022-05258-2.
87. Nkeck JR, Pelda A, Ngandeu-Singwé M. Tackling financial insecurity for autoimmune rheumatic diseases in developing countries in sub-Saharan Africa is of utmost importance. Pan Afr Med J. 2024;47:81. https://doi.org/10.11604/pamj.2024.47.81.42698.

88. Fasseeh AN, Elezbawy B, El-Fass KA, Gamal M, Seyam A, Hayek N, et al. Maximizing the benefits of using biosimilars in Egypt. J Pharm Policy Pract. 2023;16(1):79. https://doi.org/10.1186/s40545-023-00581-w.
89. Nations Émergentes. Egypt pharmaceutical survey [Internet]. Paris: Nations Émergentes; 2019 [cited 2026 Mar 15]. Available from: https://nations-emergentes.org/wp-content/uploads/2019/02/egypt-pharmaceutical-survey.pdf
90. Bassil N, Sasmaz S, El Sayah M, Akalankam A. Realizing biosimilar potential in the Middle East & Africa: the Middle East and Africa perspective [White paper] [Internet]. Dubai: IQVIA; 2020 Nov [cited 2026 Mar 15]. Available from: https://www.iqvia.com/-/media/iqvia/pdfs/mea/white-paper/biosimilar_iqvia-whitepaper_final.pdf.
91. Batran RA, Elmoshneb M, Hussein AS, Hussien OM, Adel F, Elgarhy R, et al. Biosimilars: science, implications, and potential outlooks in the Middle East and Africa. Biologics. 2022;16:161–71. https://doi.org/10.2147/BTT.S376959.
92. Supreme Council of Universities (Egypt) [Internet]. [cited 2026 Mar 15]. Available from: https://scu.eg/.
93. SCImago Journal & Country Rank. Middle East country rankings in rheumatology [Internet]. SCImago Lab; [cited 2026 Mar 15]. Available from: https://www.scimagojr.com/countryrank.php?area=2700®ion=Middle%20East.
94. Egyptian Journal of Rheumatology and Clinical Immunology. Egyptian Knowledge Bank [Internet]. Available from: https://ejrci.journals.ekb.eg/.
95. World Bank. A roadmap to achieve social justice in health care in Egypt [Internet]. Washington (DC): World Bank; 2015 [cited 2026 Mar 15]. Available from: https://www.worldbank.org/content/dam/Worldbank/Feature%20Story/mena/Egypt/Egypt-Doc/egy-roadmap-sj-health.pdf.
96. United Nations, Department of Economic and Social Affairs, population division. World population prospects 2024: Online Edition [Internet]. New York: United Nations; 2024 [cited 2026 Mar 15]. Available from: https://population.un.org/wpp/.
97. López-Medina C, Molto A, Sieper J, Duruöz T, Kiltz U, Elzorkany B, et al. Prevalence and distribution of peripheral musculoskeletal manifestations in spondyloarthritis including psoriatic arthritis: results of the worldwide, cross-sectional ASAS-PerSpA study. RMD Open. 2021;7(1):e001450.
98. Kiltz U, Van Der Heijde D, Boonen A, Bautista-Molano W, Burgos-Vargas R, Chiowchanwisawakit P, et al. Measuring impairments of functioning and health in patients with axial spondyloarthritis by using the ASAS Health Index and the Environmental Item Set: translation and cross-cultural adaptation into 15 languages. RMD Open. 2016;2(2):e000311.
99. Molto A, Gossec L, Meghnathi B, Landewé RB, van der Heijde D, Atagunduz P, et al. An assessment in SpondyloArthritis international society (ASAS)-endorsed definition of clinically important worsening in axial spondyloarthritis based on ASDAS. Ann Rheum Dis. 2018;77(1):124–7.
100. Helmy EM, Travers R. Towards the development of Egyptian medical tourism sector. Anatolia. 2009;20(2):419–39.
101. Walterová J, Vylita T, Huseynli A. Revisiting therapeutic landscapes in the spa context: toward a multisensory, evidence-based framework for healing environments. Int J Biometeorol. 2026;70(2):50. https://doi.org/10.1007/s00484-026-03137-0.
102. Protano C, Vitali M, De Giorgi A, Marotta D, Crucianelli S, Fontana M. Balneotherapy using thermal mineral water baths and dermatological diseases: a systematic review. Int J Biometeorol. 2024;68(6):1005–13. https://doi.org/10.1007/s00484-024-02649-x.
103. Egypt National Health Strategy 2024-2030 [Internet]. Ministry of Health and Population; [cited 2026 May 13]. Available from: https://www.mohp.gov.eg/UserFiles/LibraryFiles/438199.pdf?csrt=160540442788976059.

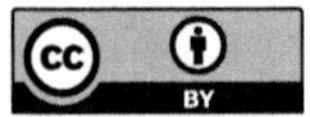
BY

Chapter 4
Rheumatic Diseases in Iraq

Nizar Abdulateef Jassim, Asal Adnan, Ziad Shafeeq Al-Rawi, and Sami Salman

Abstract Iraq, with a population exceeding 41 million, has witnessed steady development in rheumatology services over the past five decades. Rheumatology emerged as a formal specialty in the early 1970s, expanding through dedicated clinics, inpatient wards, national societies, and structured training pathways. Epidemiologic research has been ongoing since 1975, documenting the prevalence of major rheumatic diseases such as rheumatoid arthritis, systemic lupus erythematosus, ankylosing spondylitis, Behçet disease, fibromyalgia, and hypermobility in both community and hospital settings. Although the national rheumatology workforce has grown, the specialist-to-population ratio remains below international benchmarks, with uneven geographic distribution and a continuing gap in pediatric rheumatology training. Diagnostic and therapeutic capacity has advanced through broader access to laboratory testing, imaging modalities, musculoskeletal ultrasound, and multidisciplinary care, alongside increasing biosimilar uptake. The Iraqi League for Bone and Joint Health plays a central role in professional development, regional and global collaboration, and research productivity, with increasing publication output across inflammatory arthritis, connective tissue diseases, spondyloarthritis, and osteoporosis. Continued investment in workforce expansion, pediatric training, nursing certification, standardized referral pathways, and research infrastructure is expected to further strengthen rheumatology care and outcomes in Iraq.

Keywords Rheumatology · Iraq · Publications · Epidemiology · Training

N. A. Jassim · A. Adnan (✉) · Z. S. Al-Rawi · S. Salman
College of Medicine, University of Baghdad, Baghdad, Iraq
e-mail: nazarlateef@yahoo.com; asaladnan1987@gmail.com; staffmember@yahoo.com; ssshihab2@gmail.com

K. A. Alnaqbi, G. Aldabie (eds.), *Rheumatic Diseases in the Arab World*,
https://doi.org/10.1007/978-981-92-0967-5_4

4.1 Introduction

The Republic of Iraq is a country in West Asia, located in the heart of the Middle East. It shares land borders with Turkey to the north, Iran to the east, Kuwait and the Arabian Gulf to the southeast, Saudi Arabia to the south, Jordan to the southwest, and Syria to the west [1]. Iraq covers approximately 438,313 km^2 and comprises four main geographic zones: the western and southwestern deserts, the uplands between the upper Tigris and Euphrates Rivers, the mountainous Kurdish region in the north and northeast, and the alluvial plains of Lower Mesopotamia in the center and south. The two major rivers have supported irrigated agriculture for millennia. Baghdad, located on the Tigris River, is the capital and largest city [1, 2].

Iraq occupies much of ancient Mesopotamia (Land Between the Rivers), often described as the "cradle of civilization," where early urban societies such as Sumer, Akkad, Babylonia, and Assyria developed writing, law codes, and complex state structures. Specifically, King Hammurabi of Babylon, who reigned around 1792–1750 BCE, established one of the earliest systematic legal codes. After the seventh century, Iraq became a central and integral part of the Islamic world. Baghdad became the capital of the Abbasid Caliphate in the eighth century [1, 3].

Modern Iraq is one of the most ethnically and culturally diverse countries in the Middle East, home to Arabs, Kurds, Turkmen, Assyrians, Armenians, Mandaeans, Yazidis, and others. Although Iraq has faced decades of conflict, sanctions, and political turbulence, including the 2003 U.S.-led invasion, the country has continued to advance its federal parliamentary framework and pursue greater political stability.

Recently, Iraq has invested in reconstruction, infrastructure development, and health and education reforms, aiming to improve public services and rebuild essential state capacities.

This chapter will discuss the country's healthcare structure and rheumatology services, including workforce capacity, epidemiology of major rheumatic diseases, diagnostic and therapeutic resources, research output, current challenges, and future strategic priorities.

4.2 Country Demographics

Iraq had an estimated population of 41,266,109 people in 2023, reflecting relatively rapid population growth compared with many other countries in the region [2].

Iraq's population is unevenly distributed, concentrated in the north, central, and eastern regions of the country, with many of the larger urban areas situated along the Tigris and Euphrates Rivers. By contrast, much of the western and southern regions are lightly populated or uninhabited. As of 2023, approximately 71.6% of the population lives in urban areas, making Iraq a predominantly urban country. Baghdad is home to about 7.7 million people, and other major urban centers include Mosul, Basra, Kirkuk, Najaf, and Erbil [1, 2].

The median age in Iraq is 22.1 years. Iraq has a young population, with more than half (61.2%) between the ages of 15 and 64 years old, and 35.2% below the age of 15. Only about 3.6% are 65 years or older. The sex distribution is nearly balanced, with a total sex ratio of 1.01 males per female (2023 estimates) [1].

In addition to its youthful age structure, Iraq recorded a birth rate of 24.2 births per 1000 population and a death rate of 3.9 deaths per 1000 in 2023. Life expectancy at birth is 73.5 years, and health spending reached approximately 5.1% of Gross Domestic Product (GDP) in 2020, while the national literacy rate is 85.6% [1].

4.3 Country Healthcare Sectors

Access to health services is provided through two main sectors: the public and the private sectors. Public sector health services are provided through a network of primary health care centers (PHCC) and public hospitals at minimal charges. The PHCCs provide preventive and primary curative services. The main centers are located in urban areas, with smaller centers in rural areas. For secondary and tertiary care, patients are referred from PHCCs to hospitals. Most of the health sector in Iraq is financed by the government, with the private sector funded by out-of-pocket patient payments. The private sector has the potential to complement deficiencies within the public sector, particularly in curative services. In some cities like Baghdad, health services are provided through an independent network of many nationwide clinics and small private hospitals.

Other health service providers are in the semi-private sector, including public clinics operating at the PHCC in the afternoon. Such clinics provide curative services and distribute medications to patients with chronic diseases. Their fees are higher than those charged at public centers but lower than those charged by the private sector.

Electronic medical record (EMR) systems are partially implemented in governmental hospitals in Iraq, mostly in major tertiary centers, and for selected services, while most private clinics and private hospitals have already adapted EMRs to support appointments, billing, prescriptions, and patient documentation.

4.4 Rheumatology Health Services

4.4.1 Adult Rheumatology

As of November 2025, the total number of rheumatologists in Iraq is approximately 280, comprising 9 consultants, 161 specialists, 94 registrars, and 16 general practitioner rheumatologists. The sex distribution among them is 155 males and 91 females. Furthermore, there are 48 nurses working in rheumatology services; however, none of them is formally certified as a rheumatology nurse, and there are also 7 rheumatology centers recognized by the Ministry of Health (MOH). There are no internationally or regionally accredited rheumatology centers of excellence in Iraq.

4.4.2 Pediatric Rheumatology

The pediatric rheumatology specialty is still lacking in Iraq. Children with rheumatic diseases usually present to general pediatricians and adult rheumatologists who actively participate in their care. However, one tertiary center at Baghdad Teaching Hospital provides complex and comprehensive diagnostic and therapeutic services for children with rheumatic diseases and related conditions.

4.4.3 Referral System for Rheumatology Services

In practice, the referral system for rheumatology services is limited and remains underdeveloped.

Currently, there is no formalized pathway for referring patients to rheumatology, and as a result, many patients present directly to hospital services.

4.4.4 Timeline of the Iraqi Rheumatology Landscape

Rheumatology in Iraq has significantly evolved since its inception in 1972, when the first rheumatology clinic was established at Baghdad Teaching Hospital, Medical City. In 1973, the first official inpatient rheumatology ward was opened in Baghdad Teaching Hospital. By the end of 1973, the rheumatology service was established. During this period, academically active rheumatology centers emerged, and private clinics were set up. Since 1990, rheumatology has shown significant growth and advancement. Rheumatology was established as an essential subspecialty of internal medicine in 1999. The next milestone occurred in 2000 when the first national conference was held in Baghdad. The Osteoporosis Clinic and Behçet Clinic at Baghdad Teaching Hospital, Medical City, were established in 2000 and 2002, respectively.

Until 1987, no formal rheumatology degree or diploma was available. In 1988, a certificate in clinical rheumatology was instituted at the College of Medicine of the University of Baghdad.

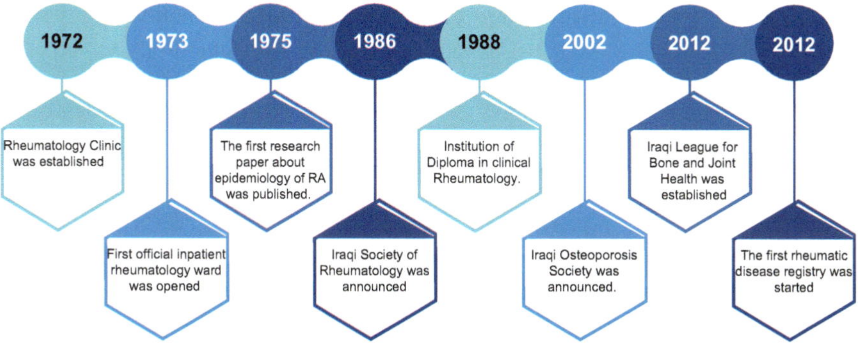

Fig. 4.1 Timeline of Rheumatology Development and Registry Establishment in Iraq

In 1978, the first research paper on epidemiology was published in Iraq [4]. The first scientific society specializing in rheumatic diseases and medical rehabilitation was established in 1986 under the Iraqi Society for Rheumatology, Medical Rehabilitation, and Care of the Handicapped.

In 2002, another association concerned with bone health was established under the Iraqi Osteoporosis Society. Building on these efforts, the Iraqi League for Bone and Joint Health was founded in 2012 and has since played an essential role in advancing and supporting the field. In the same year, the first rheumatic diseases registry was established at Baghdad Teaching Hospital, which systematically collected data on patients with various rheumatic conditions. Figure 4.1 illustrates the timeline of rheumatology services and disease registries.

4.5 Official Rheumatology Society

The Iraqi League for Bone and Joint Health is the official organization of rheumatologists in Iraq. As of November 2025, it has 265 members. It strives to propagate and consolidate rheumatology in Iraq. The league is a member of the Arab League Association for Rheumatology (ArLAR), the Asia Pacific League of Associations for Rheumatology (APLAR), the Pan Arab Osteoporosis Society (PAOS), and the International Osteoporosis Foundation (IOF). It organizes national meetings and contributes to continuing medical education through regular scientific workshops, conferences, and symposia throughout the year in different parts of the country. Every year, the league provides awards to junior rheumatologists. The league also provides a travel grant for rheumatologists to attend the conferences. Many papers, posters, and research (both basic science and clinical) are published in international journals by the league's members, as detailed in Table 4.1.

4.6 Overview of Rheumatic Diseases in Iraq

4.6.1 Epidemiology of Rheumatic Diseases

The first studies to identify rheumatic diseases at a community level started in the summer of 1975. The prevalence of rheumatoid arthritis (RA), systemic lupus erythematosus (SLE), and ankylosing spondylitis (AS) was studied [4–7].

An RA study revealed a prevalence of 1% for RA among 6999 individuals surveyed across various regions of Iraq, reflecting variations in geography and ethnicity [4].

A retrospective cohort study was carried out in Merjan Teaching Hospital in the Babylon governorate from 2001 to 2011 to assess the incidence of RA [5]. Among a total of 53,786 individuals, 1039 patients were diagnosed with RA. The incidence rate in 2001 was 1.60, increasing to 3.02 by 2011 for the same population. Additionally, the cumulative incidence in 2011 was recorded at 22.74.

The second study in Iraq screened the prevalence of AS. It was observed in 0.07% of the Iraqi population, and HLA B27 was found in 21 of 25 spondylitis patients, while it was found in only two out of 95 normal controls [6]. The observed frequency of HLA-B27 in AS and controls is less than that recorded in Britain, where the incidence was found in 96% of AS and 4% in the controls [8].

In a study published in 1983, the clinical characteristics of early cases of 67 SLE patients were reported. The disease represented 0.67% of all medical admissions and ranked as the third most common inflammatory rheumatic disease following RA and Sjogren syndrome [7]. Compared to RA, the prevalence of SLE was estimated at one case per 1867 of the population, one per 1127 of the total female population, and one per 616 women aged between 10 and 49 years.

Further community-based studies were conducted in subsequent years to better characterize the burden of other rheumatic disorders. A cross-sectional survey for Behçet disease was carried out in stages in Saglawia Town with a total population of 35,125 persons aged 16–45. The estimated prevalence was 1.7 per 10,000 inhabitants, similar to the prevalence in the other Mediterranean and Far East countries, excluding Turkey, which has a much higher prevalence of 8 per 10,000 individuals [9].

In an unpublished study, the prevalence of primary Sjogren syndrome (PSS) was studied among 1000 adult rheumatic patients attending a rheumatology clinic: 98 patients diagnosed with PSS and 165 patients diagnosed with RA. By comparing the prevalence of PSS with that of RA [4], it was found that the estimated prevalence of PSS is 0.59% of the population and is more commonly reported in elderly females, ranking next to RA in frequency among rheumatic diseases in Iraq.

The prevalence of fibromyalgia syndrome among school children and adolescents was observed to be 1.5% (2.9% for girls and 0.5% for boys) among 6471 students with a mean age of 13.1 years [10].

Other studies provided invaluable information at a community level regarding the burden of musculoskeletal (MSK) diseases in Iraq. These investigations helped identify the most common causes of impaired quality of life related to MSK complaints. Backache lifetime prevalence was 9.7% among 4079 individuals aged 15 years and over in Rawa Town, with a point prevalence of 2.9% at any time [11]. Lumbar spondylosis, a cause of backache, was reported in 58.3% of individuals [12]. More recently, a cross-sectional study among healthcare workers in Baghdad demonstrated a very high burden of low back pain, reporting prevalence rates of 92.7% (lifetime), 90.9% (past year), and 58.2% (past week). The study also showed that female sex, higher BMI, long working hours, and dentistry practice were significant risk factors and that low back pain was strongly associated with reduced quality of life and work performance [13].

In a survey conducted in 1981 among 1774 university students aged 20–24 years in Iraq, the prevalence of joint hypermobility was determined. Joint hypermobility was defined as a score of 4 out of 9 (based on the Beighton modification of the Carter and Wilkinson scoring system) and was found in 25.4% of males and 38.5% of females [14]. This study highlighted the need for further population-based research in Iraq to define the current prevalence of hypermobility and to assess its relationship with other rheumatic diseases. A more recent study revealed that joint hypermobility occurred in 32% of Iraqi asthmatic patients [15].

4.6.2 Current Country-Specific Risk Factors for Rheumatic Diseases

Considerable resources have been directed toward uncovering potential triggers for the onset of rheumatic diseases. Epidemiological research has thoroughly examined the correlation between multiple factors and the likelihood and progression of rheumatic conditions. Risk factors related to the environment include smoking, infectious agents, obesity, and other socioeconomic factors [16, 17]. Viral hepatitis is endemic in Iraq. In 2006, the World Health Organization (WHO) provided full technical and logistic support for studying viral hepatitis in Iraq [18]. Results showed that hepatitis A is hyper-endemic, with a prevalence rate of 96.4%. Hepatitis E is also endemic, with a prevalence of 20.3%; both hepatitis B and C are of low/very low endemicity (1.6% and 0.4%, respectively).

4.7 Screening Programs for Rheumatic Diseases

Formally, Iraq does not have a structured screening program for rheumatic diseases. The reasons for the lack of screening initiatives are not well-defined, underscoring the importance of developing such screening programs at the healthcare facility level and engaging in informative, educational campaigns aimed at patients to increase awareness about inflammatory arthritis.

4.8 Diagnosis of Rheumatic and Musculoskeletal Diseases

4.8.1 Availability of Laboratory Tests

Diagnostic laboratory and imaging services support effective health care delivery to patients with MSK and rheumatic diseases. A range of appropriate laboratory tests are available at each health facility level, such as complete blood count, renal and liver function tests, erythrocyte sedimentation rate (ESR), and C-reactive protein (CRP). Hepatitis serology is also available in the majority of governmental and private hospitals.

Central labs provide the necessary support for confirming specific tests, including common serological tests such as rheumatoid factor (RF), anti-cyclic citrullinated peptide (anti-CCP), and anti-nuclear antibodies (ANA). Laboratory services, including genetic analyses such as HLA-B27, HLA-B51, and Mediterranean fever gene mutation (MEFV), have limited availability.

4.8.2 Imaging Services

In the last decade, modern imaging has become increasingly integrated into rheumatology practice. Most hospitals offer standard MSK X-ray imaging, and the availability of radiology services has expanded considerably across both government healthcare facilities and the private sector. According to the latest WHO data, Iraq has a computed tomography (CT) scanner density of approximately 2.22 per million population and a magnetic resonance imaging (MRI) density of approximately 1.63 scanners per million population [19]. To the best of the authors' knowledge, positron emission tomography (PET) scanning is available in nine centers, including three in Baghdad, two in An-Najaf, two in Karbala, and two in the Kurdistan Region.

To support these expanding imaging services, an MSK radiology fellowship was created in 2019 by the Arab Board of Radiology. The program spans 2 years, and as of November 2025, three fellows have graduated from the program at Baghdad Teaching Hospital. In recent years, rheumatologists in the country have increasingly sought to acquire new skills that enable them to perform a wider range of procedures.

MSK ultrasound (MSKUS) is increasingly important in optimizing the clinical assessment of patients with rheumatic diseases and substantially improving therapeutic and diagnostic capabilities [20]. Over the last few years, it has been increasingly incorporated into Iraqi practice and is now commonly used by rheumatologists and radiologists. Many of them have attended training programs for MSKUS and have organized courses to improve their performance. MSKUS is widely available in private practice, but at present, only a limited number of governmental hospitals have fully incorporated MSKUS into their services.

Capillaroscopy, which examines microcirculatory impairment, is also becoming widely accessible for patients in both public and private sectors. To the best of the authors' knowledge, dual-energy X-ray absorptiometry (DXA) is the standard diagnostic technique for measuring bone mineral density in osteoporosis and has become more widely available in recent years. Currently, approximately 50 DXA machines operate across governmental hospitals and private clinics.

4.9 Management of Rheumatic Diseases in Iraq

4.9.1 Access to Treatment Options

The Iraqi MOH subsidized different types of disease-modifying anti-rheumatic drugs (DMARDs) to treat rheumatic diseases. Conventional DMARDs (cDMARDs) accounted for most of all DMARDs supplied through the MOH, with biological DMARDs (bDMARDs) accounting for less than 10%. cDMARDs are generally available at major hospitals in different governorates. bDMARDs are available at 13 centers: three in Baghdad and one center in each of the following governorates: Basra, Mosul, Dhi Qar, Babel, Najaf, Kirkuk, Erbil, Sulaymaniyah, Duhok, Karbala, Wasit, and Saladin. Patients need to fulfill specific eligibility criteria to begin bDMARDs for severe disease not well managed by existing, less expensive therapies and to continue biologic treatment if they demonstrate significant clinical improvement. Specialist rheumatologists have exclusive prescribing rights for these medications. These prior approval requirements have been applied to control access to high-cost medicines and are governed by the Iraqi hospital guidelines for using biologics in patients with rheumatic diseases, which were endorsed by MOH in 2010 and updated in 2020. However, targeted synthetic DMARDs are still unaffordable for the majority of patients.

4.9.2 Accessibility to Multidisciplinary Specialties

In Iraq, providing multidisciplinary (MD) care is vital for effectively managing patients with rheumatic diseases and is a key aspect of disease management and patient well-being. There are three models of MD care in place: combined clinics (MD units) with "face-to-face" consultations, MD team (MDT) meetings, and remote specialist consultations.

Combined clinics represent the first model of MD care. An example is the Behçet disease clinic, established in 2002 and initially including a dermatologist, rheumatologist, and neurologist; an ophthalmologist joined the team in 2018. These healthcare professionals (HCPs) work together in a shared clinic for half a day each week, following specific referral criteria and treatment guidelines. This coordinated approach facilitates earlier recognition of multisystem involvement and supports comprehensive care, which is associated with improved outcomes and patient satisfaction in Behçet disease.

MDT meetings represent the second model. These meetings have been regularly conducted since 2000, with rheumatologists, radiologists, and orthopedic surgeons participating weekly and more frequently in recent years. The use of virtual platforms has enhanced the effectiveness of MDT meetings in various clinical settings by improving access to specialist input and streamlining decision-making. A monthly MDT involving other specialists was established from 2020 to 2022, attended by consultants, fellows, rheumatology trainees, specialists, and pharmacists. During these sessions, challenging patient cases are discussed in detail, including history, laboratory results, and imaging, with MDT recommendations documented and shared with patients and relevant HCPs.

The third MD model involves remote specialist consultations, which are used for patients with stable chronic conditions and for newly diagnosed or active diseases requiring prompt specialty input. Collaboration between orthopedic surgeons and rheumatologists often occurs through remote consultations to discuss surgical and non-surgical treatment options. Tele-rheumatology is increasingly recognized as a valid mode of care that can improve access and continuity when implemented within defined clinical pathways [21]. However, studies examining the use and outcomes of orthopedic surgery in rheumatic diseases in Iraq remain scarce, with only a limited number of local reports available and several areas lacking national or longitudinal outcome data [22]. Challenges in MD collaboration often stem from weaker integration with rehabilitation disciplines such as occupational therapy, with key obstacles related to access, cost, and communication inefficiencies.

4.10 Research and Education

4.10.1 Rheumatology Training Programs

Iraq's first exclusive rheumatology clinic was set up at Baghdad Teaching Hospital in Medical City in 1973. The first adult rheumatology training program was started in 1988 with the establishment of a diploma center at Baghdad Teaching Hospital/Medical City. Subsequent diploma centers were established in Mosul and Erbil, providing training and promoting research. In 1999, a 3-year subspecialty training program in rheumatology and rehabilitation was introduced by the Iraqi Board of Medical Specializations, allowing entry only after completion of a specialty in medicine. Since 1988, rheumatology training and clinical services in Iraq have progressively grown in scope and capacity.

In 2013, the Iraqi Board of Medical Specializations's Rheumatology Fellowship was established, attracting candidates from different governorates of Iraq [23]. The educational program consists of 5 years and has a comprehensive curriculum covering all aspects of medicine and rheumatology. In 2013, there were less than five seats for rheumatology. Over the past 5 years, a total of 75 physicians have enrolled in the national rheumatology training program. Currently, 15 trainees are in their final year and expected to graduate shortly, reflecting ongoing growth and sustained expansion of the adult rheumatology workforce. Integrated rheumatology teaching was also introduced into the basic medical curriculum for undergraduate medical students.

At present, there is no pediatric rheumatology training program in Iraq.

4.10.2 Publications and Research Strategy in Rheumatology in Iraq

Generally, there has been quantitative and qualitative improvement in rheumatology research since 1975, as well as collaborative research work between Iraq and other countries. Table 4.1 summarizes collaborative research publications involving Iraqi and other Arab rheumatologists [24–62]. RA, SLE, vasculitis, fibromyalgia, osteoarthritis, and osteoporosis are research areas of interest in the existing literature.

Moving on to MSK manifestations of infection, the clinical features of acute brucella arthritis were reported in a prospective study of 58 patients attending the Medical City Hospital from 1981 to 1983. Brucella polyarthritis was found in 33; monoarthritis of knee or hip joints occurred in 10 patients, while the spine alone was involved in 15 [63]. Iraq's expansive geographical size prompted us to analyze data on the publishing activities of institutions from diverse regions within the country. Overall, most of the publications for the whole country were from teaching centers.

4.10.3 Rheumatology Nursing Programs

A formal rheumatology nursing program does not exist in Iraq, which presents a significant challenge in delivering rheumatology services and treating and managing different rheumatic conditions.

Table 4.1 Key rheumatology publications from Iraq

Disease/ Topic	Publication title	Year
Rheumatoid arthritis		
	Treatment satisfaction and health-related quality of life in Iraqi patients with rheumatoid arthritis receiving biologic therapy; Rituximab [24]	2025
	Anti-SSA and anti-dsDNA autoantibodies in rheumatoid arthritis patients and their association with disease severity: a case-control study in Kerbala Province [25]	2023
	Prevalence Rate of Rheumatoid Arthritis among Patients Attending Rheumatology Consultation Clinic at Baquba Teaching Hospital [26]	2023
	Incidence of Rheumatoid Arthritis at Marjan Teaching Hospital in Babylon, Iraq (2014–2019) [27]	2022
	Association of Rheumatoid Arthritis and its Severity with Human Leukocytic Antigen-DRB1 Alleles in Kurdish Region in North of Iraq [28]	2022
	Inflammatory and Bone Biomarkers/Composites as a Predictive Tool for Clinical Characteristics of Rheumatoid Arthritis Patients [29]	2022
	Lumbar Spondylolisthesis in a Sample of Iraqi Patients with Rheumatoid Arthritis [30]	2022
	Clinical Outcomes in Iraqi Patients with Rheumatoid Arthritis Following Earlier or Later Treatment with Etanercept [31]	2021
	The Belief About Medicines Among a Sample of Iraqi Patients with Rheumatoid Arthritis [32]	2021
	Demographic, clinical, and serological features of Iraqi patients with rheumatoid arthritis: evaluation of 470 patients [33]	2021
	An Estimation for the Association Between the C–RP Tests and RF Tests of Rheumatoid Condition Patients with Their Demographic Data. In Maysan Province, Iraq [34]	2020
	Assessment of renal involvement in an Iraqi cohort of rheumatoid Arthritis [35]	2020
	Galectin-8 Gene Polymorphism Among Iraqi Patients with Rheumatoid Arthritis [36]	2019
	The Influence of Rheumatoid Arthritis on Work Productivity among a Sample of Iraqi Patients [37]	2019
	Rheumatoid factor isotypes in a sample of Iraqi rheumatoid arthritis patients [38]	2018
	Some Immunological Aspects of Rheumatoid Arthritis Post Treated with Biological Treatment (Enbrel) [39]	2018
	Serum Tumor Necrosis Factor-Alpha and Gene Polymorphisms in Rheumatoid Arthritis Patients in Babylon Province, Iraq [40]	2018
Systemic lupus erythematosus		
	Hydroxychloroquine-Induced Stevens-Johnson Syndrome in the Patient with Systemic Lupus Erythematosus: A Case Report in Kurdish Region—Iraq [41]	2023
	Assessment of medication-related burden among a sample of Iraqi patients with systemic lupus erythematosus and its relationship with disease activity: a cross-sectional study [42]	2022

(continued)

Table 4.1 (continued)

Disease/ Topic	Publication title	Year
	Evaluation of Caspase-3 in Patients with Systemic Lupus Erythematous and its Connection with Disease's Activity [43]	2020
	Estimation of Some Immunological Markers of Iraqi Patients in Systemic Lupus Erythematosus with Lupus Nephritis [44]	2020
	Interleukins (4, 10, 18, 35) Immunoregulatory Systemic Lupus Erythematosus in Kerbala Province, Iraq [45]	2020
	Body composition in Iraqi Women with Systemic Lupus Erythematosus [46]	2019
	Survey of Pap Smear in Women with Systemic Lupus Erythematosus [47]	2019
Spondyloarthritis		
	The Diagnostic Value of Clinical Sacroiliac Joint Pain Provocation Tests for Detection of Sacroiliitis Identified by MRI in Sampled Iraqi Patients with Inflammatory Back Pain [48]	2022
	Raised Inflammatory Markers as Predictors of Response to Anti-Tumor Necrosis Factor Drugs (Etanercept and infliximab) in a Sample of Iraqi Patients with Ankylosing Spondylitis [49]	2021
	Polymorphism of HLA-B27 Among Ankylosing Spondylitis Patients in Basra, Iraq [50]	2020
	Effect of Smoking on Disease Activity and Functional Impairment in a Sample of Iraqi Patients with Ankylosing Spondylitis [51]	2020
Regional and international collaborative publications involving Iraq		
	The APLAR Recommendations for the Management of Psoriatic Arthritis [52]	2025
	Is the patient-perceived impact of psoriatic arthritis a global concept? An international study in 13 Arab countries (TACTIC study) [53]	2024
	An international survey of current management practices for polymyalgia rheumatica by general practitioners and rheumatologists [54]	2023
	APLAR recommendations on the practice of telemedicine in rheumatology [55]	2022
	Management of Referrals, Treatment, Strategy, and Research Challenges in Polymyalgia Rheumatica Amongst Rheumatologists Worldwide: A Questionnaire Base [56]	2022
	Acceptability of the COVID-19 Vaccine Among Patients with Chronic Rheumatic Diseases and Health-Care Professionals: A Cross-Sectional Study in 19 Arab Countries [57]	2022
	Telehealth in Rheumatology: the 2021 Arab League of Rheumatology Best Practice Guidelines [21]	2022
	The Impact of COVID-19 Pandemic on Rheumatology Practice: A Cross-Sectional Multinational Study [58]	2020
	Impact of the COVID-19 Pandemic on Patients with Chronic Rheumatic Diseases: A Study in 15 Arab Countries [59]	2020
	Anti-Tumor Necrosis Factor Biosimilars and Intended Copies in Rheumatology: Perspective from the Asia Pacific Region [60]	2019
	Biosimilars in Rheumatology: Recommendations for Regulation and use in Middle Eastern Countries [61]	2018
	Pan Arab Osteoporosis Society Guidelines for Osteoporosis Management [62]	2017

4.11 Cost-effective Care for Rheumatic Diseases

The rising cost of medications is a global concern, particularly for inflammatory rheumatic diseases. Biological medicines have revolutionized the treatment of chronic conditions like RA, but their high prices have limited patient access. In response to this issue, Iraq has taken steps to enhance access to these medications by promoting the use of biosimilars, which are biologic medicines that have been shown to be highly similar in quality, safety, and efficacy to their respective original biological reference products [64].

Before 2019, the Iraqi National Regulatory Authority (NRA) lacked clear guidelines for adopting biosimilars, leading to delays in approvals. To address this, a new committee was established within the NRA, resulting in the implementation of the first version of Iraqi guidelines for approving biosimilars. This initiative, along with improved collaboration within the Iraqi NRA, has yielded significant benefits in a short period. These include approving several vital biosimilar products, leading to estimated cost savings exceeding 50 million USD in 2020 alone [65]. Additionally, implementing the Iraqi biosimilar guidelines has resulted in the approval of six biosimilars for rheumatic diseases, including the adalimumab biosimilars Amgevita and CinnoRA, the infliximab biosimilars Remsima and Inflectra, and the rituximab biosimilars Ruxience and Truxima. This development not only enhances patient access to current and future biological products for treating severe and disabling conditions, particularly in rheumatology, but also contributes to cost savings and improved healthcare outcomes.

4.12 Key Challenges in Rheumatology Practice in Iraq

While Iraq has made meaningful progress in expanding rheumatology services and training, several systemic challenges continue to limit the full potential of rheumatology care. Recognizing these gaps provides an opportunity to refine national priorities, strengthen services, and guide future strategic planning. The key challenges identified include the following:

- *Workforce limitations*
  Despite steady improvements in training capacity, the number of certified rheumatologists (approximately 244 nationwide) remains insufficient relative to population needs, with marked geographic variation in workforce distribution across governorates. This results in uneven access to specialist care, particularly in peripheral and underserved regions. The current ratio, approximately 0.59 rheumatologists per 100,000 population, is below what is recommended for comprehensive rheumatology coverage [66].
  Pediatric rheumatology services remain absent, representing a critical unmet need, especially given the burden of juvenile idiopathic arthritis and other childhood rheumatic diseases. Moreover, the ongoing migration of experienced HCPs, including rheumatologists, continues to place additional strain on service availability.
  Workforce challenges extend beyond physicians. Nursing shortages, especially of nurses trained in rheumatology or infusion services, further impact the quality

and continuity of patient care. Strengthening interprofessional training programs would significantly help improve service capacity.

- *Health care financing and medication access*
  The major provider of rheumatic care coverage is the MOH. Traditionally, almost all services hospitals provide are free, granting easy access to rheumatologists and treatment. However, the healthcare system does not currently provide equitable access to bDMARDs with a different mode of action. Instability in medication supply chains and limited therapeutic options pose additional challenges. Evidence from Iraqi RA cohorts shows that limited drug availability contributed to failure to reach treatment targets in 10.3% of patients, while drug interruption affected 34.5% of cases [67]. These factors make it difficult to fully implement international evidence-based recommendations.
  Continued expansion of biosimilar approvals and improved procurement strategies may help reduce costs and broaden access to advanced therapies.

- *Medical tourism*
  Iraq is not currently positioned as a medical-tourism destination, particularly for the management of rheumatic diseases. Some patients, therefore, travel overseas seeking high-quality medical facilities and broader access to advanced care. Strengthening national healthcare services, improving access to advanced medications, and building multidisciplinary centers of excellence could gradually reduce outward medical tourism and keep care closer to patients' homes.

4.13 Vision and Strategic Priorities for Improving Rheumatology Care in Iraq

In order to enhance rheumatology practices and improve patient care, a comprehensive strategic plan was implemented, focusing on key areas. First, efforts were made to advance the training of HCPs through scientific workshops, conferences, and specialized groups. This included training for administrative staff and nurses in management and equipment maintenance, both locally and internationally. Second, patient education campaigns were initiated to raise awareness about MSK diseases and improve the quality of life. These campaigns, conducted through events like World Arthritis Day and World Psoriasis Day, aimed to educate the public and HCPs on the importance of early diagnosis and treatment referral systems. Additionally, a "Patient Encourage Program" was established in 2022 within the rheumatology department to enhance patient understanding and adherence to treatment plans.

Moreover, in response to the challenges posed by the COVID-19 pandemic, virtual rheumatology clinics were swiftly implemented to ensure continued access to care. This transition to remote appointments involved training clinicians and fellows in tele-consultation techniques, thereby enabling patients to receive necessary care from their homes.

Plans are also underway to address the unmet need for pediatric rheumatology care by developing a dedicated fellowship training curriculum in the future.

Furthermore, recognizing the pivotal role of physical and occupational therapy in rheumatic disease management led to the provision of board-certified specialists in medical rehabilitation. Finally, initiatives were undertaken to engage and motivate young rheumatologists, encouraging them to participate actively in ongoing medical-education activities and research in the field of rheumatic and MSK diseases.

4.14 Strategic Suggestions to Improve Rheumatic Disease Care Over the Next Decade in Iraq

Innovative approaches are essential to overcoming the challenges in rheumatology in Iraq. The authors suggest developing strategies to enhance rheumatologic care over the coming decade. First, there is a pressing need to increase the number of trained rheumatologists within Iraq to meet the rising demand. This entails the expansion of training programs for doctors and nurses to effectively share the workload. Additionally, establishing standardized referral criteria will enable earlier diagnosis and treatment, ultimately improving patient outcomes.

Next, the expansion of training centers, especially in underserved areas, and the promotion of collaborative research efforts at both national and international levels are recommended.

Education and awareness campaigns on rheumatic diseases can facilitate early detection and treatment-seeking behavior. Further, developing an EMR system for streamlined data management, initiating subspecialty rheumatology clinics within general hospitals, and formalizing advanced nursing training are crucial steps. Empowering female rheumatologists and conducting more population-based studies to assess disease burden and patient needs are also vital for enhancing rheumatologic care in Iraq. By implementing these proactive measures, the quality, accessibility, and sustainability of rheumatology services in Iraq can be significantly improved.

4.15 Conclusion

Rheumatology in Iraq has progressed from isolated early clinics to a nationally organized specialty supported by training programs, multidisciplinary services, and an active professional society. Community and hospital-based studies have shaped understanding of the local burden of rheumatic diseases, while collaborations with regional and international partners have expanded Iraq's contribution to global rheumatology literature. Despite these achievements, service delivery continues to be constrained by workforce shortages, limited pediatric rheumatology capacity, and inconsistent access to advanced therapeutics and certified nursing support. Strategic priorities for the coming years include expanding rheumatology training centers, developing pediatric fellowship pathways, strengthening rheumatology nursing education, standardizing referral systems, and enhancing national registries and research networks. With sustained policy and professional investment, Iraq is well positioned to further improve equitable access and quality of rheumatology care nationwide.

Conflict of Interest The authors declare no conflict of interest.

References

1. Encyclopaedia Britannica. Iraq [Internet]. London: Encyclopaedia Britannica. [cited 2026 Jun 14]. Available from: https://www.britannica.com/place/Iraq/Arabs.
2. Central Intelligence Agency. The World Factbook: Iraq [Internet]. Washington (DC): Central Intelligence Agency; 2023. [cited 2025 Nov 21]. Available from: https://www.cia.gov/the-world-factbook/about/archives/2023/countries/iraq/.
3. Palo Alto College. Mesopotamia: a Cradle of Civilization [Internet]. Chapter 2 of Art History. [cited 2026 Jun 14]. Available from: https://pressbooks.pub/pacarthistory/chapter/chapter-2-mesopotamia-the-cradle-of-civilization/.
4. Al-Rawi ZS, Alazzawi AJ, Alajili FM, Alwakil R. Rheumatoid arthritis in population samples in Iraq. Ann Rheum Dis. 1978;37(1):73–5. https://doi.org/10.1136/ard.37.1.73.
5. Alkazzaz AMH. Incidence of rheumatoid arthritis (2001 to 2011). Iraqi Postgrad Med J. 2013;12(4):568–72.
6. Al-Rawi ZS, Al-Shakarchi HA, Hasan F, Thewaini AJ. Ankylosing spondylitis and its association with the histocompatibility antigen HL-A B27: an epidemiological and clinical study. Rheumatol Rehabil. 1978;17(2):72–5. https://doi.org/10.1093/rheumatology/17.2.72.
7. Al-Rawi Z, Al-Shaarbaf H, Al-Raheem E, Khalifa SJ. Clinical features of early cases of systemic lupus erythematosus in Iraqui patients. Br J Rheumatol. 1983;22(3):165–71. https://doi.org/10.1093/rheumatology/22.3.165.
8. Brewerton DA, Hart FD, Nicholls A, Caffrey M, James DC, Sturrock RD. Ankylosing spondylitis and HL-A 27. Lancet. 1973;1(7809):904–7. https://doi.org/10.1016/s0140-6736(73)91360-3.
9. Al-Rawi ZS, Sharquie KE, Khalifa SJ, Al-Hadithi FM, Munir JJ. Behcet's disease in Iraqi patients. Ann Rheum Dis. 1986;45(12):987–90. https://doi.org/10.1136/ard.45.12.987.
10. Al-Rawi ZS, Kamil AN. Prevalence of fibromyalgia syndrome among school children and adolescents in Iraq. Arthritis Rheum. 2000;43(9):S212. [Abstract].
11. Al-Rawi ZS, Al-Rawi OZ, Al-Rawi AZ. Backache in population samples in Iraq. Ann Rheum Dis. 2002;61(5):157. [Abstract THU0339].
12. Al-Rawi ZS, Al-Eshahkey MH, Al-Shummari YM. Lumbar spondylosis in Iraqi people above the age of 40 years. Egypt Rheumatol. 2000;22(2):567–74.
13. Al-Bakri SHM, Al-Shuwaili SJ, Ataimish HHJ. The prevalence and risk factors of lower back pain among healthcare workers in Iraq: a cross sectional study. Rom J Rheumatol. 2024;33(1):11–4. https://doi.org/10.37897/RJR.2024.1.4.
14. Al-Rawi ZS, Al-Aszawi AJ, Al-Chalabi T. Joint mobility among university students in Iraq. Br J Rheumatol. 1985;24(4):326–31. https://doi.org/10.1093/rheumatology/24.4.326.
15. Al-Asadi I, Kazem M. Exploring joint hypermobility and hypermobility syndrome among Iraqi asthma patients. Int J Mod Med. 2024;3(09):8–13.
16. Romao VC, Fonseca JE. Etiology and risk factors for rheumatoid arthritis: a state-of-the-art review. Front Med (Lausanne). 2021;8:689698. https://doi.org/10.3389/fmed.2021.689698.
17. Belbasis L, Dosis V, Evangelou E. Elucidating the environmental risk factors for rheumatic diseases: an umbrella review of meta-analyses. Int J Rheum Dis. 2018;21(8):1514–24. https://doi.org/10.1111/1756-185X.13356.
18. Tarky AM, Akram WA, Al-Naaimi AS, Omer AR. Epidemiology of viral hepatitis B and C in Iraq: a national survey 2005–2006. Zanco J Med Sci. 2013;17(1):370–80.

19. World Health Organization. Medical devices [Internet]. Geneva: World Health Organization. [cited 2025 Nov 23]. Available from: https://www.who.int/data/gho/data/themes/topics/GHO/medical-devices.
20. Hassan S. Overview of musculoskeletal ultrasound for the clinical rheumatologist. Clin Exp Rheumatol. 2018;36 Suppl 114(5):3–9.
21. Ziade N, Hmamouchi I, El Kibbi L, Daou M, Abdulateef N, Abutiban F, et al. Telehealth in rheumatology: the 2021 Arab League of Rheumatology Best Practice Guidelines. Rheumatol Int. 2022;42(3):379–90. https://doi.org/10.1007/s00296-021-05078-w.
22. Yaseen MK, Gorial FI. An observational descriptive cross sectional multicenter study of health related quality of life among Iraqi patients after total hip replacement. Ann Med Surg (Lond). 2019;48:118–21. https://doi.org/10.1016/j.amsu.2019.10.031.
23. Iraqi Board for Medical Specializations [Internet]. (in Arabic). [cited 2026 Jun 14]. Available from: https://www.iraqiboard.edu.iq/ar.
24. Talib AF, Mohammed MM. Treatment satisfaction and health-related quality of life in Iraqi patients with rheumatoid arthritis receiving biologic therapy; Rituximab. Iraqi J Pharm Sci. 2025;33(4 SI):230–5. https://doi.org/10.31351/vol33iss(4SI)pp230-235.
25. Mahdi AF, Mohammed SH, Hadi AR. Anti-SSA and anti-dsDNA autoantibodies in rheumatoid arthritis patients and their association with disease severity: a case-control study in Kerbala Province. Al-Rafidain J Med Sci. 2023;5:105–11. https://doi.org/10.54133/ajms.v5i.169.
26. Rashid MK. Prevalence rate of rheumatoid arthritis among patients attending rheumatology consultation clinic at Baquba Teaching Hospital. Diyala J Med. 2023;24(1):970. https://doi.org/10.26505/djm.v24i1.970.
27. Al-Badran AHK, Algabri HC, Saeedi KRHA, Alqazzaz AM. Incidence of rheumatoid arthritis at Marjan teaching hospital in Babylon, Iraq (2014–2019). Med J Babylon. 2022;19(3):358–61. https://doi.org/10.4103/MJBL.MJBL_32_22.
28. Albarzinji N, Ismael SA, Albustany D. Association of rheumatoid arthritis and its severity with human leukocytic antigen-DRB1 alleles in Kurdish region in North of Iraq. BMC Rheumatol. 2022;6(1):4. https://doi.org/10.1186/s41927-021-00229-9.
29. Ali HH, Yaseen MM, AL-Rawi KF, SFT A, Al-Hakeim HK. Inflammatory and bone biomarkers/composites as a predictive tool for clinical characteristics of rheumatoid arthritis patients. Acta Biologica Szegediensis. 2022;65(2):271–83. https://doi.org/10.14232/abs.2021.2.271-283.
30. Jasim NA, Aday ZN, Derwibee FAA. Lumbar spondylolisthesis in a sample of Iraqi patients with rheumatoid arthritis. Chair, Ed Board. 2020;8(04):46–53. https://doi.org/10.37506/ijop.v8i4.1709.
31. Al-Ani N, Gorial F, Yasiry D, Al Derwibee F, Abbas Humadi Y, Sunna N, et al. Clinical outcomes in Iraqi patients with rheumatoid arthritis following earlier or later treatment with etanercept. Open Access Rheumatol. 2021;13:57–62. https://doi.org/10.2147/OARRR.S300838.
32. Faiq MK, Kadhim DJ, Gorial FI. The belief about medicines among a sample of Iraqi patients with rheumatoid arthritis. Iraqi J Pharm Sci. 2019;28(2):134–41. https://doi.org/10.31351/vol28iss2pp134-141.
33. Abdulsatar J, Mathkhor A, Abdulnasser H, Khoudhairy AS. Demographic, clinical, and serological features of Iraqi patients with rheumatoid arthritis: evaluation of 470 patients. Int J Clin Rheumatol. 2021;16(3):99–103.
34. Al-Norri MA, Hateet RR, Qasim MJ. An estimation for the association between the CRP tests and RF tests of rheumatoid condition patients with their demographic data. In Maysan Province, Iraq. Indian J Public Health Res Dev. 2020;11(2):2131.
35. Abubaker BA, Sinjari HY. Assessment of renal involvement in an Iraqi cohort of rheumatoid arthritis. Med J Babylon. 2020;17(4):353. https://doi.org/10.4103/MJBL.MJBL_29_20.
36. Muss TQ, AL-Faham M, Gorial FI, Zghair AK. Galectin-8 gene polymorphism among Iraqi patients with rheumatoid arthritis. Res J Pharm Technol. 2019;12(4):1643–5. https://doi.org/10.5958/0974-360X.2019.00274.9.
37. Gorial FI, Naema SJ, Ali HO, Hussain SA. The influence of rheumatoid arthritis on work productivity among a sample of Iraqi patients. Al-Rafidain J Med Sci. 2021;1:110–7. https://doi.org/10.54133/ajms.v1i.47.

38. Hussein RH, Al-Rayahi IBM, Taha K. Rheumatoid factor isotypes in a sample of Iraqi rheumatoid arthritis patients. J Glob Pharma Technol. 2018;10:141–5.
39. Subhi IM, Zgair AK, Al-Osami MH. Some immunological aspects of rheumatoid arthritis post treated with biological treatment (Enbrel). J Pharm Sci Res. 2018;10(11):2934–7.
40. Alanzy AK, Alta'ee AH, Alrubiae SJ. Serum tumor necrosis factor alpha and Gene Polymorphisms in Rheumatoid arthritis patients in Babylon Province, Iraq. J Glob Pharma Technol. 2018;10(3):387–95. https://doi.org/10.54133/ajms.v4i.100.
41. Al-Barzinji N, Jalal AM. Hydroxychloroquine-induced Stevens-Johnson Syndrome in the patient with systemic lupus erythematosus: a case report in Kurdish Region - Iraq. Mediterr J Rheumatol. 2023;34(4):547–9. https://doi.org/10.31138/mjr.260723.his.
42. Abbas HK, Kadhim DJ, Gorial FI, Shareef LG. Assessment of medication-related burden among a sample of Iraqi patients with systemic lupus erythematosus and its relationship with disease activity: a cross-sectional study. F1000Res. 2022;11:970. https://doi.org/10.12688/f1000research.124698.2.
43. Al-Araji AE, Ali SW. Evaluation of Caspase-3 in patients with systemic lupus erythematous and it is connection with disease's activity. Prensa Med Argent. 2020:3–5. https://doi.org/10.47275/0032-745X-S1-007.
44. Ibrahim NA, Allawi AA, Ghudhaib KK, Hammoudi FA. Estimation of some immunological markers of Iraqi patients in systemic lupus erythematosus with lupus nephritis. Medico-Legal Update. 2020;20(4):4668. https://doi.org/10.37506/mlu.v20i4.1892.
45. Alwandawi TK, Al-Saadi HA. Interleukins (4, 10, 18, 35) immunoregulatory systemic lupus erythematosus in Kerbala Province, Iraq. Biochem Cell Arch. 2020;21(01):1611–20.
46. Gorial FI, Mahmood ZA, Obaidi SA. Body composition in Iraqi Women with systemic lupus erythematosus. Global J Health Sci. 2019;11(1):63–70. https://doi.org/10.5539/gjhs.v11n1p63.
47. Muhammed A, Hazim A, Jassim NA, Hummadi J. Survey of Pap Smear in Women with Systemic Lupus Erythematosus. Iraqi Postgrad Med J. 2019;18(3):8.
48. Salman S, Jaafar F. The diagnostic value of clinical sacroiliac joint pain provocation tests for detection of sacroiliitis identified by MRI in sampled Iraqi patients with inflammatory back pain. Mediterr J Rheumatol. 2022;33(1):48–54. https://doi.org/10.31138/mjr.33.1.48.
49. Al-Shaibani SA, Jassim NA, Al-Bayati AA. Raised inflammatory markers as predictors of response to anti-tumor necrosis factor drugs (etanercept and infliximab) in a sample of Iraqi patients with ankylosing spondylitis. Med J Babylon. 2021;18(3):241. https://doi.org/10.4103/MJBL.MJBL_27_21.
50. Daekh NA, Mohammed KA, Ali NH. Polymorphism of HLA-B27 among ankylosing spondylitis patients in Basrah, Iraq. Sci J Med Res. 2020;4(13):12–6.
51. Hashim NA, Jassim NA. Effect of smoking on disease activity and functional impairment in a sample of Iraqi patients with ankylosing spondylitis. Indian J Public Health. 2020;11(02):2613.
52. Leung YY, Bird P, Haroon M, Kishimoto M, Shin K, Mathew AJ, et al. The APLAR recommendations for the management of psoriatic arthritis. Int J Rheum Dis. 2025;28(8):e70372. https://doi.org/10.1111/1756-185x.70372.
53. Ziade N, Abbas N, Hmamouchi I, El Kibbi L, Maroof A, Elzorkany B, et al. Is the patient-perceived impact of psoriatic arthritis a global concept? An international study in 13 Arab countries (TACTIC study). Rheumatol Int. 2024;44(5):885–99. https://doi.org/10.1007/s00296-024-05552-1.
54. Donskov AO, Mackie SL, Hauge EM, Toro-Gutierrez CE, Hansen IT, Hemmig AK, et al. An international survey of current management practices for polymyalgia rheumatica by general practitioners and rheumatologists. Rheumatology (Oxford). 2023;62(8):2797–805. https://doi.org/10.1093/rheumatology/keac713.
55. Ahmed S, Grainger R, Santosa A, Adnan A, Alnaqbi KA, Chen YH, et al. APLAR recommendations on the practice of telemedicine in rheumatology. Int J Rheum Dis. 2022;25(3):247–58. https://doi.org/10.1111/1756-185X.14286.
56. Overgaard Donskov A, Mackie S, Hauge EM, Toro Gutiérrez C, Hansen I, Hemmig A, et al. Management of referrals, treatment strategy, and research challenges in polymyalgia rheu-

matica amongst rheumatologists worldwide: a questionnaire-based study. Ann Rheum Dis. 2022;81(Suppl 1):1417–8. https://doi.org/10.1136/annrheumdis-2022-EULAR.1486.
57. El Kibbi L, Metawee M, Hmamouchi I, Abdulateef N, Halabi H, Eissa M, et al. Acceptability of the COVID-19 vaccine among patients with chronic rheumatic diseases and health-care professionals: a cross-sectional study in 19 Arab countries. Lancet Rheumatol. 2022;4(3):e160–e3. https://doi.org/10.1016/S2665-9913(21)00368-4.
58. Ziade N, Hmamouchi I, El Kibbi L, Abdulateef N, Halabi H, Abutiban F, et al. The impact of COVID-19 pandemic on rheumatology practice: a cross-sectional multinational study. Clin Rheumatol. 2020;39(11):3205–13. https://doi.org/10.1007/s10067-020-05428-2.
59. Ziade N, El Kibbi L, Hmamouchi I, Abdulateef N, Halabi H, Hamdi W, et al. Impact of the COVID-19 pandemic on patients with chronic rheumatic diseases: a study in 15 Arab countries. Int J Rheum Dis. 2020;23(11):1550–7. https://doi.org/10.1111/1756-185X.13960.
60. Rath PD, Chen DY, Gu J, Lee VWY, Al Ani NA, Shirazy K, et al. Anti-tumor necrosis factor biosimilars and intended copies in rheumatology: perspective from the Asia Pacific region. Int J Rheum Dis. 2019;22(1):9–24. https://doi.org/10.1111/1756-185X.13371.
61. El Zorkany B, Al Ani N, Al Emadi S, Al Saleh J, Uthman I, El Dershaby Y, et al. Biosimilars in rheumatology: recommendations for regulation and use in Middle Eastern countries. Clin Rheumatol. 2018;37(5):1143–52. https://doi.org/10.1007/s10067-018-3982-9.
62. Jassim NA, Adib G, Abdul Rahman YA, Gorial FI, Maghraoui A, Al Suhaili AR, et al. Pan Arab Osteoporosis Society guidelines for osteoporosis management. Mediterr J Rheumatol. 2017;28(1):27–32. https://doi.org/10.31138/mjr.28.1.27.
63. Al-Rawi ZS, Al-Khateeb N, Khalifa SJ. Brucella arthritis among Iraqi patients. Br J Rheumatol. 1987;26(1):24–7. https://doi.org/10.1093/rheumatology/26.1.24.
64. Smolen JS, Goncalves J, Quinn M, Benedetti F, Lee JY. Era of biosimilars in rheumatology: reshaping the healthcare environment. RMD Open. 2019;5(1):e000900. https://doi.org/10.1136/rmdopen-2019-000900.
65. Al-Kinani KK, Ibrahim MJ, Al-Zubaidi RF, Younus MM, Ramadhan SH, Kadhim HJ, et al. Iraqi regulatory authority current system and experience with biosimilars. Regul Toxicol Pharmacol. 2020;117:104768. https://doi.org/10.1016/j.yrtph.2020.104768.
66. Unger J, Putrik P, Buttgereit F, Aletaha D, Bianchi G, Bijlsma JWJ, et al. Workforce requirements in rheumatology: a systematic literature review informing the development of a workforce prediction risk of bias tool and the EULAR points to consider. RMD Open. 2018;4(2):e000756. https://doi.org/10.1136/rmdopen-2018-000756.
67. Jassim NA, Redha AA. Challenges in applying treat to target strategy in sample of Iraqi patients with rheumatoid arthritis. Mediterr J Rheumatol. 2021;32(4):331–7. https://doi.org/10.31138/mjr.32.4.331.

Chapter 5
Rheumatic Diseases in Jordan

Khaldoon Alawneh, Basel Masri, Raed Alzyoud, and Wafa Madanat

Abstract Over the past decade, rheumatology care in Jordan has significantly improved due to a rise in the number of rheumatologists and better access to advanced diagnostics and treatments. In this chapter, we review the health status and history of rheumatology care in Jordan, including statistics, infrastructure, workforce, and outcomes. We also explore the challenges faced and provide suggestions to enhance rheumatology management in Jordan.

Keywords Jordan · Rheumatology · Rheumatic diseases · Rheumatology services · Rheumatology workforce · Pediatric rheumatology · Rheumatology training · Biologic therapy · Biosimilars · Clinical research

5.1 Country Demographics

Jordan is an Arab country, located north of the Arabian Peninsula and in West Asia. To the north, Jordan borders Syria, while its eastern border borders Iraq. To the south and southeast, it shares boundaries with Saudi Arabia, and to the west, it

K. Alawneh
King Abdullah University Hospital, Department of Medicine, Jordan University of Science and Technology, Irbid, Jordan
e-mail: kalawneh@just.edu.jo; kma1234@msn.com

B. Masri
Jordan Hospital, Department of Internal Medicine, Amman, Jordan
e-mail: basel.masri@masriclinic.co

R. Alzyoud
Head of Immunology, Allergy and Rheumatology, Queen Rania Children's Hospital, Amman, Jordan
e-mail: raedalzyoud@gmail.com

W. Madanat (✉)
Private Clinic, Amman, Jordan
e-mail: w.y.madanat@gmail.com

K. A. Alnaqbi, G. Aldabie (eds.), *Rheumatic Diseases in the Arab World*,
https://doi.org/10.1007/978-981-92-0967-5_5

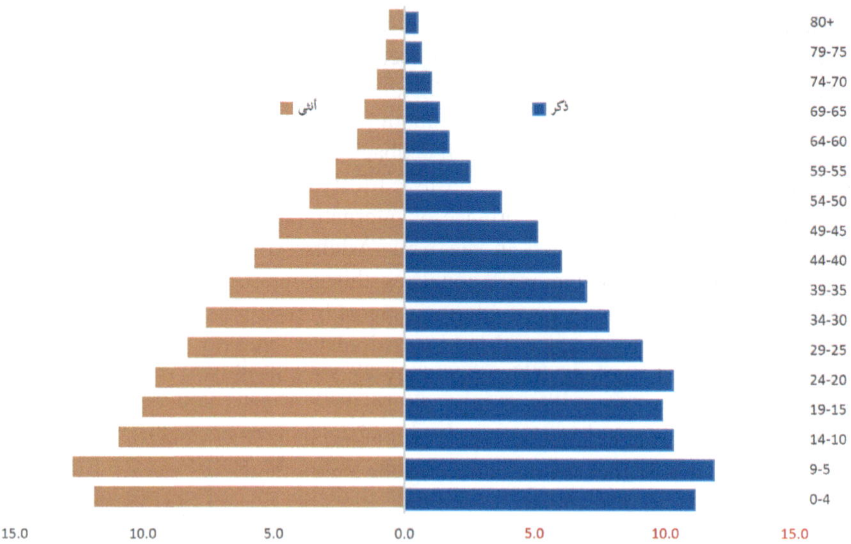

Fig. 5.1 Population pyramid of Jordan by age group (%), 2023 [1]

borders Palestine. Jordan is named for the Jordan River. The total area of the kingdom is 89.318 square kilometers. The country has 12 governorates: Amman (the capital city), Irbid, Mafraq, Jerash, Ajloun, Balqa, Zarqa, Madaba, Karak, Tafilah, Ma'an, and Aqaba [1].

In 2023, the population of Jordan was estimated at 11,516,000 people. Males represented 52.9% of the population. The male-to-female ratio was 1.12:1 (112.5 males per 100 females). The country is highly urbanized, with 90.3% of the population residing in urban areas. The median age of people in Jordan is approximately 23.8 years (Fig. 5.1) [1].

Life expectancy at birth in Jordan for both genders is 75.3 years. People under 15 make up 34.3% of the population, 62.0% are aged 15–64, and 3.7% are 65 or older [1].

5.2 Country Healthcare Sectors

The healthcare sector in Jordan comprises public, private, international, and charitable sectors.

The public sector includes the Ministry of Health (MOH), the Royal Medical Services (RMS), university hospitals (Jordan University Hospital [JUH] and King Abdullah University Hospital [KAUH]), and the Center for Diabetes, Endocrinology, and Genetics. The private sector includes private hospitals, diagnostic centers, private clinics, and private pharmacies. The international and charitable sectors providing medical services encompass United Nations Relief & Works Agency (UNRWA) clinics for Palestinian refugees in the Near East, the United Nations High

Commissioner for Refugees (UNHCR), the King Hussein Cancer Center (KHCC), and charitable organizations and association clinics.

In 2023, Jordan had 119 hospitals nationwide, reflecting a relatively stable hospital infrastructure over recent years [1].

Health policymaking in Jordan is carried out mainly by the Higher Health Council under Law No. 9 of 1999. Other institutions involved in health policy include the Jordanian Medical Council (JMC), the Supreme Council of the Population, the Jordanian Nursing Council, the National Council for Family Affairs, the Jordan Food and Drug Administration (JFDA), and the Joint Procurement Department (JPD).

JMC's primary mission is to train physicians, including both general practitioners and specialists. To accomplish this, it sets standards for teaching hospitals, certifies facilities as teaching hospitals, and supervises residency programs. JMC also plays a key role in designing, implementing, and managing scientific programs across various medical specialties, certifying physicians as general practitioners, and awarding them the Jordanian Board, the highest professional healthcare certification in Jordan. Additionally, JMC reviews continuing medical education (CME) and continuing professional development (CPD) initiatives [2].

5.3 Rheumatology Care

Rheumatology care in Jordan has gradually improved, providing comprehensive services to patients with rheumatic and musculoskeletal diseases (RMDs). Figure 5.2 illustrates the timeline of RMD care development in the country over recent decades, showing significant progress.

5.3.1 Rheumatology Manpower

Rheumatology, as a separate specialty in Jordan, was established in 1980 when two Jordanian adult rheumatologists began practicing at JUH. As of March 2026, the number of certified rheumatologists practicing in Jordan is 48 (31 males and 17 females) (Fig. 5.3), including six pediatric rheumatologists (four males and two females). Of these, 20 work full-time in the public sector, including universities and RMS, four work part-time in MOH, and the remainder work exclusively in private practice.

5.3.2 Rheumatology Nurses

There are no dedicated rheumatology nurses in Jordan. However, three nurses at the King Hussein Medical Center (KHMC), Royal Medical Services (RMS), were trained at specialized centers abroad to handle biologic therapies.

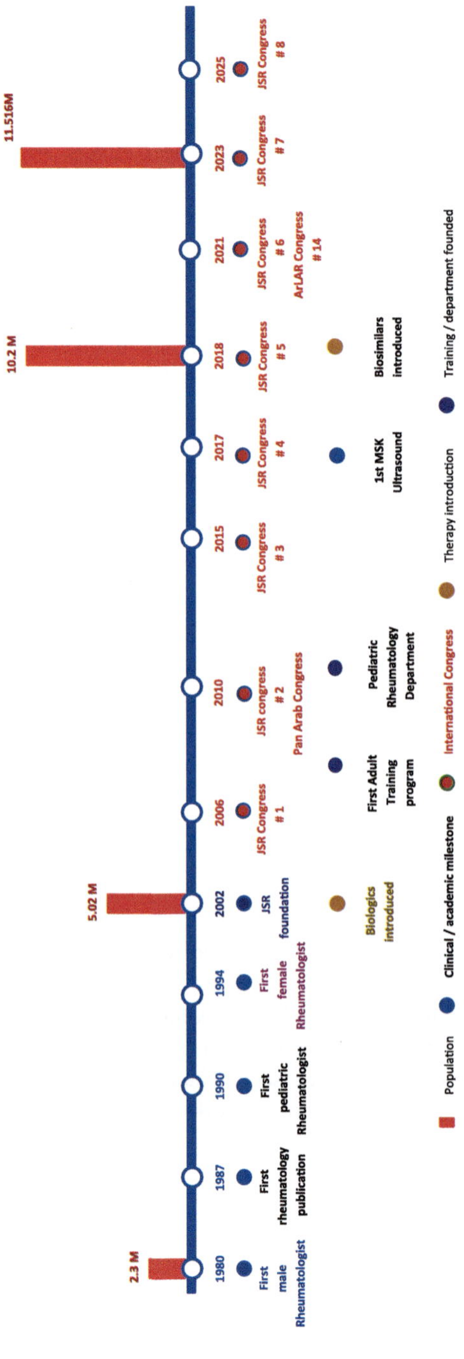

Fig. 5.2 Rheumatic diseases care growth in Jordan

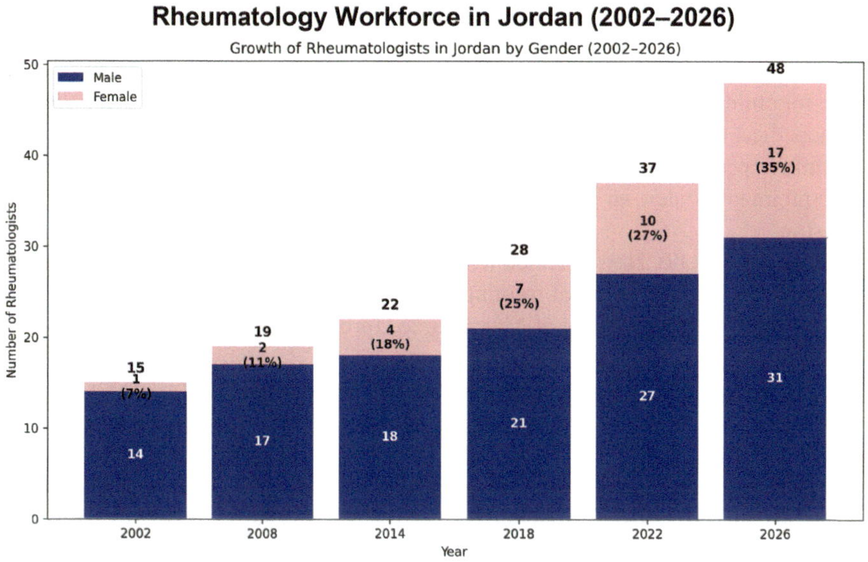

Fig. 5.3 Number of registered rheumatologists in Jordan with gender distribution, 2002–2026

5.3.3 *Accredited Center of Excellence for Rheumatology*

At present, there are no centers of excellence for rheumatology in Jordan.

5.3.4 *Pediatric Rheumatology*

The first pediatric rheumatologist (PR) began practicing in Jordan in 1991 at JUH. In 1999, a second PR established services at KHMC and RMS. However, recognition of pediatric rheumatology as a distinct specialty began in February 2010, following the inauguration of Queen Rania Children's Hospital (QRCH) at KHMC, RMS. Prior to this milestone, children with RMDs received care from various specialties, including general pediatrics, orthopedists, and adult rheumatologists.

QRCH is Jordan's first specialized medical center for children, distinguished by its modern, advanced construction, which meets the highest international standards. The hospital encompasses 22 different medical and surgical subspecialties. Within QRCH, the Pediatric Rheumatology Division (PRD) offers a comprehensive pediatric rheumatology service, including 18 inpatient beds, three clinic rooms, and a dedicated seven-bed infusion unit. Well-trained nurses provide ambulatory care for various treatments, including biologic medications, intravenous immunoglobulin, intravenous corticosteroids, pulse therapy, intra-articular steroid injections, and disease-modifying antirheumatic drugs (DMARDs).

Furthermore, PRD extends its services to include skin biopsy and educational programs for patients and their families. The hospital's unique setup, which houses various pediatric medical and surgical specialties under one roof, enhances overall care for children with rheumatological conditions. This includes access to pediatric orthopedics, physiotherapy, occupational therapy, physical and psychosocial rehabilitation, pediatric ophthalmology, a specialized uveitis clinic, nutritionists, an entertainment center, an in-house school, a laboratory, and a pediatric radiology division.

The PRD at QRCH established a structured institutional fellowship program in 2010, consisting of 3 years of training followed by 1 year of international training in a recognized program. As of March 2026, Jordan has six pediatric rheumatologists: three at Queen Rania Children's Hospital (QRCH), alongside three fellows in training; two practicing in the private sector; and one each at Al Yarmouk University, the Hashemite University, and Jordan University of Science and Technology.

Furthermore, the PRD at QRCH has been recognized by the Pediatric Rheumatology International Trials Organization (PRINTO) as a collaborative research center. The division played an essential role as a co-founder of the Pediatric Rheumatology of Arab Group (PARG), which was officially established and recognized in 2016 as a special interest group of the Arab League of Associations for Rheumatology (ArLAR). This collaboration, both within the Arab region and internationally, has been key in publishing protocols, guidelines, and consensus papers in pediatric rheumatology.

In 2020, the Jordan Medical Council (JMC) officially recognized pediatric rheumatology as a subspecialty among its certified fields, accrediting five pediatric rheumatologists. The fellowship program at QRCH is also accredited by the JMC.

5.3.5 Available System of Referrals to Rheumatology in the Country

In Jordan, patients typically access rheumatologists through referrals from primary and secondary healthcare centers, other medical specialties, or, in some cases, the private sector. Additionally, self-referral is a common practice.

5.3.6 Rheumatology Subspecialties Clinics/Programs

Unfortunately, rheumatology subspecialty clinics/programs are not available in Jordan.

5.4 Official Rheumatology Society

In 2002, the number of rheumatologists in Jordan reached 15, meeting the minimum requirement under local law for establishing a scientific society. As a result, the Jordanian Society of Rheumatology (JSR) was founded and functions under the auspices of the Jordanian Medical Association (JMA). Since its inception, the JSR has actively advanced its objectives, especially in the areas of CME and CPD. This includes hosting regular scientific meetings that cover various topics in rheumatology and increasing awareness about RMDs among medical specialists and the public.

Furthermore, the JSR has successfully organized eight international rheumatology conferences in collaboration with Arab and international societies. Additionally, the JSR hosted two Pan-Arab Rheumatology Conferences in 2010 and 2020. The latter conference was conducted virtually in 2021 due to the COVID-19 pandemic.

The JSR has also created a patient forum on social media and has initiated several awareness campaigns through mass media and face-to-face meetings to educate the public about RMDs. Moreover, the JSR is a co-founder of the ArLAR and is an active member of the Asia Pacific League of Associations for Rheumatology (APLAR).

5.5 Overview of Rheumatic Diseases in Jordan

- *Prevalence:*

Several studies analyze the prevalence of RMDs in Jordan, including Familial Mediterranean Fever (FMF), osteoporosis among postmenopausal women, Behcet disease (BD), and rheumatoid arthritis (RA).

In 1996, a paper describing FMF in children showed a high prevalence of FMF in children, 1:2600, similar to that observed in Armenians and Jews [3].

In 2007, the Osteoporosis Prevention Society reported that the prevalence of osteoporosis among postmenopausal women in Jordan was 36.5% [4]. This finding was confirmed in 2017 by another study, which showed similar results of 37.5% [5]. However, after adjusting the results of the first study to account for local peak bone mass data, which was lower than the initially reported data, the prevalence decreased to 16.7%. This figure is lower in comparison to white Caucasians in the West.

In 2017, a study on the prevalence of BD in northern Jordan was published, revealing a rate of 66 per 10,000, among the highest in the world [6]. Conversely, in 2020, a study on the prevalence of RA among hospital workers in northern Jordan reported a rate of 0.31%, similar to that observed in neighboring Arab countries [7].

- *Genetics:*

HLA and disease associations have been extensively studied in Jordan, particularly in BD and ankylosing spondylitis (AS). In patients with BD, the frequency of HLA-B-51 is significantly higher than in controls (66% vs. 15%, OR 10.9) [8].

Meanwhile, the prevalence of HLA-B27 among Jordanians with AS is notably high, with 71% compared to 2.4% in the general population [9].

In the context of FMF, researchers have examined the genotype patterns in children with the disease, analyzing 12 mutations in the Mediterranean Fever (MEFV) gene. The patients were classified into four categories based on their genotype: homozygous (24%, M694V-M694V being the most common), heterozygous (44.4%), compound heterozygous (28.1%), and a small group where no mutation could be identified (3.6%). Five mutations were the most frequent in the cohort; the most common mutations were M694V, V726A, E148Q, M680I, and M694I, detected in 50%, 21.4%, 19.4%, 15.8%, and 9.7% of cases, respectively [10]. Furthermore, Jordan participated in a multinational Arab genome-wide association study (GWAS) focused on RA. This study identified two novel genetic loci specific to Arab populations, located at 5q13 and 17p13 [11].

- *Clinical Manifestations:*

Most publications related to clinical manifestations and epidemiology of RMDs in Jordan are retrospective studies and case reports. They included data on RA, AS, systemic lupus erythematosus (SLE), myositis, vasculitis (including BD and Takayasu arteritis [TA]), juvenile idiopathic arthritis (JIA), FMF, and sarcoidosis.

FMF

Two studies conducted on children with FMF were published, one in 1999 involving data from 476 children [12] and the other in 2018 involving 196 children [13]. These studies revealed various clinical manifestations in children with FMF, including abdominal pain (81–91.8%), arthritis (14–42%), unilateral chest pain (41%), severe myalgia, and skin manifestations (6.5–12% each), scrotal swelling (4%), and recurrent episodic fever (3%). In the first study, two children developed renal complications that were successfully treated with colchicine, while in the second study, a patient developed amyloidosis and was managed with anakinra; unfortunately, the patient succumbed to septicemia.

Majeed Syndrome

In 2001, a syndrome characterized by chronic recurrent multifocal osteomyelitis and congenital dyserythropoietic anemia was first described and later named after the Jordanian physician who reported it, becoming known as Majeed syndrome [14, 15].

Juvenile Idiopathic Arthritis (JIA)

Among 210 patients with JIA, oligoarticular JIA was the most common subtype (54.7%), followed by systemic arthritis (17.1%) and polyarticular JIA (12.3%). Antinuclear antibodies (ANA) were positive in 33.6% of patients [16].

Behcet Disease (BD)

In a study of 295 patients with BD, recurrent oral ulcers were present in 99%, genital ulcers in 83%, uveitis in 43%, skin lesions in 90%, and a positive pathergy test in 50%. Arterial involvement, pleuropulmonary lesions, and gastrointestinal involvement were each rare (2%). Among the minor criteria, arthralgia was present in 41%, arthritis in 24%, deep venous thrombosis in 19%, central nervous system involvement in 16%, and superficial thrombophlebitis in 10.2% [17].

Ankylosing Spondylitis (AS)

Another study involving 70 patients with AS found that 83% had grade 4 sacroiliitis, while 17% had grade 2–3 sacroiliitis. Complete fusion of the lumbar spine was present in 76% of patients, while the remaining individuals displayed early changes or partial fusion. In 86% of patients, the cervical spine was affected. Approximately half of the patients experienced hip and peripheral arthritis [9].

Rheumatoid Arthritis (RA)

Several publications have addressed RA in Jordan. A study involving 465 patients was conducted at KAUH in northern Jordan to assess the severity of RA and its association with disease-related disabilities and comorbidities. The study revealed that the mean Disease Activity Score in 28 joints (DAS28) and Clinical Disease Activity Index (CDAI) were 5.1 ± 1.5 and 23 ± 14.2, respectively. Notably, 88% of patients were in the high or moderate disease activity category, with only 5% in remission. Despite receiving active treatment with DMARDs, including anti-TNF agents (used in 24% of patients), the remission rate remained low. Additionally, the study found that 18.3% of patients had diabetes mellitus, 24% had hypertension, and 18.3% had osteoporosis. Joint injuries were documented in 34% of patients, resulting in joint damage, while 8% underwent joint replacement [18].

Systemic Lupus Erythematosus (SLE)

Several studies on SLE were published showing that the most typical clinical manifestation was arthritis or arthralgia, followed by renal involvement. Lupus nephritis affected 50% of patients [19]. Regarding the renal involvement in SLE, class IV was the predominant type in 60% of cases, followed by class V in 12% and class III in 7% [20].

Pregnancy outcomes in 49 women with lupus were compared to those of 500 healthy women regarding preterm delivery, growth-restricted babies, and the development of pre-eclampsia. Preterm deliveries occurred in 25% of SLE patients compared to 10% of healthy controls (OR 1.97). Growth-restricted babies were observed in 20% of the SLE group versus 5% in the control group (OR 2.87), and pre-eclampsia developed in 10% of the SLE patients versus 2% in the controls (OR 5.8) [21].

In a paper published in 2020, mortality in SLE was examined. The study found a 14% mortality rate over 15 years, with a mean age at death of 35.1 ± 12 years and a mean disease duration of 7.5 ± 6.9 years. Infection and SLE-related complications contributed equally to mortality in hospitalized patients [42.5% (CI 27.5–59%) and 40% (95% CI 25–56.5%)], respectively. Most SLE-related deaths were secondary to pulmonary disease [22].

Idiopathic Inflammatory Myopathies (IIM)
A study of 30 patients with IIM found a low association with malignancy. The observed rate was lower than that reported in other countries but was similar to the expected number of malignancy cases in the general population of Jordan [23]. This was confirmed in a larger study involving 94 cases from various institutions in Jordan, in which malignancy was observed in only 4 patients (4.25%). Among them, two males were diagnosed with nasopharyngeal carcinoma at ages 51 and 59, while the remaining two were females who were found to have breast and ovarian cancer at ages 40 and 45, respectively [24].

Takayasu Arteritis (TA)
A retrospective study examined eight patients diagnosed with TA through angiography. In all patients, the aortic arch vessels were affected, while the abdominal aorta was involved in five patients and the renal arteries in four patients. Two patients experienced major clinical events, such as severe stroke and cardiac failure, which were associated with mortality [25].

Sarcoidosis
A retrospective study on 150 patients with sarcoidosis was published in 2020. Biopsy confirmation was achieved in 77% of cases. The most common site for extrapulmonary sarcoidosis was musculoskeletal (MSK) system involvement observed in 33% of patients, with cutaneous involvement being the second most common at 20%, primarily in the form of erythema nodosum (10.7%). Interestingly, females showed a statistically significantly higher prevalence of cutaneous involvement compared to males. Liver, spleen, and extra-thoracic lymph nodes were nearly equally involved, each at 16%. Liver biopsies demonstrated non-caseating granulomas in 2% of patients. Ocular involvement was identified in 14% of cases, including uveitis in 6% and orbital involvement in four patients. Additionally, heart involvement was noted in 5.3% of the cases [26]. Demographic data of patients with some RMDs in Jordan are summarized in Table 5.1 [9, 13, 16–19, 23, 25, 26].

Biologic Medications
Following the introduction of biologic therapy in Jordan, three papers were published that addressed adverse events. The first paper reported worsening osteomalacia in a BD patient treated with infliximab [27]. The second paper focused on the rate of severe infections in patients receiving anti-TNF agents in Jordan. 39 patients (19.6%) had severe infections, including respiratory tract infections (41%), urinary tract infections (30.8%), skin infections (20.5%), and extrapulmonary tuberculosis (7.7%). The only factor significantly linked to a higher infection rate was exposure to more than one anti-TNF agent [28]. Furthermore, the third paper reported the development of posterior reversible encephalopathy in an SLE patient treated with rituximab [29].

Table 5.1 Demographic data of patients with some rheumatic diseases in Jordan

	RA [18]	AS [9]	SLE [19]	IIM [23]	BD [17]	TA [25]	FMF [13]	Sarcoidosis [26]	JIA [16]
Number of patients	465	70	50	30	295	8	196	150	210
M: F	1:4.5	10:1	1:7.3	1:1.7	2.8:1	1:7	1:1.9	1:2.9	1:1.2
Mean age	47.6 ± 14.6	22 (12–40)	22 (14–48)	30	31.2 ± 9.3	–	7.8 ± 3.1	47.8 ± 11	5.33 ± 3.4
Mean disease duration	6 ± 4.45	–	3.5 (1–7.5)	–	5.5 ± 5.7	–	–	–	NA
Mean age at onset	–	22.7 ± 5	–	–	25.8 ± 8.9	–	4.9 ± 2.3	–	5.08 ± 3.4 (7 months to 14 years)
Mortality	NA	NA	14%	–	NA	25%	0.5%	1.3%	NA
Uveitis	–	26%	NA	–	43%	NA	NA	6%	14.2%
Smoking	12.5%	–	–	–	53%	–	–	13.3%	–

Abbreviations: *F* Female, *M* Male, *RA* Rheumatoid Arthritis, *SLE* Systemic Lupus Erythematosus, *IIM* Idiopathic Inflammatory Myositis, *TA* Takayasu Arteritis, *FMF* Familial Mediterranean Fever, *JIA* Juvenile Idiopathic Arthritis, *NA* Not Available

5.6 Risk Factors of Rheumatic Diseases

- *Consanguinity*

A family history of RMDs is a recognized risk factor for developing similar conditions among relatives of affected individuals. Consequently, high rates of consanguinity may contribute to the increased incidence of familial forms of these diseases. Consanguinity rates are relatively high in Jordan, with approximately 35% of marriages reported as consanguineous in 2012 [30].

Several studies from Jordan have highlighted the potential relationship between consanguinity and RMDs. For example, a positive family history of FMF was reported in 59% of affected children, and in many families, the disease was observed across three successive generations [12].

Similar observations have been reported in BD. A significantly higher frequency of family history of recurrent oral ulcers and family history of BD was observed among BD patients compared with controls (52.9% vs. 8.8%, $p < 0.001$; 17.6% vs. 2.4%, $p = 0.008$, respectively). Consanguineous marriages were also more frequent among BD patients than controls (41.2% vs. 24.8%), although this difference did not reach statistical significance ($p = 0.119$) [6].

Familial clustering has also been reported in other immune-mediated diseases. Among SLE patients, 6% reported a family history of SLE [19]. In addition, familial cases of sarcoidosis have been documented, including two sisters diagnosed with isolated pulmonary sarcoidosis 5 years apart, as well as two first cousins who developed progressive pulmonary fibrosis and ocular sarcoidosis, with orbital and sinus involvement reported in one case [26].

Evidence of familial predisposition has also been observed in JIA, where 22.5% of patients had a family history of RA, and 17.6% had parents with consanguineous marriage [16].

- *Smoking:*

Another risk factor for RMDs is smoking [31]; the overall prevalence of cigarette smoking in Jordan is high: 59.1% among males and 23.3% among females [32]. Table 5.1 shows the frequency of smoking among patients with several diseases. Smoking was more frequent among patients with BD than among controls, although the difference did not reach statistical significance ($p = 0.067$) [5]. In contrast, smoking was less frequently observed in patients with RA and sarcoidosis, in whom females outnumber males, which corresponds with patterns observed in the general population, likely reflecting social and cultural factors [7, 26].

- *Obesity:*

Obesity is another risk factor for RA [33]. Body mass index ≥30 kg/m^2 was present in 34% of RA patients [18], and this coincides with the high rate of obesity in Jordan [34].

- *Periodontal infection:*

Another environmental risk factor for RA is periodontal infection, which shows a significant association with RA as demonstrated in many systematic reviews and meta-analysis studies [35]. Statistically significant associations between periodontal infection and RA have also been reported in a study from KAUH, which found that the prevalence of having periodontitis in Jordanian RA patients was 63.7% compared to 30.0% in controls, $p < 0.005$ [36].

5.7 Screening Programs for Rheumatic Diseases

Screening programs for RMDs are not available in Jordan. This absence can be attributed to budget constraints, making it challenging to secure funding for such initiatives, as well as a shortage of healthcare professionals. As a result, the focus is primarily directed toward addressing primary healthcare concerns.

5.8 Diagnosis of Rheumatic Diseases

5.8.1 Laboratory Tests

Most of the medical laboratories in Jordan have received international accreditations.

All laboratory analyses, including routine tests, biochemistry, immunology, and other specific tests, are available in public and private health sectors.

Genetic testing for HLA-B27, HLA-B51, and MEFV mutations is available in both public and private sectors. In contrast, testing for autoinflammatory disorders and monogenic vasculitides in children is sent abroad.

5.8.2 Imaging Tests

Advanced imaging facilities and modalities, including computerized tomography (CT), CT angiography, magnetic resonance imaging (MRI), magnetic resonance angiography (MRA), magnetic resonance venography (MRV), and dual-energy X-ray absorptiometry (bone densitometry), are available. Access to MSK ultrasound in Jordan remains limited, with the first private-sector service introduced in 2017.

Positron Emission Tomography (PET) scans are available in nine centers in Jordan, including one at KAUH, one at KHCC, two in the RMS, and five in private centers.

5.9 Management of Rheumatic Disease in Jordan

5.9.1 Medications

All public and private healthcare centers providing rheumatology services have the facilities to dispense immunomodulatory treatment, including biologics.

5.9.2 Access to Multidisciplinary Specialties

- Rehabilitation

Rehabilitation services have been a part of Jordan's healthcare system for over 35 years. The MOH and RMS offer a training program for physicians specializing in rehabilitation, which is approved by the JMC. Many physicians have obtained the Jordanian Board in Rehabilitation Medicine. Additionally, five universities in Jordan offer various rehabilitation disciplines, including physiotherapy, occupational therapy, and speech-language pathology [37].

- Orthopedic surgery

In 2020, there were 584 registered orthopedic surgeons in the JMA. These orthopedic surgeons provide their services across various healthcare sectors and major cities in Jordan, with only two of them being female surgeons. A wide range of orthopedic surgical procedures is performed, including joint replacements and arthroscopic surgeries. It is noteworthy that Jordan was one of the first countries in the Middle East to offer arthroscopic surgery, performed in 1985. Additionally, some orthopedic surgeons specialize in specific joint areas such as the knee, hip, shoulder, and hand. Furthermore, dedicated pediatric orthopedic specialists are available in both the public and private healthcare sectors.

- MSK radiologists

Among 436 radiologists registered with the JMA (337 males and 99 females), only eight MSK male radiologists work across different health sectors.

5.10 Education and Research

- Rheumatology training programs:

Rheumatology training programs in Jordan commenced in 2010. The primary aim of these programs is to graduate competent rheumatologists well-versed in both the clinical and laboratory aspects of the field. The curriculum is tailored to equip physicians for various professional paths, including clinical practice, medical education, and research. This 3-year program has received approval and accreditation from the JMC. Applicants for postgraduate training in rheumatology are required to have completed a 4-year residency in internal medicine and must have obtained board certification in internal medicine. Three rheumatology fellowship programs are currently available in Jordan: one at the University of Jordan, another at the Jordan University of Science and Technology, and a third at the RMS. To date, 19 Jordanian graduates (seven males and 12 females), one fellow from Palestine, and two from Yemen have completed the fellowship and have been accredited by the JMC with the Jordanian Board of Rheumatology. In addition, 14 new candidates (12 Jordanians and two from Palestine) were recently enrolled in the program. The JMC also allows fellows trained abroad who meet the eligibility criteria to sit for the certification examination.

- Rheumatology nursing programs:

Unfortunately, programs to train nurses in rheumatology are not available in Jordan.

- Research in Rheumatology:

Jordanian rheumatologists took an active role in several local and multicenter international clinical trials of novel biologics and biosimilars, administered via intravenous, subcutaneous, and oral routes. These trials were related to RA, BD, and uveitis [38]. In this regard, Jordan stands out as one of the leading countries in the Middle East and North Africa (MENA) region for clinical trials, particularly in bioequivalence and bioavailability studies. It was one of the first Arab countries to enact legislation for clinical trials and has since become a premier location for such studies in the Arab World, supported by robust regulatory settings. In Jordan, there are 22 approved and licensed research ethics committees that operate across various academic institutions, private settings, and hospitals.

Jordan has a permanent legal framework regulating clinical research through Clinical Studies Law No. 2 of 2011, an amended version of the provisional Law No. 67 of 2001, which governs all clinical studies conducted in the country [39]. To the best of our knowledge, the first publication in rheumatology by a Jordanian rheumatologist dates back to 1987 and focused on kidney involvement in BD [40].

Rheumatologists from Jordan have contributed significantly to the field, with over 200 publications cited approximately 4270 times in both local and international journals. Most of these publications are retrospective and cross-sectional observational studies, while others are basic research papers. Some of these research endeavors have involved collaborations with international centers, while others have been conducted locally [41–54]. In addition, numerous abstracts and posters have been presented at national, regional, and international conferences, including those organized by the European Alliance of Associations for Rheumatology (EULAR) and the American College of Rheumatology (ACR).

5.11 Cost-Effective Management of Rheumatic Diseases

The Jordanian government faces significant challenges in healthcare spending, particularly in pharmaceuticals. In response, a National Medicine Policy (NMP) was introduced in 2002 with the objective of ensuring optimal healthcare delivery to the Jordanian patients. This policy's goal is to provide safe, effective, high-quality, and affordable medications to both the government and its citizens. To further manage and control governmental expenditure on medications, including those for rheumatology, the JPD was established in the same year. The JPD focuses on procuring necessary medicines at the lowest feasible cost for the public sector, without compromising product quality.

In 2015, the proportion of public health spending allocated to medications was approximately 26%, a notable reduction from 36% in 2008, prior to the JPD's establishment. In line with global trends, Jordan is increasingly turning to generic drugs to reduce health expenditure, a practice common among many governments worldwide [55]. To encourage local drug manufacture, preference is given to purchasing locally manufactured medicines.

With the introduction of biosimilars, Jordan was among the first countries in the MENA region to issue guidelines for biosimilar registration in May 2015. The JFDA has adopted the guidelines published by the European Medicines Agency (EMA) [56], recognizing that the approval of these medications is likely to lead to a significant reduction in prices. This anticipated decrease is attributed not only to the generally lower cost of these medications compared to the original (reference) biologics but also to the expected healthy competition among suppliers. Such competition is anticipated to further drive down prices. Consequently, the overall cost savings are expected to increase the number of patients who can access these treatments, ultimately having a positive impact on the nation's health status [57]. Biosimilars related to rheumatology were introduced to the Jordanian market in 2017.

5.12 Challenges and Opportunities

- Challenges in the Care of Rheumatic Disease in Jordan:

Several challenges impact the care of RMDs in Jordan. First, there is a shortage of rheumatologists. According to the latest Workforce Policy Report 2021 from the British Society for Rheumatology (BSR), it is recommended that one rheumatologist be available for every 60,000–80,000 people to meet demand and maintain reasonable waiting times [58]. Currently, the number of Jordanian rheumatologists practicing in Jordan falls far short of this recommendation, with only about 0.29 rheumatologists per 80,000 people. It is important to note that some of these rheumatologists might retire soon. Second, the financial compensation in Jordan is lower than in other countries, making it challenging to retain highly specialized Jordanian graduates. Third, there exists a significant discrepancy and inequality in the distribution of rheumatologists across health sectors and geographical regions within the country. For instance, only 24 rheumatologists are employed in the public sector, with four of them working part-time. These specialists are predominantly concentrated in the capital, Amman, Zarqa, Salt, and Irbid in the north of Jordan, serving 81.5% of the insured population. Consequently, this distribution results in heavy workloads and prolonged appointment wait times. Moreover, the unequal distribution of rheumatologists within the country, particularly in the public health sector, imposes additional burdens on patients. Even if a patient can access a rheumatologist, the indirect costs of travel and lost time from work and school make it challenging to maintain regular follow-up appointments. Fourthly, the high cost of medications, particularly the new targeted treatments, presents a significant challenge, especially for those who are uninsured.

- Human Resources

Given its status as a middle-income country with limited natural resources, Jordan has placed a strong emphasis on human resource development, considering it one of its most valuable assets and strategic pillars. The country is among the leading regional countries in terms of investment in education and manpower development.

Jordan has a literacy rate of approximately 95% among adults aged 15 years and older, reflecting a high level of educational attainment in the country [59]. In the academic year 2022/2023, the total number of undergraduate students enrolled in the 36 Jordanian universities, including both public and private institutions, reached 355,226 students. Female students accounted for 55.1% of total enrollment, while 44.9% were males. In addition, 34,502 Jordanian students were pursuing higher education abroad [1].

Human Resources for Health (HRH) represents valuable capital in the advancement and enhancement of a nation's health status. In comparison to other countries in the region, Jordan maintains a commendable density of healthcare providers, including physicians, registered nurses, and midwives, at the national level. However, this density has experienced a decline over the past 3 years. This decrease is attributed to two main factors: the rapid population growth in Jordan and the brain drain phenomenon, where physicians are attracted to more lucrative job opportunities abroad and in neighboring countries.

In 2023, the MOH employed 6737 physicians, 10,091 nurses, and 1223 pharmacists. According to the Jordanian Medical Association, a total of 39,940 physicians were registered nationwide, including 30,189 males and 9751 females, working across the public, private, and other healthcare sectors [1].

- Health Insurance Coverage:

The MOH civil health insurance fund covers 41.7% of the population, while the RMS military insurance fund covers 38%. University hospital insurance and private health insurance cover 2.5% and 12.5% of the population, respectively. UNRWA provides coverage to 2.5% of the population exclusively through primary health care services. The overall proportion of the population covered by health insurance does not exceed 78%. It is important to note that this coverage calculation excludes cases of medical exemptions provided by the non-insured patients' affairs unit at the Royal Court. These statistics pertain to rheumatology services [2].

- Medical Tourism:

Over the past decade, Jordan has become one of the most desirable destinations in the region for medical tourism because of its high-quality, affordable healthcare. Thousands of foreign patients from Arab countries received health services in Jordan. The health service sector contributed approximately 1.2 billion USD to Jordan's GDP in 2015.

This success is due to several reasons, including the competitive cost of treatment on the international level and the quality of medical services provided in Jordan [60]. Currently, 121 hospitals operate in Jordan, serving both Jordanian and non-Jordanian patients, including 71 private hospitals, 33 government hospitals, 15 affiliated with the RMS, and two university hospitals [61]. The KHCC is one of the specialized cancer treatment centers in the Middle East.

Jordan has its healthcare accreditation council, accredited by the International Society for Quality in Health Care (ISQua), ensuring that healthcare and patient safety in the country meet international standards. There are 10 Joint Commission International (JCI)-accredited and 25 Healthcare Accreditation Council (HCAC)-accredited hospitals, which ensure adherence to international standards in care and customer service.

Jordanian hospitals have made significant investments in modern technology, with equipment such as MRI, CT, nuclear medicine imaging, and PET scanners standard in most private hospitals. These facilities offer a wide range of medical specialties, including rheumatology, and are staffed by skilled physicians proficient in both Arabic and English, with relatively short waiting times.

Jordan is home to numerous drug manufacturers, and the pharmaceutical industry has experienced remarkable growth since the establishment of the first Jordanian drug factory in 1962. Many of these companies have become global exporters, producing high-quality medications, including non-steroidal anti-inflammatory drugs and non-biologic and biologic DMARDs.

Moreover, Jordan is renowned for its natural health spas, such as Ma'in Falls and the Dead Sea. The natural products extracted from the Dead Sea, rich in mineral salts, are known to aid in treating various skin and joint diseases.

5.13 Future Directions for Rheumatic Disease Care

We discuss our perspective on the future of RMD in Jordan, along with some suggestions for improving clinical care and research.

1. Addressing the Rising Burden of RMDs

With improvements in the healthcare system and the population shift toward non-communicable diseases (NCDs), Jordan is expected to see an increase in elderly populations and individuals with disabilities. However, risk factors for NCDs, including RMDs, obesity, and smoking, are also on the rise among Jordanians. The increasing prevalence of obesity, which was 60.4% among men and 75.6% among women in 2020 compared to 28.1% in men and 53.1% in women in 2008, highlights the clear need to anticipate a surge in RMDs. This surge will pose challenges to both public and private healthcare systems [34].

2. Addressing the Shortage of Rheumatology Care Providers

To address the shortage of rheumatologists, the MOH has introduced initiatives, such as scholarship programs, to encourage internal medicine specialists to pursue further training in rheumatology. Additionally, efforts to mitigate geographical discrepancies in rheumatology services have been made by the RMS, which extends its services to regions lacking rheumatologists such as Aydoun north of Jordan, Karak and Aqaba in the south of Jordan.

3. Strengthening Rheumatology Nursing Programs

The latest Workforce Policy Report of the BSR recommends a ratio of one specialist nurse for every consultant treating 60,000–80,000 people to meet the demand for rheumatology care [60]. Investing in rheumatology nursing programs will complement the workforce, improve patient care, and alleviate the workload of rheumatologists [62].

4. Addressing the Cost of Biologic Therapies

The introduction of targeted biologic therapies poses financial challenges for both public and private insurance. This should alert policymakers to plan strategies to overcome this challenge and discuss alternatives.

5. Combining Research with Integrated Clinical Care

A shift toward integrated clinical care and clinical research is essential for improving RMD care in Jordan. Government support for research initiatives and encouraging young rheumatologists, particularly at an early stage of their training, to engage in scientific research will enhance the quality of care and contribute to healthcare system improvement. Collaboration with international partners and the expansion of research networks, as advocated by the JSR, will further support research and education efforts.

6. Establishment of a National Registry for Rheumatic Diseases

The JSR's initiation of a national registry for RMDs is a positive step toward better understanding the scope of RMDs in Jordan. This registry will provide valuable data to inform future healthcare planning and decision-making.

5.14 Conclusion

Although rheumatology as a separate discipline emerged recently in Jordan, it is now a well-recognized specialty in the country. With limited resources, Jordanian rheumatologists put Jordan on the scientific map, both locally and internationally. Behcet disease and FMF seem to be highly prevalent in Jordan. The first two adult and pediatric publications were on these diseases and were confirmed in subsequent prevalence studies.

Conflict of Interest The authors declare no conflicts of interest.

References

1. Department of Statistics (Jordan). Statistical yearbook 2023 [internet]. Amman: Department of Statistics; 2023. [cited 2026 Jun 14]. Available from: https://dosweb.dos.gov.jo/databank/yearbook/YearBook2023.pdf.
2. National Strategy for Health Sector in Jordan 2016–2020 [Internet]. [cited 2026 Jun 14]. Available from: https://extranet.who.int/countryplanningcycles/sites/default/files/planning_cycle_repository/jordan/national_strategy_for_health_sector_2016-2020_jordan.pdf.
3. Rawashdeh MO, Majeed HA. Familial Mediterranean fever in Arab children: the high prevalence and gene frequency. Eur J Pediatr. 1996;155(7):540–4. https://doi.org/10.1007/BF01957901.
4. Masri B, Azar E, Faqih A, Somay-Rendou E, Duboeuf F, Delmas PD. Prevalence of postmenopausal osteoporosis in Jordan - the Fijonor study. Osteoporos Int. 2007;18(Suppl 3):245–328. https://doi.org/10.1007/s00198-007-0480-3.
5. Hyassat D, Alyan T, Jaddou H, Ajlouni KM. Prevalence and risk factors of osteoporosis among Jordanian postmenopausal women attending the National Center for diabetes, endocrinology and genetics in Jordan. Biores Open Access. 2017;6(1):85–93. https://doi.org/10.1089/biores.2016.0045.
6. Madanat WY, Alawneh KM, Smadi MM, Saadeh SS, Omari MM, Bani Hani AB, et al. The prevalence of Behcet's disease in the north of Jordan: a hospital-based epidemiological survey. Clin Exp Rheumatol. 2017;35(6 Suppl 108):51–4.
7. Alawneh KM, Madanat WY, Alawneh D, Smadi MS. Prevalence of rheumatoid arthritis among hospital workers in the north of Jordan: preliminary report of a hospital-based cohort study. Ann Med Surg (Lond). 2020;60:579–82. https://doi.org/10.1016/j.amsu.2020.11.043.
8. Verity DH, Wallace GR, Vaughan RW, Kondeatis E, Madanat W, Zureikat H, et al. HLA and tumour necrosis factor (TNF) polymorphisms in ocular Behcet's disease. Tissue Antigens. 1999;54(3):264–72. https://doi.org/10.1034/j.1399-0039.1999.540307.x.
9. Mustafa KN, Hammoudeh M, Khan MA. HLA-B27 prevalence in Arab populations and among patients with ankylosing spondylitis. J Rheumatol. 2012;39(8):1675–7. https://doi.org/10.3899/jrheum.120403.
10. Alzyoud R, Alsweiti M, Maittah H, Adayleh B, Alnobani M, Alwahadneh A, et al. Genotype pattern of pediatric familial Mediterranean fever in Jordan: a single center experience. Int J Pediatr. 2019;7(2):8935–40. https://doi.org/10.22038/ijp.2018.34530.3037.
11. Saxena R, Plenge RM, Bjonnes AC, Dashti HS, Okada Y, Gad El Haq W, et al. A multinational Arab genome-wide association study identifies new genetic associations for rheumatoid arthritis. Arthritis Rheumatol. 2017;69(5):976–85. https://doi.org/10.1002/art.40051.
12. Majeed HA, Rawashdeh M, El-Shanti H, Qubain H, Khuri-Bulos N, Shahin HM. Familial Mediterranean fever in children: the expanded clinical profile. Q J Med. 1999;92(6):309–18.

13. Alzyoud R. Familial Mediterranean fever in Jordanian children: single center experience. Mediterr J Rheumatol. 2018;29(4):211–6. https://doi.org/10.31138/mjr.29.4.211.
14. Majeed HA, Al-Tarawna M, El-Shanti H, Kamel B, Al-Khalaileh F. The syndrome of chronic recurrent multifocal osteomyelitis and congenital dyserythropoietic anemia. Report of a new family and a review. Eur J Pediatr. 2001;160(12):705–10. https://doi.org/10.1007/s004310100799.
15. Ferguson PJ, El-Shanti H. Majeed syndrome: a review of the clinical, genetic and immunologic features. Biomolecules. 2021;11(3):367. https://doi.org/10.3390/biom11030367.
16. Alzyoud RM, Alsuweiti MO, Almaaitah HQ, Aladaileh BN, Alnoubani MK, Alwahadneh AM. Juvenile idiopathic arthritis in Jordan: single center experience. Pediatr Rheumatol. 2021;19:90. https://doi.org/10.1186/s12969-021-00572-8.
17. Madanat W, Sharaiha Z, Khasawneh S, Zureikat H, Fayyad F. Gastrointestinal manifestations of Behcet's disease, proceedings of the 10th international conference on Behcet's disease. Adv Exp Med Biol. 2003;528:455–7.
18. Alawneh KM, Khassawneh BY, Ayesh MH, Smadi M. Rheumatoid arthritis in Jordan: a cross-sectional study of disease severity and associated comorbidities. Ther Clin Risk Manag. 2014;10:363–6. https://doi.org/10.2147/TCRM.S62954.
19. Al-Heresh AM. Systemic lupus erythematosus among Jordanians: a single rheumatology unit experience. JRMS. 2010;17:20–4.
20. Mustafa KN, Aladily TN, Shomaf MS, Wahbeh AM. Renal biopsy findings in lupus nephritis. Saudi J Kidney Dis Transpl. 2011;22:815–7.
21. Al Mashaaleh M, Gharaibeh A, Al Serhan A, Matar K, Burgan A, Khataybeh O, et al. Neonatal and obstetric outcome of systemic lupus erythematosus at King Hussein Medical Center, Amman, Jordan. Rawal Med J. 2014;39:449–51.
22. Adwan MH, Qasem U, Mustafa KN. In-hospital mortality in patients with systemic lupus erythematosus: a study from Jordan 2002-2017. Rheumatol Int. 2020;40(5):711–7. https://doi.org/10.1007/s00296-020-04538-z.
23. Mustafa KN, Dahbour SS. Clinical characteristics and outcomes of patients with idiopathic inflammatory myopathies from Jordan 1996-2009. Clin Rheumatol. 2010;29(12):1381–5. https://doi.org/10.1007/s10067-010-1465-8.
24. Mustafa KN, Al-Heresh AM, Khataybeh OY, Alawneh KM, Khader YS. Low prevalence of malignancy in patients with idiopathic inflammatory myopathies in Jordan. Clin Exp Rheumatol. 2015;33(5):731–3.
25. Mustafa KN, Hadidy A, Sweiss NJ. Clinical and radiological features of Takayasu's arteritis patients in Jordan. Rheumatol Int. 2010;30(11):1449–53. https://doi.org/10.1007/s00296-009-1163-5.
26. Alnaimat F, Al Oweidat K, Alrwashdeh A, Alnashrati A, Barham S, Hijaz M, et al. Sarcoidosis in Jordan: a study of the clinical phenotype and disease outcome. Arch Rheumatol. 2020;35(2):226–38. https://doi.org/10.46497/ArchRheumatol.2020.7584.
27. Madanat WY, Madanat AY. Worsening of osteomalacia in a patient successfully treated for neuro-Behcet's disease with infliximab. Clin Exp Rheumatol. 2008;26(4 Suppl 50):S128–9.
28. Alawneh KM, Ayesh MH, Khassawneh BY, Saadeh SS, Smadi M, Bashaireh K. Anti-TNF therapy in Jordan: a focus on severe infections and tuberculosis. Biologics. 2014;8:193–8. https://doi.org/10.2147/BTT.S59574.
29. Mustafa KN, Qasem U, Al-Ryalat NT, Bsisu IK. Rituximab-associated posterior reversible encephalopathy syndrome. Int J Rheum Dis. 2019;22(1):160–5. https://doi.org/10.1111/1756-185X.13427.
30. Islam MM, Ababneh FM, Khan MHR. Consanguineous marriage in Jordan: an update. J Biosoc Sci. 2018;50(4):573–8. https://doi.org/10.1017/S0021932017000372.
31. Sugiyama D, Nishimura K, Tamaki K, Tsuji G, Nakazawa T, Morinobu A, et al. Impact of smoking as a risk factor for developing rheumatoid arthritis: a meta-analysis of observational studies. Ann Rheum Dis. 2010;69(1):70–81. https://doi.org/10.1136/ard.2008.096487.
32. Abu-Helalah MA, Alshraideh HA, Al-Serhan AA, Nesheiwat AI, Da'na M, Al-Nawafleh A. Epidemiology, attitudes, and perceptions toward cigarettes and hookah smoking amongst

adults in Jordan. Environ Health Prev Med. 2015;20(6):422–33. https://doi.org/10.1007/s12199-015-0483-1.
33. Crowson CS, Matteson EL, Davis JM 3rd, Gabriel SE. Contribution of obesity to the rise in incidence of rheumatoid arthritis. Arthritis Care Res (Hoboken). 2013;65(1):71–7. https://doi.org/10.1002/acr.21660.
34. Ajlouni K, Khader Y, Batieha A, Jaddou H, El-Khateeb M. An alarmingly high and increasing prevalence of obesity in Jordan. Epidemiol Health. 2020;42:e2020040. https://doi.org/10.4178/epih.e2020040.
35. de Oliveira Ferreira R, de Brito Silva R, Magno MB, Carvalho Almeida APCPS, Fagundes NCF, Maia LC, et al. Does periodontitis represent a risk factor for rheumatoid arthritis? A systematic review and meta-analysis. Ther Adv Musculoskelet Dis. 2019;11:1759720X19858514. https://doi.org/10.1177/1759720X19858514.
36. Al Habashneh R, Alawneh K, Alshami R, Al Naji K. Rheumatoid arthritis and periodontitis: a Jordanian case-control study. J Public Health (Oxf). 2020;28(5):547–54. https://doi.org/10.1007/s10389-019-01073-5.
37. Government of Jordan, Ministry of Health. Jordan National Rehabilitation Strategic Plan 2020–2024 [internet]. Amman: Ministry of Health; 2021. [cited 2026 Jun 14]. Available from: https://reliefweb.int/report/jordan/jordan-national-rehabilitation-strategic-plan-2020-2024-enar.
38. National Library of Medicine (US). ClinicalTrials.gov [Internet]. Bethesda (MD): National Library of Medicine; [cited 2026 Mar 13]. Available from: https://clinicaltrials.gov/.
39. Association of Clinical Research Professionals (ACRP). Clinical Researcher. Vol. 28, Issue 6. December 2014 [Internet]. Alexandria (VA): ACRP; 2014 [cited 2026 Jun 14]. Available from: https://acrpnet.org/wp-content/uploads/dlm_uploads/2017/08/ACRP-Clinical-Researcher-December-2014.pdf.
40. Nasrallah N, Amr SS, Abbasi T. Kidney involvement in Behcet's syndrome: clinicopathological correlations. Arthritis Rheum. 1987;30(4):S107.
41. Saleh MM, Irshaid YM, Mustafa KN. Methylene tetrahydrofolate reductase genotypes frequencies: association with toxicity and response to methotrexate in rheumatoid arthritis patients. Int J Clin Pharmacol Ther. 2015;53(2):154–62. https://doi.org/10.5414/cp202242.
42. Oqal MK, Mustafa KN, Irshaid YM. N-acetyltransferase-2 genotypes among patients with rheumatoid arthritis attending Jordan University Hospital. Genet Test Mol Biomarkers. 2012;16(9):1007–10. https://doi.org/10.1089/gtmb.2012.0062.
43. Jaradat SA, Abujamous LA, Al-Hawamdeh AA, Alawneh KM, Rawashdeh TA, Jaradat ZM. Two novel mutations of FBN1 in Jordanian patients with Marfan syndrome. Int J Clin Exp Med. 2015;8(10):18786–92.
44. Wallace GR, Verity DH, Delamaine LJ, Ohno S, Inoko H, Ota M, et al. MIC-A allele profiles and HLA class I associations in Behcet's disease. Immunogenetics. 1999;49(7–8):613–7.
45. Mizuki N, Yabuki K, Ota M, Verity D, Katsuyama Y, Ando H, et al. Microsatellite mapping of a susceptible locus within the HLA region for Behçet's disease using Jordanian patients. Hum Immunol. 2001;62(2):186–90.
46. Verity DH, Vaughan RW, Kondeatis E, Madanat W, Zureikat H, Fayyad F, et al. Intercellular adhesion molecule-1 gene polymorphisms in Behcet's disease. Eur J Immunogenet. 2000;27(2):73–6.
47. Verity DH, Vaughan RW, Madanat W, Kondeatis E, Zureikat H, Fayyad F, et al. Factor V Leiden mutation is associated with ocular involvement in Behçet's disease. Am J Ophthalmol. 1999;128(3):352–6.
48. Ahmad T, Zhang L, Gogus F, Verity D, Wallace G, Madanat W, et al. CARD15 polymorphisms in Behçet's disease. Scand J Rheumatol. 2005;34(3):233–7.
49. Baranathan V, Stanford MR, Vaughan RW, Kondeatis E, Graham E, Fortune F, et al. The association of the PTPN22 620W polymorphism with Behcet's disease. Ann Rheum Dis. 2007;66(11):1531–3.

50. Wallace GR, Kondeatis E, Vaughan RW, Rivadeneira F, Uitterlinden A, Van Daele P, et al. IL-10 genotype analysis in patients with Behcet's disease. Hum Immunol. 2007;68(2):122–7.
51. Khabour OF, Alawneh K, Al-Kofahi E, Mesmar F. Assessment of genotoxicity associated with Behcet's disease using sister-chromatid exchange assay: vitamin E versus mitomycin C. Cytotechnology. 2015;67(6):1051–7.
52. Daoud A, Rajab W, Alawneh K, Harfiel MN. Effects of different Familial Mediterranean Fever gene mutations and in vitro Colchicine treatment on peripheral blood mononuclear cells production of IL-6. Bangladesh J Med Sci. 2013;12(4):370–7. https://doi.org/10.3329/bjms.v12i4.16659.
53. Ishigaki K, Sakaue S, Terao C, Luo Y, Sonehara K, Yamaguchi K, et al. Multi-ancestry genome-wide association analyses identify novel genetic mechanisms in rheumatoid arthritis. Nat Genet. 2022;54(11):1640–51. https://doi.org/10.1038/s41588-022-01213-w.
54. Elawi AM, Irshaid YM, Ismail SI, Mustafa KN. Thiopurine S-methytransferase gene polymorphism in rheumatoid arthritis. Arch Med Res. 2013;44(2):105–9. https://doi.org/10.1016/j.arcmed.2013.01.006.
55. Ministry of Health (Jordan). National Medicine Policy 2014 [internet]. Amman: Ministry of Health; 2014. [cited 2026 Jun 14]. Available from: https://faolex.fao.org/docs/pdf/jor180732E.pdf.
56. Malkawi RMAA, Al-Haqaish WS, Obeidat H. Biosimilar regulation and approval in Jordan. GaBI J. 2018;7(2):77–8. https://doi.org/10.5639/gabij.2018.0702.016.
57. Almaaytah A. Budget impact analysis of switching to rituximab's biosimilar in rheumatology and cancer in 13 countries within the Middle East and North Africa. Clinicoecon Outcomes Res. 2020;12:527–34. https://doi.org/10.2147/CEOR.S265041.
58. British Society for Rheumatology. Rheumatology workforce: a crisis in numbers [internet]. London: British Society for Rheumatology; 2021. [cited 2026 Jun 14]. Available from: https://www.rheumatology.org.uk/Portals/0/Documents/Policy/Reports/BSR-workforce-report-crisis-numbers.pdf.
59. World Education Statistics. UNESCO Institute for Statistics. [Internet]. Montreal: UNESCO; 2024. [cited 2026 Jun 14]. Available from: https://unesdoc.unesco.org/ark:/48223/pf0000391221.
60. Hassan V. Medical tourism in Lebanon: an analysis of tourism flows. Athens J Tourism. 2015;2(3):153–66. https://doi.org/10.30958/ajt.2-3-2.
61. Private Hospitals Association (Jordan). Hospitals sector in Jordan [Internet]. Amman; [cited 2026 Jun 14]. Available from: https://phajordan.org/EN-article-3809-
62. Uthman I, Almoallim H, Buckley CD, Masri B, Dahou-Makhloufi C, El Dershaby Y, et al. Nurse-led care for the management of rheumatoid arthritis: a review of the global literature and proposed strategies for implementation in Africa and the Middle East. Rheumatol Int. 2021;41(3):529–42. https://doi.org/10.1007/s00296-020-04682-6.

Chapter 6
Rheumatic Diseases in Kuwait

Ahmed Thuweni Alenizi, Eman Haji Hasan, Muna Almutairi, and Adel Alawadhi

Abstract This chapter explores the country's demographics, healthcare sectors, rheumatology health services and provides an overview of rheumatic diseases in Kuwait, comparing their burden on the health system to other specialties through relevant statistics and showing available data on prevalence, incidence, and mortality. The chapter goes through rheumatic diseases, including risk factors, screening programs, diagnosis, and management. It also discusses the research and education related to rheumatic diseases, highlighting the current national rheumatic disease registries and published studies, besides the activities of the rheumatology community in Kuwait. Finally, we cover the cost-effectiveness of rheumatic disease care, challenges, and areas of improvement in this subspecialty.

Keywords Demography · Rheumatic Diseases · Healthcare · Kuwait

6.1 Demographics of Kuwait

The state of Kuwait is a developed country with a population of 4,881,254 people, 68% of whom were foreigners in 2025 [1]. There are 1,893,283 million women and 2,987,971 million men. The percentage of the female population is 38.79%

A. T. Alenizi
Rheumatic Disease Unit, Al-Jahra Hospital, Ministry of Health, Al Jahra, Kuwait
e-mail: bohmaid@yahoo.com

E. H. Hasan
Rheumatic Disease Unit, Amiri Hospital, Ministry of Health, Kuwait City, Kuwait
e-mail: eman14doctor@yahoo.com

M. Almutairi
Rheumatic Disease Unit, Al-Adan Hospital, Ministry of Health, Hadiya, Kuwait
e-mail: dr.monakw@hotmail.com

A. Alawadhi (✉)
Department of Medicine, Faculty of Medicine, Kuwait University, Kuwait City, Kuwait
e-mail: adel.alawadhi@yahoo.com; adel.alawadhi@ku.edu.kw

K. A. Alnaqbi, G. Aldabie (eds.), *Rheumatic Diseases in the Arab World*,
https://doi.org/10.1007/978-981-92-0967-5_6

compared to the 61.21% male population. Kuwait is located in the northern section of the Arabian Gulf. It shares its border with Saudi Arabia and Iraq and has a land area of 17,828 km^2. It has a chilly climate in the winter and exceedingly hot and dry in the summer. Administratively, it is divided into six governorates or health regions: Mubarak Al-Kabeer, Capital, Ahmadi, Hawalli, Farwaniya, and Jahra.

6.2 Healthcare Sectors in Kuwait

The health system is governed by the Ministry of Health (MOH) of Kuwait, which is the body that regulates and monitors both the public and private sectors. The MOH is also the primary service provider in the public sector, a more significant health sector than the private sector.

Seven major governmental hospitals provide tertiary healthcare. The main healthcare centers are Al-Adan, Al-Amiri, Al-Farwaniya, Al-Jahra, Jaber Al-Ahmed, Mubarak Al-Kabeer, and Al-Sabah Hospitals.

The National Centre for Health Information (NCHI) has published annual health reports since 1958, serving as an official source of healthcare statistics and system development in Kuwait [2]. Based on the latest published annual health report 2022 by the National Centre for Health Information Kuwait (NCHI) [3], MOH had 21 hospitals; 6 general hospitals (one in each health region besides Jaber Al-Ahmad hospital), plus Sabah medical center and 14 specialized hospitals, besides 111 primary health care clinics and 102 diabetic clinics. The number of physicians working in MOH is 11,417, with 2819 dentists and 22,890 nurses. The total bed capacity was 8735 beds. The population/bed ration have increased from 637 in 2018 to 511 in 2022 in public hospitals and from 2991 to 2810 in the private sector. MOH's total expenses for medical services in the public sector for 2021–2022 were 2.11 billion Kuwaiti Dinar (6.9 billion USD). The expenditure on drugs, equipment, laboratories, and instruments in 2022 was 520.9 million KD (1.7 billion USD).

Thirteen private hospitals and three owned by oil firms were incorporated into the private health sector in 2022, with a total bed capacity of 1589 beds and 2207 physicians, 1010 dentists, and 7905 nurses. The private sector also included independently run 31 medical centers, 221 polyclinics, and 168 solo clinics.

6.3 Rheumatology Services in Kuwait

Since opening the first rheumatology clinic in Kuwait in 1980, the rheumatology services, manpower, educational and research activities have been growing, especially over the last 15 years, Fig. 6.1.

Currently, all Kuwait's major public hospitals have rheumatology units. Each unit has senior and junior staff members who provide care for rheumatology patients in their hospital's particular district.

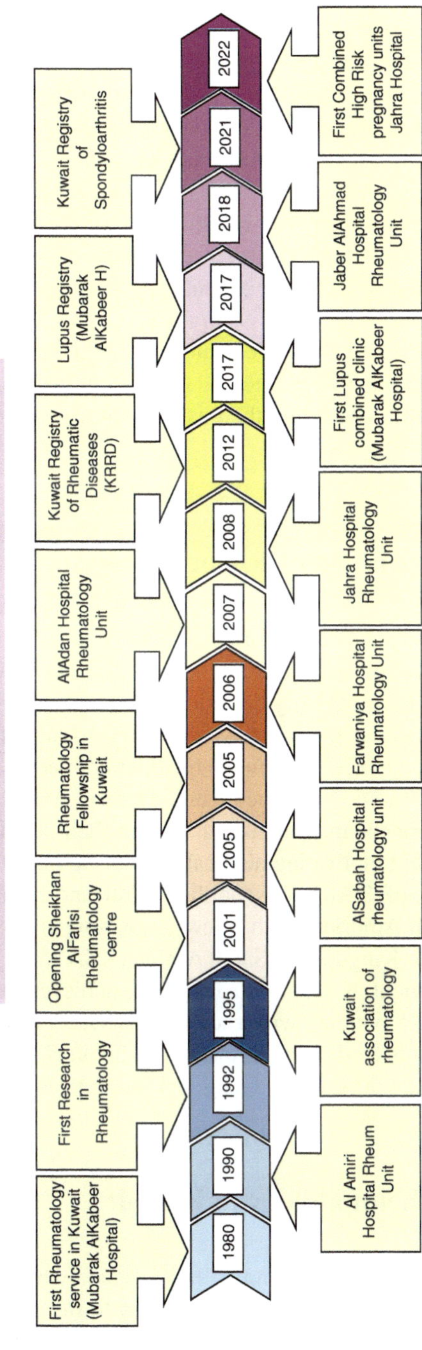

Fig. 6.1 Evolution of Rheumatology Services in Kuwait

The referral system to rheumatology services at the government hospitals for patients with suspected rheumatic disease is through polyclinics distributed all over the districts of the governorates. General practitioners or family physicians assigned to these polyclinics are the first to see these patients. They refer suspected patients to the hospital belonging to that governorate. Then, patients are screened by an internal medicine specialist and referred to rheumatic disease clinics as tertiary referrals. There are also referrals from other subspecialties, such as dermatology, ophthalmology, orthopedic surgery, gastroenterology, neurology, nephrology, and rehabilitation medicine. Self-referral system to rheumatology occurs in private hospitals/clinics.

The number of registered and certified adult rheumatologists is 31 (19 males, 12 females), and 8 certified pediatric rheumatologists (2 males, 6 females) in Kuwait as of September 2025.

The number of registered nurses dedicated to the rheumatology service is around 24. There are seven hospitals accredited by Accreditation Canada. Each hospital has a rheumatic disease unit. Currently, there is no accredited Center of Excellence for Rheumatology in Kuwait.

6.4 Kuwait Association of Rheumatologists

The Kuwait Association of Rheumatologists (KAR), founded in 1995, is the official rheumatology organization in Kuwait. Its vision is to raise awareness of rheumatic illnesses globally and promote early detection, effective management, research funding, and educational advancement. KAR's mission is to support rheumatologists and trainees while advancing excellence in the treatment of people with rheumatic disorders. Its goals include improving rheumatology care, providing access to clinical guidance, and assisting rheumatologists in raising their standard of care across all levels of healthcare, and motivating medical students to pursue rheumatology.

The vast majority of KAR's 39 qualified adult and pediatric rheumatologists were trained in North America, with a few graduating from the United Kingdom (UK), Kuwait, and the Kingdom of Saudi Arabia (KSA).

Since its establishment, KAR has made notable achievements, including improving standard of care to patients with rheumatic disease, educating the public and healthcare professionals from various specialties about rheumatic diseases through awareness campaigns, workshops, educational sessions, and publications.

6.5 Pediatric Rheumatology in Kuwait

An official referral to pediatric rheumatology is made when a general pediatrician suspects rheumatic disease, with patients directed to the appropriate health sector. Pediatric rheumatology services in Kuwait began in 1990 at Mubarak Al-Kabeer Hospital.

Currently, five main hospitals provide pediatric rheumatology services across the country. Mubarak Al-Kabeer Hospital in the Hawalli sector is the largest unit, serving a dense population. Al-Adan Hospital in the Ahmadi sector was established in 2013, followed by Al-Sabah Children's Hospital in 2015. More recently, services were introduced in Farwaniya Hospital (2024) and Al-Amiri Hospital (2025).

There are six females and two males certified in pediatric rheumatology. These rheumatologists collaborate across the hospitals and with colleagues in the Gulf region to exchange expertise and conduct research aimed at improving care for children and adolescents with rheumatic diseases.

Juvenile idiopathic arthritis (JIA) is the most common pediatric rheumatic disease in Kuwait. The Ministry of Health (MOH) provides pediatric rheumatologists with essential medications, including biologics, and ensures access to comprehensive laboratory and diagnostic services. Non-Kuwaiti children can also receive biologic therapies with the support of patient funds, while csDMARDs are available to them at a minimal cost.

Pediatric rheumatology services in Kuwait's private sector are limited, with only two specialized clinics staffed by a certified pediatric rheumatologist.

6.6 Overview of Rheumatic Diseases in Kuwait

Rheumatic diseases and musculoskeletal (MSK) pain are widespread in Kuwait, and the rheumatology service is very busy, especially in the outpatient clinics, where the waiting time to see a rheumatologist for new cases and referrals may take, on average, several months. Indeed, the word "rheumatism" in Kuwait is closely connected to aging and is misused for chronic pain, making rheumatologists the target referred physicians for such complaints. In a local survey for general practitioners and family medicine physicians, the need for training in rheumatic diseases comes second after asthma, reflecting common MSK-related pain encountered in the primary health care sector.

To have an overview of rheumatic diseases in Kuwait, and based on available data, we will highlight the burden of rheumatic diseases on the health system in Kuwait, incidence and prevalence, and other epidemiological data.

6.7 The Burden of Rheumatic Diseases in Kuwait

Based on the latest published Annual Health Report 2022 by the National Centre for Health Information, Kuwait (NCHI) [3], the burden of rheumatic diseases in Kuwait, when comparing rheumatology services to services provided by other specialties, is shown in Table 6.1. The Genetic Centre and Islamic Centre are part of governmental hospitals.

Table 6.1 Burden of rheumatic diseases in Kuwait

		Public				Private		
	Number	%*	F:M	Yr	Number	%	F: M	Yr
Outpatient visits: Rheumatology Cases	58,703	0.8%	1.4:1	2022	7651	0.2%	1.6:1	2022
Osteoporosis	40,328	0.5%		2022				
Physical Medicine	78,881	2.0%		2022				
Physiotherapy	196,161	2.7%		2022				
Hospital discharges of all rheumatic cases	144.4/ year		1.2:1	2016–2020	34	<0.1%	0.9:1	2022
Genetic Center visits for all related rheumatic diseases	981/9851	10%	1.2:1	2022				
Islamic Center visits all related rheumatic diseases	140/5223	2.6%	1.9:1	2022				

Abbreviations: % percentage of a sum of all visits for other diseases (total for the public sector is 3,906,173 visits, for the private sector is 3,681,640 visits), *F:M* female-to-male ratio, *Yr* Year

Based on the annual health report 2022 [3], the total number of outpatient visits for the rheumatology specialty in the MOH of Kuwait was 58,703 visits in 2022, representing 1.5% (3,906,173 visits) of all outpatient visits for the same year. Compared to 2020 annual health report statistics, the total number of outpatient visits for the rheumatology specialty in the MOH of Kuwait has almost tripled as it was 18,000 visits approximately, which may reflect not only increased number of qualified rheumatologists but also increased awareness of rheumatic diseases among other medical specialties and probably among the public as well. New patients referred to rheumatology services were 18,936 visits with a female-to-male ratio of 2:1. For a comparison with other specialties, the highest total number of visits was for dermatology (9%), orthopedics (7.8%), physiotherapy (5%) followed by cardiology (4.9%). The total number of outpatient visits for osteoporosis in the MOH of Kuwait was 40,325 in 2022, representing 1.0% of all outpatient visits for the same year.

The total number of outpatient visits for physical medicine rehabilitation in the MOH was 78,881 in 2022, representing 2% of all outpatient visits for the same year.

Based on recent NCHI data [2], the average hospital discharges per year for rheumatoid arthritis (RA) and other inflammatory polyarthropathies between 2016 and 2020 is 144.4 discharges/year. For females, 79 discharges/year, and for males, 66.6 discharges/year, with a female-to-male ratio of 1.2:1.

In 2022, the Medical Genetic Center recorded 9851 visits. Of these, 9 involved pure immunological genetic diseases, 3 connective tissue diseases, 415 skeletal genetic disorders, and 554 muscular or neuromuscular genetic diseases. Altogether, rheumatic and immune disorders accounted for about 10% of all visits [3].

According to the annual health report 2022, out of 5223 visits to the Islamic Medical Center, there were 140 RA visits, compared to 4485 visits for hyperlipidemia and 312 for diabetes.

In the private sector, the total number of outpatient visits for the rheumatology specialty of major hospitals was 7651 visits in 2022, representing 0.2% of all outpatient visits, which are 3,681,640 visits for the same year. The new rheumatology cases in these hospitals were 3950 cases with a female-to-male ratio of 1.6:1. Compared to other specialties in the same sector, the highest total number of visits in these hospitals was emergency room representing 14% of all visits followed by obstetrics and gynecology, representing 12.9% and internal medicine 12.2%. Of note, the private sector also has other health organizations like medical centers, polyclinics, and solo clinics that may cover rheumatology practice and are not included in these statistics.

The total number of outpatient visits for physical medicine rehabilitation in private sector hospitals was 162,223 in 2022, representing 4.4% of all outpatient visits for the same year.

In 2022, the total number of discharges from private sector hospitals for all rheumatology cases was 34 cases, with an almost equal female-to-male ratio.

6.8 Prevalence and Incidence of Rheumatic Diseases

The epidemiological data on rheumatic diseases, in general, are limited. However, some data on the major diseases like MSK pain, rheumatoid arthritis, osteoarthritis (OA), and a few others [4–7] may give a view of rheumatology diseases in Kuwait (Table 6.2).

The WHO-ILAR Community Oriented Program for Control of Rheumatic Diseases (COPCORD) primarily aims to estimate the burden of MSK symptoms/disorders. It was adopted for the first community-based COPCORD study in Kuwait to estimate the incidence of adult MSK pain in 2005 [4]. Out of the 3,341 respondents, 220 reported having recently developed MSK pain, making up a total incidence of 6.6%. Age, body mass index (BMI), and marital status (i.e., being married) increased the incidence rate. The age and sex-adjusted incidence rate for females were 7.2% and 6.1% for males. There were 106 females and 114 males in the complainant group, making a male-to-female ratio of 1.1:1. The average age of the complainers was 36.9 ± 16.1 years; 16.1% significantly higher than non-complainers (30.0 ± 12.7 years). In addition, 64% of the complainers were married, and 35.2% were unemployed. In comparison to non-complainers, complainers' BMI was substantially higher. Knee, low back, shoulder, and leg pain were the most frequently mentioned MSK pain sites in the phone calls.

Only 29 of the 220 people attended clinical assessments, and all of them had rheumatic diseases with a female-to-male ratio of 1.6 (18 females and 11 males). Women were, on average, 47 years old, while men were 43.5 years old. The most prevalent type of soft tissue rheumatism was low back pain (30%), followed by regional myofascial pain syndrome (24%), peri-shoulder arthritis (18%), and fibromyalgia (12%). Nine cases (31%) of OA were found, all in the knees. One patient had osteoid osteoma, while two patients had patellofemoral syndrome.

Table 6.2 Prevalence of different MSK/rheumatic diseases and risk factors of rheumatic diseases [4–7]

Rheumatic disease	Prevalence	F: M	Associated factors	Year
Osteoarthritis	16.1% (Kuwaitis), 6.3% (non-Kuwaitis) 32%.1% (Crude)	2.2:1	Age, female sex	2013 2004
MSK pain	26.9%	1.6:1	Age, female sex, BMI	2004
Regional LBP	37%			2004
Shoulder periarthritis	37% (crude)			2004
Neck Pain	12% (crude)			2004
Rheumatoid arthritis	1.3% (crude)			2004
Gout	0.8% (crude)			2004
Trauma pain	18%			2004
Risk factor				
Smoking	20.5%	1:11.8		2015
Alcohol intake	2.1%	All Males		2015
Overweight	77.2	1:1		2015
Obesity	40.2%	1.2:1		2015
Diabetes mellitus/ impaired glucose tolerance	14.6%	1:1.1		2015

MSK musculoskeletal, *F:M* female-to-male ratio, *BMI* body mass index, *Crude Prevalence* prevalence rate of the selected population

To estimate the prevalence of such disorders, another community-based COPCORD study was conducted in 2004, investigating MSK pain, disability, and health-seeking behavior [5]. A total of 7670 adults were interviewed, and 2057 had MSK pain unrelated to trauma. The most common locations of pain were the shoulders, back, and knees. The majority of the patients described their pain as moderate to severe. In addition, 39.1% of the patients reported functional impairment. With an overall prevalence of MSK pain at 26.8%, the age-sex population-adjusted prevalence rate for females was 35.7%, and that for men was 20.2%.

Compared to the non-sufferers, who had a mean age of 31.1 (±12.8) years, the sufferers' mean age was 42.5 years (±15.9), which was significantly higher. Compared to non-sufferers (25.7 ± 4.8 kg/m^2), sufferers' BMI was significantly higher at 29.0 ± 6.3 kg/m^2. Knee pain (66.3%), back pain (43.8%), shoulder pain (37.8%), and ankle pain (26.3%) had the highest prevalence rates. Hospital physicians (68.8%) and general practitioners (30.4%) were the most frequent sources of treatment advice. Eighty-two percent of patients had prescriptions, while 19.4% self-prescribed their pills.

Of the 2057 respondents who had MSK pain, 238 respondents showed up for appointments and clinical examinations. All but one had rheumatic diseases (82 males and 155 females with a male-to-female ratio of 1:1.9).

Women were, on average, 44.4 years old, while men were 47.5 years old. The most prevalent type of soft tissue rheumatism ($n = 130$) was regional low back pain (37%), followed by peri-arthritis of the shoulder (15%), neck pain (12%), and fibromyalgia (7.7%). With a crude frequency of 32.1%, 76 cases of OA were found; more than half of these patients had OA of the knee, 8 had OA of the spine, one had OA of the hip, and one had generalized OA. Gout frequency was 0.8%, and rheumatoid arthritis prevalence was 1.3%.

In the COPCORD Core questionnaire, 88% (2511/7670) of participants reported MSK pain, of whom 18.1% (454) associated the pain to trauma. Among these trauma survivors, motor vehicle accidents accounted for 20.3%, falls for 28.7%, strain for 13.2%, fractures for 3.4%, and other trauma for 34.4%.

The Arabic version of the COPCORD survey uses a mannequin to indicate the pain sites. The percentage of painful areas marked by the sufferers on the mannequin was highest in the knee (66.1%) and lower back (35.6%). Women reported a significantly higher prevalence of pain at most sites. Factors associated with MSK pain were female sex, advancing age, marriage, non-working status, physical inactivity, and high BMI. Pain in the lower limb was statistically and significantly correlated with BMI.

According to the 2013 World Health Survey in Kuwait, on 28,157 population of all age groups and Kuwaiti citizens, representing 79.4% of the whole surveyed household population [6], the prevalence of OA was 16.1% for Kuwaiti respondents, and 65.1% said to have sought treatment during 2 weeks before the survey's administration. Females were more likely than males to report having OA (20.3% vs. 9.6%), and they were also more likely to report having recently undergone treatment (66.7% vs. 59.7%). The proportion of people reporting the need for therapy increased with age, as predicted, emphasizing how severe OA was. Only 6.3% of non-Kuwaiti respondents claimed they had OA, and 58% said they had received treatment. Once more, females were more likely to experience OA (9.4% vs. 4.5%, respectively) and more likely to seek therapy (60.7% vs. 54.8%). However, the reduced prevalence observed in non-Kuwaitis may be the result of selection bias. Rates of OA are greater in Jahra and Mubarak Al-Kabeer regions when age and gender are considered in the six governorates.

6.9 Mortality Data

Based on the available data from the MOH [2, 3], mortality may differ based on the format used for collecting these data (Table 6.3).

Based on data collected directly from NCHI, through hospital registries in Kuwait, the overall mortality rate of any rheumatological disease was 18.8 deaths/year between 2016 and 2020. The mortality rate for females was 12.8 deaths/year, and for males, 6 deaths/year. The cause-specific death rates (using pre-specified ICD-10 codes: major categories) for diseases of the blood and blood-forming organs and immune disorders were reported in the 2020 annual health report [2] and were

Table 6.3 Mortality rates related to rheumatic diseases according to ICD-10 mortality tabulation, Kuwait, 2022 [2, 3]

	Mortality rate	Source	F:M	Year
Rheumatic disease	18.8 death/year	Hospital registries*	2.1:1	2016–2020
Rheumatology cause-specific	0.6 death/100,000	AHR		2020
MSK and CTD	0.2 death/100,000	AHR	2.5:1	2022
Rheumatic fever and RHD	0.0 death/100,000	AHR		2022
Co-Morbidities: TB Viral hepatitis COVID-19 infection	0.6 death/100,000 0.1 death/100,000 19.4 death/100,000	AHR		2022

F:M Female-to-male ratio, *MSK* Musculoskeletal, *CTD* Connective Tissue Disease, *RHD* Rheumatic heart disease, *AHR* Annual Health Report, *TB* Tuberculosis
* Unpublished data acquired directly from the National Center for Health Information and permitted to be used

as follows: 0.4 deaths/100,000 population, 0.5 deaths/100,000 population for females, and 0.4 deaths/100,000 population for males. The overall mortality rates ranged between 0.3 and 0.5 deaths/100,000 population for the years between 2016 and 2019.

The cause-specific death rate for diseases of musculoskeletal and connective tissue diseases was 0.5 deaths/100,000 population and 0.2 deaths/100,000 population in 2020 and 2022, respectively [3]. The reduction of mortality may reflect the advantageous increase in the number of qualified rheumatologists as well as the treatment options of rheumatic diseases in Kuwait. For females, the mortality rate is 0.45/100,00 population and for males 0.05/100,000 population. The overall mortality rate is 0.3 deaths/100,000 population between 2016 and 2019. The mortality of acute rheumatic fever and chronic rheumatic heart disease is 0.1 deaths/100,000 population. For comparison, the total mortality rate for all causes in 2020 was 219.4 deaths/100,000, out of which 0.6% are related to rheumatic diseases [3].

Mortalities of diseases may be considered as important as co-morbidities to rheumatic diseases, especially autoimmune diseases subject to immunosuppressive therapy. The respiratory TB mortality rate in 2020 was 0.2 deaths/100,000 population, viral hepatitis 0.1 deaths/100,000 population, and COVID-19 19.4 deaths/100,000 population [3].

6.10 Risk Factors of Rheumatic Diseases in Kuwait

The WHO STEP-wise approach to surveillance (STEPS), a second national cross-sectional survey on non-communicable disease (NCD) risk factors, was undertaken and published in 2015 [7] under the umbrella of the Eastern Mediterranean Approach for control of non-communicable diseases (EMAN). Using a straightforward sample technique, 4391 people between 18 and 69 were randomly chosen. In this survey, a number of significant risk factors for rheumatic diseases will be emphasized, including smoking, obesity, alcohol usage, diabetes, and poor physical health habits.

Of a total number of respondents ($n = 3918$), 20.5% reported being current smokers, and 18% said they smoked daily. The mean number of cigarettes smoked (daily) among daily smokers was 18.9 cigarettes/day. Men smoked more than women (39.2% vs. 3.3%). The mean age of starting smoking was 17.1 years for both sexes (16.9 years for men and 21.2 years for women). Manufactured cigarettes are used in 88.5% of cases. The vast majority (97.9%) of respondents were lifetime alcohol abstainers, whereas 0.8% were past 12-month abstainers. Past 30-day drinkers amounted to 0.8% of respondents, and only 0.3% were episodically heavy drinkers, all were men. Three-fifths (62.6%) did not meet WHO recommendations on physical activity for health [with a significant difference between men (51.49%) and women (72.8%)]. The highest percentage of those not meeting WHO recommendations were identified in the 60–69 years age group (78.8%). The total median time spent carrying out physical activity constituted 1.4 min per day [higher among men (17.1 min) than women (0.0 min)].

More than half of respondents reported receiving healthy lifestyle advice from a doctor or a health worker during the past 3 years regarding reducing fat in the diet (51.3%), starting or practicing physical activity (54.6%), and maintaining a healthy body weight or reducing weight (52.4%).

As a result of physical measurements, about 8 in every 10 respondents (77.2%) were overweight or obese (BMI $\geq$ 25 kg/m^2), with no differences between sexes. Two-fifths of respondents (40.2%) were obese (BMI =30 kg/m^2), and the proportion of obese women (44.0%) was 1.2 times higher than that of men (36.3%). The mean BMI recorded was 29.4 kg/m^2, and the mean waist circumference was 88.4 cm for women and 93.6 cm for men. The waist–hip circumference ratio was equal to 0.9 for men and 0.8 for women, at the lower limit of obesity.

Fruit and vegetable consumption was generally low: 83.8% of respondents reported consumption of fewer than five servings of fruit and vegetables per day, thus being at higher risk for NCD. The proportion was higher for women in comparison with men (86.0% vs. 81.4%). Consumption of both fruit and vegetables was less frequent in younger age groups. Households most often used vegetable oil for the preparation of meals (93.0%).

The survey revealed that the proportion of respondents with impaired fasting glycemia (26.1 mmol/L and $<$7.0 mmol/L) was 6.1% and this proportion was higher among men (7.6%) than women (4.7%). Mean fasting blood glucose was 5.7 mmo/L, with no difference between men and women. More than 1 in 10 individuals (14.6%) had diabetes or reduced tolerance to glucose (fasting blood glucose $\geq$7.0 mmol/L or taking antidiabetic medication), and this proportion was higher among men (15.8%) than women (13.4%). It was also established that just more than half (55.9%) had a raised total cholesterol level ($\geq$5 mmol/L or taking medication for hypercholesterolemia), with a significant difference between men and women (58.6% vs. 53.5%). In conclusion, the survey showed that about three-fifths of respondents (57.9%) had three or more risk factors for NCDs, and this increases proportionally with age (51.6% of 18–44 years old and 74.79% for 45–69 years old). Based on these results, the Kuwait population has an increased risk of rheumatic diseases and MSK pain. Only 1.2% of the population studied had none of the five risk factors for NCD.

Based on the 2020 and 2022 annual health report from NCHI [2, 3], the number of reported cases of hepatitis B virus (HBV) and hepatitis C virus (HCV) in 2016 was 420 and 433, respectively. However, these rates fell dramatically to 103 and 87 in 2022, likely due to more restrictions in the policies of work permits and residency health rules for expatriates, and because of the routine compulsory HBV vaccine for newborns since 1996 and the availability of the vaccine for all adults in Kuwait. In addition, the introduction of cure treatment of HCV infection, free of charge for all citizens, may also have significantly reduced newly reported HCV cases.

6.11 Screening Programs for Rheumatic Diseases

There are no current official active screening programs for rheumatic diseases in Kuwait. However, KAR is one of the most active rheumatology associations under the Kuwait Medical Association (KMA) umbrella. Activities target both the public and other health professionals related to rheumatic diseases. Targeting the public by having different types of gatherings allow people to communicate directly with healthcare professionals, including rheumatologists, outside the health organizations, like in parks and major shopping malls, where they provide educational brochures, lectures, screening MSK ultrasound, and allow direct communications with patient support groups like the RA group and SLE group. In addition, KAR celebrates World Arthritis Day annually, which is usually held in October.

During scientific awareness activities, general practitioners, family physicians, orthopedics, internists, and other subspecialties are invited to participate.

KAR is also very approachable to the public by having active social media programs connecting the public with rheumatologists and patient groups.

Under the same umbrella of KAR, or directly under the umbrella of internal medicine departments in the public and private sectors, different rheumatology units in the six health regions may also have much wider awareness coverage through frequent activities all over year targeting both the public and other health professionals.

Despite these efforts, there is still a need for more official national screening programs. For instance, in a local sub-analysis of a global axial spondyloarthritis (SpA) observational study of 32 patients in Kuwait, the median time for making the final diagnosis was 6.4 years, where most of the delay came from the primary health care sector [8]. This may not give an accurate estimate of the diagnosis delay, given the small number of patients in this analysis, but it at least provides a rough idea of that burden.

There is an ongoing effort to reduce the time to see rheumatologists by opening a new case rheumatology clinic in almost all rheumatology divisions in Kuwait, where patients have relatively quick access to rheumatology services, where they can be screened for rheumatic diseases.

6.12 Diagnostic Tests for Rheumatic Diseases

All routine and autoimmune laboratory tests are widely available in public and private health sectors, with a relatively acceptable time for results and tracking. All also have access to genetic testing, like HLA subtypes. In addition, genetic tests like Mediterranean Fever mutation and all other mutations for autoinflammatory diseases are also available. Still, they may take longer to get the results back as they may be sent abroad through official health channels.

MSK ultrasound is available and accessible to all rheumatology divisions, where it has become a basic clinic service. In addition, all seven rheumatology divisions in their health regions have local access to advanced imaging facilities and modalities like computed tomography (CT) scans, CT angiography, magnetic resonance imaging, and magnetic resonance angiography. The positron emission tomography (PET) scan is available in all seven general hospitals and is an essential tool for helping the diagnosis of vasculitis; however, nuclear studies and PET scans are not yet available in the private sector. Unfortunately, in the public sector, a relatively small number of MSK radiologists practice in some public health regions.

6.13 Management of Rheumatic Diseases in Kuwait

In public health sectors, all seven general hospitals have standard tertiary care, including seven rheumatology divisions. All these seven units provide immunomodulatory treatment, including conventional, targeted, and biologic DMARDs. The infusion day case units are also available in almost all hospitals. Unfortunately, biologic agents and targeted synthetic DMARDs are only available free of charge for Kuwaiti citizens, Gulf Cooperation Council (GCC) residents, and those working in the MOH. In the private sector, these options are still limited. For those who cannot afford biological treatment, the Patient Help Fund Society and Nama'a Charity Society provide huge support. Both societies cover at least 80% and up to 100% of the cost, regardless of the patient's financial status. These societies provide most of the biologics and targeted synthetic DMARDs (tsDMARDs).

In the private sector, rheumatologists work individually, and treatment options are somewhat limited compared to the public services; however, because all are working part-time in the private sector and have access to public hospitals when needed, patients will be referred in a timely fashion to the necessary treatment facility. Furthermore, almost all therapeutic options are available in the oil companies' hospitals, like public hospitals.

Regarding accessibility to rheumatic drugs, most anti-rheumatic drugs are available in Kuwait. A non-formulary medication that is required for a patient can be ordered only in the MOH hospitals on a case-by-case basis. The following DMARDs are registered in Kuwait:

- csDMARDs: methotrexate, sulfasalazine, cyclosporin, hydroxychloroquine, azathioprine, mycophenolate mofetil, mycophenolate sodium.
- tsDMARDs/small molecules: JAK inhibitors (tofacitinib, baricitinib, upadacitinib), apremilast.
- Biological originator DMARDs:
  - Tumor necrosis factor inhibitors: adalimumab (humira), etanercept (enbrel), golimumab, certolizumab, infliximab (intravenous remicade)
  - IL-1 inhibitor: anakinra
  - IL-12/23 inhibitor: ustekinumab
  - IL-6 inhibitor: tocilizumab (intravenous, subcutaneous)
  - CTLA4-Ig inhibitor: abatacept (intravenous, subcutaneous)
  - IL-17 inhibitors: secukinumab, ixekizumab, bimekizumab
  - IL-23 inhibitors: guselkumab, risankizumab
  - Other biologic DMARDs: rituximab (MabThera), belimumab (intravenous, subcutaneous), canakinumab, denosumab, romosozumab, anifrolumab
- Biosimilars: infliximab biosimilar (intravenous remsima), adalimumab biosimilar (amgevita, hyrimoz)
- Others: cyclophosphamide, intravenous immunoglobulin, teriparatide, bisphosphonates

6.14 Accessibility to Multidisciplinary Specialties

Over the past few years, there has been a significant improvement in the services available for patients with rheumatic diseases, marked by the establishment of numerous multidisciplinary team clinics within government hospitals. These include high-risk pregnancy clinics combining rheumatology and obstetric medicine (currently three clinics), rheumatology-dermatology clinics (four), rheumatology-nephrology clinics (two), and rheumatology-respiratory clinics (three).

All rheumatology units have direct access to physical medicine, physiotherapy, and occupational therapy, available in all seven general hospitals. These services are also widely available in the private sector.

Surgery services, including orthopedic surgery, are available in almost all the hospitals and are easily accessible by rheumatology units, except the Kuwait Orthopedic Hospital (Al-Razi Hospital), in which all the orthopedic subspecialty units and services are easily accessible throughout the public health system. In the private sector, orthopedic surgeons outnumber rheumatologists and are easily accessible.

6.15 Research and Education

Kuwait Institute for Medical Specialization (KIMS) is responsible for post-graduate training and programs. In 2005, a rheumatology program was established, and two candidates graduated in 2008. Unfortunately, the program was not sustained due to a lack of funding. However, it is now set to restart, with the program opening again in October 2026.

In recent years, the pathway to becoming a rheumatologist typically involves completing an internal medicine residency followed by a rheumatology fellowship abroad, usually lasting 2 to 3 years in countries, such as Canada, the United States, the UK, or KSA. This approach helps meet the increasing demand for such specialties once they graduate and return to Kuwait.

In Kuwait, currently, there are four active registries under the umbrella of KAR: Adult RA, SLE, and SpA registries, in addition to the Pediatric JIA Registry. The RA registry has been established and has been running since 2013, contributing to more than 22 published local studies and numerous conference posters. A more recent SLE registry was established in 2018, followed by the SpA registry in 2021, and the pediatric JIA registry in 2024.

Rheumatologists from Kuwait have been involved in many national/international clinical trials. These studies were published in prestigious, international, peer peer-reviewed, and indexed journals. Publications included basic/clinical [9–13], epidemiological [4, 5, 14], registry [15–17], and recommendation studies [18–22].

Unfortunately, the availability of formal rheumatology nursing programs in Kuwait is lacking.

This is because we do not have a college of nursing at Kuwait University that can graduate nurses of a highly specialized caliber.

6.16 Cost-Effective Rheumatic Diseases Care

There are no studies in Kuwait assessing the cost-effectiveness of expensive medications, such as biologics. Such studies are timely and highly recommended. From our personnel observations, immunomodulators reduced the expenses of inpatient admissions and care. MOH continues putting pressure on rheumatologists to reduce the costs of these expensive medications, especially since many new medications are being introduced in the field of rheumatology. Luckily, rheumatic medications are free of charge to Kuwaiti nationals. Furthermore, the MOH's vision is to introduce more biosimilars if their costs are 40–50% less than the original biologics.

This initiative has been planned formally through the Medical Council to reduce prescriptions of the originator biologics by 20–30%.

6.17 Opportunities and Specific Challenges to Rheumatic Care

Currently, the total number of adult rheumatologists in Kuwait is 31, in addition to 8 pediatric certified rheumatologists, keeping in mind that the entire population is 4.8 million. Therefore, there is a need for more rheumatologists. In addition, we lack specialized rheumatology nurses, research assistants, and basic immunologists.

Although few rheumatologists underwent rheumatology sub-specialty fellowships, such as SLE, psoriatic arthritis, axial SpA, vasculitis, and RA in accredited programs abroad, no official subspecialty clinics have structured care programs and incorporate patient-reported outcomes. This is most likely due to the low number of rheumatologists in our country and the high number of patients visiting our clinics.

The government of Kuwait, presented by MOH, is paying for the care and treatment, including immunomodulator and biological drugs, for Kuwaiti nationals. Expatriates are required to pay approximately 50 KD in insurance to the government for basic care. Costly drugs are arranged via private insurance or patient charities.

Due to the availability of qualified rheumatologists, medical tourism for rheumatic diseases to foreign countries has diminished tremendously. Few patients travel mostly for rehabilitation purposes.

Our suggestions for improving rheumatic disease care over the next decade in our country are as follows:

- Expand the number of combined specialized clinics, such as high-risk pregnancy (rheumatology and obstetrics), nephritis for lupus or vasculitis (rheumatology and nephrology), and psoriatic arthritis (rheumatology and dermatology).
- Establishing subspecialty rheumatic disease clinics.
- Implementation of electronic medical records across all hospitals.
- Improving primary care clinics and providing more authority to family physicians in refilling rheumatic medications. This will minimize the patient's load in rheumatology clinics.
- Establishing a team approach to care for patients with rheumatic disease. This team comprises rheumatologists, physiotherapists, occupational therapists, social therapists, psychiatrists, immunologists, and orthopedic surgeons.
- Collaboration with basic scientists and immunologists in meetings and conducting research studies combining clinical with basic science.
- Collaboration with international centers for conducting studies on rheumatic diseases.

6.18 Conclusion

In Kuwait, rheumatic diseases are common, and the rheumatologist community has rapidly grown over the last 15 years. Yet, more is needed to match the service demands and to establish more subspecialized and combined clinic care. The rheumatology community in Kuwait is very active in education and research, with four active national registries, besides tens of activities every year covering scientific and public awareness activities, whether under KAR's umbrella or local health organizations.

In this chapter, we have revealed the heavy burden of rheumatic diseases on the health system, besides the considerable common risk factors. This has created multiple areas of improvement, as heightened above, to optimize rheumatology care, especially in diagnosis delay and combined care.

Conflict of Interest The authors have no conflicts of interest to declare.

References

1. Public Authority for Civil Service. Kuwait Civil Service Bureau [Internet]. [cited 2026 Jun 14]. Available from: https://www.csb.gov.kw/.
2. National Centre for Health Information (NCHI), Ministry of Health, Kuwait. Annual health report 2020 [Internet]. 57th ed. Kuwait: Ministry of Health; 2020. [cited 2026 Jun 14]. Available from: https://www.moh.gov.kw/en/NCHI/Policies/2011-2020/2020.pdf.
3. National Centre for Health Information (NCHI), Ministry of Health, Kuwait. Annual health report 2022 [Internet]. 50th ed. Kuwait: Ministry of Health; 2022. [cited 2026 Jun 14]. Available from: https://www.moh.gov.kw/en/NCHI/Policies/2022.pdf.
4. Al-Awadhi A, Olusi S, Al-Saeid K, Moussa M, Shehab D, Al-Zaid N, Al-Herz A, Al-Jarallah K. Incidence of musculoskeletal pain in adult Kuwaitis using the validated Arabic version of the WHO-ILAR COPCORD Core Questionnaire. Ann Saudi Med. 2005;25(6):459–62.
5. Al-Awadhi A, Olusi S, Moussa M, Shehab D, Al-Zaid N, Al-Herz A, Al-Jarallah K. Musculoskeletal pain, disability and health-seeking behaviour in adult Kuwaitis using a validated Arabic version of the WHO-ILAR COPCORD Core Questionnaire. Clin Exp Rheumatol. 2004;22:177–83.
6. World health survey in Kuwait, State of Kuwait, Ministry of Health. Main Report 2013.
7. Eastern Mediterranean approach for control of non-communicable diseases. Survey of risk factors for chronic non-communicable diseases. State of Kuwait 2015.
8. Al-Enizi A, Dalle H. Interim results from PROOF- a 5-year observational study of long-term disease outcome in axial spondyloarthritis Sub-analysis from Kuwait. ARLAR 2017, Abstract Code ABS180.
9. Al-Awadhi A, Haider MZ, Sharma PN, Hasan EA, Botaiban F, Al-Herz A, Nahar I, Al-Enezi H, Al-Saeid K. Angiotensin-converting enzyme gene polymorphism in Kuwaiti patients with systemic lupus erythematosus. Clin Exp Rheumatol. 2007;25:437–42.
10. Al-Awadhi A, Hasan EA, Sharma PN, Haider MZ, Al-Saeid K. Angiotensin-converting enzyme gene polymorphism in patients with psoriatic arthritis. Rheumatol Int. 2007;27:1119–23.
11. Al-Awadhi A, Olusi S, Hasan EA, Abdullah A. Frequency of abnormal thyroid function tests in Kuwaiti Arabs with autoimmune diseases. Med Princ Pract. 2008;17:61–5.

12. Shehab D, Al-Jarallah K, Al-Awadhi A, Al-Herz A, Nahar I, Haider M. Association of angiotensin-converting enzyme (ACE) gene insertion-deletion polymorphism with spondylarthropathies. J Biomed Sci. 2008;15:61–7.
13. Shehab D, Al-Jarallah K, Al-Awadhi A, Al-Herz A, Nahar I, Haider M. Prevalence of angiotensin-converting enzyme (ACE) gene insertion-deletion polymorphism in patients with primary knee osteoarthritis. Clin Exp Rheumatol. 2008;26:305–10.
14. Al-Awadhi A, Olusi S, Moussa M, Al-Zaid N, Shehab D, Al-Herz A, Al-Jarallah K, Al-Salem IH, Pedro A. Validation of the Arabic version of the WHO-ILAR COPCORD Core Questionnaire for community screening of rheumatic diseases in Kuwaitis. J Rheumatol. 2002;29:1754–9.
15. Al-Herz A, Alawadhi A, Saleh K, Al-Kandari W, Hasan E, Ghanem A, Abutiban F, Alenizi A, Hussain M, Ali Y, Khadrawy A, Fazal A, Mokaddem K, Aftab B, Haider N, Zaman A, Mazloum G, Bartella Y, Hamed S, Al-Saber A. Comparison of rheumatoid arthritis patients in Kuwait with other populations: results from the KRRD registry. Br J Med & Med Res. 2016;14(9):1–11.
16. Al-Herz A, Alawadhi A, Saleh K, Al-Kandari W, Hasan E, Ghanem A, Abutiban F, Alenizi A, Hussain M, Ali Y, Khadrawy A, Fazal A, Mokaddem K, Aftab B, Haider N, Zaman A, Mazloum G, Bartella Y, Hamed S, Al-Saber A. Prevalence of nodules in rheumatoid arthritis patients in Kuwait: a description and comparison of patients from the Kuwait Registry for rheumatic diseases. Med Princ Pract. 2017;26:152–6.
17. Alsaber A, Pan J, Al-Herz A, Alkandary D, Al-Hurban A, Setiya P. Influence of ambient air pollution on rheumatoid arthritis disease activity score index. Int J Environ Res Public Health. 2020; https://doi.org/10.3390/ijerph17020416.
18. Haraoui B, Smolen JS, Aletaha D, Breedveld FC, Burmester G, Codreanu C, Da Silva JP, de Wit M, Dougados M, Durez P, Emery P, Fonseca JE, Gibofsky A, Gomez-Reino J, Graninger W, Hamuryudan V, Jannaut Peña MJ, Kalden J, Kvien TK, Laurindo I, Martin-Mola E, Montecucco C, Santos Moreno P, Pavelka K, Poor G, Cardiel MH, Stanislawska-Biernat E, Takeuchi T, van der Heijde D, Al Awadhi A, AlShehhi WY, Babic-Naglic D, Michel BA, Galarza C, Hammoudeh M, Harrison M, Kolarov Z, Lee SK, Nash P, Otsa K, Sokka T, Tate GA, Tomsic M, Uthman I, Venalis A, Villegas de Morales S. Treating Rheumatoid Arthritis to Target: multinational recommendations assessment questionnaire. Ann Rheum Dis. 2011;70(11):1999–2002.
19. El Zorkany B, Al Wahshi H, Hammoudeh M, Al Emadi S, Benitha R, Al-Awadhi A, Bouajina E, Laatar A, El Badawy S, Al Badi M, Al-Maini M, Al Saleh J, Alswailem R, Moosa M, Mahomed Ally T, Batha W, Djoudi H, El Garf A, El Hadidi K, El Marzouqi M, Hadidi M, Maharaj A, Masri A, Mofti A, Nahar I, Pettipher C, Spargo C, Emery P. Suboptimal management of rheumatoid arthritis in the Middle East and Africa: could the EULAR recommendations be the start of a solution? Clin Rheumatol. 2013;32:151–9.
20. Al-Enizi A, AlSaeid K, Alawadhi A, Hasan E, Husain EH, AlFadhli A, Ghanem A, Abutiban F, Ali Y, Al-Herz A, Saleh K, Alkandari W, Aldei A, Alhajeri H, Dehrab A, Hayat S. Kuwait recommendations on vaccine use in people with inflammatory rheumatic diseases. Int J Rheumatol. 2018;2018:5217461.
21. Alhajeri H, Abutiban, Al-Adsani W, Al-Awadhi A, Aldei A, AlEnizi A, Alhadhood N, Al-Herz A, Alkandari W, Dehrab A, Ghanem A, Hasan E, Hayat S, Saleh K, Tarakmeh H, Ali Y. Kuwait Association of Rheumatology 2018 treatment recommendations for patients with rheumatoid arthritis. Rheumatology Int. 2019;39:1483–97.
22. Baron F, Alhajeri H, Abutaiban F, Al-Murtairi M, Ali Y, Alawadhi A. Rheumatologic aspects of the COVID-19 pandemic: a practical resource for physicians in Kuwait and the Gulf region based on recommendations by the Kuwait Association of Rheumatology (KAR). Curr Rheumatol Rev. 2021;18:108–16.

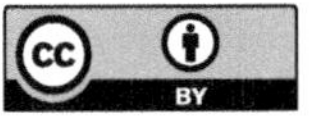

Chapter 7
Rheumatic Diseases in Lebanon

Georges El Hasbani, Kamel Mroue, and Imad Uthman

Abstract Lebanon is one of the Arab countries historically known for its multiple regional referral hospital centers. With several principal investigators leading international randomized clinical trials, several Lebanese researchers have been devoted to advancing the quality of practice in the Arab world, ultimately improving patients' quality of life. Rheumatology is not a stranger to these descriptions. Since the 1950s, the number of rheumatology providers has been substantially increasing. The Lebanese Society of Rheumatology was established in 1961 to attract ideas and organize collaborations. The prevalence of rare autoimmune/autoinflammatory diseases, such as Behcet's disease and familial Mediterranean fever, partly shapes Lebanon's research and clinical practice. Despite having no dedicated basic science autoimmune facilities, many groups work on the genetic and immunological aspects of systemic autoimmune rheumatic diseases. From a clinical research perspective, Lebanese rheumatologists collaborate on regional and international projects.

Regarding clinical practice, the availability of serological and imaging facilities is an asset for rheumatologists. One of the significant challenges is the cost of novel antirheumatic therapies, such as biological agents. While national and private services try to aid dependent patients, the burden is still significant. Future challenges lie in attracting more expertise, making research funding available to investigators, and establishing dedicated centers of excellence, which frequently incorporate patient-reported outcomes.

Keywords Rheumatology practice · Lebanon · History · Diagnostics · Research · Challenges

---

G. El Hasbani
Division of Rheumatology, Department of Medicine, Mayo Clinic, Rochester, MN, USA
e-mail: elhasbani.georges@mayo.edu

K. Mroue
Department of Internal Medicine, Al Zahra University Medical Center, Beirut, Lebanon
e-mail: khmroue@gmail.com

I. Uthman (✉)
Department of Internal Medicine, American University of Beirut Medical Center, Beirut, Lebanon
e-mail: iuthman@aub.edu.lb

K. A. Alnaqbi, G. Aldabie (eds.), *Rheumatic Diseases in the Arab World*,
https://doi.org/10.1007/978-981-92-0967-5_7

7.1 Country Demographics

Lebanon is a Middle Eastern country located along the eastern border of the Mediterranean basin. Despite its West Asian location, it is centralized at the intersection of the three continents of the ancient world. Physiographically, Lebanon is divided into four distinct regions: the coastal plain, the Lebanon Mountain Range, the Beqaa Valley, and the Anti-Lebanon Mountains [1]. Geographically, Lebanon is divided into nine governorates, further subdivided into 25 districts. These districts constitute several municipalities, each enclosing a group of villages or cities. Lebanon's capital is Beirut, the largest city in the country. Other major cities include Tripoli, Jounieh, Zahle, Saida, Tyre, Byblos, and Baalbak.

According to the 2025 United Nations Population Fund, Lebanon's population is estimated at 5.9 million. Approximately 26% of the population is aged 0–14 years, 64% are between 15 and 64 years, and 10% are aged 65 years and above. The life expectancy at birth is 76 years for males and 80 years for females [2]. The estimated male-to-female ratio at birth is around 1.05, and the median age is approximately 36.3 years [3].

7.2 Country Healthcare Sectors

Lebanon has more than 950 infirmaries and primary healthcare centers. There are around 110 private hospitals and 29 public hospitals in Lebanon. All these hospitals are accredited by the Lebanese Ministry of Public Health (MoPH). Besides, many of these hospitals, especially private ones, participate in internationally renowned accreditation systems [4]. Indeed, the Lebanese healthcare system is primarily constituted by the private sector. Lebanese citizens without private medical insurance rely upon the MoPH and the National Social Security Fund (NSSF) to reimburse a portion of their medical bills. Although there is a need to enhance the healthcare administration, monitor the workflow at the hospitals and primary healthcare centers, and encourage the appropriate use of grievance systems [4], patient satisfaction with primary healthcare services is remarkably high [5].

7.3 Rheumatology Health Services

Although the exact number of adult rheumatologists in Lebanon is unknown, there is a limited number of rheumatologists for the diagnosis of many patients suffering from rheumatic conditions [6]. Most of the adult rheumatologists in Lebanon encounter a variety of rheumatological disorders, and despite that, some have specialized in a specific domain, such as vasculitis or spondyloarthritis (SpA). According to a latest update on the rheumatology workforce in the Arab world, there are currently 51 rheumatologists in Lebanon, 18 (35.3%) of whom are females [7].

Additionally, many rheumatologists encounter both adult and pediatric cases. There are a few pediatric rheumatologists who also currently practice general pediatrics. Some rheumatologists are members of major international organizations such as the Royal College of Physicians or the American College of Rheumatology. The major private hospitals have dedicated rheumatology services. These services or divisions have multiple rheumatologists along with nurses. The nurses working in the rheumatology services have experience with multispecialty clinics.

Because of the availability of electronic medical records, providers can send referrals to each other along with a detailed sign-out on cases. Notably, there is no accredited center of excellence for rheumatology or autoimmunity in Lebanon yet.

7.4 Lebanese Society of Rheumatology

The Lebanese rheumatologists also collaborate via the Lebanese Society of Rheumatology (LSR), founded in 1961. As part of the Lebanese Order of Physicians and a member of the Arab League of Associations for Rheumatology (ArLAR) and the European Alliance of Associations for Rheumatology (EULAR), the LSR is dedicated to organizing scientific meetings throughout the year. Currently, the LSR comprises 53 rheumatologists. Four of the seven board members of LSR are females [8].

The significant milestones in rheumatology practice in Lebanon were established in the 1950s and 1960s (Fig. 7.1) [9].

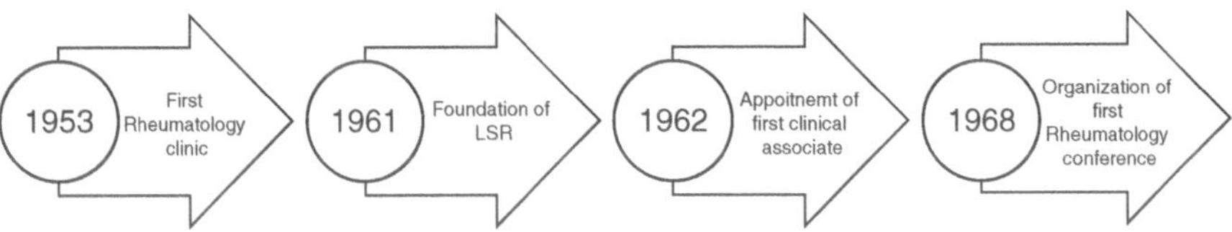

Fig. 7.1 Major Milestones in the Establishment of Rheumatology Services in Lebanon

7.5 Overview of Rheumatic Diseases in Lebanon

Lebanon has a rapid demographic transition, with 7.4% of the population aged 65 years or older [10]. Certain rheumatic diseases have been assessed throughout the years in Lebanon. For example, the incidence of SpA was 8.6%, and that of rheumatoid arthritis (RA) was 5.5% in 1995, being assessed among a specific patient population [11]. With time, more data have been elaborated on the incidence and prevalence of rheumatic diseases in Lebanon. Lebanon's first population-based estimate of rheumatic diseases was published in 2012 [12]. Mechanical rheumatic diseases constituted most of the rheumatic diseases, namely soft-tissue rheumatism and osteoarthritis. On the other hand, RA and SpA formed the most common inflammatory disorders. The prevalence of rheumatic diseases in the general population was 14.3%, with 1% for RA and 0.3% for SpA. Interestingly, the prevalence of rheumatic diseases was higher in women than in men and was concentrated away from the coastal regions [12]. Among patients with rheumatic diseases, the most frequent comorbidities are cardiovascular risk factors and conditions, osteoporosis, and depression [13].

7.6 Risk Factors of Rheumatic Diseases

Cigarette smoking has been related to an increased risk of the development of autoimmunity [14]. In Lebanon, cigarette and waterpipe (shisha) smoking have been significantly high [15]. Smoking is closely related to stroke [16] and coronary artery disease [17]. Likewise, smoking is associated with autoimmunity. For example, oxidative stress, inflammation, autoantibody formation, and epigenetic changes in RA patients have been affected by smoking [18]. As a result, adequate sleep hygiene and smoking reduction/cessation among Lebanese patients had positive effects in terms of disease progression and related outcomes [19].

Obesity has an increased risk of RA, multiple sclerosis, psoriasis, and psoriatic arthritis (PsA) [20]. The Eastern Mediterranean region, including Lebanon, has high obesity rates, exceeding at times those reported from obesity rates and those reported in developed countries such as the USA and Europe [21]. Notably, there has been a significant increase in the prevalence of obesity among Lebanese youth [22]. Despite the proposed theoretical association between obesity and autoimmunity, no study has assessed that relationship in Lebanon specifically.

Consanguinity is a known risk factor for autoinflammation, autoimmunity, and immunodeficiency [23]. For example, consanguinity significantly increases the risk of Hashimoto's thyroiditis [24]. In Lebanon, children born to consanguineous couples are at risk of chronic diseases, intellectual disability, thalassemia, and psychological problems [25]. There has been no reported association with any autoimmune rheumatic diseases in Lebanon.

7.7 Screening Programs for Rheumatic Diseases

Unlike the osteoporosis screening program in Lebanon [26], there is no active screening program for rheumatic diseases. Patients undergo screenings per protocol when in time to initiate specific immunosuppressive regimens. In addition, certain autoantibodies are ordered based on the patient's symptomatology.

7.8 Laboratory Tests for Rheumatic Diseases

Several laboratories have advanced techniques in immunology and serology. Therefore, ordering autoantibody profiles is not a limiting step. HLA-B27 has been linked with a severe axial SpA [27]. It is commonly detected by a flow cytometry assay. However, a sequence-based genetic testing enables the distinction of allelic variants [28]. Both flow cytometry and sequence-based genetic testing are present in Lebanon. Among SpA patients in Lebanon, the prevalence of HLA-B27 ranges from 26% to 41.1% (Table 7.1) [29–32].

Like HLA-B27, HLA-B51 is another important genetic factor that might predispose to certain autoinflammatory diseases, specifically Behcet's disease (BD). To date, there has been no comprehensive study to assess the exact prevalence of BD among the Lebanese population. However, the prevalence among the Lebanese population located in Germany was 101.3/per 100,000 [33]. Furthermore, there have been a few studies describing BD characteristics among Lebanese cohorts. For example, half of the patients in one cohort had an ocular disease [34]. Among 48 Lebanese patients diagnosed with BD, 36.4% were HLA-B51 positive [35].

Pathogenic variations in the Mediterranean fever (MEFV) gene are responsible for FMF, a common disease in Lebanon [36]. More than 370 MEFV gene sequence variants have been reported in the literature [37]. MEFV molecular analysis among a Lebanese population with FMF showed that 63.79% were heterozygotes for an MEFV mutation, 9.20% were homozygotes, and 27.01% carried two variants or more [36]. M694I was the most common variant among homozygotes, E148Q was the most common variant among heterozygotes, and E148Q/M694V was the most frequent in the compound heterozygous/complex genotype group [36]. Multiple laboratories in Lebanon have the core facilities to detect MEFV variants.

Table 7.1 HLA-B27 prevalence among spondyloarthritis patients (axial and peripheral) and the general population in Lebanon

Study	Normal population, HLA-B27 (%)	SpA
Awada et al. [29]	$N = 139$, 1.4%	$N = 65$, 13.8%
Serre et al. [30]	$N = 315$, 1.7%	NA
Abdelnoor et al. [31]	$N = 461$, 2%	NA
Ziade et al. [32]	NA	$N = 141$, 41.1%

Abbreviations: N, number; NA, not available; SpA, spondyloarthritis

Additionally, certain genetics basic science laboratories have published on the different variants of MEFV in Lebanon.

7.9 Imaging Tests for Rheumatic Diseases

Many rheumatological conditions require imaging modalities, such as computed tomography (CT), magnetic resonance imaging (MRI), and positron emission tomography (PET) for diagnosis and disease activity monitoring. For example, simple radiographs and MRI can be used to monitor structural joint damage in RA [38]. Ultrasound can assess superficial joints, such as the metacarpophalangeal, proximal interphalangeal, and distal interphalangeal joints of the hands for joint effusion, synovial proliferation, and synovitis [39]. There are multiple Lebanese facilities that possess different musculoskeletal (MSK) radiological modalities. Some of these facilities are independent of an academic institution. The exact number of these facilities has not been evaluated yet. In addition, certain radiologists have undergone formal training in MSK radiology, making it easier for rheumatologists to streamline the process of diagnosis and follow-up.

7.10 Management

Disease-modifying antirheumatic drugs (DMARDs) are the basis for treating rheumatological conditions. Conventional or classical synthetic DMARDs (csDMARDs), including methotrexate and hydroxychloroquine, are based on targeting the inflammatory and infectious pathologies of autoimmune diseases [40]. In Lebanon, the available csDMARDs include chloroquine, hydroxychloroquine, sulfasalazine, methotrexate, and leflunomide. With further understanding of the pathophysiology of several autoimmune rheumatic diseases, biologic DMARDs (bDMARDs) were introduced [41]. These bDMARDs target specific cytokines, such as tumor necrosis factor-α (TNF) or minor cellular antigens. Infliximab, a TNF inhibitor, has been used in Lebanon for multiple autoimmune diseases with minimal severe adverse events [42]. Rituximab, an anti-CD20 agent, has been used for autoimmune, neurological, and oncological diseases [43–45]. Patients in Lebanon have access to analgesics, steroids, csDMARDs, or bDMARDs. The National Social Security Fund (NSSF) tends to cover a portion of the price of these agents for patients. Besides, pharmaceutical companies sometimes can willingly cover a part of the price of these expensive agents. Otherwise, private insurers have certain processes for financial coverage. In addition to pharmacotherapy, patients with autoimmune rheumatic diseases may need multi-disciplinary specialties such as physiotherapy and occupational therapy. For that, numerous centers exist in Lebanon, whether belonging to academic institutions or privately owned.

Furthermore, surgical treatment of some forms of chronic arthritis is feasible in the presence of several orthopedic surgery referral centers.

7.11 Research and Education

There are a total of three rheumatology training programs in Lebanon. Major universities in the country, namely the American University of Beirut, Balamand University, and the University of Saint Joseph, drive these programs and are primarily based on referral hospitals where complex cases are encountered. Each fellowship program tends to graduate one or two rheumatologists annually. Besides, rheumatology divisions or departments offer rotations for medical students and residents. This opportunity provides experience in outpatient clinics and inpatient consults. Nevertheless, rheumatology fellows often have to interact with medical and nursing students by delivering presentations on the basics of musculoskeletal and autoimmune rheumatic diseases. However, there is no formal rheumatology nursing program.

As rheumatology is a research-driven field, rheumatologists tend to engage in research projects [46]. Lebanon plays a major part in regional research on rheumatology topics. For example, studies on the disease activity of RA and PsA among Middle Eastern patients were led by Lebanese rheumatologists and researchers with a significant contribution of Lebanese study subjects [47, 48]. Nevertheless, many Lebanese rheumatologists are part of prestigious international committees and groups. For example, several Lebanese researchers authored the 2021 American College of Rheumatology guideline for treating RA [49].

Additionally, a major university hospital in Lebanon, and the only one in the Arab world, is a part of the international network to launch clinical antiphospholipid syndrome studies worldwide—APS ACTION—with recent participation in the position statement and management guidance on COVID-19 and antiphospholipid antibodies [50]. For basic science research, no dedicated facility or laboratory is purely focused on autoimmune rheumatic diseases. Still, immunological and basic genetic science research can sometimes involve autoimmunity. For example, some Lebanese research groups assessed genome sequencing and oxidative stress profile among FMF patients [51, 52]. Other groups assessed BD patients' neutrophil extracellular traps and TNF polymorphisms [35, 53].

7.12 Cost-Effective Rheumatic Diseases Care

While traditional DMARDs are affordable medications in Lebanon, biologics are quite expensive, especially for uninsured or NSSF-dependent patients. Therefore, cost considerations influence the use of biological guidelines. In addition, the choice of the biologic agent is affected by the availability of facilities or resources. Adequate objective economic long-term evaluations with prospective efficacy plans are still lacking. Nevertheless, one of the major challenges is identifying patients who will respond to a single or a combination of classical DMARDs instead of initiating a biological agent. The Lebanese government, through the Ministry of Health, tries to work closely with pharmaceutical companies to cover a portion of certain expensive medications.

7.13 Opportunities and Specific Challenges

Lebanon is unique in terms of the high prevalence of certain rare autoinflammatory/autoimmune diseases such as FMF and BD. The availability of human and facility resources is also valuable. Many of the rheumatologists in Lebanon have specialized in prestigious fellowship programs in the United States, Canada, France, United Kingdom, and Belgium. Interestingly, some providers have sub-specialized and worked under the supervision of experts in lupus and SpA. These providers still currently pursue research in their areas of interest.

The rheumatology clinics in Lebanon are mostly part of subspecialty clinics that incorporate patient-reported outcomes to improve overall survival [54]. Besides, rheumatology clinics in Lebanon are in direct contact with NSSF offices and pharmaceutical companies' representatives who frequently financially help patients in need. In addition, rheumatology clinics have been a target for many patients presenting from regional countries, such as Syria, Jordan, and Iraq, for consultations.

7.14 The Future of Rheumatic Disease Care

In the expanding field of rheumatic diseases, the Lebanese healthcare sector and the pharmaceutical market aim to import the latest U.S. Food and Drug Administration (FDA)-approved medications. It is a real challenge for the whole healthcare sector to monitor the indications of the use of such medications. However, the presence of substantial expertise gives relief for staying up-to-date with pharmacological advancements. Expanding and broadening the rheumatology expertise is another challenge. Current rheumatologists practicing abroad might find it challenging to return to Lebanon to practice in a diverse healthcare model setting. Therefore, rheumatologists living in the country should provide reassurance to their colleagues. Although rheumatology is a fascinating diagnostic specialty, medical students might frequently find it puzzling. Rheumatologists must simplify the basics of rheumatic diseases whenever approaching millennials. Similarly, rheumatologists should try different approaches that encourage residents to pursue rheumatology as a specialty by engaging them in patient care and research. As funding of investigator-initiated randomized clinical trials in Lebanon is a significant problem, rheumatologists should try working with pharmaceutical companies to recruit Lebanese centers in international trials.

7.15 Conclusion

Lebanon, a Middle Eastern Mediterranean country, has a healthcare system that is primarily constituted by the private sector. Major university hospitals are considered regional referral centers for various specialties, including rheumatology. Rheumatology practice started back in the 1950s. With the growing number of practicing rheumatologists, an official society for rheumatology was established, which currently organizes frequent educational events and annual conferences attended by internationally renowned speakers. Lebanon is unique in terms of rare autoimmune/autoinflammatory diseases such as familial Mediterranean fever and Behcet's disease. This uniqueness shapes the clinical and research encounters of rheumatologists practicing in Lebanon. Rheumatology providers are not usually challenged regarding serological or imaging diagnostics, as multiple facilities can perform what is requested. However, similar to other countries, the cost of certain antirheumatic agents, especially biologicals, presents a major challenge for practice. The national, as well as private services in Lebanon, can cover a portion of the high cost of such agents. In the expanding field of rheumatology, Lebanon needs research funding, more human resources, and dedicated rheumatology centers of excellence to improve patient satisfaction and climb up the institutional ranking ladder.

Conflict of Interest The authors declare that they have no conflicts of interest.

References

1. Etheredge L. Syria, Lebanon, and Jordan (Middle East: region in transition). The Rosen Publishing Group; 2011. p. 85–159.
2. IBP I. Lebanon labor laws and regulations handbook – strategic information and basic Laws. International Business Publications USA; 2016.
3. Central Intelligence Agency. The World Factbook [Internet]. Edition Oct 16 2025 [cited 2025 Oct 22]. Available from: https://www.cia.gov/the-world-factbook/.
4. Saleh SS, Bou Sleiman J, Dagher D, Sbeit H, Natafgi N. Accreditation of hospitals in Lebanon: is it a worthy investment? Int J Qual Health Care. 2013;25(3):284–90.
5. Hemadeh R, Hammoud R, Kdouh O, Jaber T, Ammar L. Patient satisfaction with primary healthcare services in Lebanon. Int J Health Plann Manag. 2019;34(1):e423–e35.
6. Slim ZF, Uthman I. The state of rheumatic diseases in Lebanon. A call for research and education. Rheumatology (Oxford). 2012;51(11):1929–30.
7. Ziade N, Hmamouchi I, El Kibbi L. Women in rheumatology in the Arab league of associations for rheumatology countries: a rising workforce. Front Med (Lausanne). 2022;9:880285.
8. Lebanese Society of Rheumatology [Internet]. [cited 2026 Jun 14]. Available from: https://lsrheumatology.lopbeirut.org/history-of-lsr/.

9. Uthman I, Kassak K, Sanjakdar R, Mendelek V, Masri A, Nasr FJR. Letter from Lebanon. 1997;36(7):806–7.
10. Sibai AM, Sen K, Baydoun M, Saxena P. Population ageing in Lebanon: current status, future prospects and implications for policy. Bull World Health Organ. 2004;82(3):219–25.
11. Awada H, Baddoura R, Okais J, Habis A, Attoui S, Abi Saab M, editors. Lippincott-Raven rheumatology practice. Arthritis and rheumatism. Philadelphia (PA): Lippincott-Raven Publishers; 1995.
12. Chaaya M, Slim ZN, Habib RR, Arayssi T, Dana R, Hamdan O, et al. High burden of rheumatic diseases in Lebanon: a COPCORD study. Int J Rheum Dis. 2012;15(2):136–43.
13. Ziade N, El Khoury B, Zoghbi M, Merheb G, Abi Karam G, Mroue K, et al. Prevalence and pattern of comorbidities in chronic rheumatic and musculoskeletal diseases: the COMORD study. Sci Rep. 2020;10(1):7683.
14. Kiyohara C, Washio M, Horiuchi T, Asami T, Ide S, Atsumi T, et al. Cigarette smoking, alcohol consumption, and risk of systemic lupus erythematosus: a case-control study in a Japanese population. J Rheumatol. 2012;39(7):1363–70.
15. Speyer CB, Costenbader KH. Cigarette smoking and the pathogenesis of systemic lupus erythematosus. Expert Rev Clin Immunol. 2018;14(6):481–7.
16. El-Hajj M, Salameh P, Rachidi S, Al-Hajje A, Hosseini H. Cigarette and waterpipe smoking are associated with the risk of stroke in Lebanon. J Epidemiol Glob Health. 2019;9(1):62–70.
17. Almedawar MM, Walsh JL, Isma'eel HA. Waterpipe smoking and risk of coronary artery disease. Curr Opin Cardiol. 2016;31(5):545–50.
18. Chang K, Yang SM, Kim SH, Han KH, Park SJ, Shin JI. Smoking and rheumatoid arthritis. Int J Mol Sci. 2014;15(12):22279–95.
19. Chehade L, Jaafar ZA, El Masri D, Zmerly H, Kreidieh D, Tannir H, et al. Lifestyle modification in rheumatoid arthritis: dietary and physical activity recommendations based on evidence. Curr Rheumatol Rev. 2019;15(3):209–14.
20. Versini M, Jeandel PY, Rosenthal E, Shoenfeld Y. Obesity in autoimmune diseases: not a passive bystander. Autoimmun Rev. 2014;13(9):981–1000.
21. Mehio Sibai A, Nasreddine L, Mokdad AH, Adra N, Tabet M, Hwalla N. Nutrition transition and cardiovascular disease risk factors in Middle East and North Africa countries: reviewing the evidence. Ann Nutr Metab. 2010;57(3–4):193–203.
22. Nasreddine L, Naja F, Chamieh MC, Adra N, Sibai AM, Hwalla N. Trends in overweight and obesity in Lebanon: evidence from two national cross-sectional surveys (1997 and 2009). BMC Public Health. 2012;12:798.
23. Al-Herz W, Aldhekri H, Barbouche MR, Rezaei N. Consanguinity and primary immunodeficiencies. Hum Hered. 2014;77(1–4):138–43.
24. Zaghlol RY, Haghighi A, Alkhayyat MM, Theyab OF, Owaydah AM, Massad MM, et al. Consanguinity and the risk of Hashimoto's thyroiditis. Thyroid. 2017;27(3):390–5.
25. Barbour B, Salameh P. Consanguinity in Lebanon: prevalence, distribution and determinants. J Biosoc Sci. 2009;41(4):505–17.
26. Bassatne A, Harb H, Jaafar B, Romanos J, Ammar W, El-Hajj Fuleihan G. Disease burden of osteoporosis and other non-communicable diseases in Lebanon. Osteoporos Int. 2020;31(9):1769–77.
27. Coates LC, Baraliakos X, Blanco FJ, Blanco-Morales EA, Braun J, Chandran V, et al. The phenotype of axial spondyloarthritis: is it dependent on HLA-B27 status? Arthritis Care Res (Hoboken). 2021;73(6):856–60.
28. Skalska U, Kozakiewicz A, Maśliński W, Jurkowska M. HLA-B27 detection – comparison of genetic sequence-based method and flow cytometry assay. Reumatologia. 2015;53(2):74–8.
29. Awadia H, Baddoura R, Naman R, Klayme S, Mansour I, Tamouza R, et al. Weak association between HLA-B27 and the spondylarthropathies in Lebanon. Arthritis Rheum. 1997;40(2):388–9.
30. Serre JL, Lefranc G, Loiselet J, Jacquard A. HLA markers in six Lebanese religious subpopulations. Tissue Antigens. 1979;14(3):251–5.

31. Abdelnoor A, Abdelnoor M, Heneine W, Khauli R, Kobeissy F, Mansur S, et al. Major histocompatibility complex class I and II antigens frequencies in selected groups of Lebanese. Transplant Proc. 2001;33(5):2839–40.
32. Ziade N, Abi Karam G, Merheb G, Mallak I, Irani L, Alam E, et al. HLA-B27 prevalence in axial spondyloarthritis patients and in blood donors in a Lebanese population: results from a nationwide study. Int J Rheum Dis. 2019;22(4):708–14.
33. Papoutsis N, Abdel-Naser M, Altenburg A, Orawa H, Kötter I, Krause L, et al. Prevalence of Adamantiades-Behcet's disease in Germany and the municipality of Berlin: results of a nationwide survey. Clin Exp Rheumatol. 2006;24(5 Suppl 42):S125.
34. Hamdan A, Mansour W, Uthman I, Masri AF, Nasr F, Arayssi T. Behçet's disease in Lebanon: clinical profile, severity and two-decade comparison. Clin Rheumatol. 2006;25(3):364–7.
35. Arayssi TK, Hamdan AR, Touma Z, Shamseddeen W, Uthman IW, Hourani HB, et al. TNF polymorphisms in Lebanese patients with Behçet's disease. Clin Exp Rheumatol. 2008;26(4 Suppl 50):S130–1.
36. El Roz A, Ghssein G, Khalaf B, Fardoun T, Ibrahim J-N. Spectrum of MEFV variants and genotypes among clinically diagnosed FMF patients from southern Lebanon. Med Sci (Basel). 2020;8(3):35.
37. Infevers—Registry of hereditary auto-inflammatory disorder mutations [internet]. Montpellier (FR): UMAI & ISSAID; [cited 2026 Jun 14]. Available from: https://infevers.umai-montpellier.fr/web/.
38. Tins BJ, Butler R. Imaging in rheumatology: reconciling radiology and rheumatology. Insights Imaging. 2013;4(6):799–810.
39. Spencer SP, Ganeshalingam S, Kelly S, Ahmad M. The role of ultrasound in the diagnosis and follow-up of early inflammatory arthritis. Clin Radiol. 2012;67(1):15–23.
40. Firestein GS, McInnes IB. Immunopathogenesis of rheumatoid arthritis. Immunity. 2017;46(2):183–96.
41. Kerrigan SA, McInnes IB. Reflections on 'older' drugs: learning new lessons in rheumatology. Nat Rev Rheumatol. 2020;16(3):179–83.
42. Nahra V, Hasbani GE, Chaaya M, Uthman I. The use of infliximab (Remicade®) for the treatment of rheumatic diseases at a Tertiary Center in Lebanon: a 17-year retrospective chart review. Mediterr J Rheumatol. 2020;31(4):400–5.
43. Amhaz G, Ibrahim A, Usta U, El Cheikh J, Bazarbachi A, Abou Dalle I. First-line treatment of hairy cell leukemia with cladribine followed by rituximab consolidation significantly improves leukemia-free survival. Clin Lymphoma Myeloma Leuk. 2021;21(8):564–6.
44. Moussa H, Sawaya RA. Rituximab treatment for chronic idiopathic axonal polyneuropathy. J Clin Neuromuscul Dis. 2021;22(4):214–9.
45. Yamout BI, El-Ayoubi NK, Nicolas J, El Kouzi Y, Khoury SJ, Zeineddine MM. Safety and efficacy of rituximab in multiple sclerosis: a retrospective observational study. J Immunol Res. 2018;2018:9084759.
46. Kelly A, Tymms K, Fallon K, Sumpton D, Tugwell P, Tunnicliffe D, et al. Qualitative research in rheumatology: an overview of methods and contributions to practice and policy. J Rheumatol. 2021;48(1):6–15.
47. Ziadé N, Saad S, Al Mashaleh M, El Kibbi L, Elzorkany B, Badsha H, et al. Perceptions of patients with rheumatoid arthritis about self-assessment of disease activity after watching an educational video: a qualitative pilot study from the AUTO-DAS in Middle Eastern Arab countries project. Rheumatol Int. 2021;41(4):733–40.
48. Ziade N, El Hajj J, Rassi J, Hlais S, Lopez-Medina C, Gamal SM, et al. Root joint involvement in spondyloarthritis: a post hoc analysis from the international ASAS-PerSpA study. Rheumatology (Oxford). 2022;61(2):667–78.
49. Fraenkel L, Bathon JM, England BR, St Clair EW, Arayssi T, Carandang K, et al. 2021 American College of Rheumatology Guideline for the treatment of rheumatoid arthritis. Arthritis Care Res (Hoboken). 2021;73(7):924–39.

50. Wang X, Gkrouzman E, Andrade DCO, Andreoli L, Barbhaiya M, Belmont HM, et al. COVID-19 and antiphospholipid antibodies: a position statement and management guidance from AntiPhospholipid Syndrome Alliance for Clinical Trials and InternatiOnal Networking (APS ACTION). Lupus. 2021;30(14):2276–85.
51. Umar M, Megarbane A, Shan J, Syed N, Chouery E, Aliyev E, et al. Genome sequencing unveils mutational landscape of the familial Mediterranean fever: potential implications of IL33/ST2 signalling. J Cell Mol Med. 2020;24(19):11294–306.
52. Ibrahim JN, Jounblat R, Jalkh N, Abou Ghoch J, Al Hageh C, Chouery E, et al. RAC1 expression and role in IL-1β production and oxidative stress generation in familial Mediterranean fever (FMF) patients. Eur Cytokine Netw. 2018;29(4):127–35.
53. Safi R, Kallas R, Bardawil T, Mehanna CJ, Abbas O, Hamam R, et al. Neutrophils contribute to vasculitis by increased release of neutrophil extracellular traps in Behçet's disease. J Dermatol Sci. 2018;92(2):143–50.
54. Eid R, Haddad FG, Kourie HR, Kattan J. Electronic patient-reported outcomes: a revolutionary strategy in cancer care. Future Oncol. 2017;13(27):2397–9.

Chapter 8
Rheumatic Diseases in Libya

Khaled Elmuntaser and Soad Hashad

Abstract Rheumatic and musculoskeletal diseases (RMDs) represent a significant burden in Libya. Certain conditions, including systemic lupus erythematosus, Behçet disease, and familial Mediterranean fever, appear more prevalent than in Western countries, while polymyalgia rheumatica and spondyloarthritis appear less common. Epidemiological data remain scarce due to the absence of a national RMD registry.

Rheumatology services began in the early 1990s and have since expanded to include adult and pediatric departments in Tripoli and Benghazi. The Libyan Rheumatology Society plays a central role in education and specialty development since its founding in 2002. Despite these advances, the ongoing political instability following the 2011 revolution has severely disrupted healthcare infrastructure, contributed to a significant brain drain of rheumatologists, and prevented the establishment of formal training programs, national screening initiatives, and accredited centers of excellence. Key genetic diagnostic tests remain unavailable locally. Access to biologic therapies is confined to a few major cities, requiring patients from other regions to travel for treatment.

Political stabilization and targeted investment in rheumatology infrastructure, training, and research are essential to improving outcomes for RMD patients in Libya.

Keywords Rheumatic diseases · Rheumatology care · Libya · Pediatric rheumatology · Epidemiology · Health care system · Armed conflict

K. Elmuntaser (✉)
Kadisia Clinic, Tripoli, Libya
e-mail: kelmunt@hotmail.com

S. Hashad
Peditratic Rheumatology, University of Tripoli, Tripoli, Libya
e-mail: soadhashad@hotmail.com

K. A. Alnaqbi, G. Aldabie (eds.), *Rheumatic Diseases in the Arab World*,
https://doi.org/10.1007/978-981-92-0967-5_8

8.1 Country Demographics

Libya is situated in the Maghreb area of North Africa. It shares its borders with various countries and geographic features, including the Mediterranean Sea to the north, Egypt to the east, Sudan to the southeast, Chad to the south, Niger to the southwest, Algeria to the west, and Tunisia to the northwest. It has maritime borders with Malta, Greece, and Turkey in the eastern Mediterranean [1].

Libya comprises three historical regions: Tripolitania, Fezzan, and Cyrenaica. Covering an area of nearly 1.8 million square kilometers, it ranks as the fourth-largest country in both Africa and the Arab world, and the 16th globally. The country's largest city and capital, Tripoli, is situated in the Western part of Libya [1]. The terrain is predominantly flat and largely covered by the Sahara Desert, which is mostly uninhabitable. The Mediterranean Coast serves as its most well-known geographical feature. As of 2023, the population was estimated at 7.305 million [2].

Libya has a vast land area with a relatively modest population. Population density is much higher in the northern coastal regions of Tripolitania and Cyrenaica, while the desert interior is sparsely populated with fewer than one person per square kilometer in many areas. Approximately 90% of the population lives in a narrow coastal strip that represents less than 10% of the country's land area. Urbanization is high, with the majority of the population residing in cities, particularly in the two largest urban centers, Tripoli and Benghazi [1].

In 2023, Libya's population was predominantly of working age, with 80.6% aged 15–64 years, while 13.6% were younger than 15 years and 5.8% were aged 65 years or older. The population pyramid of Libya in 2023 reflects a predominantly young population structure, with larger proportions in the younger and working-age groups and smaller proportions in the elderly population and a generally balanced distribution between males and females across most age groups [2].

Indigenous Libyans are predominantly of Arab and Berber (Amazigh) ancestry. Smaller ethnic groups include the Tuareg and Tebu communities located mainly in the southern regions of the country, many of whom have historically practiced nomadic or semi-nomadic lifestyles. Libya also hosts foreign residents, particularly migrant workers from neighboring North African countries such as Egypt and Tunisia, as well as individuals from Sub-Saharan African nations [1]. In addition to demographic characteristics, several health indicators provide insight into the overall health status of the Libyan population.

8.2 Health Indicators

Life expectancy at birth in Libya declined slightly over the past two decades, decreasing from approximately 74 years in 2000 to 72.2 years in 2021. In 2021, life expectancy was higher among females (74.2 years) than among males (70.2 years) [2].

In 2021, the leading cause of death in Libya was ischemic heart disease, accounting for 102.4 deaths per 100,000 population, followed by COVID-19 (85.9 per 100,000) and stroke (43.1 per 100,000). Other major causes included road injuries, kidney diseases, hypertensive heart disease, diabetes mellitus, tuberculosis, cirrhosis of the liver, and respiratory cancers [2].

The maternal mortality ratio in Libya was estimated at 59.5 deaths per 100,000 live births in 2023, with an improving trend observed since 2019 [2].

8.3 Country Healthcare Sectors

Libya's healthcare system follows a mixed model that incorporates both public and private healthcare components. The system includes teaching hospitals, general hospitals, rural hospitals, specialized hospitals, polyclinics, and primary healthcare centers distributed across the country. Additionally, there are specialized tertiary care hospitals to address specific healthcare needs. However, political instability and armed conflict since the Libyan Revolution in 2011 have significantly affected the functionality of many health facilities. According to the Health Sector Libya Annual Report (2020), more than 300 public healthcare facilities, including primary healthcare centers and hospitals, required operational support, and reliable nationwide data on the total number of hospitals and healthcare facilities remain limited. Major tertiary hospitals and referral centers are located in Tripoli and Benghazi, while private hospitals and clinics operate mainly in urban areas such as Tripoli, Misrata, and Benghazi [3].

In 2021, domestic general government health expenditure in Libya represented 6.9% of total government spending. In 2022, development assistance for medical research and basic health sectors was estimated at US$2.43 per capita. The health workforce density included 20.42 physicians, 63.8 nurses and midwives, 5.8 dentists, and 4.1 pharmacists per 10,000 population, indicating moderate availability of healthcare professionals [3].

8.4 Rheumatology Health Services

Rheumatology is a relatively recent specialty in Libya. In the early 1990s, a European-trained internist and rheumatologist started providing rheumatology services through the internal medicine unit, emphasizing a special interest in rheumatology and establishing an outpatient department dedicated to rheumatic and musculoskeletal diseases (RMDs).

In 1997, the first rheumatology unit was opened in the new Tripoli Medical Center, which later became a department. Many young physicians were trained in the department and became experienced in managing RMDs. These physicians went to Europe, the USA, and Canada to pursue their postgraduate studies, but most of them did not come back because of the civil war and unstable political situation in Libya.

As of January 2024, both Tripoli and Benghazi each have a dedicated rheumatology department and unit, offering comprehensive rheumatology services. Additionally, pediatric rheumatology units operate in the teaching pediatric hospitals of both cities. The combined rheumatology workforce comprises approximately 26 specialists, including 8 consultants, 8 specialists, and 10 registrars, with a female-to-male ratio of 2 to 1.

8.4.1 Pediatric Rheumatology

Rheumatology in Libya is a relatively new specialty, especially in the field of pediatric rheumatology. Before 2002, pediatric rheumatology patients were primarily treated by adult rheumatologists or general practitioners. In February 2002, the first pediatric rheumatology clinic was established at Tripoli Children's Hospital, a tertiary referral center and teaching hospital that serves a wide range of pediatric subspecialties. This clinic was initiated by two pediatric consultants who had received specialized training in Italy for the rheumatology subspecialty. It is the only clinic caring for pediatric rheumatology patients in Libya.

Initially, referrals to the clinic were limited because it was newly established and not yet widely recognized and because awareness of pediatric RMDs was low among both physicians and patients. As awareness increased, thanks in part to online resources providing information about the clinic, there was a noticeable improvement in referrals. Over the subsequent years, the growing number of patients and the increasing interest in the subspecialty attracted young physicians to join the rheumatology unit. As a result, a well-established unit now exists, with more than 1500 registered patients diagnosed with various RMDs (unpublished data), referred by orthopedic surgeons, emergency physicians, general practitioners, adult rheumatologists, and ophthalmologists (Table 8.1). The pediatric rheumatology staff consists of four consultants, three specialists, four pediatric rheumatology fellows who

Table 8.1 Diagnoses of 1500 registered pediatric rheumatology cases in 2022 at Tripoli Children's Hospital

Diagnosis	Percentage
Juvenile idiopathic arthritis	70%
Autoinflammatory syndromes	8%
Vasculitis	6%
Systemic lupus erythematosus	5%
Chronic idiopathic uveitis	5%
Behçet disease	3%
Juvenile dermatomyositis	1%
Scleroderma	0.60%
Polymyositis	0.20%

undergo specialized training in pediatrics on a rotational basis, with changes occurring every 6 months, and two nurses.

The outpatient clinics are open for follow-up 5 days a week, seeing around 100 new cases each year. About 30% of the patients registered are from Tripoli, and the rest are from different parts of the country.

The department further operates specialized clinics for pediatric uveitis and transition care, alongside a dedicated infusion clinic for the administration of intravenous biologic therapy, accommodating up to two patients daily. This clinic benefits from the expertise of a specialist physician, a fellowship trainee, and a registered nurse, ensuring comprehensive and efficient care delivery.

There are 2 days dedicated for giving biological therapies and intra-articular injections. During the period of civil war and the COVID-19 pandemic, video calls were used to follow up with the patients. Several publications from the clinic were published in journals or presented at conferences.

In 2022, approximately 500 transient cases, including IgA vasculitis, acute arthritis, Kawasaki disease, and transient synovitis, were seen in the pediatric department.

8.4.2 Rheumatology Nurses

At present, there are no registered nurses with specialized training or certification in rheumatology. However, each rheumatology unit has four nurses who collaborate with rheumatologists and gain valuable experience in managing patients with RMDs, totaling 20 nurses.

8.4.3 Accredited Center of Excellence for Rheumatology

At present, there are no accredited centers of excellence for rheumatology in Libya.

8.4.4 Available System of Referrals to Rheumatology

There is currently no well-established system for directing patients to rheumatology services. Typically, patients are referred from polyclinics or smaller hospitals to the rheumatology clinics of teaching hospitals. In certain instances, patients may be directly referred to rheumatologists in the private sector. Rheumatologists commonly split their work between government hospitals in the morning and private clinics in the afternoon.

8.5 Official Rheumatology Society

The Libyan Rheumatology Society (LRS), the first in the country, was founded on January 3, 2002. Since its launch, LRS has actively promoted continuing medical education in rheumatology by organizing a variety of events, including symposia, meetings, and lectures.

8.6 Overview of Common Rheumatic Diseases in Libya

Due to the absence of a registry for RMDs in Libya, there is a lack of epidemiological data, such as incidence, prevalence, mortality rates, and gender-specific patterns. Based on the authors' three decades of experience in the field of rheumatology in Libya, certain trends have been observed. Some diseases appear to be more prevalent in Libya compared to Western countries, while others are less common. Specifically, polymyalgia rheumatica and spondyloarthritis (SpA) are less frequently encountered, whereas systemic lupus erythematosus (SLE) appears to be more prevalent. Behçet disease and familial Mediterranean fever (FMF) are relatively common and exhibit higher incidence rates compared to Western countries. Rheumatoid arthritis (RA) appears to be the most prevalent autoimmune RMD, while osteoarthritis is also common and predominantly affects the knees, with less frequent involvement of the hip.

8.6.1 Gout

Gout is the most common inflammatory RMD in Libyan men, and its incidence appears to have increased over the last few decades. Several factors are likely responsible for this rise in gout cases, including urbanization; the adoption of a Western lifestyle; increased consumption of purine-rich foods; as well as the growing incidence of obesity, hypertension, diabetes mellitus, and renal disease within the Libyan population. Epidemiological data on the prevalence of hyperuricemia and gout are scarce. In one study, it was shown that the serum uric acid levels in all patients with hypertension increased significantly when compared to controls [4]. Clinical and radiographic surveys were not conducted.

Currently, no studies have explored the relationship between genetics and gout in Libyans. This genetic study is needed due to the wide genetic diversity among Libyans. Based on the author's experience, there is a notable variation in the sex distribution of gout patients, with a predominance of males. Most patients with primary gout exhibit a monoarticular or oligoarticular presentation, with only a few having polyarticular involvement. The joints most frequently affected include the first metatarsophalangeal joints, followed by larger joints like the knees and ankles. The available treatment options for acute attacks encompass non-steroidal anti-inflammatory drugs, colchicine, glucocorticoids, and allopurinol for urate-lowering therapy. In recent years, febuxostat has also become available, while drugs like pegloticase, rilonacept, and canakinumab remain unavailable.

8.6.2 Rheumatoid Arthritis (RA)

RA is the most common inflammatory autoimmune RMD in females and the second most common inflammatory RMD among Libyan males. Currently, there are no available epidemiological data regarding the prevalence of RA in Libya. Limited observational studies with small participant numbers have been published, shedding some light on the clinical manifestations and treatment of RA in Libyans [5]. Furthermore, early genetic studies to determine susceptibility to RA, including different alleles of HLA-DRB1, have not been conducted. Similarly, genome-wide association studies exploring susceptibility loci, which can vary among different Libyan ethnic groups, have yet to be conducted.

Some environmental risk factors for RA include smoking, which is linked to the development and severity of RA [6]. Periodontal infection is another environmental risk factor significantly associated with RA [7]. Based on the author's experience, RA manifestations in Libya often involve an earlier age of onset, a lower prevalence of subcutaneous nodules and extra-articular symptoms, and milder disease with less severe radiographic changes compared to Western countries.

RA is more prevalent in women than men, with a ratio of approximately 3–4 to 1, similar to the ratio observed in patients in Mediterranean countries [8]. Delays in referral to rheumatology specialists are common, particularly in smaller cities and villages. These delays often result in untreated or inadequately treated active disease, leading to higher disease activity, increased functional impairment, and more severe joint damage. In the authors' experience, common extra-articular manifestations include subcutaneous nodules, scleritis, and pulmonary involvement. Approximately 60–70% of RA patients have rheumatoid factor and anti-cyclic citrullinated peptide (CCP) antibodies. Methotrexate is the most commonly used disease-modifying anti-rheumatic drug (DMARD) for RA treatment in Libya, with effective outcomes observed since its introduction in the early 1990s. In cases resistant to methotrexate, the addition of leflunomide has shown promising results. Many biologic DMARDs are available in teaching hospitals that offer rheumatology services, and they are provided free of charge to Libyan patients.

8.6.3 Spondyloarthritis (SpA)

SpA is frequently reported in North African countries like Egypt, Morocco, Tunisia, and Algeria [9]. However, there is a lack of specific data regarding SpA prevalence in Libya. Egypt, for instance, has reported an overall SpA prevalence of 0.15% [10].

It is suspected that the prevalence in Libya is similar, falling below the rates observed in European countries, which range from 0.3% to 1.9% [11]. Notably, the genetic risk factor HLA-B27, associated with certain SpA types, is less prevalent in North Africans at 3–5% compared to 8% in individuals of European ancestry [12]. For patients with ankylosing spondylitis, HLA-B27 prevalence is 90–95% in those of European ancestry but only 29–64% in North African patients from Algeria, Egypt, Morocco, and Tunisia with the disease [13–16]. A similar trend is expected in Libya. Based on the authors' experiences, most of the SpA patients are in their twenties, with a male-to-female ratio of 8:1. Inflammatory back pain is a common symptom, whereas peripheral oligoarthritis and dactylitis were rare. Extra-musculoskeletal manifestations like uveitis, psoriasis, and inflammatory bowel disease are infrequently seen. Notably, there is often a significant delay in diagnosis as patients initially seek orthopedic surgeons and neurosurgeons for their symptoms. Raising awareness of SpA in Libya is needed, along with further research into genetic diversity among various ethnic groups.

8.6.4 Systemic Lupus Erythematosus (SLE)

While there is a lack of specific data on the incidence and prevalence of SLE in Libya, it appears to be the second most common inflammatory RMD among females in the country, surpassing its occurrence in some Western countries, based on the authors' experience. Many patients referred to rheumatology clinics for joint-related symptoms are diagnosed with SLE. Consanguinity in Libyan society may play an important role in the development of SLE. The most prevalent clinical manifestation is arthritis, followed by mucocutaneous symptoms. Renal involvement is observed in approximately 50% of patients. The majority of SLE patients test positive for antinuclear antibodies (ANA), while about half of them have double-stranded DNA (dsDNA) antibodies. Other antibodies, such as anti-Ro, anti-La, and anti-Sm, are not routinely tested in Libya and must be sent abroad at the patients' expense. Renal biopsies, used to classify lupus nephritis, are available. Treatment options include antimalarials, glucocorticosteroids, mycophenolate mofetil, and cyclophosphamide. However, the biologic drugs belimumab and anifrolumab are not utilized due to their unavailability.

8.6.5 Behçet Disease

Behçet disease is relatively common in Libya, a Mediterranean country, particularly among young males. However, there is a lack of statistical data regarding its prevalence and incidence. Data on Behçet disease in Libya are limited; however, small clinical series from Tripoli have described the clinical characteristics of patients with the disease. In a study of 23 patients, the disease showed a marked male predominance, with males accounting for 82.6% of cases and females 17.4%, corresponding to a male-to-female ratio of approximately 3.4:1 [17]. The most common age of onset was between 21 and 30 years, observed in about 70% of patients. Recurrent oro-genital ulcers were present in all patients. Ocular involvement was reported in 10 cases, while joint involvement occurred in six cases. Other manifestations included erythema nodosum, thrombophlebitis, epididymitis, deep vein thrombosis, central nervous system involvement, and esophageal ulcers, each occurring in a smaller number of patients. Elevated erythrocyte sedimentation rate was observed during active phases of the disease. Most patients responded to treatment with oral prednisolone, while colchicine was effective in controlling mucocutaneous and skin manifestations in several cases.

8.7 Risk Factors for Rheumatic Diseases

8.7.1 Infections

Viral and bacterial infections remain relatively common in Libya. For instance, in one study, the incidence rate of rotavirus diarrhea in children aged 5 and below was estimated at 640 per 100,000 [18].

A national sero-epidemiological survey involving more than 65,000 individuals across Libya reported a prevalence of hepatitis B surface antigen (HBsAg) of approximately 2.2%, while hepatitis C virus infection was detected in about 1.3% of the population [19].

In 2023, the incidence of tuberculosis in Libya was estimated at approximately 57 cases per 100,000 population [2]. It is worth noting that infections can potentially contribute to the disruption of immune tolerance and the onset of autoimmune reactions in RMDs [20].

8.7.2 Smoking

Tobacco use remains an important public health concern in Libya. In 2022, an estimated 975,000 adults were smokers, including 961,000 men and 14,000 women, highlighting a marked gender disparity in smoking prevalence. This poses a persistent and serious public health concern [21]. Tobacco smoking has been associated with the development of RMDs, such as SLE and RA, and has been shown to interact with genetic factors, significantly increasing the risk of these diseases. Additionally, smoking can impact the course and outcome of RMDs [22].

8.7.3 Vitamin D Deficiency

Vitamin D deficiency is a significant concern in Libya. Factors contributing to this problem include cultural practices of body covering, dark skin color in certain areas, prolonged breastfeeding without vitamin D supplementation, low dietary calcium intake, limited outdoor activity, obesity, and a lack of government regulation for vitamin D fortification in food. A retrospective study conducted in Benwalied and Sirte cities found that 63% of patients had suboptimal vitamin D levels. Among 133 of these patients, 70.7% had a deficiency, and 29.3% had insufficiency. Being female was identified as a risk factor for vitamin D deficiency [23]. Vitamin D deficiency may play a role in autoimmune RMDs, impacting both their development and severity [24].

8.7.4 Consanguinity

High rates of consanguineous marriages were reported in the Arab countries, including Libya, with a rate of 46.5% of all marriages in 2009 [25]. For instance, it has been shown that a family history of SLE is a risk factor for the development of the disease, and the risk increases with the increasing number of relatives affected. This might explain the high incidence of SLE in Libya observed by the authors.

8.8 Screening Programs for Rheumatic Diseases

There are no screening programs for RMDs in Libya. Due to the ongoing unstable political situation and civil war, state authorities are primarily focused on managing basic healthcare and cannot expand their activities to include screening programs. Additionally, the Libyan Rheumatology Society lacks financial support to initiate such programs. If the political situation stabilizes, there is hope for improvements in the healthcare system and other areas.

8.9 Diagnostic Tests for Rheumatic Diseases

In Libya, genetic tests such as HLA-B27, HLA-B51, and MEFV (*Mediterranean fever* gene) mutations are not available. Rheumatologists rely on their clinical expertise for related diagnoses. Occasionally, these tests are sent abroad at the patient's expense if they can afford it.

Advanced imaging services such as computed tomography (CT), CT angiography, magnetic resonance imaging (MRI), and magnetic resonance angiography

(MRA) are available but are more commonly found in private facilities than in teaching hospitals. PET scans are not available anywhere in the country.

There are two musculoskeletal (MSK) radiologists, and some rheumatologists have acquired MSK ultrasound skills through practice. Teaching hospitals are equipped with ultrasound machines and probes for the MSK system to diagnose and monitor RMDs.

8.10 Management of Rheumatic Diseases

In Tripoli, there are three hospitals providing immunomodulatory treatment, including conventional synthetic DMARDs, biologic originators, and biosimilars. Two hospitals in Benghazi and one in Misrata offer similar services. This treatment is also provided in private clinics under the supervision of the responsible rheumatologist. Patients from other areas needing such treatment are referred to these cities.

8.11 Access to Multidisciplinary Care

Physiotherapy and rehabilitation services are available in numerous public centers and the private sector, distributed throughout the country. Orthopedic surgery is available in all public hospitals and is properly functioning. In the private sector, there are many well-equipped orthopedic surgery clinics offering good service for the patients at affordable costs.

8.12 Access to Cost-effective Rheumatic Diseases Care

The ongoing political instability in Libya has significantly disrupted the ability to provide cost-effective healthcare services, including the management of RMDs. Unfortunately, due to these persistent challenges, there has been a lack of long-term planning for the healthcare system.

8.13 Education and Research

8.13.1 Rheumatology Training Programs

Young physicians are trained in rheumatology without formal fellowship programs. Training for adult patients takes place in Tripoli and Benghazi, while pediatric training occurs at the Children's Hospital.

8.13.2 Rheumatology Nursing Program

At present, there are no nursing programs in Libya that offer training or certification in rheumatology.

8.13.3 Research in Rheumatology

Rheumatologist-driven research initiatives are conducted individually on a small scale, resulting mainly in case reports or studies from single centers [26–32]. A few collaborative studies and international initiatives have included investigators from North Africa and the broader Arab region, reflecting growing interest in RMD research and regional cooperation [33–36]. Despite these efforts, there are no well-organized national multicenter studies or clinical trials, and basic research related to RMDs has not yet been established.

8.14 Opportunities and Specific Challenges

Many Libyan medical specialists, including rheumatologists, have not returned to the country after their training abroad or have left for other countries like the Gulf countries, Europe, Canada, and the USA. This shortage of practicing rheumatologists in Libya has hindered the establishment of training programs for physicians and nurses in rheumatology and has contributed to the lack of specialized rheumatology clinics. One way to solve this problem is to raise awareness and enhance the education and training of healthcare professionals. This will enable early diagnosis and treatment of patients, ultimately improving their outcomes.

Patients with RMDs, like others, aim to access free diagnostic and treatment services in the public healthcare system, but sometimes they have to cover the costs themselves, which can lead to poor outcomes. Only a small portion of the population has medical insurance that covers private sector healthcare expenses.

Due to low confidence in the local healthcare system and the lack of adequate facilities, some patients seek medical care in countries like Tunisia, Jordan, and Turkey.

8.15 Future Directions

Currently, there are no specific plans in place to enhance the care and outcomes of RMDs. The healthcare authorities are primarily focused on providing basic healthcare services. However, it is expected that as political stability returns to the country, the overall healthcare system in Libya will improve. This improvement may pave the way for the implementation of future programs aimed at enhancing RMD management.

These potential future programs may include specialized training for physicians and nurses in rheumatology to address the shortage of qualified professionals in this field.

Collaboration with international organizations and neighboring countries with advanced healthcare systems may also play a role in shaping the future of rheumatology care in Libya. However, to support these initiatives, the government and relevant authorities will need to allocate adequate resources and funding.

Rebuilding the healthcare infrastructure and improving confidence in the medical system are essential steps toward a more promising future for RMD management in Libya.

8.16 Conclusion

RMDs are prevalent in Libya and significantly impact the quality of life and survival of affected individuals. However, providing adequate care for these conditions remains a considerable challenge. The ongoing civil conflict has disrupted numerous health programs, adversely affecting all aspects of healthcare, including rheumatology. These conflicts have resulted in mass displacements and extensive damage to critical infrastructure, including healthcare facilities.

Despite these challenges, rheumatologists and their teams in Libya continue to make every effort to provide patients with the care they need, even in the face of limited diagnostic and therapeutic resources. Clinical experience, therefore, plays a crucial role in the management of RMDs under these circumstances. Continued efforts to strengthen rheumatology services, training, and research will be important to improve patient care in the future.

There is hope that with political stability, Libyan rheumatologists currently abroad may return to their home country to contribute to the development of medical care for RMD patients and the training of more healthcare professionals in diagnosis and management.

Conflict of Interest The authors declare that there is no conflict of interest.

References

1. Demographics of Libya. Wikipedia, The Free Encyclopedia [Internet]. [cited 2026 Mar 12]. Available from: https://en.wikipedia.org/wiki/Demographics_of_Libya.
2. World Health Organization. Libya: health data overview [Internet]. Geneva: World Health Organization; [cited 2026 Mar 12]. Available from: https://data.who.int/countries/434.

3. World Health Organization. Health sector Libya annual report 2020 [Internet]. Geneva: WHO; 2021. [cited 2026 Mar 12]. Available from: https://data.who.int/countries/434.
4. Jarari AM. Uric acid levels in patients with hypertension in Benghazi. Libyan J Med Res. 2009;6(2):14.
5. Basma E. Health-related quality of life in Libyan patients with rheumatoid arthritis. Afr J Rheumatol. 2013;1(2).
6. Ishikawa Y, Terao C. The impact of cigarette smoking on risk of rheumatoid arthritis: a narrative review. Cells. 2020;9(2):475. https://doi.org/10.3390/cells9020475.
7. Bingham CO III, Moni M. Periodontal disease and rheumatoid arthritis: the evidence accumulates for complex pathobiologic interaction. Curr Opin Rheumatol. 2013;25(3):345–53. https://doi.org/10.1097/BOR.0b013e32835fb8ec.
8. Carmona L, Villaverde V, Hernández-García C, Ballina J, Gabriel R, Laffon A, EPISER Study Group. The prevalence of rheumatoid arthritis in the general population of Spain. Rheumatology. 2002;41:88–95.
9. Adelowo O, Mody GM, Tikly M, et al. Rheumatic diseases in Africa. Nat Rev Rheumatol. 2021;17:363–74. https://doi.org/10.1038/s41584-021-00603-4.
10. Chopra A. The COPCORD world of musculoskeletal pain and arthritis. Rheumatology. 2013;52:1925–8.
11. Torre-Alonso JC, Queiro R, Comellas M, Lizán L, Blanch C. Patient-reported outcomes in European spondyloarthritis patients: a systematic review of the literature. Patient Prefer Adherence. 2018;12:733–44.
12. Amroun H, Djoudi H, Busson M, Allat R, El Sherbini SM, Sloma I, et al. Early-onset ankylosing spondylitis is associated with a functional MICA polymorphism. Hum Immunol. 2005;66:1057–61.
13. Tayel MY, Soliman E, El Baz WF, El Labaan A, Hamaad Y, Ahmed MH. Registry of the clinical characteristics of spondyloarthritis in a cohort of Egyptian population. Rheum Int. 2012;32:2837–42.
14. Kchir MM, Hamdi W, Laadhar L, Kochbati S, Kaffel D, Saadellaoui K, et al. HLA-B, DR and DQ antigens polymorphism in Tunisian patients with ankylosing spondylitis (a case–control study). Rheum Int. 2010;30:933–9.
15. El Mouraghi I, Ouarour A, Ghozlani I, Collantes E, Solana R, El Maghraoui A, et al. Polymorphisms of HLA-A,-B,-Cw and DRB1 antigens in Moroccan patients with ankylosing spondylitis and a comparison of clinical features with frequencies of HLA-B* 27. Tissue Antigens. 2015;85:108–16.
16. Davatchi F, Assaad-Khalil S, Calamia KT, Crook JE, Sadeghi-Abdollahi B, Schirmer M, et al. The International Criteria for Behcet's Disease (ICBD): a collaborative study of 27 countries on the sensitivity and specificity of the new criteria. J Eur Acad Dermatol Venerol. 2014;28(3):338–47.
17. Khatri ML, Shafi M. Behcet's disease (a study of 23 cases from Tripoli, Libya). Indian J Dermatol Venereol Leprol. 1987;53(5):282–5.
18. Alkoshi S, Ernst K, Maimaiti N, Dahlui M. Rota viral infection: a significant disease burden to Libya. Iran J Public Health. 2014;43(10):1356–63.
19. Elzouki AN, Smeo MN, Sammud M, Elahmer O, Daw M, Fararah A, et al. Prevalence of hepatitis B and C virus infections and their related risk factors in Libya: a national seroepidemiological survey. East Mediterr Health J. 2013;19(7):589–99.
20. Sakkas LI, Bogdanos DP. Infections as a cause of autoimmune rheumatic diseases. Auto Immun Highlights. 2016;7(1):13. https://doi.org/10.1007/s13317-016-0086-x.
21. Tobacco Atlas. Libya [Internet]. [cited 2026 Mar 12]. Available from: https://tobaccoatlas.org/factsheets/libya/.
22. Harel-Meir M, et al. Tobacco smoking and autoimmune rheumatic diseases. Nat Clin Pract Rheumato. 2007;3(12):707–15. https://doi.org/10.1038/ncprheum0655.
23. Nasef A, Hassan M, El-Taguri A, Nagi AA. Prevalence of vitamin D deficiency in the central region of Libya. Int J Adv Res. 2020;8:988–94. https://doi.org/10.21474/IJAR01/11009.

24. Gatenby P, Lucas R, Swaminathan A. Vitamin D deficiency and risk for rheumatic diseases: an update. Curr Opin Rheumatol. 2013;25(2):184–91. https://doi.org/10.1097/BOR.0b013e32835cfc16.
25. United Nations Development Programme. Consanguinity and early marriage 2009 in the Arab World. Report 2009.
26. Basma E, Rajab T, Manal E. Adalimumab effect in a cohort of Libyan patients with rheumatic diseases. Afr J Rheumatol. 2017;5(2).
27. Ahmed AM, Ibkhatra SA, Elbraki FM, Ehsouna HF, Alsaeiti KD. Clinical presentations of Sjogren's syndrome in Benghazi. Libya Ibnosina J Med Biomed Sci. 2020;12:195–9.
28. Etaher NA, Saeed NM, Elmejrab MM, Sherif RF, Sherif FM. Prescribing patterns of methotrexate in Libyan patients with rheumatoid arthritis. J Pharmacol Res Dev. 2021;3(1):21–7.
29. Zaid FE. Clinical patterns of psoriatic arthritis and the relationship between psoriasis skin severity and joint activity in Libya. J Rheum Dis Treat. 2021;7:089. https://doi.org/10.23937/2469-5726/1510089.
30. Moustafa HM. Rheumatoid arthritis (RA) in Libyan patients. Al-Azhar Assiut Med J 2013;11(4).
31. Hashad S, Zletni MA, Al-Mayouf SM, Etayari H, Ibrahim E, Etfil M, et al. The Libyan Arabic version of the Juvenile Arthritis Multidimensional Assessment Report (JAMAR). Rheumatol Int. 2018;38(Suppl 1):267–74. https://doi.org/10.1007/s00296-018-3962-z.
32. Zaid FE, Elaish E. Correlation between radiological score and prognostic markers in rheumatoid arthritis in Libya. J Arthritis. 2019;8:286.
33. Alasmari A, Aldakhil H, Almutairi A, Nashawi M, Basahl E, Abushhaiwia A, et al. Utility of pan-immune-inflammation value as a predictor of the prognosis of childhood lupus. Lupus. 2024;33(12):1365–72. https://doi.org/10.1177/09612033241275227.
34. Caggiano V, Vitale A, Hinojosa-Azaola A, Guaracha-Basañez GA, Ruscitti P, Cipriani P, et al. Development and implementation of the international AIDA network spondylarthritis registry. Front Med (Lausanne). 2025;12:1509357. https://doi.org/10.3389/fmed.2025.1509357.
35. Gaggiano C, DE-LA-Torre A, Guerriero S, Tierradentro-Alape R, Ragab G, Forero-Uribe A, et al. Reproductive life stages and female sex-specific patterns in uveitis activity: data from the AIDA network uveitis registry. Am J Ophthalmol 2026;282:292–304. https://doi.org/10.1016/j.ajo.2025.11.009.
36. Hassan W, Mosa DM, Faleye A, Libe TT, Palalane E, Migowa A, et al. PAFLAR guidelines for oligoarticular juvenile idiopathic arthritis. Clin Rheumatol. 2026;45(2):1323–36. https://doi.org/10.1007/s10067-025-07792-3.

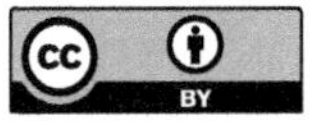

Chapter 9
Rheumatic Diseases in Mauritania

Mohamed Khattry Ahmed Ghassem, Saleck Ahmed Vall, Noura Biha, and Sidi El Wafi Baba

Abstract In northwest Africa, the Islamic Republic of Mauritania is the 27th largest country in the world, with economic opportunities for sustainable healthcare system development, particularly in rheumatology. However, many challenges need to be overcome in the short and long term, like the need for dedicated rheumatic disease infrastructure, qualified personnel, and the absence of a national approach to combating rheumatic diseases. The frequency of risk factors for rheumatic diseases is already high in the country and probably underestimated, predominantly obesity and physical inactivity. However, current data support the significant prevalence of rheumatic diseases in Mauritania. Spinal diseases, such as low back pain, and osteoarthritis, such as knee osteoarthritis, are common in the country. Rheumatoid arthritis, systemic lupus erythematosus, and osteoporosis also exist, as well as juvenile idiopathic arthritis. The management of rheumatic diseases remains suboptimal, leading to frequent encounters with advanced and disabling disease forms in daily practice.

Keywords Rheumatic diseases · Mauritania · Rheumatology · Drug cost · Osteoarthritis · Healthcare

M. K. Ahmed Ghassem (✉)
Department of Internal Medicine, National Hospital Centre (CHN), Nouakchott, Mauritania
e-mail: m.ahmedghassem@gmail.com

S. Ahmed Vall
Cheikh Zayed Hospital (HCZ), Nouakchott, Mauritania
e-mail: drsalek@yahoo.fr

N. Biha
Department of Internal Medicine, Military Hospital, Nouakchott, Mauritania
e-mail: nourabiha80@gmail.com

S. E. W. Baba
Faculty of Medicine, University Al Aasriya, Nouakchott, Mauritania
e-mail: siwamed@gmail.com

K. A. Alnaqbi, G. Aldabie (eds.), *Rheumatic Diseases in the Arab World*,
https://doi.org/10.1007/978-981-92-0967-5_9

9.1 Mauritania Demographics

Mauritania is an Islamic Republic in the northwest of Africa, bordered in the west by the Atlantic Ocean, to the northwest by Western Sahara, to the north by Algeria, to the east and southeast by Mali, and to the southwest by Senegal. Halfway between the Sahara and the Sahel, Mauritania is the 27th largest country in the world, with an area of 1,030,700 km^2, divided into 13 regions (*Wilaya*) subdivided into 52 *Mougahtaa* [1, 2]. The World Health Organization (WHO) estimates the population at 5,170,000 in 2024 [3]. There are 2,591,838 people over the age of 18. Nouakchott, the country's capital, was home to 1,077,169 inhabitants in 2016, with a male/female sex ratio of 1.07. Administratively, the city of Nouakchott is subdivided into three regions: Nouakchott West, Nouakchott North, and Nouakchott South [4].

9.2 Mauritania Healthcare Sectors

The healthcare system in Mauritania is structured as a three-tier pyramidal model, with health posts and health centers at the peripheral (Moughataa) level, three types of hospitals in the regional capitals at the intermediate level, and four public reference institutions concentrated in Nouakchott at the tertiary level (Table 9.1).

Alongside the public system is a private healthcare system, mainly located in the main urban centers (Nouakchott, Nouadhibou), which is experiencing growth [5].

Table 9.1 Public Hospitals in Nouakchott

Hospital name	Location	Specialized activity
National Hospital Centre (CHN)	Nouakchott West	Multi-purpose hospital
Cheikh Zayed Hospital (HCZ)	Nouakchott North	Multi-purpose hospital
Amitié Hospital Centre	Nouakchott South	Multi-purpose hospital
Military Hospital	Nouakchott West	Multi-purpose hospital
National Specialty Centre	Nouakchott West	Head and neck care
National Institute of Hepato-Virology	Nouakchott West	Gastroenterology and hepatology care
Mother and Child Hospital	Nouakchott West	Gynecology and pediatric care
National Oncology Centre	Nouakchott West	Oncology care
National Cardiology Centre (CNC)	Nouakchott West	Cardiovascular care

9.3 Rheumatology Health Services

Mauritania has only seven rheumatologists, including two assistant professors at the University of Nouakchott and one professor, and they are all practicing in Nouakchott.

Mauritania currently has no accredited rheumatology centers of excellence or a dedicated rheumatology nursing workforce. However, specialized rheumatology outpatient consultations are available at the five major multi-purpose public hospitals in the capital city. Within these hospitals, rheumatology practice is seamlessly integrated into the internal medicine departments, ensuring each department has at least one rheumatologist.

Data from the Cheikh Zayed Hospital (HCZ) Rheumatology Consultation Registry [6] reveals that pediatric rheumatology cases represent around 1.7% of general rheumatology practice, even in the absence of a specialist in this field. This highlights the necessity for enhanced epidemiological data and the establishment of a dedicated comprehensive care center specifically for pediatric rheumatology.

The traditional referral system to rheumatology involves family doctors and other specialists referring patients to rheumatologists. However, there has been a recent trend where patients seek referrals directly from the community without going through the healthcare system.

9.4 Overview of Rheumatic Diseases in Mauritania

While there is a need for high-quality data on the prevalence of rheumatic diseases in Mauritania, the available, although limited and often low-quality, data still provide valuable insights into these conditions in the country.

The percentage of patients with arthritis increases slightly with age. According to the Mauritania Demographic and Health Survey 2019–2021 [7], 3% of women aged 15–49 years and 1% of men aged 15–59 years reported that a health provider had informed them that they had arthritis. In the *Wilaya* of *Tagant*, with a population of 80,962 [4], 11% of men were informed by a health provider that they had arthritis [7].

To better understand the rheumatological situation in Mauritania, we present unpublished registry data from the rheumatology outpatient consultation at Cheikh Zayed Hospital (HCZ) and the National Hospital Centre (CHN). These data are unpublished and not available online. Non-specific spinal diseases and osteoarthritis are the most frequent rheumatic diseases. Rheumatoid arthritis is the most frequent inflammatory rheumatic disease in Mauritania. Osteoarticular infections are managed in hospitals by surgeons, which explains the low rate of rheumatological consultations for these cases. Systemic lupus erythematous exists in Mauritania (Fig. 9.1).

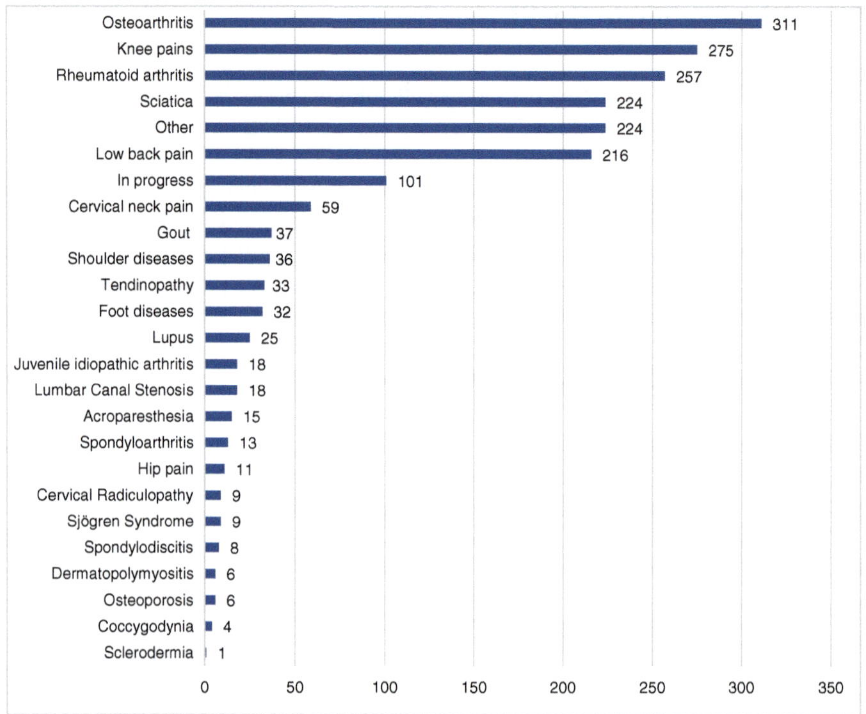

Fig. 9.1 Distribution of rheumatic diseases seen at the Cheikh Zayed Hospital (HCZ) from June 2021 to May 2022

From June 2021 to May 2022, 1860 patients were seen at the HCZ rheumatology consultation [6]. Children aged 5–16 years represented 1.70% of these patients. The sex ratio of women to men is 3.16 (Fig. 9.1). The label "in progress" in the figure refers to cases in which the final diagnosis had not been established at the time of data collection.

At the CHN, from April 2021 to May 2022 [8], 1367 patients presented for rheumatology consultation. The average age was 46.8 ± 14.3 years. The female/male sex ratio is 2.80.

Figure 9.2 shows the distribution by month of the number of patients with a marked increase in cases in the first half of 2022 compared to the second half of 2021 [8].

Figure 9.3 shows the distribution of rheumatic diseases in the CHN cohort [8]. Non-specific spinal diseases and osteoarthritis account for 35.1% and 21.6% of cases, respectively. Low back pain is the most frequent reason for consultation, accounting for 82.44% of mechanical spinal diseases. Knee osteoarthritis represents 5.02% of the CHN cohort. Shoulder diseases represent 2.77% of cases, dominated by rotator cuff tendinopathy, accounting for 63.15% of shoulder diseases.

300
250
200
150
100
50
0
April 2021
May 2021
June 2021
July 2021
August 2021
September 2021
October 2021
November 2021
December 2021
January 2022
February 2022
March 2022
April 2022
May 2022

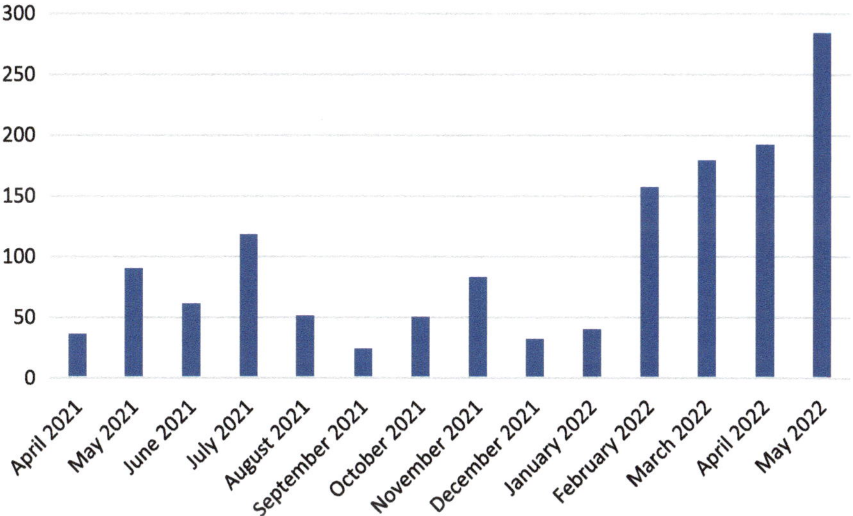

Fig. 9.2 Distribution of the number of patients per month at the National Hospital Centre (CHN) from April 2021 to May 2022

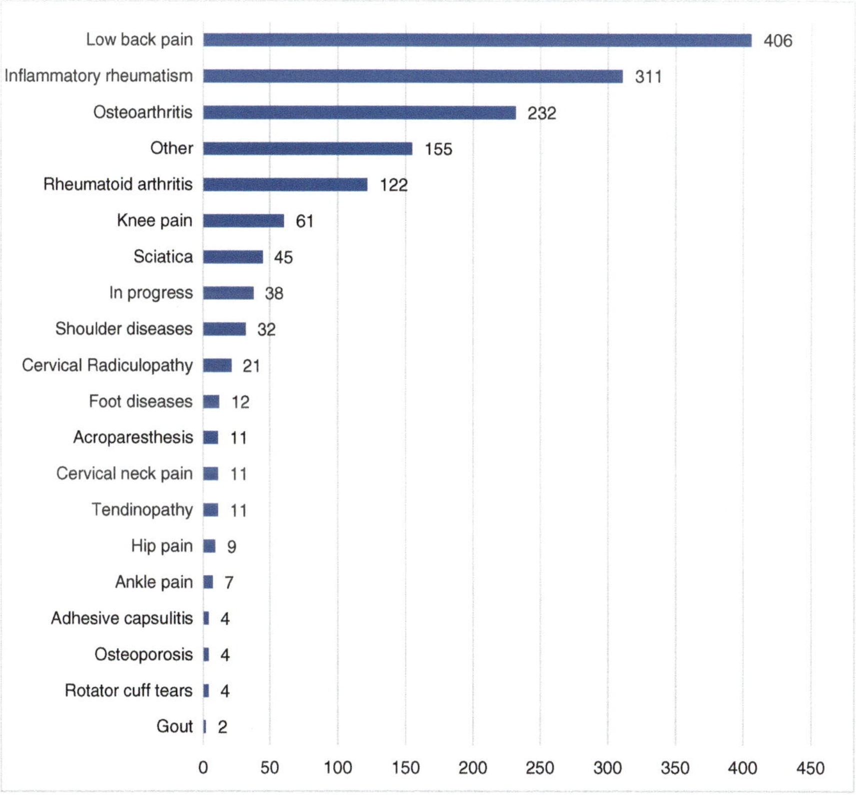

Low back pain 406
Inflammatory rheumatism 311
Osteoarthritis 232
Other 155
Rheumatoid arthritis 122
Knee pain 61
Sciatica 45
In progress 38
Shoulder diseases 32
Cervical Radiculopathy 21
Foot diseases 12
Acroparesthesis 11
Cervical neck pain 11
Tendinopathy 11
Hip pain 9
Ankle pain 7
Adhesive capsulitis 4
Osteoporosis 4
Rotator cuff tears 4
Gout 2
0
50
100
150
200
250
300
350
400
450

Fig. 9.3 Number of rheumatic diseases in the National Hospital Centre (CHN)

Rheumatoid arthritis accounts for approximately 8% of cases (122 patients) in the CHN cohort.

According to a study of 134 patients assessed in Mauritania's first dual-energy X-ray absorptiometry (DXA) unit, the prevalence of osteoporosis was 39.6%, indicating a significant burden of disease [9].

A recent Mauritanian study looked at 25 patients with lupus nephritis. The average age was 35.6 years [10]. Kidney function was often impaired: the mean serum creatinine level was 46.4 mg/L (±53.2), ranging from 5 to 229 mg/L, and it was elevated in about two-thirds of the patients (64%). Antinuclear antibodies were positive in 52% of cases, and anti-double-stranded DNA antibodies were found in 64%. Kidney biopsies most commonly showed class IV lupus nephritis (11 patients) and class III (six patients). Four patients had a combination of class IV and class V disease, while five had mainly vascular and/or tubulointerstitial lesions. Among the 22 patients who were followed regularly, three achieved complete remission, and five achieved partial remission. Among the 22 patients who were followed over time, three achieved complete remission, and five showed partial improvement. Nine patients progressed to end-stage kidney disease, and five died.

9.5 Risk Factors of Rheumatic Diseases

9.5.1 Smoking

In Mauritania, the adult smoking prevalence is approximately 15%, with a strong male predominance (14.8% men vs. 1.4% women) [11]. Tobacco use is also a concern among adolescents. According to the 2009 Global Youth Tobacco Survey (GYTS), 22.6% of students aged 13–15 years reported current tobacco use. Among them, 11.6% smoked cigarettes and 13.1% used other tobacco products [12]. According to the 2006 STEP-Wise survey [13], this prevalence is 4.9% among females and 32% among males. A systematic review of the Global Burden of Disease Study (GBD) 2015 found a prevalence of smoking in Mauritania of 2.4% among women and 14.9% among males [14]. According to a 2016 study among students at the Faculty of Medicine in Nouakchott, the prevalence of smoking is 10.6%, of which 92.3% are men [15].

9.5.2 Obesity

According to the 2006 STEP-Wise survey, 20.9% of Mauritanians were classified as obese, with a marked difference between women (31.5%) and men (8.6%) [13]. Cultural factors may help explain this gap. For many years, higher body weight in women was associated with beauty and social status, although this view has become less common. More recent data point to a continuing rise in obesity. A 2019 study of 150 elderly hypertensive patients from the CNC found that 58% were overweight or obese [16]. Similar findings were reported in a cardiology outpatient cohort, where among 666 patients, 227 were obese (34.08%), of whom 82.4% were women and 17.6% men, with an average weight of 84.6 kg [17].

9.5.3 Physical Inactivity

The 2006 STEP-WISE survey found that 50.7% of people have a low level of physical activity, and 95.7% do not engage in high-intensity physical activity [13]. In Mauritanian society, cultural norms discourage sports participation, particularly among women. A systematic review of cardiovascular risk in the Maghreb reported that 50.6% of the Mauritanian population had insufficient physical activity [18].

9.5.4 Viral Hepatitis

In Mauritania, very few studies have been published on the prevalence of viral hepatitis. Available data suggest that the prevalence of hepatitis B surface antigen ranges from 10% to 24% across different study populations and that hepatitis B and hepatitis D co-infection is present in 31.3% of individuals infected with hepatitis B [19–21]. The prevalence of chronic hepatitis C in the general population is estimated at 0.75% in 2022 [22]. A prospective study of chronic hemodialysis patients at the CHN found a hepatitis B prevalence of 24.3%, hepatitis C prevalence of 5.8%, and hepatitis B–hepatitis C co-infection in 1.9% of cases [23].

9.5.5 Periodontitis

A study on periodontitis in Africa, in which Mauritania was included, found that the prevalence of periodontitis in Africa was among the highest in the world [24]. According to the WHO 2022 Oral Health Country Profile for Mauritania, oral diseases are highly prevalent, with untreated dental caries and periodontal disease affecting a substantial proportion of the population [25].

9.5.6 Menopause

A recent report found 80% of Mauritanian women aged 30–49 were in menopause. The proportion of menopausal women increases with age: from 2% among those aged 30–34, it reaches 6% at 40–41 and 43% at the end of the childbearing period at 48–49 [7].

9.6 Screening Programs for Rheumatic Diseases

Mauritania currently lacks a screening program for rheumatic diseases due to several obstacles. First, there is no dedicated rheumatology service; patients are dispersed across multiple hospitals, making referral from peripheral or intermediate levels difficult in the absence of a central reference centre. Second, the shortage of rheumatologists presents a significant challenge, as each practitioner manages a substantial workload, serving approximately 700,000 inhabitants. Third, access to bone densitometry is extremely limited: there are only three DXA machines available in the private sector, severely restricting osteoporosis detection and management. Fourth, high costs of immunological testing hinder early diagnosis of autoimmune rheumatic conditions, often resulting in delayed diagnosis.

To address these challenges, we propose establishing a well-equipped public rheumatology service in Mauritania that includes at least one DXA machine to assess osteoporosis and serves as the national reference for rheumatic diseases. The rheumatology department has already planned an extension to the CHN, which has been officially inaugurated.

Equally important is investment in human resources; training a cadre of rheumatology specialist nurses is an urgent priority. In addition, screening programs should be designed to be financially accessible, for example, by reducing or waiving the cost of key tests, in order to encourage participation, enable earlier diagnosis, and improve outcomes for patients with rheumatic diseases.

9.7 Diagnosis

Diagnosis of rheumatic diseases in the country involves clinical examination, basic laboratory tests like inflammatory markers, and standard radiography. These so-called essential diagnostic tools are available throughout the country at the intermediate and tertiary levels of the health system. Synovial fluid analysis, including cell count and culture, is limited to a few hospitals in the capital, such as the CHN and some private medical laboratories. The search for crystals in synovial fluid is not available in the public sector, nor are immunological and genetic tests for rheumatological purposes. Some private laboratories can do the immunological tests necessary to diagnose autoimmune diseases on the spot or send genetic tests abroad. However, their high cost makes them inaccessible to most of the population.

Ultrasound machines with lunar probes that could diagnose and monitor rheumatic diseases are available in all hospitals in the capital. One private institution has a musculoskeletal ultrasound machine with a high-frequency "golf club" probe and a General Electric (GE) Lunar Prodigy Advance-type DXA machine.

According to the WHO's Global Health Observatory, Mauritania had 1.53 computed-tomography (CT) units per one million population in 2013 [26]. Two 1.5

tesla MRI machines, which can diagnose spinal and sacroiliac diseases, are available in Nouakchott at the CHN and the HM. Positron-emission tomography (PET) scans are not currently available in Mauritania. Furthermore, to our knowledge, there are no radiologists specializing in musculoskeletal diseases in the country, further limiting diagnostic capacity in rheumatology.

9.8 Management

9.8.1 Pharmacological Treatment

Analgesics WHO classifies analgesics into three levels based on pain intensity: non-opioids (Level 1), weak opioids (Level 2), and strong opioids (Level 3). WHO level 1 and 2 analgesics, including paracetamol, non-steroidal anti-inflammatory drugs (NSAIDs), and weak opioids such as tramadol, are available in Mauritania in standard formulations and dosages similar to those used in other French-speaking countries. WHO level 3 analgesics (strong opioids such as morphine) are available, but only at the National Oncology Centre. The Central Purchasing Office for Medicines, Equipment, and Medical Consumables (CAMEC) supplies these drugs to health facilities across the country [27].

Corticosteroids Prednisone is the corticosteroid of choice for Mauritanian rheumatologists and is marketed as a scored tablet in doses of 5 mg and 20 mg. Hydrocortisone is available in doses of 10 mg and 100 mg and is often used for corticosteroid tapering. Betamethasone injectable suspension is available and is often used for local peri-articular or intra-articular procedures. Methylprednisolone is available in the form of 20 mg, 40 mg, and 120 mg intravenous solution.

Conventional DMARDs (csDMARDs) All three major csDMARDs (methotrexate, leflunomide, and sulfasalazine) are available in Mauritania. Methotrexate is available in the form of a 2.5 mg tablet and a 5 0 mg/2 mL injectable solution. Hydroxychloroquine is also available in a 200 mg dose.

Biological DMARDs (bDMARDs) In Mauritania, the availability of bDMARDs is limited to rituximab (anti-CD20), supplied in 100 mg and 500 mg vials, and adalimumab (anti-TNFα) available as a 40 mg subcutaneous injection. However, the high cost of these medications and the low rate of patient coverage pose significant barriers for rheumatic patients in accessing this type of therapy. Additionally, because of the high prevalence of infectious diseases, particularly tuberculosis, and the low literacy rate in Mauritania (62.2% of women and 71.8% of men [28]), healthcare providers are often hesitant to prescribe adalimumab.

9.8.2 Non-pharmacological Treatment

Rehabilitation In Mauritania, physical rehabilitation is provided by the National Centre for Orthopaedics and Functional Rehabilitation (CNORF), located in Nouakchott. Regional functional rehabilitation units exist in three regional hospitals in the 12 regions of the country outside Nouakchott. In recent years, several privately available rehabilitation centers have also opened in Nouakchott.

Surgery Joint replacement surgery exists in Mauritania, but its high cost and the cultural reluctance toward surgery pose major barriers to access. Furthermore, to our knowledge, there is no hand surgery specialist in the country.

9.9 Research and Education

A core teaching rheumatology program is part of the medical training at the Faculty of Medicine in Nouakchott; however, rheumatology specialization can only be pursued abroad. There are currently seven certified rheumatologists in Mauritania: one trained in Switzerland, two in Senegal, three in Tunisia, and one in Morocco.

Basic research on rheumatic diseases and national/international clinical trials are nonexistent in Mauritania. Medical publications in rheumatology are few; there are a few case reports, most of which concern spinal diseases, published by our fellow surgeons [29–32], and a few by rheumatologists and other physicians [33]. A national training program for rheumatology nurses has yet to be available in Mauritania.

9.10 Cost-Effective Rheumatic Diseases Care

There is no specific national strategy for rheumatic diseases. Instead, Mauritania follows a broader health policy aimed at making care available and accessible to the entire population. Universal health insurance is one of Mauritania's commitments in the framework of the 2030 development objectives [34]. In line with this, 100,000 low-income families have already been insured through the General Delegation for National Solidarity and the Fight against Exclusion "T*aazour*" [35]. More recently, a national system called "El-Mouyassar" was introduced [36]. This initiative aims to provide essential medicines at affordable prices across public health facilities, while also improving both physical and geographical access to care for citizens.

9.11 Opportunities and Challenges

Only 17% of the population is covered by the Caisse Nationale d'Assurance Maladie (CNAM), the national public health insurance Scheme [37], while private insurance covers only 5% of the population. This leaves the majority of Mauritanians without formal insurance coverage.

Despite this gap, the country's economic potential, including its long coastline with one of the world's richest fisheries, as well as its oil, gas, and iron resources, creates opportunities to support the sustainable development of the healthcare system, especially in disciplines such as rheumatology.

Mauritania is not currently a destination for medical tourism. Instead, many Mauritanian patients travel abroad to seek medical care, especially to neighboring countries such as Senegal and Tunisia. This outward medical travel is often driven more by cultural and social factors than by purely medical ones, and paradoxically, it is sometimes practiced by the poorest segments of the population. This phenomenon deserves further study. This phenomenon deserves further study. The nomadic (Bedouin) tradition of Mauritanian society may help explain this pattern, since travel has long been part of daily life, including for health reasons.

Rheumatic patients often face dissatisfaction and inadequate care when their treatment is repeatedly interrupted or prematurely discontinued due to funding constraints. This dissatisfaction is often linked to the chronic nature of the disease and the high cost of diagnostic procedures.

In Mauritania, chronic inflammatory rheumatic disease is often diagnosed at a late stage due to the lack of dedicated infrastructure, low patient income, the high cost of care, and the small number of rheumatologists. The lack of transport facilities, often uncomfortable for rheumatic patients, also contributes to diagnostic delay.

No rheumatology subspecialists are available in Mauritania, nor are there any official subspecialty clinics in rheumatology.

9.12 The Future of Rheumatic Disease Care

There has yet to be an official plan to improve rheumatic disease care in the country. We therefore suggest the following recommendations for strengthening rheumatology care in Mauritania over the next decade.

- Open a rheumatology department in major hospitals that provides care for all rheumatic diseases and is equipped with the necessary diagnostic and therapeutic tools, including at least one ultrasound machine, one DXA machine, a technical platform dedicated to interventional rheumatology, and a pharmacy unit. This service will be modern with an electronic and secure management system (shared medical files, receipts, etc.) and capable of providing ambulatory care, with a functional rehabilitation unit located nearby.

- Create an official society that brings together all the country's rheumatologists and other specialists who care for rheumatic diseases and that is responsible for coordinating and leading the various areas of improvement in Mauritanian rheumatology.
- Train dedicated rheumatology nurses, mainly rheumatology radiology technicians (standard radiography and absorptiometry), through the National School of Health Sciences. Within this broader training strategy, establishing a National Diploma in Rheumatology within the Faculty of Medicine in Nouakchott is required to improve the care of rheumatic diseases in the country. Continuous and postgraduate training should be considered a key pillar in this context.
- Conduct research on the epidemiology of rheumatic diseases in Mauritania, particularly low back pain, osteoarthritis, and osteoporosis. In addition to its steering center based in the rheumatology department, this research should be supported by mobile radiography and DXA units, allowing access to almost the entire population, with periodic medical campaigns carried out to cover nearly the whole country. The main objectives of this project are to assess the exact burden of rheumatic diseases in Mauritania and to promote free care to the population in their communities.
- Provide non-medical transport for rheumatic patients to access the hospital and integrate the cost of this transport into the overall cost so that it can be reimbursed by social security.
- Improve media coverage of rheumatology in Mauritania to increase patient engagement. This can be achieved through local television channels, press coverage, social networks, and establishing a dedicated website. The aim is to raise awareness and encourage more individuals to seek hospital treatment.
- Identify and engage national partners, such as the government, and international partners to finance the care of rheumatic diseases in Mauritania.

9.13 Conclusion

The lack of funding, infrastructure, and qualified personnel in rheumatology poses challenges to providing adequate care for rheumatic patients in Mauritania, a resource-limited country. To overcome these obstacles, it is essential to establish a dedicated rheumatology department and develop training programs for physicians, nurses, and radiology technicians. Although current services remain limited, growing national interest in chronic disease care and improved health planning offer an opportunity to strengthen rheumatology services in the coming years.

Conflict of Interest The authors declare they have no conflicts of interest.

References

1. Trésor Économie. Mauritanie - Présentation générale [Internet]. Paris: Ministère de l'Économie, des Finances et de la Souveraineté industrielle et numérique; [cited 2026 May 11]. Available from: https://www.tresor.economie.gouv.fr/Pays/MR/mauritanie-presentation-generale
2. Larousse. Mauritanie. In: Encyclopédie Larousse en ligne [Internet]. Paris: Larousse; [cited 2026 May 11]. Available from: https://www.larousse.fr/encyclopedie/pays/Mauritanie/132366
3. World Health Organization Regional Office for Africa. Mauritania [Internet]. Brazzaville: WHO Regional Office for Africa; [cited 2026 May 11]. Available from: https://www.afro.who.int/fr/countries/mauritania
4. Agence Nationale de la Statistique et de la Démographie. ANSADE [Internet]. Mauritania: Agence Nationale de la Statistique et de la Démographie; [cited 2026 May 11]. Available from: https://ansade.mr/
5. World Health Organization Regional Office for Africa. Mauritania Plan National De Developpement Sanitaire 2012–2020 [Internet]. Brazzaville: WHO Regional Office for Africa; [cited 2026 May 11]. Available from: https://extranet.who.int/countryplanningcycles/planning-cycle-files/mauritania-plan-national-de-developpement-sanitaire-2012-2020
6. Procédures et Formalités Administratives. Hôpital Cheikh ZAYED (HCZ), Nouakchott [Internet]. Registry 2021-2022; [cited 2026 May 11]. Available from: https://procedures.gov.mr/fr/procedures/categorie/122
7. Agence Nationale de la Statistique et de l'Analyse Démographique et Économique (ANSADE). Enquête Démographique et de Santé de la Mauritanie (EDSM) 2019–2021 [Internet]. Nouakchott: ANSADE; [cited 2026 May 11]. Available from: https://dhsprogram.com/pubs/pdf/FR373/FR373.pdf
8. Procédures et Formalités Administratives. Centre Hospitalier National (CHN), Nouakchott [Internet]. Registry 2021–2022. 2022. [cited 2026 May 11]. Available from: https://procedures.gov.mr/fr/procedures/categorie/121
9. Ould Khatry M. [Bone status of 134 patients received in Mauritania's first bone densitom]. Thesis:Medicine: Cheikh Anta Diop University of Dakar; 2016, p. 141.
10. Lemrabott M, Mah SM, Awa J, Sidi Hamoud MY, Meyine M, Abed A, El Atigh A, Ehbibi B, Izidbih Y, Sidi Aly A. Lupus nephropathy in Mauritania: A clinical and longitudinal study from the National Hospital Center of Nouakchott. Cureus. 2025;17(8):e90636. https://doi.org/10.7759/cureus.90636.
11. The Tobacco Atlas. Mauritania — country factsheet [Internet]. Atlanta (GA): Vital Strategies; 2022 [cited 2026 May 11]. Available from: https://tobaccoatlas.org/factsheets/mauritania/
12. World Health Organization. Global youth tobacco survey (GYTS) fact sheet—Mauritania [Internet]. Geneva: World Health Organization; [cited 2026 May 11]. Available from: https://www.who.int/publications/m/item/2009-gyts-fact-sheet-mauritania
13. World Health Organization. STEPwise approach to surveillance (STEPS)—Mauritania [Internet]. Geneva: World Health Organization; [cited 2026 May 11]. Available from: https://www.who.int/publications/m/item/2006-steps-country-report-mauritania
14. GBD 2015 Tobacco Collaborators. Smoking prevalence and attributable disease burden in 195 countries and territories, 1990–2015: a systematic analysis from the Global Burden of Disease Study 2015. Lancet. 2017;389:1885–906.
15. Sidi Mohamed Mohamed Saleh A. Smoking among students at the Faculty of Medicine in Nouakchott. Thesis: Medicine: University of Nouakchott Al Aasriya; 2016. p. 21.
16. Ba H, Yahia F, Ba F, Camara S, Kane A, Sarr SA, et al. Epidemiological, clinical and progressive aspects of arterial hypertension in older patients in Nouakchott (Mauritania). Tunis Med. 2019;97:1219–23.
17. Ba ML. Obesity in Mauritania: epidemiologic aspects. Tunis Med. 2000;78:671–6.
18. Mrabet HE, Mlouki I, Nouira S, Hmaied O, Ben Abdelaziz A, El Mhamdi S. Cardiovascular risk factors in the Maghreb. A systematic review. Tunis Med. 2021;99:120–8.

19. Lahlali M, Abid H, Lamine A, Lahmidani N, El Yousfi M, Benajah D, et al. Epidemiology of viral hepatitis in the Maghreb. Tunis Med. 2018;96:606–19.
20. Rui WZ, Lo Baïdy B, N'Diaye M. Hepatitis B virus infection in the school milieu of Kiffa and Selibaby, Mauritania. Bull Soc Pathol Exot. 1998;91:247–8.
21. Salem MLO, Abdalla AS, Mohamed GS. Hepatitis B and delta co-infection: prevalence and serological characteristics in Mauritania. J Gen Med Clin Pract. 2022;5(1):1–9. https://doi.org/10.31579/2639-4162/062.
22. Coalition for Global Hepatitis Elimination. Mauritania—data profile [Internet]. Atlanta (GA): Coalition for Global Hepatitis Elimination; 2022 [cited 2026 May 11]. Available from: https://www.globalhep.org/data-profiles/countries/mauritania
23. Salem MLO, Bellamech ME, Mohamed MS, Mohamed GS. Prevalence and clinico-biological characteristics of viral hepatitis B and C in chronic hemodialysis patients at the National Hospital Center of Nouakchott, Mauritania. Arch Nephrol Urol. 2023;6(1):1–7. https://doi.org/10.31579/2690-4861/228.
24. Franklin ER. Periodontal diseases are a grave socio-economic problem in Black Africa. Odontostomatol Trop. 1978;1:16–28.
25. World Health Organization. Global database on the implementation of food and nutrition action [Internet]. Geneva: World Health Organization; [cited 2026 May 11]. Available from: https://cdn.who.int/media/docs/default-source/country-profiles/oral-health/oral-health-mrt-2022-country-profile.pdf?sfvrsn=47da0e6b_6&download=true
26. World Health Organization. Medical device: computed tomography units (per million population), Total density [internet]. Geneva: World Health Organization; [cited 2026 May 11]. Available from: https://www.who.int/data/gho/data/indicators/indicator-details/GHO/total-density-per-million-population-computed-tomography-units
27. Centrale d'Achat des Médicaments, Equipements et Consommables Médicaux (CAMEC). Les diverses sources d'approvisionnement [Internet]. Nouakchott: CAMEC; [cited 2026 May 11]. Available from: http://camec.mr/
28. UNESCO Institute for Lifelong Learning (UIL). GAL country profiles: Mauritania [Internet]. Hamburg: UIL; 2022 [cited 2026 May 11]. Available from: https://www.uil.unesco.org/sites/default/files/medias/files/2022/11/gal_country_profiles_mauritania.pdf
29. Biha N, Ghaber SM, Hacen MM, Collet C. Osteoporosis-Pseudoglioma in a Mauritanian child due to a novel mutation in LRP5. Case Rep Genet. 2016;2016:9814928.
30. Boushab BM, Kone N, Basco LK. Contribution of computed tomography scan to the diagnosis of spinal tuberculosis in 14 cases in Assaba, Mauritania. Radiol Res Pract. 2019;2019:7298301. https://doi.org/10.1155/2019/7298301.
31. Diagana M, Traore H, Badiane SB. Tuberculosis spondylodiscitis in a neurological service in Nouakchott. Dakar Med. 2000;45:185–7. French
32. Noukhoum K, Outouma S, Ahmed-Salem KSS-M, Daouda Sissoko AH. Staged lumbar spondylolysis: report of two cases. Rev Mar Rhum. 2018;44:65–7.
33. Ahmed Ghassem M, Biyi A, Djossou JH, Hamza T, Majjad A, Achemlal L. Hypertrophic osteoarthropathy associated with probable smear-negative pulmonary tuberculosis. Case Rep Rheumatol. 2022;2022:5429138. https://doi.org/10.1155/2022/5429138.
34. International Labour Organization. Politique nationale de santé à l'horizon 2030. [Internet]. Geneva: International Labour Organization; [cited 2026 May 11]. Available from: https://libguides.ilo.org/2030-agenda-fr
35. Primature. The President of the Republic supervises the distribution of health insurance cards for the benefit of 100,000 needy families. [Internet]. Nouakchott: Primature; [cited 2026 May 11]. Available from: https://www.primature.gov.mr/ar/node/339

36. Agence Mauritanienne d'Information (AMI). Création d'un système national d'accès aux soins et aux médicaments essentiels de qualités dénommé « EL MOUYASSAR ». [Internet]. Nouakchott: AMI; [cited 2026 May 11]. Available from: https://fr.ami.mr/Depeche-64712.html
37. Al-Mahboubi M, Atigh S. Right to health in Mauritania. Nouakchott: Arab NGO Network for Development (ANND); 2023 [cited 2026 May 11]. Available from: https://annd.org/uploads/publications/Right_to_health_in_Mauritania_Mohamed_Al-Mahboubi_Sidina_Atigh_En.pdf

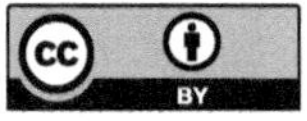

Chapter 10
Rheumatic Diseases in Morocco

Ihsane Hmamouchi, Bouchra Amine, Ibtissam Bentaleb, Abir Souissi, Salma Zemrani, and Rachid Bahiri

Abstract Morocco has approximately 400 registered rheumatologists serving a population of 37.7 million, corresponding to a low workforce density of about one rheumatologist per 100,000 inhabitants. This shortage is particularly concerning in the context of population aging and the anticipated increase in the burden of rheumatic diseases. The Moroccan health system includes both public and private sectors, with the private sector expanding rapidly, particularly in regions such as Casablanca-Settat and Rabat-Salé-Kénitra.

Rheumatology practice is represented nationally by the Moroccan Society of Rheumatology (SMR), which brings together specialists and practitioners interested in musculoskeletal diseases. The SMR plays a central role in advancing clinical practice, education, research, and advocacy and has progressively strengthened its organizational structure and strategic capacity. Key initiatives include training

I. Hmamouchi (✉)
Faculty of Medicine, Health Sciences Research Center (CReSS), International University of Rabat (UIR), Rabat, Morocco

Rheumatology Unit, Temara Hospital Center, Temara, Morocco
e-mail: ihsane.hmamouchi@gmail.com

B. Amine · R. Bahiri
Department of Rheumatology A, El Ayachi Hospital, Ibn Sina University Hospital, Salé, Morocco
e-mail: amine_bouchra@yahoo.fr; bahirirachid@yahoo.fr

I. Bentaleb
Faculty of Medicine and Pharmacy of Rabat, Rabat, Morocco
e-mail: ibtissam.bentaleb1718@gmail.com

A. Souissi
Rheumatology Unit, Mohammed VI Hospital Center, Al Hoceima, Morocco
e-mail: souissi.abir12@gmail.com

S. Zemrani
Department of Rheumatology A, El Ayachi Hospital, Ibn Sina University Hospital, Salé, Morocco
e-mail: medsalma3@gmail.com

K. A. Alnaqbi, G. Aldabie (eds.), *Rheumatic Diseases in the Arab World*,
https://doi.org/10.1007/978-981-92-0967-5_10

programs in musculoskeletal ultrasound; the Moroccan Registry of Biological Therapies in Rheumatoid Diseases (RBSMR), one of the earliest registries of its kind in Africa; patient education programs to improve long-term disease management; and national public awareness campaigns.

Despite substantial progress over the past two decades, important challenges remain. Priority areas for future development include increasing the rheumatology workforce, establishing centers of excellence, and expanding research programs tailored to the specific epidemiological and health care needs of the Moroccan population.

Keywords Morocco · Rheumatology · Rheumatic Diseases · Arthritis · Registry · Health Workforce · Registries · Health Services Accessibility · Biological Therapy

10.1 Country Demographics

Morocco, officially the Kingdom of Morocco, is a North African country strategically located at the crossroads of Europe and Africa. It covers approximately 711,000 km^2 and has a coastline of 3466 km along both the Atlantic Ocean and the Mediterranean Sea. Islam is the predominant religion, and Arabic and Amazigh are the official languages according to the 2011 Constitution [1]. This geographic and sociolinguistic positioning has implications for population diversity, mobility, and health system organization.

The population reflects a complex historical and genetic background, predominantly of Arab and Amazigh origin, with additional Mediterranean, European, African, and Jewish influences resulting from long-standing population mixing in the region [1, 2]. As of 2026, the population is estimated at approximately 36.8 million, with a slight female predominance (51%). Morocco is undergoing a demographic transition characterized by a declining fertility rate (2.26 births per woman) and a reduced annual population growth rate of around 1%. Despite these changes, the population remains relatively young, with a median age of 29.8 years. Urbanization is increasing, with 63% of the population living in urban areas, highlighting evolving patterns of health needs and service utilization [3].

Administratively, Morocco is divided into 12 regions, further subdivided into 75 prefectures and provinces, and 1538 municipalities, including both urban and rural communes. This territorial organization plays a critical role in the decentralization of health services and in shaping regional disparities in access to care.

10.2 Country Healthcare System

The Moroccan health system is characterized by a mixed public–private structure. The public sector encompasses institutions, infrastructure, and human resources dedicated to health promotion, disease prevention, and the delivery of care. It includes seven university hospital centers located in Rabat, Casablanca, Fez, Oujda, Tangier, Marrakech, and Agadir, as well as 149 public hospitals and approximately 12,000 physicians. In parallel, a separate military health system comprises six hospitals and one medical center. Public healthcare delivery is organized across three levels: primary care, mainly provided by general practitioners and nurses in regional health centers; secondary care, delivered in regional hospitals offering a broad range of medical specialties, including rheumatology; and tertiary care, concentrated in university hospitals and academic medical centers in major urban areas.

In the context of health system strengthening, Morocco is undertaking a substantial expansion of its hospital infrastructure. This includes the construction of 29 new hospitals, including university-affiliated facilities, with a projected capacity of 3354 beds. Additionally, 21 regional and provincial hospital centers, representing an extra capacity of 3254 beds, are currently under construction or undergoing rehabilitation, reflecting ongoing efforts to improve territorial equity in access to care.

The private sector has experienced rapid growth and now comprises more than 360 private clinics, predominantly concentrated in the Casablanca-Settat and Rabat-Salé-Kénitra regions. It employs approximately 13,500 physicians and accounts for an estimated capacity of over 10,000 beds, playing an increasingly important role in healthcare provision, particularly in urban and peri-urban settings.

Health financing in Morocco has undergone major reform with the implementation of universal health coverage (UHC). The Mandatory Health Insurance scheme assurance maladie obligatoire (AMO) has been progressively extended to cover the entire population, including previously uninsured and vulnerable groups. This reform has led to the integration of populations formerly covered under the Medical Assistance Scheme Régime d'Assistance Médicale (RAMED) into the AMO framework, marking a shift from a fragmented system to a more unified model. The AMO now covers both private sector employees through the National Social Security Fund (CNSS) and public sector employees through the National Fund of Social Welfare Organizations (CNOPS), while its extension aims to improve financial protection, reduce out-of-pocket expenditures, and enhance equitable access to healthcare services across the country [4].

10.3 Rheumatology Health Services

10.3.1 Rheumatology Workforce

Morocco faces a severe shortage of rheumatology specialists. The country has approximately 400 qualified rheumatologists, of whom 59% are women, serving a population of more than 37 million people. This corresponds to a very low workforce density of approximately one rheumatologist per 100,000 inhabitants. This shortage is particularly concerning given the aging population and the expected increase in the burden of rheumatic diseases, which is expected to generate growing demand for specialized care [5].

Currently, nationally representative data are insufficient to draw firm conclusions regarding pediatric rheumatology services and disease burden in Morocco.

10.3.2 Availability of Specialized Rheumatology Nurses

At present, Morocco does not have formally trained rheumatology nurses, and rheumatology care is primarily delivered by physicians without specialized nursing support.

10.3.3 Accreditation and Center of Excellence for Rheumatology

Currently, Morocco does not have accredited centers of excellence for rheumatology that follow the guidelines established by international bodies such as the European Alliance of Associations for Rheumatology (EULAR).

10.3.4 Referral System for Rheumatology Care

Morocco operates a universal public referral system; however, it is not structured by medical specialty. As a result, there is no formal referral pathway for patients with rheumatic diseases, and access to rheumatology care mostly depends on general practitioner recognition and local practice patterns.

10.3.5 Academic Rheumatology in the Public and Private Sectors

More than 30 rheumatology professors are currently affiliated with university hospitals in Morocco, and about one-third of them are military rheumatologists. The rest of the faculty are mainly based in public university hospitals. Teaching positions in rheumatology in the private sector have only recently been established.

10.4 Official Rheumatology Society and Associations

The Moroccan Society of Rheumatology (Société Marocaine de Rhumatologie, SMR) is the only national professional society representing rheumatologists in Morocco [6]. Founded in 1980, the SMR brings together Moroccan rheumatologists and practitioners interested in musculoskeletal (MSK) diseases. Its mission includes advancing the study of rheumatic and MSK disorders, promoting scientific knowledge, providing expert input on epidemiology, prevention, legislation, and patient information, and responding to requests from national and international organizations.

With more than 400 members, nearly all of whom are practicing rheumatologists in Morocco, the SMR serves as a central platform for professional exchange and collaboration. Over time, the society has progressively strengthened its organizational structure to support the development of the specialty. Academic, hospital-based, and private sector rheumatologists are represented by an executive board comprising five elected members, who are responsible for implementing strategic and administrative decisions.

The SMR's primary objectives include promoting scientific progress in rheumatology and supporting education, training, and continuing professional development. The society works in close coordination with regional rheumatology associations, including the Moroccan Association dedicated to Rheumatoid Arthritis (AMP), the Moroccan Association for Research in Rheumatology and Social Assistance to Rheumatic Patients (AMRAR), the Group of Imaging in Rheumatology (GIRHUM), the Association of Rheumatologists of the Public Health Sector of the North (ARNP), the Association of Private Rheumatologists of Rabat (ARR), and the Association of Rheumatology of Marrakech (ARM).

In recent years, the SMR has undertaken substantial efforts to modernize its governance and activities. These initiatives include the recruitment of full-time administrative staff, establishment of a permanent office, revision of its statutes, creation of a board of directors with biennial elections, and expansion of collaborations with international societies, including the French Society of Rheumatology (SFR), the Arab League of Associations for Rheumatology (ArLAR), and the Tunisian League Against Rheumatism (LITAR). Digital activities have been strengthened through webinars, online meetings, and educational courses, and the annual national SMR congress has been significantly upgraded. The congress now attracts more than 300 participants annually and includes plenary lectures, oral presentations, and poster sessions, bringing together rheumatologists across generations and practice settings.

In addition, the SMR has initiated and supported several innovative projects, some of which are completed and others are ongoing. These include the nationwide implementation of MSK ultrasound training for rheumatologists; the Moroccan Registry of Biological Therapies in Rheumatoid Diseases (RBSMR), a large multicenter national registry and one of the earliest initiatives of its kind in Africa; publication of the Revue Marocaine de Rhumatologie, the society's official journal with over 20 years of continuous activity; modernization of the SMR website; creation of a national college of rheumatology educators (CORUM) to harmonize academic training across university hospitals; development of regular webinars and monthly online courses for rheumatology residents; a multicenter therapeutic education program aimed at improving the management and follow-up of patients with chronic rheumatic diseases; and annual national media campaigns to raise public awareness of rheumatic conditions.

10.5 Diagnostic Services for Rheumatic Diseases in Morocco

10.5.1 Laboratory Services

In Morocco, laboratory services are provided by both public and private sectors. At the national level, reference institutions such as the National Institute of Hygiene and the Pasteur Institute play a key role in performing advanced immunological and genetic tests. However, there are noticeable differences in laboratory practices, particularly regarding the reagents and assays used across public and private laboratories. Genetic tests relevant to rheumatology, including HLA-B27 typing and Mediterranean fever (MEFV) gene analysis, are available in the country. All immunological tests and HLA antigen tests are available in Morocco for patients with health insurance or with a government-issued indigence card.

10.5.2 Imaging Services

Morocco has seven public university hospitals equipped with radiology departments. Within the public sector, available imaging resources include approximately 129 computed tomography (CT) scanners, 24 magnetic resonance imaging (MRI) units, 14 bone densitometry (DXA) scanners, and two positron emission tomography (PET) scanners. In addition, the private sector includes more than 283 radiology centers distributed across the country.

In recent years, Morocco has made substantial progress in the use of MSK ultrasound (MSUS) for the diagnosis and monitoring of rheumatic diseases. The Moroccan College of Rheumatology has developed a structured national training program in MSUS and has organized regular national symposia and courses to expand rheumatologists' expertise in this technique [7]. The national RHUMECHO certification program, established in Rabat in 2010, provides training to approximately 25 rheumatologists annually.

Currently, nearly 70% of Moroccan rheumatologists have received formal training in MSUS, and more than 50% use MSK ultrasound devices in their clinical practice.

10.6 Management of Rheumatic Diseases in Morocco

10.6.1 Availability of and Access to Antirheumatic Medications

In Morocco, the therapeutic landscape for chronic inflammatory diseases has expanded substantially with the availability of a broad range of conventional synthetic disease-modifying anti-rheumatic drugs (DMARDs), biologics, biosimilars, and targeted synthetic agents. Conventional synthetic DMARDs available in clinical practice are methotrexate, azathioprine, leflunomide, hydroxychloroquine, sulfasalazine, cyclosporine, tacrolimus, and cyclophosphamide. Several originator biologic agents are available, such as golimumab, certolizumab, tocilizumab, ustekinumab, secukinumab, ixekizumab, and guselkumab. Biosimilars comprise three adalimumab products (Hulio, Amjevita, and Yuflyma), one etanercept biosimilar (Nepexto), one infliximab biosimilar (Remsima), and one rituximab biosimilar (Zelva). In addition, targeted synthetic DMARDs include Janus kinase (JAK) inhibitors such as tofacitinib, baricitinib, and upadacitinib. These therapies are available in both public and private healthcare facilities, although their use may vary across institutions.

Although the cost of biologic therapies remains high, access is partially supported through national funding mechanisms. A proportion of biologic treatments is allocated to patients covered by the Medical Assistance Scheme (Régime d'Assistance Médicale, RAMED) and distributed across university hospital centers. Furthermore, social health insurance funds in Morocco provide reimbursement for biologic therapies and targeted therapies, allowing broad coverage for eligible patients.

10.6.2 Access to and Collaboration with Other Specialties

As of 2022, Morocco had more than 500 registered orthopedic surgeons practicing across both public and private sectors, in addition to numerous physiotherapy and occupational therapy centers nationwide. While these services are generally accessible to patients with rheumatic diseases, they often operate independently. Formal multidisciplinary care pathways involving coordinated collaboration between rheumatologists, orthopedic surgeons, physiotherapists, and occupational therapists remain limited.

10.7 Overview of Rheumatic Diseases

10.7.1 Juvenile Idiopathic Arthritis (JIA)

Data on the epidemiology of JIA in Morocco remain limited, with only a small number of hospital-based studies available. JIA accounted for 2.2% of inflammatory rheumatic diseases seen in consultation or hospitalization [8]. Reported mean age at diagnosis ranges from 6 to 15 years, with sex distribution varying according to JIA subtype. Diagnostic delay has been reported and appears to be influenced by socioeconomic factors and geographic barriers affecting access to specialized rheumatology care [8–13].

Within these Moroccan cohorts, polyarticular and oligoarticular JIA are the most frequently observed clinical subtypes [9, 13, 14]. Structural joint damage is a major concern. In a cross-sectional study of 112 patients, hip involvement was reported in 33% of cases, predominantly bilateral (85%), and present at disease onset in 11%. Hip involvement was more frequent in polyarticular, enthesitis-related, and systemic JIA, with radiographic erosions or joint space narrowing observed in nearly half of affected patients. Growth abnormalities and ankylosis were also reported in a subset of patients [14].

Extra-articular manifestations have been described, particularly uveitis. In a Moroccan series of 30 children with JIA, uveitis was identified in four patients, often bilateral and associated with severe ocular complications, including cataract, glaucoma, elevated intraocular pressure with vision loss, band keratopathy, and bilateral posterior synechiae. No significant association was observed between uveitis and disease activity or quality of life in this cohort [10].

MSK imaging plays an important role in disease assessment, particularly for detecting subclinical synovitis [15]. While clinical evaluation of joint damage in JIA is challenging, Moroccan studies have highlighted the value of advanced imaging. MRI of the wrist demonstrated a higher prevalence of bone erosions and synovitis in children with JIA compared with healthy controls, with synovitis correlating strongly with disease activity and functional impairment [16].

Although more Moroccan studies are needed to comprehensively explore comorbidities and disease impact in JIA, available data highlight a substantial burden [17]. Overweight and obesity were common, affecting more than 60% of children in one cohort, and were associated with higher disease activity and functional limitation [8]. Reduced bone mineral density has also been reported, particularly in patients with systemic JIA and higher cumulative corticosteroid exposure [13].

The impact of JIA on quality of life has been well documented in Moroccan cohorts. In particular, validated Moroccan versions of the Childhood Health Assessment Questionnaire (CHAQ) and the Juvenile Arthritis Quality-of-Life Questionnaire (JAQQ) have demonstrated good psychometric properties [18, 19]. Nearly half of children in one series reported impaired health-related quality of life, with disease activity, hip involvement, and diagnostic delay being key determinants [12, 20]. School absenteeism and sleep disturbances were also significantly more frequent among children with JIA compared with healthy controls and were closely linked to pain and disease activity [9, 11].

Biologic therapies are available in Morocco, but access remains limited. In a single-center Moroccan study, tocilizumab was the most frequently prescribed biologic agent, followed by etanercept and adalimumab. After 1 year of treatment, approximately one-third of patients achieved inactive disease. However, lymphopenia and infectious complications, including tuberculosis, were reported, highlighting the need for careful monitoring [21]. Access to biologic therapy is influenced by hospital availability, health insurance coverage, and geographic proximity to tertiary care centers [21].

Beyond clinical outcomes, JIA also has a significant psychosocial impact on families.

In a Moroccan cross-sectional study of parents caring for children with JIA, caregiving was associated with substantial negative impacts, including disruption of daily activities, financial strain, and health problems, particularly among mothers who were predominantly unemployed and had low literacy levels. Despite these challenges, caregiving was also reported to enhance caregivers' self-esteem [22].

Data on the direct medical costs of JIA management in Morocco are limited. In a retrospective study conducted between January 2017 and December 2017 and focused on 118 cases of the infantile form of rare diseases at the Children's Hospital of Rabat, JIA had an annual cost of 3,684,193.17 Moroccan Dirhams (MAD), i.e., an average cost of 56,978.22 MAD.

In summary, Moroccan data highlight the substantial burden of JIA in terms of joint damage, comorbidities, and quality-of-life impairment, while emphasizing ongoing challenges related to delayed diagnosis, limited access to advanced therapies, and the need for broader national data.

10.7.2 Rheumatoid Arthritis (RA)

Data on the epidemiology of RA in Morocco remain limited, and population-based incidence or prevalence studies are lacking. The prevalence of RA is estimated at 1% in developed countries and 0.3–0.5% in developing countries [23, 24]. Epidemiological studies conducted on the African continent have reported an estimated prevalence of 0.36% in 1990 [25]. Based on expert estimates and hospital-based cohorts, the number of patients with RA in Morocco is estimated to range from 200,000 to 250,000, although mortality data are unavailable [23–26].

Moroccan studies consistently report a female predominance, with women representing approximately 80–88% of affected patients. The mean age at disease onset ranges from 45 to 55 years across cohorts, including the IPSOS survey, the QUEST-RA study, the ESPRIM and COMORA studies, and data from the Moroccan biotherapy registry (RBSMR) [23–29].

Clinical characteristics vary according to serological status. In a Moroccan cross-sectional study, seropositive RA was associated with more severe disease, including higher rates of synovitis, joint deformities, and radiographic damage compared with seronegative RA [30]. Genetic susceptibility has also been suggested, with an association between RA and HLA-DRB1*04 reported in Moroccan patients with rheumatoid factor–positive disease [31].

Several Moroccan studies have examined modifiable factors that influence disease severity. Obesity has been associated with higher disease activity and greater structural damage, particularly among women [27]. In contrast, smoking appears to play a limited role in Moroccan cohorts, likely reflecting the low prevalence of tobacco use among women [30, 32, 33]. In a post hoc analysis of the COMORA database, which included 3439 patients with RA, no association was observed between smoking status and seropositivity among the 200 Moroccan participants ($p = 0.63$; OR = 0.67, 95% CI = 0.13–3.42). This finding may be explained by the marked female predominance and very low smoking rates in this population [33].

Seasonal and environmental factors have also been explored. It has been hypothesized that the winter onset of RA may be associated with greater disease severity and joint damage, potentially mediated by seasonal infections and enhanced protein citrullination. In a Moroccan retrospective longitudinal study of 117 patients with RA, no association was found between weather parameters and objective disease activity measures across seasons. However, pain intensity during summer was negatively correlated with minimum temperature and atmospheric pressure, suggesting that meteorological factors, particularly extreme temperatures, may influence pain perception rather than inflammatory activity [34].

In conclusion, available data highlight a substantial burden of RA in Morocco, characterized by female predominance, middle-aged onset, and significant disease severity. However, the absence of population-based studies underscores the need for national epidemiological data to better inform healthcare planning and resource allocation.

10.7.3 Spondyloarthritis (SpA)

SpA represents a significant cause of disability in young adults and is associated with substantial functional, socioeconomic, and quality-of-life burden. Early diagnosis and appropriate management are essential to improve long-term outcomes [35].

In North Africa, including Morocco, epidemiological data on SpA remain limited, and population-based incidence or prevalence studies are lacking. Nevertheless, SpA is widely recognized as a public health concern due to its apparent frequency and clinical severity [36–38]. Available data suggest geographic variation in disease expression, with ankylosing spondylitis (AS) remaining the predominant SpA subtype in Morocco. In recent multicenter studies from Morocco, axial forms accounted for approximately 65–80% of SpA cases [39, 40]. Mortality data specific to SpA in Morocco are currently unavailable. In a multinational multicenter study of patients with inflammatory back pain, the prevalence of non-radiographic axial spondyloarthritis varied by region, with the lowest prevalence in Africa (16.0%) and the highest in Europe (29.5%) and Asia (36.5%) [39].

SpA typically affects young adults, with most Moroccan studies reporting disease onset in the third or fourth decade of life and a mean age at diagnosis between 38 and 40 years [39, 41, 42]. Earlier studies demonstrated a marked male predominance; however, more recent Moroccan data suggest a narrowing sex gap, with female patients increasingly recognized, particularly in non-radiographic and peripheral disease forms [41–44]. Women tend to present with more peripheral symptoms and fewer radiographic spinal changes. However, there are no notable differences between the two sexes, neither in the prevalence of extra-articular manifestations nor in the activity of the BASDAI and BASFI diseases [44].

Genetic susceptibility plays an important role in SpA [45]. The prevalence of HLA-B27 in the general North African population is estimated at approximately 4% [46]. In Moroccan SpA cohorts, HLA-B27 positivity ranges from about 45% to 65%, with variation related to regional and ethnic composition [39, 40, 46, 47]. For example, cohorts from Marrakesh, which include a higher proportion of Sahrawi and Berber populations, report HLA-B27 frequencies different from those in cohorts from Rabat, where Arab and Caucasian ancestries are more prevalent [46, 47]. In Moroccan patients, HLA-B27 positivity has been associated with earlier disease onset, higher disease activity, increased frequency of uveitis and hip involvement, and greater use of biologic therapy [39, 41].

Among environmental and lifestyle factors, smoking and obesity have been explored in Moroccan cohorts. Smoking is more prevalent among male patients and has shown inconsistent associations with disease activity and functional impairment across studies [48, 49]. Obesity, however, appears more consistently linked to higher disease activity, functional limitation, and inflammatory burden, in line with international data [50–52].

Overall, Moroccan studies highlight SpA as a disabling condition predominantly affecting young adults, with axial and peripheral disease forms, significant genetic contribution, and modifiable lifestyle factors influencing disease severity. The lack of national epidemiological data emphasizes the need for population-based studies to better guide healthcare planning and optimize patient care.

10.8 Screening Programs for Rheumatic Diseases

For the moment, Morocco has no official screening programs for patients with chronic inflammatory rheumatic diseases (RA, SpA) due to the current health situation, but the project is still under discussion with the medical societies.

10.9 Research and Education

10.9.1 Rheumatology Training Programs

In Morocco, there are currently seven university hospital departments providing rheumatology training, collectively graduating approximately 30 rheumatologists each year. A rheumatologist is a physician who, after completing 6 years of medical school and 1 year of internship, enters a four-year postgraduate training program in rheumatology. This specialty training also includes multidisciplinary rotations in neurology, internal medicine, and intensive care.

10.9.2 Rheumatologist-Driven Research Initiatives

Rheumatology in Morocco has demonstrated steady progress in clinical expertise, research activity, and scientific output over the past two decades. Moroccan rheumatologists have contributed substantially to the international literature across a wide range of rheumatic diseases, mainly through investigator-initiated studies, hospital-based cohorts, and national registries.

More than 120 publications have addressed RA, including real-world data from the Moroccan Biotherapy Registry (RBSMR), such as studies evaluating the first biologic choice in RA and the prevalence of latent tuberculosis before starting biologic therapy [29, 53, 54]. SpA, particularly AS, has also been widely studied, with more than 70 publications covering clinical and radiologic phenotypes, late-onset disease, difficult-to-treat SpA, diagnostic and therapeutic strategies, and the real-world effectiveness, treatment retention, and safety of biologic therapies [55–62].

Osteoporosis is another major area of research, with approximately 90 publications addressing bone mineral density, cardiovascular comorbidities, and quality-of-life assessment tools validated in Arabic-speaking populations, including the European Foundation for Osteoporosis quality-of-life questionnaire [63, 64]. Additional national research efforts include more than 20 publications on gout, such as the Moroccan Society of Rheumatology national survey on gout management [65], and over 70 publications on osteoarthritis, including studies evaluating predictors of clinically meaningful improvement using validated outcome measures [66].

In summary, these rheumatologist-driven research initiatives reflect a sustained academic commitment and have generated valuable region-specific evidence.

10.9.3 Rheumatology Nursing Programs

There are no formal rheumatology nursing programs in Morocco.

10.10 Economic Burden of Biologic Therapies in Rheumatic Disease Care

A Moroccan study using data from the Moroccan Biotherapy Registry (RBSMR) evaluated the annual direct costs of biologic therapies among patients with RA. The total expenditure on biologic agents was substantial, amounting to approximately €one million for the treatment of 197 patients. The median annual cost per patient was €1665, with reported costs ranging from €1472 to €9879 per patient per year [67].

To estimate the annual direct costs of biologic therapies in SpA and to identify factors associated with these expenses, another Moroccan study analyzed one-year data from 89 patients with SpA enrolled in the RBSMR. The findings were similarly high, with a mean annual biologic therapy cost of €9569.39 per patient and a total annual cost of €851,675.98 for this cohort [68].

These costs are particularly high in the context of a developing country such as Morocco and are disproportionate to national income levels. The Moroccan inter-professional guaranteed minimum wage (SMIG) is approximately €263 per month, while the average monthly salary across sectors is estimated at €222 [68]. This economic disparity has prompted the development of national strategies to improve the governance and sustainability of biologic therapy expenditures. One of the most important ongoing initiatives is the expansion of universal health coverage to ensure equitable access to biologic therapies for all eligible patients [68].

10.11 Conclusion

Despite considerable progress over the past two decades, significant challenges remain in improving care for patients with rheumatic diseases in Morocco. Continued efforts are needed to expand the rheumatology workforce, strengthen formal continuing medical education, establish accredited centers of excellence, broaden social security coverage, and enhance access to comprehensive care services. In addition, the development and support of locally relevant research programs are essential to generate evidence tailored to the needs of the Moroccan population.

Conflict of Interest Declaration The authors declared no conflict of interest.

References

1. Morocco. In: Wikipedia: The Free Encyclopedia [Internet]. [cited 2026 Jan 5]. Available from: https://en.wikipedia.org/wiki/Morocco.

2. Kingdom of Morocco Government, Kingdom of Morocco. Constitution of the Kingdom of Morocco. Rabat: Official Bulletin; 2011. [cited 2026 Jun 14]. Available at: https://www.constituteproject.org/constitution/Morocco_2011.
3. U.S. Department of Commerce. Healthcare Resource Guide: Morocco [Internet]. Washington (DC); 2024 [cited 2026 Jun 14]. Available from: https://www.trade.gov/healthcare-resource-guide-morocco.
4. Universal Healthcare in Morocco. New York: SDG16+; 2024. [cited 2026 Jun 14]. Available from: https://www.sdg16.plus/policies/universal-healthcare-morocco/.
5. The World Bank. Morocco—Country Data [Internet]. 2025 [cited 2025 Nov 3]. Available from: https://data.worldbank.org/country/morocco.
6. Société Marocaine de Rhumatologie (SMR). Official website [Internet]. Rabat (Morocco): Société Marocaine de Rhumatologie; [cited 2026 Jan 5]. Available from: https://smr.ma/.
7. Bouhouche L, Tazi LH, Rostom S, Amine B, Bahiri R. Current state of musculoskeletal ultrasound training and implementation among rheumatologists in Arab countries. J Rheumatol Arthritic Dis. 2017;2(4):1–5.
8. Amine B, Ibn Yacoub Y, Rostom S, Hajjaj-Hassouni N. Prevalence of overweight among Moroccan children and adolescents with juvenile idiopathic arthritis. Joint Bone Spine. 2011;78(6):584–6. https://doi.org/10.1016/j.jbspin.2011.02.001.
9. Bouaddi I, Rostom S, El Badri D, Hassani A, Chkirate B, Amine B, et al. Impact of juvenile idiopathic arthritis on schooling. BMC Pediatr. 2013;13:2. https://doi.org/10.1186/1471-2431-13-2.
10. Ezzahri M, Amine B, Rostom S, Rifay Y, Badri D, Mawani N, et al. The uveitis and its relationship with disease activity and quality of life in Moroccan children with juvenile idiopathic arthritis. Clin Rheumatol. 2013;32(9):1387–91. https://doi.org/10.1007/s10067-013-2262-y.
11. Shyen S, Amine B, Rostom S, El Badri D, Ezzahri M, Mawani N, et al. Sleep and its relationship to pain, dysfunction, and disease activity in juvenile idiopathic arthritis. Clin Rheumatol. 2014;33(10):1425–31. https://doi.org/10.1007/s10067-013-2409-x.
12. Ezzahri M, Amine B, Rostom S, Badri D, Mawani N, Gueddari S, et al. Factors influencing the quality of life of Moroccan patients with juvenile idiopathic arthritis. Clin Rheumatol. 2014;33(11):1621–6. https://doi.org/10.1007/s10067-014-2489-2.
13. El Badri D, Rostom S, Bouaddi I, Hassani A, Chkirate B, Amine B, et al. Bone mineral density in Moroccan patients with juvenile idiopathic arthritis. J Arthritis. 2014;3:3. https://doi.org/10.4172/2167-7921.1000131.
14. Rostom S, Amine B, Bensabbah R, Abouqal R, Hajjaj-Hassouni N. Hip involvement in juvenile idiopathic arthritis. Clin Rheumatol. 2008;27(6):791–4. https://doi.org/10.1007/s10067-008-0853-9.
15. Devauchelle-Pensec V. Quels sont les critères d'évaluation de la destruction articulaire dans l'arthrite juvénile idiopathique? Rev Rhum Monogr. 2010;77(2):89–92. https://doi.org/10.1016/j.monrhu.2010.02.001.
16. Eddaoudi M, Rostom S, Amine B, Bahiri R. Assessment of disease activity and carpal erosions by MRI of the wrist in children. Beyond Rheumatol. 2022;4(1):e381. https://doi.org/10.53238/br_20223_381.
17. Hamdi O, Bouden S, Saidane O, Tekaya R, Mahmoud I. Comorbidités chez les patients atteints de polyarthrite rhumatoïde. Rev Rhum. 2020;87:A111–2. https://doi.org/10.1016/j.rhum.2020.10.192.
18. Rostom S, Amine B, Bensabbah R, Chkirat B, Abouqal R, Hajjaj-Hassouni N. Psychometric properties evaluation of the childhood health assessment questionnaire (CHAQ) in Moroccan juvenile idiopathic arthritis. Rheumatol Int. 2010;30(7):879–85. https://doi.org/10.1007/s00296-009-1069-2.
19. Singh G, Athreya BH, Fries JF, Goldsmith DP. Measurement of health status in children with juvenile rheumatoid arthritis. Arthritis Rheum. 1994;37(12):1761–9. https://doi.org/10.1002/art.1780371209.

20. Amine B, Rostom S, Benbouazza K, Abouqal R, Hajjaj-Hassouni N. Health related quality of life survey about children and adolescents with juvenile idiopathic arthritis. Rheumatol Int. 2009;29(3):275–9. https://doi.org/10.1007/s00296-008-0672-y.
21. Bouayed K, Hamraoui D, Mikou N, Sakhi A, Hilmi W. Biotherapy in juvenile idiopathic arthritis Moroccan patients: a single-center experience. Pan Afr Med J. 2022;41:135. https://doi.org/10.11604/pamj.2022.41.135.27377.
22. Mawani N, Amine B, Rostom S, El Badri D, Ezzahri M, Moussa F. Moroccan parents caring for children with juvenile idiopathic arthritis: positive and negative aspects of their experiences. Pediatric Rheumatol. 2013;11(1):39. https://doi.org/10.1186/1546-0096-11-39.
23. Guillemin F. Évolution récente de l'épidémiologie des maladies rhumatismales. Rev Rhum. 2016;83:A21–5. https://doi.org/10.1016/S1169-8330(16)30200-9.
24. Minichiello E, Semerano L, Boissier MC. Évolution dans le temps de la polyarthrite rhumatoïde: incidence, prévalence, gravité—revue systématique de la littérature. Rev Rhum. 2017;84(1):9–16. https://doi.org/10.1016/j.rhum.2016.05.015.
25. Brunier L, Bleterry M, Merle S, Derancourt C, Polomat K, Dehlinger V, et al. Prévalence de la polyarthrite rhumatoïde aux Antilles françaises: Résultats de l'étude EPPPRA en Martinique. Rev Rhum. 2018;85(4):346–52. https://doi.org/10.1016/j.rhum.2017.07.052.
26. Hajjaj-Hassouni N. Rheumatoid arthritis in Morocco: past and present. Int J Med Surg. 2017;4(1) https://doi.org/10.15342/ijms.v4is.139.
27. Jawaheer D, Olsen J, Lahiff M, Forsberg S, Lähteenmäki J, da Silveira IG, et al. Gender, body mass index and rheumatoid arthritis disease activity: results from the QUEST-RA Study. Clin Exp Rheumatol. 2010;28(4):454–61.
28. Dougados M, Soubrier M, Antunez A, Balint P, Balsa A, Buch MH, et al. Prevalence of comorbidities in rheumatoid arthritis and evaluation of their monitoring: results of an international, cross-sectional study (COMORA). Ann Rheum Dis. 2014;73(1):62–8. https://doi.org/10.1136/annrheumdis-2013-204223.
29. Eddaoudi M, Rostom S, Hmamouchi I, Binoune IE, Amine B, Abouqal R, et al. The first biological choice in patients with rheumatoid arthritis: data from the Moroccan register of biotherapies. Pan Afr Med J. 2021;38:183.
30. Salma K, Nessrine A, Krystel E, Khaoula EK, Noura N, Khadija E, et al. Rheumatoid arthritis: seropositivity versus seronegativity; a comparative cross-sectional study arising from Moroccan context. Curr Rheumatol Rev. 2020;16(2):143–8. https://doi.org/10.2174/1573397115666191018115337.
31. Atouf O, Benbouazza K, Brick C, Bzami F, Bennani N, Amine B, et al. HLA polymorphism and early rheumatoid arthritis in the Moroccan population. Joint Bone Spine. 2008;75(5):554–8. https://doi.org/10.1016/j.jbspin.2008.01.027.
32. Akasbi N, Tahiri L, Houssaini GS, Harzy T. Les facteurs associés à l'infection au cours de la polyarthrite rhumatoïde. Pan Afr Med J. 2013;16:35. https://doi.org/10.11604/pamj.2013.16.35.2571.
33. Elzorkany B, Mokbel A, Gamal SM, Hmamouchi I, Dougados M. Does smoking affect level of seropositivity in RA? Post-hoc analysis of the COMORA cohort. Rheumatol Int. 2021;41(4):699–705. https://doi.org/10.1007/s00296-021-04791-w.
34. Azzouzi H, Ichchou L. Seasonal and weather effects on rheumatoid arthritis: myth or reality? Pain Res Manag. 2020;2020:5763080. https://doi.org/10.1155/2020/5763080.
35. Braun J, Sieper J. Ankylosing spondylitis. Lancet. 2007;369(9570):1379–90. https://doi.org/10.1016/S0140-6736(07)60635-7.
36. Slimani S, Hamdi W, Nassar K, Kalla AA. Spondyloarthritis in North Africa: an update. Clin Rheumatol. 2021;40(9):3401–10. https://doi.org/10.1007/s10067-021-05630-w.
37. Shirazy K, Hajjaj-Hassouni N, Hammond C, Jones H, Ladjouze Rezig A, Pedersen R, et al. The prevalence of non-radiographic axial spondyloarthritis among patients with inflammatory back pain from Northwest and South Africa: data from a noninterventional, cross-sectional study. Rheumatol Ther. 2018;5:437–45. https://doi.org/10.1007/s40744-018-0122-6.

38. Burgos-Vargas R, Wei JC-C, Rahman MU, Akkoc N, Haq SA, Hammoudeh M, et al. The prevalence and clinical characteristics of nonradiographic axial spondyloarthritis among patients with inflammatory back pain in rheumatology practices: a multinational, multicenter study. Arthritis Res Ther. 2016;18:132. https://doi.org/10.1186/s13075-016-1027-9.
39. Arabi H, Mougui A, Sahimi H, Takhrifa N, Mouhcine S, Bentaleb I, et al. Profile of spondyloarthritis in the Moroccan population: results of a multicenter study. Ann Rheum Dis. 2022;81(Suppl 1):1549. https://doi.org/10.1136/annrheumdis-2022-eular.3831.
40. Bentaleb I, Rostom S, Amine B, El Binoune I, El Bouchti I, Ghozlani I, et al. Prevalence of HLA-B27 antigen in Moroccan patients with spondyloarthritis (SpA): a multicenter study. Ann Rheum Dis. 2022;81(Suppl 1):1552. https://doi.org/10.1136/annrheumdis-2022-eular.4081.
41. Essouiri J, Abourazzak FE, Kona I, Harzy T. Profile of patients with spondyloarthritis in Morocco. Curr Rheumatol Rev. 2018;14(3):258–63. https://doi.org/10.2174/1573397113666170406125338.
42. Mboussi PC, Baba Z, Chekkouri FE, Rafi A, Mougui A, El Bouchti I. Factors associated with a delayed diagnosis of spondyloarthritis in a population of the south of Morocco. Ann Rheum Dis. 2022;81(Suppl 1):1538. https://doi.org/10.1136/annrheumdis-2022-eular.3124.
43. Ibn Yacoub Y, Amine B, Laatiris A, Hajjaj-Hassouni N. Gender and disease features in Moroccan patients with ankylosing spondylitis. Clin Rheumatol. 2012;31(2):293–7. https://doi.org/10.1007/s10067-011-1819-x.
44. Nihad S, Nessrine A, Sofia Z, Salma G, Khadija EK, Taoufik H. Distinctive features in spondyloarthritis between women and men in Moroccan context: disease beginning, clinical manifestations, disease activity and function scores. Curr Rheumatol Rev. 2021;17(1):95–100. https://doi.org/10.2174/1573397115666190626113230.
45. Liu K, Lin H, Ying J, Luo P, Wang M, He Z, et al. Modifiable lifestyle factors, genetic susceptibility, and incident radiographic axial spondyloarthritis. J Rheumatol. 2025;52(9):893–901. https://doi.org/10.3899/jrheum.2025-0042.
46. Akassou A, Yacoubi H, Jamil A, Dakka N, Amzazi S, Sadki K, et al. Prevalence of HLA-B27 in Moroccan healthy subjects and patients with ankylosing spondylitis and mapping construction of several factors influencing AS diagnosis by using multiple correspondence analysis. Rheumatol Int. 2015;35(11):1889–94. https://doi.org/10.1007/s00296-015-3342-x.
47. El Mouraghi I, Ouarour A, Ghozlani I, Collantes E, Solana R, El Maghraoui A. Polymorphisms of HLA-A, -B, -Cw and DRB1 antigens in Moroccan patients with ankylosing spondylitis and a comparison of clinical features with frequencies of HLA-B*27. Tissue Antigens. 2015;85(2):108–16. https://doi.org/10.1111/tan.12515.
48. Bouayad S, Rostom S, Hmamouchi I, El Binoune I, Amine B, Abouqal R, et al. Evaluation of the impact of smoking on spondyloarthritis: data from the Moroccan Biotherapy Register (RBSMR). Saudi J Pathol Microbiol. 2021;6(3):e004. https://doi.org/10.36348/sjpm.2021.v06i03.004.
49. Kaut IK, Abourazzak FE, Jamila E, Sènami FA, Diketa D, Taoufik H. Axial spondyloarthritis and cigarette smoking. Open Rheumatol J. 2017;11:53–61. https://doi.org/10.2174/1874312901711010053.
50. Wilson Zingg R, Kendall R. Obesity, vascular disease, and lumbar disk degeneration: associations of comorbidities in low back pain. PM R. 2017;9(4):398–402. https://doi.org/10.1016/j.pmrj.2016.09.011.
51. Ortolan A, Lorenzin M, Felicetti M, Ramonda R. Do obesity and overweight influence disease activity measures in axial spondyloarthritis? A systematic review and meta-analysis. Arthritis Care Res (Hoboken). 2021;73(12):1815–25. https://doi.org/10.1002/acr.24416.
52. Chennouf F, Azzouzi H, Boutaibi H, Linda I. Body composition in spondyloarthritis: is there any impact on disease activity? Ann Rheum Dis. 2022;81(Suppl 1):1541. https://doi.org/10.1136/annrheumdis-2022-eular.3333.
53. Oulkadi L, Rostom S, Hmamouchi I, El Hassani Sbai S, El Binoune I, Amine B, et al. Prevalence of latent tuberculosis before biotherapy initiation in rheumatoid arthritis and spondyloarthritis: data from the Moroccan biotherapy registry. Rheumatol Int. 2021;41(9):1625–31. https://doi.org/10.1007/s00296-021-04929-w.

54. El Ouardi N, Hmamouchi I, Abouqal R, Allali F, Bahiri R, El Bouchti I, et al. Real-world evidence of biological treatments in rheumatoid arthritis and spondyloarthritis in Morocco: results of the RBSMR registry. BMC Rheumatol. 2025;9(1):62. https://doi.org/10.1186/s41927-025-00510-1.
55. Hmamouchi I, Bahiri R, Hajjaj-Hassouni N. Clinical and radiological presentations of late-onset spondyloarthritis. ISRN Rheumatol. 2011;2011:840475. https://doi.org/10.5402/2011/840475.
56. El Mansouri L, Bahiri R, Abourazzak FE, Abouqal R, Hajjaj-Hassouni N. Two distinct patterns of ankylosing spondylitis in Moroccan patients. Rheumatol Int. 2009;29(12):1423–9. https://doi.org/10.1007/s00296-009-0873-z.
57. Zemrani S, Amine B, ElBinoune I, Rostom S, Bahiri R. Difficult-to-treat spondyloarthritis in Morocco: a real-world study. Mediterr J Rheumatol. 2024;35(Suppl 3):549–56. https://doi.org/10.31138/mjr.290124.dtt.
58. Zemrani S, Amine B, El Binoune I, Rostom S, Tahiri L, Allali F, et al. The retention rate and safety of secukinumab as a first-line biologic agent in axial spondyloarthritis compared to a first tumor necrosis factor (TNF) inhibitor: a real-world, longitudinal study. Cureus. 2024;16(9):e70365. https://doi.org/10.7759/cureus.70365.
59. Bentaleb I, Oulkadi L, Jaouad N, Maghraoui AE, Niamane R, Bouchti IE, et al. Recommendations of the Moroccan Society of Rheumatology (SMR) for Diagnostic Management of Spondyloarthritis (SpA) and Psoriatic Arthritis (PsA). Mediterr J Rheumatol. 2023;34(3):302–14.
60. Jaouad N, Oulkadi L, Bentaleb I, Bezza A, Maghraoui AE, Niamane R, et al. Recommendations of the Moroccan Society of Rheumatology (SMR) for the Therapeutic Management of Spondyloarthritis (SpA) including Psoriatic Arthritis (PsA). Mediterr J Rheumatol. 2023;34(2):139–51.
61. Zemrani S, Amine B, Elbinoune I, Charoui C, Rostom S, Hmamouchi I, et al. Tuberculosis under biotherapy in patients with Spondyloarthritis: data from the Moroccan biotherapy registry (RBSMR) during 3 years of follow up. Mediterr J Rheumatol. 2025;36(1):79–85. https://doi.org/10.31138/mjr.210324.tub.
62. Taoubane L, Maghraoui AE, Niamane R, Hmamouchi I, Allali F, Bahiri R, et al. What are the characteristics of paradoxical effects in the biotherapies registry of the Moroccan Society of Rheumatology? Reumatologia. 2025;63(4):244–50. https://doi.org/10.5114/reum/205366.
63. Rostom S, Allali F, Bahiri R, Abouqal R, Hajjaj-Hassouni N, et al. Psychometric properties evaluation of the quality of life questionnaire of the European Foundation for Osteoporosis in Arabic population. Rheumatol Int. 2012;32(7):2037–49. https://doi.org/10.1007/s00296-011-1910-2.
64. Hmamouchi I, Allali F, Khazzani H, Bennani L, EL Mansouri L, Ichchou L, et al. Low bone mineral density is related to atherosclerosis in postmenopausal Moroccan women. BMC Public Health. 2009;9:388. https://doi.org/10.1186/1471-2458-9-388.
65. Moulay Berkchi J, Rkain H, Benbrahim L, Aktaou S, Lazrak N, Faiz S, et al. Management of gout by Moroccan rheumatologists: a Moroccan Society for Rheumatology national survey. Rheumatol Int. 2020;40(9):1399–408. https://doi.org/10.1007/s00296-020-04599-0.
66. Hmamouchi I, Allali F, Tahiri L, Khazzani H, Mansouri LE, Ali Ou Alla S, et al. Clinically important improvement in the WOMAC and predictor factors for response to non-specific non-steroidal anti-inflammatory drugs in osteoarthritic patients: a prospective study. BMC Res Notes. 2012;5:58. https://doi.org/10.1186/1756-0500-5-58.
67. Fellous S, Rkain H, Ahid S, Abouqal R, Tahiri L, Hmamouchi I, et al. One-year direct costs of biological therapy in rheumatoid arthritis and its predictive factors: data from the Moroccan RBSMR registry. Rheumatol Int. 2021;41(4):787–93. https://doi.org/10.1007/s00296-020-04762-7.
68. Bahloul S, Rkain H, Fellous S, Ahid S, Abouqal R, Latifa T, et al. AB0486 One-year direct costs of biological therapy in ankylosing spondylitis and its predictive factors: data from the Moroccan RBSMR registry. Ann Rheum Dis. 2021;80:1270. https://doi.org/10.1136/annrheumdis-2021-eular.4117.

Chapter 11
Rheumatic Diseases in the Sultanate of Oman

Nasra K. Al Adhoubi, Zakariya Alismaeili, and Maha Ali

Abstract The Sultanate of Oman's healthcare services have evolved significantly, and rheumatology has become an essential component of this progress. Among 94 healthcare facilities, eight governmental hospitals provide rheumatology care. These hospitals include the following: Royal Hospital, Al-Nahda Hospital, Sultan Qaboos Hospital, Salalah, Sultan Qaboos University Hospital, Sohar Hospital, Al Burami Hospital, Nizwa Hospital, and Armed Forces Hospital. Several facilities are part of a rheumatology unit, offering inpatient and outpatient services, as well as daycare.

There are no formally certified rheumatology nurses, and the number of trained rheumatology nurses in Oman is limited. A total of 22 adult rheumatologists and five pediatric rheumatologists currently practice across major hospitals.

Rheumatologists face several challenges in delivering optimal patient care, including the shortage of specialists, long waiting times for radiological procedures, and limited access to musculoskeletal ultrasound equipment in several regions. Daycare services for intravenous therapies are lacking, and biologic treatments remain restricted in some regions. In addition, poor medication adherence, limited disease awareness among patients, and insufficient rehabilitation facilities further hinder quality care.

To meet the growing demand, it is essential to establish national rheumatology fellowship programs and strengthen multidisciplinary teams by increasing the number of specialized nurses, physical therapists, and musculoskeletal radiologists. Furthermore, enhanced screening, early diagnosis, and equitable access to care across all regions are required.

N. K. Al Adhoubi (✉)
Rheumatology Unit, Royal Hospital, Muscat, Oman
e-mail: nasrak2004@yahoo.com

Z. Alismaeili
Rheumatology Unit, Nizwa Hospital, Nizwa, Oman
e-mail: zakismaeili@gmail.com

M. Ali
Rheumatology Unit, Al Nahdha Hospital, Muscat, Oman
e-mail: alimaha@hotmail.com

K. A. Alnaqbi, G. Aldabie (eds.), *Rheumatic Diseases in the Arab World*,
https://doi.org/10.1007/978-981-92-0967-5_11

Lastly, greater emphasis on rheumatology research is needed to support evidence-based practice and improve healthcare outcomes for patients with rheumatic diseases in Oman.

Keywords Rheumatic diseases · Rheumatology services · Oman · Health services accessibility · Rheumatology workforce · Biologic therapy · Rheumatology training · Fellowship program · Oman rheumatology society · Arab world

11.1 Country Demographics

The Sultanate of Oman is an Arab country in the southern part of the Arabian Peninsula and is one of the largest in the region.

Oman is located in the middle of the Middle East, bordered on the west by the Kingdom of Saudi Arabia and the United Arab Emirates (UAE), on the south by the Republic of Yemen, on the north by the Strait of Hormuz, and on the east by the Arabian Sea. From the Strait of Hormuz in the north to the Republic of Yemen, the coast stretches 3165 kilometers and overlooks three seas: the Sea of Oman, the Arabian Sea, and the Arabian Gulf. Various topographic areas make up the Sultanate. It comprises plains, wadis (dry river beds), and mountains. With a percentage of about 3% of the total area, the plain overlooking the Oman Sea and the Arabian Sea is considered the most important. Nearly 15% of Oman's land is covered by mountain ranges. Approximately 82% of the remaining area comprises deserts and wadis [1].

The climate varies significantly by location. In the coastal region, it is hot and humid during the summer, while in the interior, it is hot and dry during the winter, except in the higher mountains and Dhofar Governorate [2].

Administratively, Oman is divided into 11 governorates and 61 wilayats. As a result of this, the following governorates are included: Muscat Governorate, Al Batinah North Governorate, Al Batinah South Governorate, Al Buraymi Governorate, Dakhliyah Governorate, Ash Sharqiyah South Governorate, Ash Sharqiyah North Governorate, Adh Dhahirah Governorate, Al Wusta Governorate, Dhofar Governorate, and Musandam Governorate [3].

In December 1993, the Sultanate of Oman undertook a general census of population, housing, and establishments, the first of its kind for the Sultanate. Over 2 years, detailed results of the General Census were published. The census reported that about two million people were living in Oman, of which about 27% were non-Omani. Before 1993, demographic information and population estimates derived from surveys such as the 1985 "Demographic Survey" and 1988 "Child Health Survey" were used to derive demographic and population estimates and projections [3, 4].

According to the National Center for Statistics and Information (NCSI), Oman's total population was estimated at 5,203,674 in 2024, comprising 2,955,171 Omanis

(56.8%) and 2,248,503 non-Omanis, representing around 43.2% of the total population. This represents a steady population increase since the 2020 electronic census, which recorded 4.47 million inhabitants. More recent projections in the middle of 2025 indicate that the population has risen further to approximately 5.3 million. The demographic structure reflects a youthful population and a balanced sex distribution. Maintaining a ratio close to 102 males for every 100 females [4].

11.2 Country Health Care Sectors

The Ministry of Health (MOH) serves as the governing body responsible for healthcare provision and is committed to ensuring universal healthcare access for all citizens. However, a significant challenge encountered during the implementation of health development initiatives was aligning the organizational framework with the strategies and objectives established in 1990. These objectives encompass decentralizing health services and enhancing regional decision-making processes, emphasizing the importance of strategic planning, investing in health systems research, highlighting the roles of local governments and international partnerships, and executing educational and training initiatives within the healthcare sector. Health services in the Sultanate of Oman have grown immensely in recent decades.

At the beginning of the 1970s, there were only two hospitals with 12 beds and 10 outpatient clinics. Currently, there are more than 211 health centers in the country, 94 of which are equipped with beds. In addition, there are 21 extended health centers under MOH [5].

Health Institutes in the Sultanate of Oman utilize a comprehensive health information network called Al Shifa, a system developed by the MOH Information Technology in consultation with different hospital administrations, doctors, nurses, and paramedics. This system is designed to manage healthcare facilities effectively. It has been installed in over 200 healthcare facilities of various sizes and capabilities, including non-MoH caregiver facilities. It offers a range of inpatient and outpatient services, capturing all clinically significant aspects of a patient's health, from referral or walk-in to discharge [5].

The most recent version of the system, Al Shifa 3 Plus, can manage diverse institutes, ranging from primary health centers to tertiary care facilities. Since the program is developed in-house, any requested user changes can be implemented in real time. The software adheres to widely accepted standards in the healthcare industry worldwide. This software codes diagnoses according to international standards, such as ICD-10, ICD-9CM, and SNOMED. It also supports interoperability standards, including ASTM and HL7. Compared to its predecessor, Al Shifa 3 Plus provides several advantages. Still, its primary advantage is its ability to be implemented by smaller institutes and higher levels since it can be parameterized entirely. As part of the Al Shifa health system, various rheumatology units offer services to patients referred from other hospitals or departments within the same hospital [6].

11.3 Rheumatology Health Services

Rheumatology services are an essential component of the healthcare system in Oman. Generally, the rheumatology division functions as a separate unit within the Department of Internal Medicine. Among the 94 hospitals in the country, only eight governmental hospitals have dedicated rheumatology units: Royal Hospital, Al Nahdha Hospital, Sultan Qaboos Hospital, Salalah; Sultan Qaboos University Hospital; Sohar Hospital; Al Buraimi Hospital; Nizwa Hospital; and Armed Forces Hospital. The first rheumatology unit was established at the Royal Hospital in 1982 (Fig. 11.1). The rheumatology unit usually has inpatient and outpatient care and daycare units.

A total of 27 adult rheumatologists are currently practicing in Oman, three of whom work exclusively in the private sector. In addition, there are five pediatric rheumatologists based in the pediatric departments of the Royal Hospital and Sultan Qaboos University Hospital. The distribution of rheumatologists across hospitals is as follows:

- Royal Hospital: six rheumatologists
- Sultan Qaboos University Hospital: five rheumatologists
- Al-Nahda Hospital: two rheumatologists
- Sohar Hospital: three rheumatologists
- Al Burami Hospital: two rheumatologists
- Nizwa Hospital: two rheumatologists
- Armed Forces Hospital: one rheumatologist
- Medical City Rheumatology Unit: two rheumatologists
- Sultan Qaboos Hospital, Salalah: one rheumatologist

The authors estimate that approximately 83.3% of rheumatologists in Oman are employed in government institutions, while the private sector accounts for the remaining 16.7%. Among all rheumatologists, about 44.5% conduct a minimum of three clinics per week, and 39% have at least two clinics per week.

The Oman Medical Specialty Board (OMSB) and the Ministry of Higher Education have been facilitating local and international training programs, including those in rheumatology, due to the absence of a rheumatology fellowship training program in Oman. Physicians seeking specialization in this field must pursue training abroad after completing their internal medicine board. Over the years, there has been a progressive increase in physicians participating in these fellowship programs. Between 1990 and 1995, only one physician was sent abroad for this purpose. This number slightly increased, with three physicians sent for rheumatology training in each of the following periods: 1996–2001, 2002–2007, and 2008–2013. Notably, six physicians were sent for the rheumatology fellowship from 2014 to 2019. At present, Oman has no formally certified rheumatology nurses (i.e., no one holds a recognized rheumatology-nursing certification). Only a few nurses have received any level of rheumatology-specific training (informal or on-the-job). Currently, three hospitals each employ a dedicated rheumatology nurse.

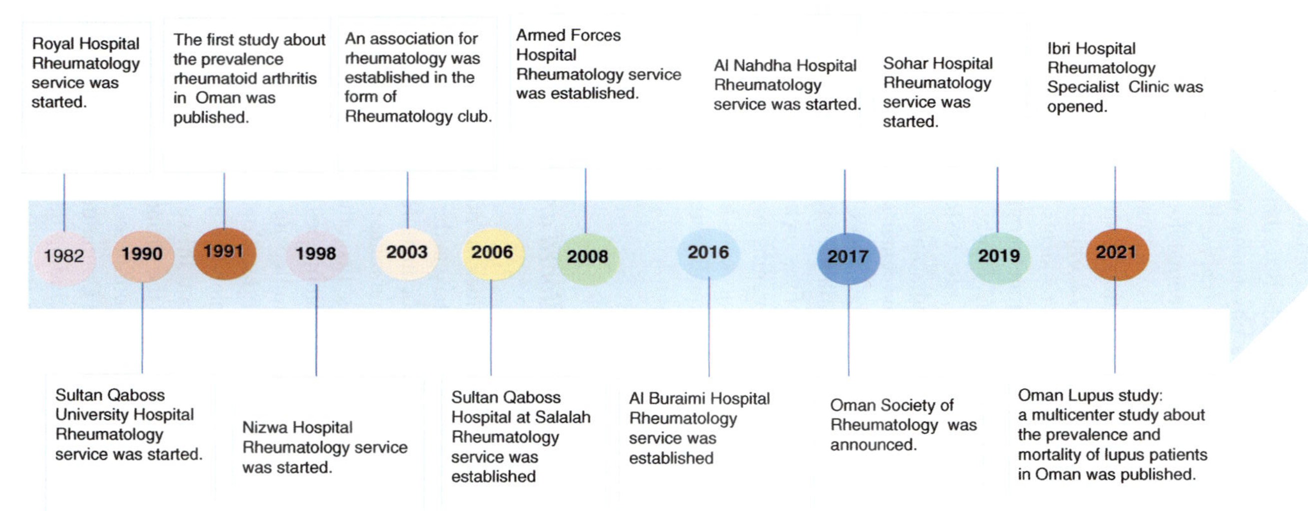

Fig. 11.1 Timeline of milestones in rheumatology services in the Sultanate of Oman

11.4 Official Rheumatology Society

Early in the 2000s, the rheumatology community in Oman had no society or association; instead, clinicians met regularly to share information under the name of the Rheumatology Club. Numerous physicians were members of the Rheumatology Club, including rheumatologists, internal medicine physicians interested in rheumatology, and general practitioners. Rheumatology Club members participated in regular education activities about various rheumatic conditions.

Under the Oman Medical Association (OMA) umbrella, the Oman Rheumatology Society (OSR) was established on 22 March 2017. The members of this society include rheumatologists, internists, residents, nurses, and medical students interested in rheumatology. Many educational programs have been conducted for OMSB residents, including internal medicine, family medicine, and other programs.

As part of its mission statement, the OSR was committed to promoting early detection, effective management, education, research, and raising awareness of rheumatic diseases in the country. The center's vision of OSR was to provide teaching and training for rheumatology health professionals and trainees, emphasizing patient outcomes as it promoted excellence in rheumatology care [7].

Additionally, the Society's objectives include supporting rheumatologists with clinical advice and resources, encouraging medical trainees to enter the specialty, facilitating the exchange of scientific knowledge, advancing continuing medical education, helping clinicians meet quality standards, and promoting national and international research collaborations.

11.4.1 The OSR Executive Board and Committees

There are three regular members besides the president, vice president, treasurer, and OSR Executive Board general secretary in the OSR.

The society comprises several subcommittees, including a scientific committee, an advisory committee, a finance committee, and an information and technology committee. In addition to the forums, two other committees are being established: the research and patient advocacy committees.

The duties of the Scientific Committee are to organize the society's educational programs and Continuous Medical Education (CME) activities and ensure that all CME activities comply with the society's objectives and mission. It also provides that these educational activities support the strategic priorities of society.

The finance committee oversees the finances, investments, and budget. It also serves as the society's yearly audit committee, working closely with the treasurer.

The Information and Technology Committee is responsible for coordinating all of the Society's online activities, including its public web pages, which are accessible to all members. It also aids in recruiting members from residency program directors and general practitioners in different health services. Moreover, there is a plan to seek out new ideas for enhancing the design of the society's website to maximize user-friendliness and provide members with the greatest possible benefit and utility.

The number of members of OSR was around 20 in the first year of its foundation. OSR now encompasses more than 70 members, and the number grows yearly. Regarding gender distribution, females represent the majority, with a female-to-male ratio of approximately 5:2. Within the OSR board, representation remains balanced, with a female-to-male ratio of about 4:3, reflecting the society's commitment to diversity and inclusivity in leadership.

The OSR's funding comes from several sources, including annual membership fees, sponsorship from pharmaceutical companies for educational activities, and additional income through grants, donations, and other channels.

11.4.2 Oman Rheumatology Society Achievements and Challenges

The OSR has achieved much in the last 5 years; its standout achievement was hosting the Arab League Against Rheumatism (ArLAR) Congress in Oman in 2018. Rheumatologists from Arab countries and the Asia-Pacific region attended this congress, one of the largest in the region.

The society has achieved several other milestones, including involvement in various educational programs to enhance community awareness of rheumatic diseases among patients. Numerous scientific meetings with rheumatologists have been conducted as part of continuous medical education initiatives. The society has established a presence on social media platforms like Instagram, Facebook, and X (formerly Twitter) and has created educational videos to educate the public about different rheumatic diseases. Collaborative efforts with the Omani Women's Association have been made to raise awareness of rheumatic diseases among women through lecture series.

Additionally, a WhatsApp group in Oman has been established for systemic lupus erythematosus (SLE) patients for health education and disease awareness. Collaborative scientific research projects among OSR members, such as the Oman Lupus Study and investigations into COVID-19 mortality in patients with rheumatic diseases, have been undertaken. The second Gulf Conference for Rheumatology in 2022 was planned to be held in Oman but was conducted virtually due to the COVID-19 pandemic.

In its initial stages, OSR struggled with several issues, including securing financial support for its activities and achieving its aims. The society successfully addressed its financial challenges by securing support from several pharmaceutical companies and through membership contributions.

11.4.3 *Future Plans of the Oman Rheumatology Society*

The OSR's upcoming goals include enhancing local research in rheumatology and strengthening the connections with rheumatologists in other Arab countries. It plans to increase the number of campaigns and activities dedicated to patient awareness. Additionally, it aims to organize scientific conferences actively in partnership with various societies. It also focuses on setting up annual lectures in different regional hospitals for general practitioners to broaden their understanding of rheumatic diseases. An additional crucial initiative is to initiate a rheumatology fellowship program within Oman and establish the OSR Rheumatology Journal.

11.5 Rheumatic Diseases in Oman

Over 200 rheumatic conditions, primarily affecting joints, connective tissues, cartilage, and tendons, can also impact other organs due to their autoimmune characteristics [8].

In Oman, the incidence of these diseases is not well-documented and appears to vary across regions. More research is needed to collect accurate data, track disease patterns, and better understand their underlying causes. Table 11.1 presents the findings from various epidemiological studies on rheumatic diseases in Oman [9–12].

In 1991, the estimated prevalence of rheumatoid arthritis (RA) in Omani adults aged 16 and above was approximately 8.4 cases per 1000 individuals, based on the criteria set by the American College of Rheumatology (ACR) in 1987 [9].

According to a report by Abdwani et al., the prevalence of juvenile idiopathic arthritis (JIA) was 20 cases per 100,000 inhabitants. The incidence of JIA was estimated to be two cases per 100,000. Among girls, the prevalence of JIA was 28 cases per 100,000, while among boys, it was 12 cases per 100,000. The most common subtype of JIA in this cohort was polyarticular JIA rheumatoid factor positive.

Table 11.1 Epidemiological studies of various rheumatic diseases in Oman

	Prevalence per 100,000	Incidence per 100,000	Female: male ratio	Mortality rate	5-year survival rate	10-year survival rate
Rheumatoid arthritis	840	—	—	—	—	—
Systemic lupus erythematosus	38	—	7:1	5%	100%	100%
Juvenile idiopathic arthritis	20	2	2.5:1	—	—	—
Polymyositis	2.2	—	2:1	5.6%	94.4%	67%
Dermatomyositis	2.2	—		8.3%	91.7%	69%
Juvenile dermatomyositis	1.14	—		11.1%	89%	83.3%

Table 11.2 The prevalence rate of SLE patients of different age groups in the Oman Lupus Cohort

Age group	Lupus patients/total population	The prevalence (per 100,000 inhabitants)
Pediatric patients up to 12 years	39/771,780	5.05
Adolescent patients 13–18 years	90/284,826	31.6
Adult patients		
Adult 19–24 years	136/387,448	35.1
Adult 25–29 years	154/475,403	32.4
Adult 30-39 years	403/639,636	63.01
Adult 40-49 years	212/352,632	60.12
Adult >49 years	103/262,192	39.28
Mean for all adult patients	**45.96**	
Oman Lupus Cohort overall mean	**38.08**	

Reproduced from Al-Adhoubi et al. [11]. © 2021 John Wiley & Sons. Reproduced with permission

Polyarticular JIA rheumatoid factor negative cases accounted for 39.2% of the cases, followed by oligoarthritis (31.8%), systemic (17.8%), and rheumatoid factor positive polyarticular JIA (7.5%). Notably, uveitis was not observed in this cohort [10].

In 2021, Al-Adhoubi et al., collaborating with the Oman lupus study group, reported a prevalence of SLE of approximately 38 cases per 100,000 inhabitants. Among the pediatric group (up to 12 years of age), the prevalence of lupus was about 5.1 cases per 100,000 inhabitants, while among adolescents, it was 31.6 cases per 100,000 inhabitants. The highest prevalence was observed in the 30–49 age group, with a prevalence of up to 62 cases per 100,000 inhabitants (Table 11.2) [11].

The same group found that male patients with lupus had a significantly higher mortality rate than female patients (7.6% vs. 5.4%, $p = 0.04$). There were several risk factors for mortality, but sepsis was the most common reason for mortality (63%), followed by kidney disease (35%), respiratory system illness (31%), CNS involvement (24%), and cardiovascular diseases (22%). It is important to note that the analysis of survival rates within the lupus group demonstrated encouraging results. Over 10 years, the survival rate was found to be 100%, while at the 20-year mark, it was 99%, and at 40 years, it stood at 90%. These findings suggest that advancements in the management and the increased awareness of lupus positively impact the quality of life of individuals with the disease [11].

11.5.1 Risk Factors of Rheumatic Diseases in Oman

Rheumatic diseases might share genetic and environmental factors. While specific clinical risk factors for developing inflammatory diseases have been identified, more comprehensive studies are needed to compare these risk factors across multiple inflammatory conditions. Furthermore, there is a gap in research examining whether the risk factors for rheumatic diseases have similar associations with other related disorders. This highlights the need for further investigation in this area [13].

Despite the substantial evidence that lifestyle factors such as smoking, obesity, and alcohol consumption are linked to a wide variety of rheumatic diseases, the strength of these associations varies from one disease to another and from one study to another. For example, tobacco use has been closely associated with the development of RA over the years, whereas there is a mixed association with psoriatic arthritis (PsA) [13–15].

In Oman, studies are limited in investigating the association between environmental and behavioral factors and the risk of developing rheumatic diseases. However, the prevalence of common risk factors identified in other studies has been reported. A recent study by Al Mawali et al. utilized a cross-sectional, prospective, observational, community-based survey as part of the World Health Organization STEPwise approach to surveillance (STEPS). The survey involved 6582 individuals in Oman. The study aimed to gather comprehensive information on demographic, behavioral, and physical characteristics related to health in adults aged 18 and older. The prevalence of various behavioral risk factors was observed in the study. Tobacco use was found to be prevalent in 9% of participants, while alcohol consumption was reported by 2% of individuals [16].

Additionally, a significant proportion of the population, approximately 61%, reported not consuming fruits or vegetables regularly. Insufficient physical activity was also a prevalent risk factor, with 39% of participants failing to meet the recommended activity levels. Among the biological risk factors, overweight and obesity were observed in 66% of cases, high blood pressure in 33% of cases, high blood sugar in 16%, and high blood cholesterol in 36% of cases. Additionally, the study found that 95% of the population had multiple risk factors. Specifically, 33% of adults aged 18 and above had three or more risk factors, which increased to 45% among adults aged 45 and above (Table 11.3) [16].

The results from this study indicate the high prevalence of non-communicable disease risk factors in Oman. These findings highlight the importance of implementing health promotion, education, and policy initiatives to address these risk factors and mitigate their impact on public health [16].

Table 11.3 Prevalence of risk factors of non-communicable diseases in Oman

Risk Factor	% ($N = 6582$)
Obesity	30.7%
Overweight	66.1%
Raised total cholesterol	35.5%
Raised blood pressure	33.3%
Raised blood glucose	15.7%
Insufficient physical activity	38.6%
Insufficient fruit/vegetable consumption	60.7%
Current tobacco smoking	8.5%
Current daily tobacco smoking	7.1%
Alcohol consumption	2.4%

11.6 Screening Programs for Rheumatic Diseases

Early identification of autoimmune rheumatic disease through structured screening programs is crucial, as timely diagnosis can significantly reduce morbidity and mortality and optimize patient outcomes within the narrow therapeutic window. Therefore, establishing systematic screening initiatives is essential for early intervention and disease control. General practitioners are ideally positioned to lead such programs within the primary care setting [17, 18]. However, similar nationwide screening initiatives for rheumatic diseases have not yet been established in the Sultanate of Oman. Hence, it is imperative for the rheumatology community to work in close partnership with governmental bodies and non-profit organizations to develop and implement effective early detection strategies nationwide.

11.7 Diagnosis and Management

11.7.1 Laboratory Tests

In Oman, essential laboratory investigations are available, including anti-nuclear antibodies, extractable nuclear antigens, anti-cyclic citrullinated peptides, antiphospholipid antibodies, and other serological testing. Accessing genetic testing for HLA-B27, HLA-B51, and MEFV mutations in Oman requires sending samples overseas, resulting in a longer turnaround time for receiving the test results.

11.7.2 Imaging

Plain X-rays and ultrasounds are available at all rheumatology centers in Oman. However, there is limited availability of musculoskeletal ultrasound. Computed tomography (CT) scans are available in most large secondary and tertiary care hospitals, and magnetic resonance imaging (MRI) machines are only accessible in tertiary care hospitals. There are only three centers nationwide that offer positron emission tomography (PET) scans. There are only five musculoskeletal radiologists in Oman: three working at Khoula Hospital, the country's only tertiary care center for orthopedics and trauma, and one at the Royal Hospital and another one at the Armed Forces Hospital.

11.7.3 Management

In Oman, conventional disease-modifying anti-rheumatic drugs (cDMARDs) are widely available across all healthcare institutions. These include methotrexate, sulfasalazine, hydroxychloroquine, leflunomide, tacrolimus, cyclosporine, and cyclophosphamide.

In contrast, the availability of biologic and targeted synthetic DMARDs is limited to rheumatology specialists and requires formal approval through a special request process. Among biologics, anti-TNF agents such as etanercept, adalimumab, golimumab, infliximab, and certolizumab are the most commonly used. Interleukin inhibitors (anakinra, canakinumab, secukinumab, ustekinumab, guselkumab, and risankizumab) are also accessible, along with other biologics such as rituximab and abatacept, and lupus-specific therapies including belimumab, anifrolumab, and obinutuzumab.

Targeted synthetic DMARDs, such as tofacitinib, upadacitinib, and baricitinib, are available as oral options, whereas filgotinib is not yet registered, similar to the situation in other Gulf countries. Additionally, the phosphodiesterase inhibitor, apremilast, is available and provides an oral alternative, particularly beneficial for patients with Behçet's disease.

For osteoporosis management, agents such as alendronate, zoledronic acid, pamidronate, denosumab, and teriparatide are available nationwide, ensuring comprehensive coverage for bone health across the country.

11.7.4 Rheumatology Subspeciality Clinics

In Oman, rheumatology offers a range of subspecialty clinics dedicated to conditions like SLE, scleroderma, spondyloarthritis, inflammatory arthritis, vasculitis, and more. These clinics collaborate with other healthcare professionals to provide comprehensive care for patients with complex conditions. The routine use of patient-reported outcome measures in these clinics has not been systematically reported.

Specialized rheumatology clinics also include osteoporosis, musculoskeletal ultrasound, obstetrics and rheumatology, multidisciplinary pulmonary hypertension, and combined interstitial lung disease clinics. These clinics are run by local rheumatologists who specialize in specific diseases and have received formal training or have a particular focus on managing these conditions.

11.8 Cost-Effective Care for Rheumatic Diseases

11.8.1 Health Insurance Coverage for Rheumatic Diseases in Oman

Oman's MOH is the primary government agency responsible for providing healthcare services to its citizens. The system consists of hospitals and health centers at national, regional, sub-regional, and local levels, all of which are integrated into a network of referrals that run through the entire system [5].

Private clinics and hospitals also provide medical services, which have become increasingly important in health care delivery. These clinics are connected to the MOH system through a network of referrals.

It is worth mentioning that the Sultanate requires all non-Omani nationals and visitors to have health insurance to establish, maintain, or restore health coverage for diverse diseases during their stay, except for citizens of Gulf Cooperation Council (GCC) member states and citizens entitled to free or discounted treatment.

In an era when biological therapies are widely available, expatriate patients with rheumatic diseases often face significant challenges due to the high cost of treatment. Coverage for biologic therapies is frequently denied because of financial constraints, limiting access to optimal disease control. The introduction of biosimilar therapies offers a cost-effective alternative with comparable efficacy and safety to originator biologics. Their wider adoption within the healthcare system could reduce expenditure on high-cost medications and support more efficient resource allocation.

11.9 Medical Tourism and Rheumatic Diseases in Oman

Medical tourism refers to seeking medical services in a foreign country to improve, maintain, or restore a person's physical or mental well-being. Patients consider various factors when pursuing medical tourism, including affordability, availability, and acceptability of treatment options [19]. In the Middle East, individuals feel a personal obligation and responsibility to spend significant amounts of money on the health of their family members. The emotional attachment to doctors and hospitals is crucial in motivating patients to travel to specific destinations. For example, Omani patients often seek treatment in Shiraz, Iran, due to its Islamic heritage and cultural familiarity [19, 20].

In Oman, there is a need to develop the rheumatology medical tourism sector and gather statistics on patient travel destinations for rheumatic diseases. A small study conducted in Oman in 2011, which included 45 patients, revealed that orthopedic ailments were the most common reason for Omani patients seeking medical treatment abroad. Thailand emerged as the most popular destination (50%), followed by India (30%) [19, 21].

In addition to Thailand and India, our observations have shown that patients with rheumatic diseases also travel for medical tourism to countries such as China, Iran, Turkey, Germany, Singapore, the United Kingdom, Malaysia, the UAE, and Jordan.

Increasing research efforts in the GCC region and throughout the Middle East are crucial to better understanding treatment trends abroad. Additionally, establishing a national registry and database for medical tourism that provides comprehensive information on facts, costs, implications, issues, and patient rights is necessary. This registry should be publicly available and protected by regulatory, advisory, and governmental agencies [19].

11.10 Rheumatic Diseases: Challenges and Opportunities

Rheumatic diseases represent a major public concern, posing both clinical and systemic challenges that demand sustained quality improvement efforts. It is important to recognize that rheumatology covers many quality initiatives, some of which may present implementation challenges. Moreover, managing rheumatic diseases can be financially burdensome, mainly when health insurance coverage is inadequate, and individuals face escalating healthcare expenses, resulting in higher out-of-pocket costs [22].

11.10.1 Challenges

System-Based challenges

Rheumatology services in Oman face several system-level limitations that affect the delivery of optimal care. These include a shortage of rheumatologists compared with countries of similar population size and prolonged waiting times for radiological investigations due to a limited number of musculoskeletal radiologists and ultrasound machines.

Furthermore, unequal access to biologic therapies across regions can delay disease control and increase long-term healthcare expenditures.

Other systemic issues include the lack of specialized immunology laboratories in some facilities, the absence of specialized rheumatology nurses, and insufficient infusion services for intravenous therapies in several hospitals. In addition, the limited availability of rehabilitation centers further restricts the provision of comprehensive multidisciplinary care.

Patient-Level challenges

At the patient level, the main barriers include limited awareness and understanding of rheumatic diseases, which adversely affect adherence to treatment and follow-up. In addition, financial constraints related to out-of-pocket expenses for advanced therapies can further hinder consistent access to care.

11.10.2 Opportunities

Several opportunities exist to improve rheumatology care in Oman. These include encouraging medical students and residents to specialize in rheumatology and increasing the recruitment and training of nurses interested in this field. Another focus is identifying and implementing cost-effective therapy methods and medical investments to manage the high costs of rheumatic diseases.

Conducting epidemiological studies on various rheumatic diseases and establishing disease registries is crucial for understanding and addressing these diseases' unique characteristics in Oman. It is also essential to ensure equal access to advanced treatments, workforces, and radiological imaging across the Sultanate, promoting equity in healthcare quality and enabling the decentralization of health services.

Raising awareness about rheumatic diseases among patients, physicians, and the wider community is another key goal. This goes hand in hand with encouraging research into diagnosing and treating these diseases, which calls for enhanced research methodologies and high-quality research facilities.

Developing regional recommendations, guidelines, and treatment pathways specifically tailored to the unique characteristics of Omani patients is essential. Additionally, fostering collaboration and exchanging expertise with rheumatologists from the GCC, the Middle East, and globally is beneficial.

Empowering OSR to engage with stakeholders about the challenges rheumatologists face in Oman is vital. Finally, once the OSR journal is launched, this will encourage rheumatologists to publish their research and promote a research culture within the rheumatology field.

11.11 Rheumatology Fellowship Programs

Currently, there is no rheumatology training program in Oman, and most rheumatologists have received their training in accredited centers outside the country, including the United Kingdom, Canada, Ireland, the Kingdom of Saudi Arabia, France, and Australia. Upon passing the internal medicine board, physicians must travel overseas for training. OSR plans to initiate a fellowship program in rheumatology in Oman. This will be one of society's most vital priorities in the coming years.

11.12 Research

The field of rheumatology in Oman began with the publication of the first article in 1991, which focused on the prevalence of RA [9]. Since then, the number of rheumatology articles published by Oman in well-known national, regional, and international journals has steadily increased, with over 45 articles published by rheumatologists from Oman in recent years [23–42]. This increase can be attributed to the growing number of rheumatologists working in the country. However, there is still room for improvement in the research field, and efforts and collaboration are needed to enhance the viability of research in Oman.

11.13 Future of Rheumatic Diseases Care

It is expected that the prevalence of rheumatic diseases will continue to rise. Improving awareness about different types of rheumatic diseases at various levels, including the community level, medical professionals, and stakeholders, is essential. This will ultimately enhance the quality of care for patients suffering from these diseases and facilitate early detection. Moreover, there is a need for more research and development in the country's rheumatology field. Rheumatic disease research should aim to assess the prevalence of rheumatic diseases in the region while exploring more diagnostic tests to aid in earlier detection. Furthermore, it is essential to encourage research that aims to identify therapeutic alternatives that have a better safety profile, are highly effective, and are economically viable.

Although risk factors for rheumatic diseases are multifactorial, studies identifying genetic, behavioral, and environmental contributors are essential for primary prevention, particularly in addressing modifiable factors.

In recent years, rheumatology has undergone rapid advances, making the introduction of a rheumatology fellowship program in Oman crucial for keeping up with these rapid advancements and to meet the needs of its rheumatology community.

11.14 Conclusion

Continuous advancement requires sustained efforts to strengthen healthcare delivery. The rheumatology community in Oman should focus on enhancing services for patients with rheumatic diseases across all regions. This can be achieved by increasing the number of rheumatologists, specialist rheumatology nurses, physical therapists, and musculoskeletal radiologists. Improving screening, diagnosis, and treatment methods for these diseases is crucial, along with ensuring equitable access to quality care nationwide. Furthermore, expanding research and training in rheumatology is essential to build local expertise and sustain progress in this field.

Acknowledgments Our sincere appreciation is extended to all our colleagues who have provided us with the information and resources necessary for the book chapter. We also thank the Statistics Department at the Ministry of Health and the Royal Hospital Library for their support and assistance.

Authors' Conflict of Interest Declaration The authors declare that they have no conflicts of interest.

References

1. OmanInfo. Page 572 [Internet]. OmanInfo; [cited 2026 Jun 15]. Available from: https://www.omaninfo.om/en/pages/161/show/572.
2. Encyclopaedia Britannica. Oman [Internet]. Chicago: Encyclopaedia Britannica; [cited 2026 Jun 14]. Available from: https://www.britannica.com/place/Oman.
3. National Centre for Statistics and Information. Home - NCSI Portal [Internet]. Muscat: National Centre for Statistics and Information; [cited 2025 Oct 30]. Available from: https://www.ncsi.gov.om/ar.
4. National Center for Statistics and Information [Internet]. Oman: Oman Government; [cited 2026 Jun 15]. Available from: https://gov.om/en/national-center-for-statistics-and-information.
5. Ministry of Health, Oman. Annual Health Report 2024 [Internet]. Muscat: Ministry of Health; [cited 2026 Jun 15]. Available from: https://moh.gov.om/media/b3unoywd/annual-health-report-2024.pdf.
6. Khan SF, Ismail MY. Al-Shifa: case study on Sultanate of Oman's National Healthcare Information System. Indian J Sci Technol. 2017;10(17):1–4. https://doi.org/10.17485/ijst/2017/v10i17/113060.
7. Oman Society of Rheumatology. Oman Society of Rheumatology [Internet]. Muscat: OSR; [cited 2026 Jun 15]. Available from: https://www.omanrheumatology.org.
8. Altorok N, Nada S, Nagaraja V, Kahaleh B. Epigenetics in bone and joint disorders. Med Epigenet. 2016;8:295–314.
9. Pountain G. The prevalence of rheumatoid arthritis in the Sultanate of Oman. Br J Rheumatol. 1991;30(1):24–8. https://doi.org/10.1093/rheumatology/30.1.24.
10. Abdwani R, Abdalla E, Al Abrawi S, Al-Zakwani I. Epidemiology of juvenile idiopathic arthritis in Oman. Pediatr Rheumatol Online J. 2015;13:33. https://doi.org/10.1186/s12969-015-0030-z.
11. Al-Adhoubi NK, Al-Balushi F, Al Salmi I, Ali M, Al Lawati T, Al Lawati BSH, et al. A multicenter longitudinal study of the prevalence and mortality rate of systemic lupus erythematosus patients in Oman: Oman Lupus study. Int J Rheum Dis. 2021;24(6):847–54. https://doi.org/10.1111/1756-185X.14130.
12. Al Adhoubi NK, Liyanage P, Al Salmi I, Abdul Hameed Z, Al Abrawi S, Al Lawati T, et al. The prevalence, epidemiological characteristics and mortality trends of inflammatory myopathies patients in Oman: the prevision study. Clin Exp Rheumatol. 2024;42(7):1333–42. https://doi.org/10.55563/clinexprheumatol/o78ssl.
13. Meer E, Thrastardottir T, Wang X, Dubreuil M, Chen Y, Gelfand JM, et al. Risk factors for diagnosis of psoriatic arthritis, psoriasis, rheumatoid arthritis, and ankylosing spondylitis: a set of parallel case-control studies. J Rheumatol. 2022;49(1):53–9. https://doi.org/10.3899/jrheum.210006.
14. Deane KD, Demoruelle MK, Kelmenson LB, Kuhn KA, Norris JM, Holers VM. Genetic and environmental risk factors for rheumatoid arthritis. Best Pract Res Clin Rheumatol. 2017;31:3–18.
15. Nguyen USDT, Zhang Y, Lu N, Louie-Gao Q, Niu J, Ogdie A, et al. Smoking paradox in the development of psoriatic arthritis among patients with psoriasis: a population-based study. Ann Rheum Dis. 2018;77:119–23.
16. Al-Mawali A, Jayapal SK, Morsi M, Al-Shekaili W, Pinto AD, Al-Kharusi H, et al. Prevalence of risk factors of non-communicable diseases in the Sultanate of Oman: STEPS survey. PLoS One. 2021;16(10):e0259239.
17. Chien SY, Chuang MC, Chen IP. Why people do not attend health screenings: factors that influence willingness to participate in health screenings for chronic diseases. Int J Environ Res Public Health. 2020;17(10):3495. https://doi.org/10.3390/ijerph17103495.
18. Xiang L, AHL L, Leung YY, Fong W, Gandhi M, Xin X, et al. Improving the sensitivity of the connective tissue disease screening questionnaire: a comparative study of various scoring methods. Lupus. 2021;30(1):35–44. https://doi.org/10.1177/0961203320966378.

19. Mehdi I, Al Bahrani BJ. Medical tourism in Oman. Cancer Rep Rev. 2020;4:1000212. https://doi.org/10.15761/CRR.1000212.
20. Khan MJ, Chelliah S, Haron MS. International patients' travel decision making process: a conceptual framework. Iran J Public Health. 2016;45:134–45.
21. Al-Hinai SS, Al-Busaidi AS, Al-Busaidi IH. Medical tourism abroad: a new challenge to Oman's health system—Al Dakhiliya region experience. Sultan Qaboos Univ Med J. 2011;11(4):477–84.
22. Soriano E. Current status and future challenges in the treatment of rheumatic diseases. Front Drug Saf Regul. 2022;2:1–5.
23. Abdwani R, Abdalla E, Al Masilhi B, Shalaby A, Al-Maawali A. Novel mutation in interleukin 1 receptor antagonist associated with chronic diarrhea in infancy. J Paediatr Child Health. 2022;58(1):186–8.
24. Al Lawati T, Hassan B. Mixed connective tissue disease with severe axonal polyneuropathy: a case report. Oman Med J. 2022;37(3):e376.
25. Al-Adhoubi NK, Ali M, Al Wahshi HA, Al Salmi I, Al-Balushi F, Al Lawati T, et al. COVID-19 mortality in patients with rheumatic diseases: a real concern. Curr Rheumatol Rev. 2022;
26. Mahdi AS, Nasr IH, Al Jahdhami S, Kamona A, Al Wahshi HA. Eosinophilic fasciitis responds well to steroids and methotrexate. Oman Med J. 2019;34(6):564–7.
27. Al-Adhoubi NK, Al Salmi I. Safety of denosumab in patients with chronic kidney disease. Saudi J Kidney Dis Transpl. 2021;32(5):1235–42.
28. Al-Adhoubi NK, Bystrom J. Systemic lupus erythematosus and diffuse alveolar hemorrhage: etiology and novel treatment strategies. Lupus. 2020;29(4):355–63.
29. Metry AM, Al Salmi I, Al Balushi F, Yousef MA, Al Ismaili F, Hola A, et al. Systemic lupus erythematosus: symptoms and signs at initial presentations. Antiinflamm Antiallergy Agents Med Chem. 2019;18(2):142–50. https://doi.org/10.2174/1871523018666181128161828.
30. Abdwani R, Abdalla E, Al-Zakwani I. Unique characteristics of prepubertal onset systemic lupus erythematosus. Int J Pediatr. 2019;2019:9537065. https://doi.org/10.1155/2019/9537065.
31. Abdalla E, Jeyaseelan L, Ullah I, Abdwani R. Growth pattern in children with systemic lupus erythematosus. Oman Med J. 2017;32(4):284–90. https://doi.org/10.5001/omj.2017.56.
32. Al-Busaidi T, Wali U, Al-Shirawi A, Al-Mujaini A. Dacryoadenitis as first presenting feature in systemic lupus erythematosus. Lupus. 2013;22(13):1431–2. https://doi.org/10.1177/0961203313498804.
33. Alkaabi JK, Alkindi S, Riyami NA, Zia F, Balla LM, Balla SM. Successful treatment of severe thrombocytopenia with romiplostim in a pregnant patient with systemic lupus erythematosus. Lupus. 2012;21(14):1571–4. https://doi.org/10.1177/0961203312463621.
34. Al-Saleh JA, Saab MA, Negm A, Balushi F, Namas R, Ziade N. Predictors of not achieving remission or low disease activity in axial spondyloarthritis patients from Middle Eastern countries: a prospective, multicenter, real-world study. Oman Med J. 2022;37(3):e375. https://doi.org/10.5001/omj.2022.69.
35. Al-Jabri AA, Al-Gahdani AK, Al-Shuaili I. High frequency of Smith autoantibodies in Omani patients with systemic lupus erythematosus. Rheumatol Int. 2009;30(1):51–6. https://doi.org/10.1007/s00296-009-0909-4.
36. Abdwani R, Al-Abrawi S, Sharef SW, Al-Zakwani I. Geographical clustering of juvenile onset systemic lupus erythematosus within the Sultanate of Oman. Oman Med J. 2013;28(3):199–203. https://doi.org/10.5001/omj.2013.54.
37. Moghadam EA, Hamzehlou L, Moazzami B, Mehri M, Ziaee V. Increased QT interval dispersion is associated with coronary artery involvement in children with Kawasaki disease. Oman Med J. 2020;35(1):e88. https://doi.org/10.5001/omj.2020.06.
38. Alkaabi JK, Gravell D, Al-Haddabi H, Pathare A. Haemostatic parameters in patients with Behçet's disease. Sultan Qaboos Univ Med J. 2014;14(2):e1906.
39. Al-Adhoubi NK, Al Salmi I, Al Kaabi J, Al-Balushi F, Ali M, Al Lawati T, et al. Diving deep into lupus: gastrointestinal involvement insights from the Oman lupus study. Lupus. 2024;33(14):1637–44. https://doi.org/10.1177/09612033241292704. Epub 2024 Oct 14

40. Al Hosni F, Abdwani R, Al Flaiti AH, Rafei MA, Al Zuhaibi S, Mal M, et al. Adherence to screening recommendations for uveitis in juvenile idiopathic arthritis (JIA) patients: a retrospective cohort study from a tertiary referral hospital in Oman. Oman J Ophthalmol. 2025;18(2):121–5. https://doi.org/10.4103/ojo.ojo_388_24.
41. Al Rawahi A, Awlad Thani S, Alriyami M, Al Furqani A, Al-Abrawi S. Pericardial effusion as the first presentation of systemic lupus erythematosus in a 22-month-old infant: a case report and literature review. Cureus. 2025;17(3):e80042. https://doi.org/10.7759/cureus.80042.
42. Al-Battashy A, Al Ghaithi H, Al Lawati BS, Al-Mujaini AS. Ptosis: an uncommon manifestation of autoimmune disease activity in systemic lupus erythematosus. BMC Ophthalmol. 2025;25(1):537. https://doi.org/10.1186/s12886-025-04384-2.

Chapter 12
Rheumatic Diseases in Palestine

Sima Abu Al-Saoud, Nezam Altorok, and Muaath Itmaizeh

Abstract Rheumatology care has witnessed notable progress in Palestine over the past two decades, a trajectory detailed in this chapter. The Palestinian territories encompass the West Bank and the Gaza Strip, the latter of which is one of the most densely populated areas in the world. However, beyond the pervasive economic and political instability and its ramifications, optimal rheumatology care faces a number of distinct obstacles. These include a shortage of practicing rheumatologists and rheumatology services, as well as challenges in providing advanced therapies, such as biologics, for rheumatic diseases. Developing realistic strategies is essential to address these barriers and establish multidisciplinary services to improve patient outcomes. Concurrent efforts are needed to create educational and research initiatives, which remain scarce at this stage due to limited resources. It is also important to allocate more financial resources to develop national screening and diagnostic programs and to improve access to advanced therapies for rheumatic diseases in Palestine.

Keywords Palestine · Palestinian territories · West bank · Gaza strip · Rheumatology · Rheumatic diseases · Rheumatology services · Rheumatology workforce · Health services accessibility · Armed conflicts

S. Abu Al-Saoud (✉)
Department of Pediatrics, Division of Pediatric Rheumatology, Al-Quds University, Faculty of Medicine, Makassed Hospital, Jerusalem, Palestine
e-mail: ssaud@staff.alquds.edu

N. Altorok
Division of Rheumatology, Department of Internal Medicine, University of Toledo, Toledo, OH, USA
e-mail: Nezam.Altorok@utoledo.edu

M. Itmaizeh
Department of Internal Medicine, Division of Rheumatology, Makassed Hospital, Faculty of Medicine, Al-Quds University, Jerusalem, Palestine
e-mail: muaath.t2016@gmail.com

K. A. Alnaqbi, G. Aldabie (eds.), *Rheumatic Diseases in the Arab World*,
https://doi.org/10.1007/978-981-92-0967-5_12

12.1 Introduction

Rheumatic and musculoskeletal diseases (RMDs) represent a major cause of chronic morbidity, disability, and reduced quality of life worldwide. According to global burden estimates, musculoskeletal (MSK) conditions affect more than 1.7 billion people and are among the leading contributors to years lived with disability (YLDs) globally, reflecting their substantial impact on individuals, health systems, and societies [1]. In the Middle East and North Africa (MENA) region, the burden of MSK disorders has increased over recent decades, with RMDs contributing significantly to disability and healthcare needs [2].

While data on the epidemiology of RMDs in Palestine are limited, available community and clinical surveys indicate that a proportion of the population reports MSK diagnoses, with prevalence increasing with age, and that prevalent RMDs include seronegative spondyloarthropathy, rheumatoid arthritis (RA), and systemic lupus erythematosus. In addition, the ongoing challenges of the healthcare environment, including political instability, resource constraints, workforce shortages, and fragmented service delivery, shape access to specialist care and long-term management for individuals living with RMDs.

This chapter provides a comprehensive overview of RMDs in Palestine, with a focus on demographics, healthcare structure, workforce capacity, diagnostic and therapeutic resources, and research and education.

12.2 Demographics of Palestine

12.2.1 Geography

Palestine is located in the Levant region, along the eastern coast of the Mediterranean Sea, south of Lebanon and west of the Jordan River. The region has been historically significant as a crossroads of civilization, religion, culture, and commerce, linking Africa, Asia, and the Mediterranean since ancient times. The area is recognized as the birthplace of Judaism and Christianity and is also known as the Holy Land, held sacred by Jews, Christians, and Muslims [3]. The current administrative reality reflects the politically fragmented territories of the West Bank, East Jerusalem, and the Gaza Strip. As of today, these areas are divided into 16 governorates (muhafazat): 11 in the West Bank (Tulkarem, Jenin, Nablus, Tubas, Qalqilya, Salfit, Ramallah and Al-Bireh, Jericho and the Jordan Valley, Bethlehem, Hebron, and East Jerusalem) and five in the Gaza Strip (North Gaza, Gaza City, Deir al-Balah, Khan Yunis, and Rafah). This administrative division has a significant impact on rheumatologic care, contributing to challenges in patient access, specialist mobility, and continuity of healthcare delivery across regions.

12.2.2 Population

The estimated Palestinian population worldwide by mid-2025 is approximately 15.2 million. This includes the 5.61 million residing in the West Bank and Gaza Strip (3.4 million in the West Bank), 1.9 million in the 1948 territories, and nearly 7.8 million in the diaspora (with a majority of 6.5 million living in Arab countries). The population in Gaza has seen a decline from pre-war projections, currently estimated at 2.1 million, due to the devastating 2023–2025 war [4].

The refugee population remains a central demographic feature, with around 2.5 million registered refugees living in Gaza, the West Bank, and East Jerusalem. This is particularly salient in the Gaza Strip, where the majority of the population has undergone internal displacement in the last 2 years. Internationally, more than 3.4 million refugees are registered abroad [4–6].

The population growth rate is currently estimated at 1.71% annually, with a high density of around 889 people per square kilometer by mid-2022. There is a stark contrast between the West Bank (563 per sq. km) and the Gaza Strip (5936 per sq. km), consistently ranking the Palestinian territories among the most densely populated globally [7, 8]. Palestinian society is predominantly young, with about 37% of the population under the age of 15 and about 65% under the age of 30 [4]. The average life expectancy at birth was estimated at 73.1 years in 2023 [4], and the sex ratio shows a slight male majority, with 102.4 males for every 100 females [9].

Key economic indicators reveal profound challenges. Unemployment remains a critical issue, with rates approximating 34% in the West Bank and nearly 80% in the Gaza Strip, reflecting the profound economic fragility and the impact of the latest war [10]. It is important to note that while these figures present the latest data from official sources, the ongoing extreme conditions and logistical constraints in Gaza limit the availability of real-time data, and actual figures may differ substantially from reported estimates.

12.3 Palestine Healthcare Sectors

The Palestinian Ministry of Health (MoH) has managed the Palestinian health system since 1994, following the Oslo Accords. Health care services across primary, secondary, and tertiary health care levels were primarily made available by four main providers: the Palestinian MoH, Palestinian non-governmental organizations (NGOs), the UN Relief and Works Agency (UNRWA), and the private sector [11, 12].

The distribution of these providers varied significantly between regions. The MoH was the main provider of primary health care in the West Bank, accounting for more than 71% of clinics. In the Gaza Strip, however, UNRWA and the non-governmental sectors played a more substantial role than the MoH, which accounted for nearly a third of the primary healthcare clinics [11].

The government sector was dominant overall, operating primary health care clinics and government hospitals. It also managed a referral system for tertiary care to centers in East Jerusalem and private hospitals in the West Bank, Israel, Jordan, and Egypt [11]. Data from 2022 indicated that approximately 9.73% of Palestine's *Gross Domestic Product (GDP)* was allocated to the healthcare sector, which aligns more closely with the international benchmark of 10% [13].

The framework outlined previously provided a struggling yet operational healthcare system for decades. However, the war in Gaza that began in October 2023 shattered this foundational system, severely degrading its functionality and replacing it with a desperate struggle for basic medical provision through an overwhelmed emergency response [14, 15].

12.3.1 Health Insurance

Prior to the 2023–2025 war, approximately 79% of Palestinians in the West Bank and Gaza Strip had some form of health insurance coverage, while 20% lacked any coverage, according to the 2017 census by the Palestinian Central Bureau of Statistics (PCBS) [16].

In Palestine, four main health insurance schemes operate: the governmental health insurance system, UNRWA health insurance for refugees (many living in overcrowded camps with poor conditions), military-service insurance, and private health insurance. The government health insurance scheme, established in 2004 with mandatory enrollment for public sector employees and voluntary enrollment for any Palestinian citizen, and UNRWA together accounted for over 90% of total coverage, with a significant overlap in their beneficiary populations [17].

Despite this relatively high insurance coverage, households still faced considerable financial strain. Out-of-pocket payments represented approximately 45.5% of total health financing, mostly for pharmaceutical costs [17]. The government health insurance program provided comprehensive benefits, covering all primary healthcare services (including maternal and child health), secondary care, medications on the essential drug list, and tertiary care services not available in MoH facilities, often purchased from non-MoH facilities [17].

Re-establishing a functional health insurance system in Gaza remains a long-term goal, dependent on a rebuilt healthcare infrastructure within a stable, secure environment.

12.3.2 Hospitals in Palestine

As of 2024, the Palestinian healthcare system comprised 83 hospitals. Of these, 60 were located in the West Bank, seven in East Jerusalem, and 16 were partially functioning in the Gaza Strip. Together, these facilities had a total capacity of approximately 7126 beds. This overall figure comprises 2614 beds in the Gaza Strip, including 519 beds in field hospitals, 718 in East Jerusalem, and the remainder in the West Bank [18].

In the West Bank, the number of beds per 10,000 population was 13.4, while the number of hospitals per 100,000 population was 1.8, with the highest rates concentrated in the Bethlehem governorate in the West Bank. Hospital ownership was distributed across four main providers: MoH hospitals representing (42.7%) of the total number of beds in the West Bank, NGOs (37.3%), the private sector (18.7%), and UNRWA (1.3%) [18].

Hospitals in the West Bank are classified by specialty. General hospitals, providing secondary and some tertiary care, accounted for 69.4% of all beds. Specialized hospitals constituted 23.4%, offering advanced and comprehensive secondary and tertiary care. Maternity hospitals comprised 4.6%, while rehabilitation and physiotherapy centers—all owned by NGOs—accounted for the remaining 2.6% [18].

The distribution of beds in governmental hospitals across key specialties reflects the priorities of the system's service. In the West Bank, internal medicine constituted the largest share at *26.3% (498 beds),* followed by surgery at *25.5% (483 beds),* pediatrics at *17% (323 beds),* intensive care units at 16.9% (320 beds), and obstetrics/gynecology at *14.3% (271 beds).* MoH hospitals in the West Bank operated under heavy strain, with an overall bed occupancy rate of 93.2%, reaching 117% at Alia Hospital in Hebron and Beit Jala Hospital in Beit Jala [18].

The healthcare situation in Gaza has undergone catastrophic change. While 35 hospitals were operational in 2022, the war has devastated the infrastructure. By the end of 2024, only 16 hospitals remained partially functional, supported by 10 field hospitals, bringing the total inpatient beds in Gaza to 1967 [18]. As of May 2025, over 94% of hospitals in Gaza had been damaged or destroyed. The few remaining facilities, such as Al-Shifa and Al-Ahi hospitals in Gaza City, were overwhelmed, operating at nearly 300% over capacity, crippled by critical shortages of supplies, staff, and security [19].

12.4 Rheumatology Health Services in Palestine

12.4.1 Rheumatology Workforce in Palestine

Palestine's rheumatology workforce is critically insufficient and unevenly distributed, especially considering the national physician density of 2.8 per 1000 population [20]. With only 19 practicing specialists serving a population of over five million, the density falls far below the global desirable benchmark of 1–2 rheumatologists per 100,000 people [21]. Geographically, the disparity is substantial: the West Bank and East Jerusalem are served by 15 adult and two pediatric rheumatologists, while the Gaza Strip has just one adult specialist.

Pediatric rheumatology is a more recent development, with services formally introduced in 2017, and is currently provided by two pediatric rheumatologists (one female and one male). The field is marked by a significant gender disparity in adult rheumatology, where only one female practices among a predominantly male cohort, a contrast to the Arab region, where women comprise 56% of the rheumatology workforce [22].

The severely limited workforce in Gaza has historically relied on internal referral pathways for specialized care. Until October 2023, patients requiring advanced management were referred to centers in East Jerusalem and the West Bank; a critical pathway has now been severed. The training pathway for future specialists is another pressing concern, as no rheumatology fellows are currently in training within Palestine, though some may be pursuing training abroad.

Furthermore, the multidisciplinary team remains incomplete, with the lack of dedicated rheumatology nurses representing a significant gap. This challenge has been recognized as a key obstacle for rheumatology services across the African and Middle Eastern regions [21]. These professionals play a pivotal role in long-term patient management, contributing to patient education, self-injection training for methotrexate and biologics, and providing psychosocial support [23].

12.4.2 Patient Referrals

To address the shortfalls in government health services, including specialist shortages, equipment limitations, full bed occupancy, and waiting lists exceeding 6 months, the Palestinian MoH has developed a medical referral system. This system enables the ministry to expand patient access by purchasing medical services from non-MoH facilities, including private sector institutions, NGOs, and charitable institutions, primarily located in the West Bank and East Jerusalem. When necessary services are unavailable locally, referrals are made abroad [24]. With World Bank financing, the Palestinian MoH launched an electronic eReferrals database in 2019 to improve the recording and tracking of outside medical referrals and enhance access to specialized care services not available within MoH facilities [25].

Due to the limited number of rheumatologists, both adult and pediatric specialists receive a high volume of referrals, primarily from the public sector, particularly government hospitals. They also receive referrals from the private sector and self-referrals from patients and families, though to a lesser extent. Referrals are primarily initiated by general practitioners, internists, pediatricians, and other specialties such as orthopedics and ophthalmology.

12.5 Official Rheumatology Society of Palestine

The Palestinian Rheumatology Society was officially established in 2012 as a branch of the Palestinian Medical Association. The society promotes connections with the global Palestinian medical diaspora by awarding honorary memberships to some rheumatologists practicing in the occupied Palestinian territory and abroad, such as the United States of America and the United Kingdom.

The society's leadership and activities have also been recognized at the regional level through participation in Arab and regional rheumatology meetings, including collaborations with neighboring national rheumatology societies [26, 27].

A key function of society is to encourage continuous medical education for healthcare professionals in Palestine. Its activities include organizing national rheumatology conferences, facilitating journal clubs, conducting scientific workshops, and developing consensus guidelines for local practice, targeting rheumatologists, internists, pediatricians, and general practitioners.

The society's president is democratically elected by the members of the society and serves a three-year term.

12.6 Overview of Rheumatic Diseases in Palestine

12.6.1 Prevalence of Rheumatic Diseases in Palestine

Documenting the incidence and prevalence of RMDs in Palestine is challenging due to several obstacles and limitations. These include the absence of a national disease registry capable of capturing cases of RMDs, as well as the lack of a unified electronic medical record system (EMR), or even a robust institution-assigned EMR that is capable of filtering out these cases. Additionally, many patients with rheumatic complaints establish care with orthopedic surgeons or internists rather than rheumatologists, further complicating efforts to determine the exact epidemiology of rheumatic conditions.

Due to the historically high rate of consanguineous marriage, particularly first-cousin marriage among Palestinians, many hereditary disorders, especially those with an autosomal recessive mode of inheritance, are common. While data from the Gaza Strip indicates a consanguinity rate of 39.9%, this reflects a significant decline from 45.2% in the previous generation, a trend observed in other Palestinian communities as well [28]. A 2023 study in the West Bank found the rate among married participants was 18.7%, compared to 28.8% among their parents [29]. Familial Mediterranean Fever (FMF), for instance, is one of the most common RMDs in Palestine, with an estimated incidence of at least 1:2000 [30, 31]. The most frequently detected mutations are M694V, V726A, M694I, and M680I, which together account for more than 80% of identified mutations [32], a genotypic profile similar to that seen in neighboring countries.

Table 12.1 Distribution of rheumatic diseases at Makassed Hospital's rheumatology outpatient clinic in 2019

Rheumatic disease	Male	Female	Total
Rheumatoid arthritis	170	280	450
Ankylosing spondylitis	70	10	80
Systemic lupus erythematosus	15	25	40
Vasculitis of any type	27	30	57
Inflammatory myopathy	10	15	25
Scleroderma	15	25	40
Sjogren disease	50	250	300

12.6.2 Retrospective Overview of Rheumatic Diseases in a Single Center in Palestine

In 2019, we conducted a retrospective analysis of patient visits to the rheumatology clinic at Makassed Hospital. This hospital is the home to the only rheumatology training program in Palestine and serves as a tertiary referral center for other health facilities across the West Bank and Gaza Strip. Makassed Hospital is one of the largest hospitals in East Jerusalem, with 250 beds, more than 60 of which are intensive care unit beds. Annually, the hospital records approximately 42,272 outpatient visits and 15,597 inpatient admissions. Table 12.1 (based on unpublished data) presents the distribution of RMDs among patients aged 14 years and older who visited the rheumatology outpatient clinic at Makassed Hospital in 2019, including sex distribution.

Our findings indicate that RA was the most commonly encountered RMD at the clinic, consistent with regional data from the Middle East and North Africa showing RA to be a major and prevalent inflammatory rheumatic condition [33, 34]. Sjogren's disease also appeared frequently and is often associated with other RMDs. Less commonly encountered diseases included vasculitis, systemic sclerosis, and inflammatory myopathies.

12.7 Risk Factors for Rheumatic Diseases

Several modifiable and non-modifiable risk factors are known to be associated with an increased incidence of RMDs. In Palestine, the prevalence of these risk factors is high. Tobacco smoking, a well-established risk factor for diseases such as RA, has an estimated prevalence of 47.7% in Palestine, with a concerning trend of initiation at a very young age, particularly among males [35].

Obesity has also been linked to the development of autoimmune and inflammatory conditions, as adipose tissue serves as a reservoir for inflammatory mediators that may initiate or worsen RMDs. A study of an urban Palestinian population found that 49% of women and 30% of men were obese [36].

Furthermore, vitamin D deficiency, which is associated with increased disease activity and flares in certain RMDs [37, 38], is common among the Palestinian population. A 2022 study found that 78.8% of adult participants had vitamin D deficiency [39].

As detailed in the previous section, consanguineous marriage is a non-modifiable risk factor for hereditary RMDs, including periodic fever syndromes, other monogenic auto-inflammatory disorders, and monogenic forms of lupus [40, 41].

12.8 Screening Programs for Rheumatic Diseases

Non-communicable diseases (NCDs) are the leading cause of mortality in Palestine, posing substantial challenges to healthcare development and accounting for a significant portion of health expenditures. This reality necessitates strategic interventions targeting key modifiable risk factors such as tobacco use, unhealthy diet, and physical inactivity that are linked to urbanization and societal changes [42].

For RMDs, where early diagnosis is critical to prevent irreversible damage and disability, the absence of effective national screening programs represents a major gap in care. This stems from several interconnected constraints. The fragmentation of the Palestinian territories by checkpoints and the separation wall disrupts geographic continuity and severely impedes the consistent movement of patients and health workers required for a screening system. Additionally, screening programs impose a significant financial burden on an already strained healthcare budget. The implementation of such initiatives also requires trained personnel and technical infrastructure, which remain largely unavailable at this stage.

In response, increasing public awareness about RMDs, particularly the importance of early diagnosis and timely follow-up with rheumatologists, has become increasingly crucial. The Palestinian Rheumatology Society has taken several steps to raise awareness through broadcast media, but reaching a wider audience through diverse media channels and community engagement remains an ongoing need.

12.9 Diagnostic Tools for Rheumatic Diseases in Palestine

12.9.1 Laboratory Test

A core panel of laboratory tests essential for the classification and diagnosis of RMDs is accessible within the West Bank and East Jerusalem. These include routine immunological tests such as anti-nuclear antibodies (ANA), anti-double-stranded DNA antibodies (anti-dsDNA), extractable nuclear antigen antibodies (ENA), antiphospholipid antibodies, anti-neutrophil cytoplasmic antibodies (ANCA), anti-cyclic citrullinated peptide (anti-CCP), and rheumatoid factor (RF), as well as genetic testing such as HLA-B27, HLA-B51, and MEFV gene mutations.

However, many specialized tests are not readily available. These include monitoring tests like serum amyloid A, a crucial test for monitoring amyloidosis risk in a country where FMF is prevalent. Additionally, more advanced serological and immunological panels, such as the full myositis antibody panel, type I interferon signature testing, soluble IL-2 receptor (sCD25), soluble CD163, and broader cytokine panels, are unavailable entirely.

While all of the available core tests are widely accessible, they are offered mainly through private laboratories, although most rheumatologists can order them when needed. In fact, most are also available in the major government hospitals. Genetic testing for the 10 most common MEFV gene mutations has recently become available in governmental hospitals. This represents a key advancement, offering faster, more accessible, and cost-effective diagnosis of FMF.

For more advanced genetic testing, including whole exome sequencing (WES), services are available at two non-governmental hospitals, but typically at the patient's expense. For many, cost remains the primary barrier to accessing these necessary diagnostic tests, which impacts both initial diagnosis and ongoing disease monitoring.

12.9.2 Imaging for Diagnosis of Rheumatic Diseases in Palestine

Most practicing rheumatologists in the West Bank and East Jerusalem have access to imaging facilities such as X-rays, computed tomography (CT) scans, computed tomography angiography (CT angiography), magnetic resonance imaging (MRI), and magnetic resonance angiography (MRA). These imaging facilities are available in almost every specialized hospital. However, access to specific scans remains limited. For example, sacroiliac joint MRI is available in only a few government hospitals. The capacity is insufficient to meet demand, as rheumatology patients compete with others for appointments and are not prioritized. Consequently, the wait time for this scan can exceed 6 months.

Positron emission tomography (PET) was introduced in 2018 and is now available at three centers outside the MoH. These are located in the north of the West Bank at a private diagnostic center, in the south at a general hospital, and in East Jerusalem at Augusta Victoria Hospital, a comprehensive cancer center [43]. However, there is a shortage of local experts; the images used to be sent abroad for review and reporting. These centers are already overwhelmed by the needs of oncology patients, making PET scans effectively inaccessible for rheumatology cases.

A major challenge is the severe shortage of specialized radiologists. MSK radiology is a critically needed subspecialty. Only two radiologists in the country have formal training in MSK radiology, and their services are primarily available through the private sector. The situation is particularly difficult for pediatric patients, as there is only one pediatric radiologist in the entire country; this frequently requires adult radiologists to interpret pediatric scans.

MSK ultrasound is a relatively low-cost modality that can be used to diagnose and monitor RMD activity [44]. It is available primarily through a few private centers. However, most practicing rheumatologists in Palestine are not yet familiar with its use and application in clinical rheumatology practice.

The diagnostic landscape described above primarily reflects services in the West Bank and East Jerusalem. In the Gaza Strip, the situation is severely compromised. The destruction of healthcare infrastructure has severely limited access to even the most basic diagnostic tests. Laboratory services are disrupted by resource depletion, power cuts, and the inability to replenish supplies, all compounded by a severe lack of specialized personnel. Critical medical equipment—including X-ray machines, CT scanners, and MRI machines—is scarce due to both damage and import restrictions [45]. While specific data on rheumatology is unavailable, this systemic collapse makes specialized investigations and advanced imaging for chronic diseases exceptionally difficult to access, if not entirely unavailable, as the remaining health services are overwhelmingly directed toward emergency care.

12.10 Management of Rheumatic Diseases in Palestine

The management of RMDs has witnessed a revolutionary shift over the past decades worldwide, as our understanding of the mechanisms involved in the pathogenesis of these diseases has advanced. The introduction of disease-modifying anti-rheumatic drugs (DMARDs) that target specific immune pathways, such as biologics and Janus kinase (JAK) inhibitors, has significantly improved outcomes for patients with RMDs [46–49].

12.10.1 Availability of Conventional DMARDs and Biologic DMARDs in Palestine

In the West Bank, most conventional DMARDs (cDMARDs) are available at the main health clinics of government hospitals in cities including Jenin, Nablus, Tulkarm, Ramallah, Jericho, Bethlehem, and Hebron. For patients with medical insurance, these medications are provided at a nominal patient share. However, even when available at this low cost, there is a persistent risk of medication shortages. When shortages occur, patients must pay for their medications out-of-pocket or stop treatment altogether.

Access to biological DMARDs is more limited. Only a few are routinely available with an affordable patient share, namely etanercept, adalimumab, rituximab, and secukinumab. Other agents, such as infliximab, tocilizumab, tofacitinib, and, more recently, updacitinib, require a special request. Approval is not always guaranteed, and these medications are not routinely stocked in MoH pharmacies, which can delay treatment initiation by several months, sometimes over a year. Even when approved, the remaining patient share can be costly, and any supply shortages typically cause treatment interruptions.

The situation in the Gaza Strip was markedly worse even prior to 2023, with chronic shortages of essential medicines and very low availability of treatment supplies that left many therapeutic drugs out of reach for patients with chronic conditions. A 2025 survey of remaining health facilities found essential medicine availability far below World Health Organization (WHO) targets, highlighting systemic scarcity [50]. Following the latest war and intensification of the blockade, the collapse of pharmaceutical supply has deepened, with the MoH reporting zero stock for more than half of essential drugs and most medical disposables. Reports from health authorities also describe severe overall shortages of medicines and supplies critical for patient care [51, 52]. In this context, access to advanced therapies in Gaza is severely constrained, with chronic shortages affecting cDMARDs, biologic agents, and intravenous immunoglobulin (IVIG), reflecting the extreme limitations in delivering specialized rheumatologic care locally.

12.10.2 Accessibility to Multidisciplinary Specialties

Optimal management of RMDs requires the collaboration of multidisciplinary teams. Beyond pharmacotherapy, physiotherapy, occupational therapy, and comprehensive rehabilitation are crucial for addressing the physical and psychological aspects of these chronic conditions [53].

The need for these services in Palestine is significant. According to the WHO Rehabilitation Need Estimator, approximately two in seven Palestinians experience conditions that could benefit from rehabilitation [54]. This demand is reflected in the high volume of care provided, with outpatient visits to physiotherapy departments in the hospitals of the Palestinian MoH reaching 2,245,471 visits in 2020 alone [55]. However, this need is exacerbated by the scarcity of rehabilitation services, which have been described as few in number, unevenly distributed, and city-centered [56].

Table 12.2 (based on unpublished data) below outlines the main rehabilitation centers operating in the West Bank and Gaza Strip in 2022. These facilities provide a range of services, including physiotherapy, occupational therapy, and psychological therapy; some also offer specialized services such as hydrotherapy, as well as visual and speech therapy. A significant barrier for patients accessing these services is cost, as rehabilitation services are relatively expensive and are often paid for out-of-pocket. For those with medical insurance, patients can apply to the MoH for coverage with a reasonable patient share, if accepted.

For patients with advanced chronic arthritis, orthopedic surgeries such as total hip or knee arthroplasty are often necessary to restore function and relieve pain in severely damaged joints. In the West Bank, these procedures are accessible and performed by qualified surgeons in both the public and private sectors. However, in the Gaza Strip, such operations were rarely performed locally. Historically, patients

Table 12.2 Rehabilitation centers in Palestine (2022)

Rehabilitation center name	Location	Date of establishment	Number of beds	Service
Bethlehem Arab Society for Rehabilitation	Bethlehem	1961	118	Inpatient/ outpatient care (adult and pediatric rehabilitation center)
Al-Amal for Physical Therapy	Nablus		12	Inpatient/ outpatient care
Abu-Rayya Rehabilitation Center	Ramallah	1991	39	Inpatient/ outpatient (spinal cord injuries, orthopedic injuries)
Al-Mizan Hospital	Hebron		12	Inpatient/ outpatient
Jerusalem Princess Basma Center	East Jerusalem	1965	31	Inpatient/ outpatient (pediatric rehabilitation center- centered on family education)
American University of Jenin	Jenin		NA	Outpatient care
Palestinian Center of Excellence for Brain Development (Takween)	Ramallah	2019	NA	Outpatient care (pediatric rehabilitation center)
Al-Amal Rehabilitation Center	Gaza- Khan Younis	2013	55	Inpatient/ outpatient care
Al-Wafa Rehabilitation Center	Gaza	1980	40	Inpatient/ outpatient care (rebuilt after damage to healthcare infrastructure during the 2022 Gaza conflict)
Sheikh Hamad Hospital for Rehabilitation and Prosthetics	Gaza	2016	100	Inpatient/ outpatient care

NA, not available

required referrals outside Gaza or relied on sporadic delegations of orthopedic surgeons as part of medical missions. Although arthroplasty was recently introduced as a local service, the European hospital in the Gaza Strip was the only center in Gaza performing these procedures in-house until at least 2019, underscoring the extreme limitations in surgical capacity even prior to the recent escalation [57].

The war in Gaza has rendered most rehabilitation centers non-operational. By late 2025, the WHO reported that over 94% of hospitals in Gaza had been destroyed or damaged. This coincides with a massive surge in need, with an estimated 42,000 people sustaining life-threatening injuries, including over 5000 amputations. The situation is further crippled by severe shortages of specialized staff and essential equipment. Gaza's only dedicated limb reconstruction and rehabilitation center is currently non-functional, and only a handful of prosthetists remain. Consequently, the ongoing needs of people with chronic conditions and disabilities are being overlooked [19, 58].

12.11 Rheumatology Research and Education in Palestine

12.11.1 Education

Nearly 85% of practicing Palestinian rheumatologists received their specialty training abroad, particularly in Europe, North America, and other Arab countries. A major milestone was the establishment of Palestine's first and only rheumatology training program in 2017, based at Makassed Hospital in Jerusalem.

This 2-year program includes 1 year of clinical training at Makassed Hospital, followed by a second year at Jordan University Hospital in Amman, Jordan. The program's capacity is limited by funding and typically recruits only one fellow per year, operating intermittently depending on available resources. To date, four rheumatologists have graduated from the program, all of whom successfully passed the Palestinian Board of Rheumatology examination and currently practice in the West Bank and East Jerusalem.

Furthermore, the multidisciplinary team remains incomplete; the country has no specialized rheumatology nurses, and there are no formal training programs for rheumatology nursing or physician assistants.

12.12 Cost-Effective Rheumatology Care in Palestine

The global burden of MSK diseases is rising significantly, a challenge particularly pronounced in resource-limited countries like Palestine [59]. In response to the economic burden imposed by the growing demand for biological medications, the Palestinian MoH has recently begun transitioning toward the use of biosimilars, which are considered cheaper alternatives (to some extent) compared to originator biologic agents [60].

The high cost of external referrals also places a major strain on the healthcare system. In 2018 alone, the Palestinian MoH spent over 34% of its expenditures on purchasing services unavailable in its own hospitals. That year, the MoH issued 71,923 referrals from the West Bank and 30,944 from the Gaza Strip to non-MoH facilities [17, 61]. Rheumatology patients have been part of this referral pattern due to gaps in specialized services.

To address this issue, the Palestinian MoH has appointed a rheumatologist to most of its major hospitals. Another key development has been the local manufacturing of some anti-inflammatory medications and cDMARDs by Palestinian pharmaceutical companies, which in turn has contributed to easing the financial burden caused by the high cost of imported medications.

12.13 Opportunities and Specific Challenges

There is no doubt that rheumatology care in Palestine has witnessed remarkable development in recent years, despite enduring significant economic and political obstacles. However, the challenges are still enormous, and the situation in Gaza has deteriorated to a catastrophic level since 2023.

A global rheumatology workforce shortage exists, particularly in developing countries, and is expected to worsen with the rising prevalence of RMDs due to population aging [62]. In Palestine, only 16 board-certified adult rheumatologists and two pediatric rheumatologists serve a population of approximately five million, equating to just 0.32 rheumatologists per 100,000 people, well below global recommendations. The field also lacks rheumatology subspecialists and subspecialty clinics. Consequently, most rheumatologists work full-time in clinical practice, with very limited time for research, limiting opportunities for research advancement.

Furthermore, many patients seek medical care at an advanced stage of their disease, having missed the critical 'window of opportunity' for early treatment. Initiating therapy during this window is essential to achieve disease remission, prevent long-term complications, and improve patient outcomes. This delay is partly due to a lack of a developed referral system to rheumatology and the inappropriate intrusion of other specialties, such as orthopedics and neurosurgery, to name a few, into rheumatology care. This leads to delays in diagnosis, disease progression, and a higher risk of complications. Additional factors contributing to delayed diagnosis include low public awareness of RMDs, limited knowledge among general physicians, and financial barriers, as patients often must pay out-of-pocket to see a private rheumatologist or face long waits to see a rheumatologist in MoH clinics.

Transportation is a significant obstacle for patients, particularly those traveling between the West Bank, the Gaza Strip, and East Jerusalem for medical care. Patients commonly face multiple checkpoints when traveling between cities. The separation wall around Jerusalem makes transit impossible without a special permit from the Israeli authorities, which is often hard to obtain [63]. The situation has been severely compounded by the latest war, with a significant proportion of patient permit applications being denied by Israeli authorities and the approval process causing critical delays that worsen patient outcomes [64]. Since 2023, all patient referrals from the Gaza Strip to the West Bank or East Jerusalem have been stopped.

To address the lack of services, the Palestinian MoH has historically referred patients to hospitals in East Jerusalem, Israel, Egypt, and Jordan, a practice which has exhausted financial health resources [17, 64]. For instance, in April 2022, 7426 referrals were issued, with 46% to West Bank hospitals, 38% to East Jerusalem hospitals, 7% inside the Gaza Strip, 6% to Israeli hospitals, 3% to Egypt, and 0.2% to Jordan [64]. Notably, rheumatology has not been among the top specialties requiring external referrals. Referrals for rheumatology patients to non-MoH facilities, especially abroad, have been significantly reduced. This can be attributed to the approval of more biological DMARDs through the MoH, the increased capacity for major laboratory investigations within major governmental hospitals, and the appointment of rheumatologists to most major governmental hospitals. Furthermore, with the introduction of the pediatric rheumatology subspecialty in Palestine in 2017, there is no longer a need to refer pediatric patients abroad. In Gaza today, however, the destruction of infrastructure and the overwhelming focus on emergency trauma and infectious disease outbreaks have made specialized rheumatology care virtually inaccessible.

12.14 Future Directions for Rheumatic Disease Care in Palestine

Over the past years, rheumatology has grown in popularity, becoming a more appealing career choice for medical students and graduating physicians. According to the U.S. National Resident Matching Program, fellowship applicants increased by 49% from 2015 to 2019, with rheumatology among the most competitive subspecialties [65]. This has also been the case among Palestinian graduating physicians.

The prevailing stereotype about RMDs is that they are incurable diseases and that patients suffering from them will live their lives with inevitable disabilities. However, appropriate early management of patients with RMDs can lead to excellent outcomes, refuting this myth and reducing the physical, psychological, and economic burden associated with delayed diagnosis. This has undoubtedly helped change the MoH's approach to the rheumatology specialty, with greater attention now paid to RMDs. However, it is still a lower priority for the Palestinian government. Rheumatology care should be advanced; more specialized training should be offered to healthcare workers, especially nurses, due to the lack of specialized rheumatology nurses and physician assistants. More immunomodulatory therapies must be made available, and strategies should be implemented to guarantee their sustainability and prevent persistent shortages. The Palestinian Rheumatology Society is currently working with the responsible authorities to implement national guidelines and protocols for treating RMDs.

Research in Palestine is another area that deserves tremendous support. Promoting and supporting research will be essential to improving rheumatology care by developing national clinical trials and participating in regional and international ones. In recent years, hospitals have switched to using electronic medical records, a step that will hopefully facilitate research and the establishment of national registries.

The establishment of the first Palestinian rheumatology training program was a much-needed step to address the shortage of rheumatologists, despite its very limited trainee capacity. Education about RMDs is vital to overcoming the shortage of rheumatologists and preventing delayed diagnosis. Such education is most effective when introduced early, beginning with medical students and residents. In this aspect, one of the primary medical schools in the country has included rheumatology education in the curricula of internal medicine and pediatrics. For a while, rheumatology was among the elective courses offered to fifth-year medical students and was particularly popular. The Palestinian Rheumatology Society recognizes its important role in raising awareness about RMDs. Various lectures, workshops, and conferences have been organized for internists, general practitioners, rheumatologists, and other specialists. Increasing public awareness is just as important. The Arab Adult Arthritis Awareness Group is an important initiative launched under the umbrella of the Arab League of Associations for Rheumatology (ArLAR). It is the first group of its kind in the Arab world, aiming to raise awareness about RMDs, primarily in Arabic, but also in English and French [66]. The group consists of 19 rheumatologists from 17 Arab countries, including Palestine.

12.15 Conclusion

Rheumatology is a rapidly advancing specialty, with substantial progress achieved in the understanding and management of RMDs. These conditions remain a major cause of disability and morbidity worldwide, contributing to a growing global health burden. In Palestine, prolonged conflict and persistent economic constraints further complicate the delivery of equitable and sustainable healthcare.

Despite these challenges, the healthcare system has taken important steps to address existing gaps and to keep pace with scientific developments in order to provide appropriate rheumatology care. Nevertheless, significant work remains. Continued progress will require coordinated efforts from healthcare professionals, policymakers, and stakeholders to identify realistic opportunities, strengthen services, and overcome ongoing challenges in the years ahead.

Acknowledgments We would like to thank the members of the Palestinian Rheumatology Society for their valuable support in providing relevant information. We also acknowledge Dr. Anas Muhanna for his pioneering role in advancing rheumatology in Palestine, particularly through the establishment of the national rheumatology fellowship program.

Conflict of Interest The authors have no conflict of interest to declare.

References

1. World Health Organization. Musculoskeletal health: fact sheet. Geneva: World Health Organization; 2022. [cited 2026 Jun 15]. Available from: https://www.who.int/news-room/fact-sheets/detail/musculoskeletal-conditions.
2. Al-Ajlouni YA, Al Ta'ani O, Mushasha R, Lee JL, Capoor J, Kapadia MR, et al. The burden of musculoskeletal disorders in the Middle East and North Africa (MENA) region: a longitudinal analysis from the global burden of disease dataset 1990-2019. BMC Musculoskelet Disord. 2023;24(1):439. https://doi.org/10.1186/s12891-023-06556-x.
3. Palestine [Internet]. Encyclopædia Britannica; 2025. [cited 2026 Jun 15]. Available from: https://www.britannica.com/place/Palestine.

4. Palestinian Central Bureau of Statistics. The Palestinian Central Bureau of Statistics (PCBS) presents the conditions of the Palestinian population on the occasion of World Population Day. Ramallah: Palestinian Central Bureau of Statistics; 2025. [cited 2026 Jun 15]. Available from: https://www.pead.ps/files/image/2025/Pdf/2025710.pdf.
5. United Nations Relief Works Agency for Palestine Refugees in the Near East (UNRWA). Where we work - West Bank [Internet]. Amman: UNRWA; 2024. [cited 2026 Jun 15]. Available from: https://www.unrwa.org/where-we-work/west-bank.
6. United Nations Relief Works Agency for Palestine Refugees in the Near East (UNRWA). Where we work - Gaza Strip [Internet]. Amman: UNRWA; 2024. [cited 2026 Jun 15]. Available from: https://www.unrwa.org/where-we-work/gaza-strip.
7. Palestinian Central Bureau of Statistics. Summary of demographic indicators in Palestine by region. Ramallah (PA): PCBS; 2022. [cited 2025 Oct 30]. Available from: https://www.pcbs.gov.ps/statisticsIndicatorsTables.aspx?lang=en&table_id=1228.
8. World Bank Group. West Bank and Gaza—towards economic sustainability: a country economic memorandum [internet]. Washington, D.C.: The World Bank Group; 2023. [cited 2026 Jun 15]. Available from: https://documents1.worldbank.org/curated/en/099102023064581959/pdf/P50039206405f9090ac360e24acb1624cf.pdf.
9. Palestinian Central Bureau of Statistics. Women and men in Palestine - issues and statistics 2025 [Internet]. Ramallah: Palestinian Central Bureau of Statistics; 2025. [cited 2026 Jun 15]. Available from: https://www.palestine-australia.com/highlights/news/2025/women-and-men-in-palestine-issues-and-statistics-2025/.
10. Palestinian Central Bureau of Statistics. The Palestinian Central Bureau of Statistics (PCBS) issues a press release on the occasion of World Statistics Day, 20/10/2025 [Internet]. Ramallah: Palestinian Central Bureau of Statistics; 2025. [cited 2025 Oct 30]. Available from: https://www.pcbs.gov.ps/default.aspx.
11. Health Annual Report: Palestine 2017 [Internet]. Ramallah: Palestinian Health Information Center; 2018. [cited 2026 Jun 15]. Available from: https://site.moh.ps/Content/Books/38pf7Q9KpsHKGjWZxroQEuJ1OZeOJw8mhssgDKBJGnoAu5C4oKFpoW_kUFGingMuntf-G2fm4rVu2grDremJD77xH9P5xgfSFQPvvxcOPgeyD7.pdf.
12. Mataria A, Khatib R, Donaldson C, Bossert T, Hunter D, Alsayed F, et al. Health in the Occupied Palestinian Territory 5: the health-care system: an assessment and reform agenda. Lancet. 2009;373:1207–17. https://doi.org/10.1016/S0140-6736(09)60111-2.
13. The World Bank. Current health expenditure (% of GDP) - West Bank and Gaza [Internet]. Washington, D.C.: The World Bank Group; 2025. [cited 2026 Jun 15]. Available from: https://data360.worldbank.org/en/indicator/WB_WDI_SH_XPD_CHEX_GD_ZS?view=trend&average=LCN.
14. Abuelaish I, Musani A. Reviving and rebuilding the health system in Gaza. East Mediterr Health J. 2025;31(2):56–8. https://doi.org/10.26719/2025.31.2.56.
15. Asmar I. The devastating effects of Gaza war on healthcare. East Mediterr Health J. 2025;31(2):77–8. https://doi.org/10.26719/2025.31.2.77.
16. Palestinian Central Bureau of Statistics. Statistical yearbook of Palestine, 2022 [Internet]. Ramallah: Palestinian Central Bureau of Statistics; 2022. [cited 2026 Jun 15]. Available from: http://www.pcbs.gov.ps/Downloads/book2637.pdf.
17. World Health Assembly, 72. Health conditions in the Occupied Palestinian Territory, including East Jerusalem, and the occupied Syrian Golan: report by the Director-General. World Health Organization [Internet]. 2019. [cited 2026 Jun 15]. Available from: https://apps.who.int/iris/handle/10665/328758.
18. Ministry of Health. Health annual report: Palestine 2024 [Internet]. Ramallah: Ministry of Health; 2025. [cited 2025 Oct 30]. Available from: https://ghdx.healthdata.org/series/palestine-health-annual-report.
19. World Health Organization. Health system at breaking point as hostilities further intensify in Gaza, WHO warns [Internet]. 2025 [cited 2026 Jun 15]. Available from: https://www.who.

int/news/item/22-05-2025-health-system-at-breaking-point-as-hostilities-further-intensify%2D%2Dwho-warns.
20. Palestinian Central Bureau of Statistics (PCBS) [Internet]. [cited 2026 Feb 1]. Available from: https://www.pcbs.gov.ps/site/881/default.aspx
21. Ziade N, Hmamouchi I, Haouichat C, Baron F, Al Mayouf S, Abdulateef N, et al. The rheumatology workforce in the Arab countries: current status, challenges, opportunities, and future needs from an ArLAR cross-sectional survey. Rheumatol Int. 2023;43:2281–92. https://doi.org/10.1007/s00296-023-05427-x.
22. Ziade N, Hmamouchi I, El Kibbi L. Women in rheumatology in the Arab league of associations for rheumatology countries: a rising workforce. Front Med (Lausanne). 2022;9:880285. https://doi.org/10.3389/fmed.2022.880285.
23. Miloslavsky EM, Bolster MB. Addressing the rheumatology workforce shortage: a multifaceted approach. Semin Arthritis Rheum. 2020;50(4):791–6. https://doi.org/10.1016/j.semarthrit.2020.05.009.
24. Coalition for Accountability and Integrity – AMAN. Integrity and transparency in medical referrals outside the Ministry of Health institutions: assessment report. Ramallah (Palestine): AMAN Coalition; 2024. [cited 2026 Jun 15]. Available from: https://www.aman-palestine.org/cached_uploads/download/2024/10/30/integrity-and-transparency-in-medical-referrals-1730291903.pdf.
25. World Bank. Improving the efficiency of outside medical referrals in Palestine: eReferrals system [Internet]. Washington, DC: World Bank; 2021. [cited 2026 Jun 15]. Available from: https://documents1.worldbank.org/curated/en/099050003292220485/pdf/P17354106933170e08f75037bb896706d0.pdf.
26. JSR – Jordanian Society of Rheumatology Website [Internet]. [cited 2026 Jun 15]. Available from: https://www.jsr-jo.org/jsr25-welcomemessage.
27. Arab League of Associations for Rheumatology (ArLAR). ArLAR Members—National Rheumatology Societies in the Arab World [Internet]. 2026. [cited 2026 Jun 15]. Available from: https://www.arabrheumatology.org/national-societies.
28. Sirdh MM. Consanguinity profile in the Gaza strip of Palestine: large-scale community- based study. Eur J Med Genet. 2014;57(2–3):90–4. https://doi.org/10.1016/j.ejmg.2014.01.003.
29. Ghanim M, Mosleh R, Hamdan A, Amer J, Alqub M, Jarrar Y, et al. Assessment of perceptions and predictors towards consanguinity: a cross-sectional study from Palestine. J Multidiscip Healthc. 2023;16:3443–53. https://doi.org/10.2147/JMDH.S433506.
30. Majeed HA, Rawashdeh M, El-Shanti H, Qubain H, Khuri-Bulos N, Shahin HM. Familial Mediterranean fever in children: the expanded clinical profile. QJM Int J Med. 1999;92(6):309–18. https://doi.org/10.1093/qjmed/92.6.309.
31. Barakat MH, Karnik AM, Majeed HW, Fenech FF. Familial Mediterranean fever (recurrent hereditary polyserositis) in Arabs — a study of 175 patients and review of the literature. QJM. 1986;60(3):837–47. https://doi.org/10.1093/oxfordjournals.qjmed.a068041.
32. Ayesh SK, Nassar SM, Al-Sharef WA, Abu-Libdeh BY, Darwish HM. Genetic screening of familial Mediterranean fever mutations in the Palestinian population. Saudi Med J. 2005;26(5):732–7.
33. Mousavi SE, Nejadghaderi SA, Khabbazi A, Alizadeh M, Sullman MJM, Kaufman JS, et al. The burden of rheumatoid arthritis in the Middle East and North Africa region, 1990-2019. Sci Rep. 2022;12(1):19297. https://doi.org/10.1038/s41598-022-22310-0.
34. Almoallim H, Al Saleh J, Badsha H, Ahmed HM, Habjoka S, Menassa JA, et al. A review of the prevalence and unmet needs in the management of rheumatoid arthritis in Africa and the Middle East. Rheumatol Ther. 2021;8(1):1–16. https://doi.org/10.1007/s40744-020-00252-1.
35. Abu Seir R, Kharroubi A, Ghannam I. Prevalence of tobacco use among young adults in Palestine. East Mediterr Health J. 2020;26(1):75–84. https://doi.org/10.26719/2020.26.1.75.
36. Abdul-Rahim HF, Abu-Rmeileh NM, Husseini A, Holmboe-Ottesen G, Jervell J, Bjertness E. Obesity and selected co-morbidities in an urban Palestinian population. Int J Obes Relat Metab Disord. 2001;25(11):1736–40. https://doi.org/10.1038/sj.ijo.0801799.

37. Arshad A, Mahmood SBZ, Ayaz A, Al Karim Manji A, Ahuja AK. Association of vitamin D deficiency and disease activity in systemic lupus erythematosus patients: two-year follow-up study. Arch Rheumatol. 2020;36(1):101–6. https://doi.org/10.46497/ArchRheumatol.2021.8178.
38. Mouterde G, Gamon E, Rincheval N, Lukas C, Seror R, Berenbaum F, et al. Association between vitamin D deficiency and disease activity, disability, and radiographic progression in early rheumatoid arthritis: the ESPOIR cohort. J Rheumatol. 2020;47(11):1624–8. https://doi.org/10.3899/jrheum.190795.
39. Abukhalil AD, Falana H, Hamayel R, Yasser F, Nasser A, Naseef H, et al. Vitamin D deficiency association with comorbid diseases in Palestine: a cross-sectional observation study. Int J Gen Med. 2022;15:8033–42. https://doi.org/10.2147/IJGM.S389190.
40. AlSaleem A, Al-Mayouf SM. Consanguinity and rare monogenic systemic autoinflammatory disorders: implications for prevalence and genetic variability. Pediatr Rheumatol Online J. 2025;23(1):83. https://doi.org/10.1186/s12969-025-01133-z.
41. Souali M, Sakhi A, Benbrahim Ansari G, Mikou N, Bousfiha AA, Bouayed K. Spectrum of auto-inflammatory diseases in Morocco: a monocentric experience. Rheumatol Adv Pract. 2023;7(1):rkad001. https://doi.org/10.1093/rap/rkad001.
42. Massad S, Isbeih M, Owess M, Fouad H, Saman KA, Issawi S, et al. Noncommunicable diseases: a silent epidemic in occupied Palestine: results from the World Health Organization STEPS survey 2022. BMC Public Health. 2025;25(1):2726. https://doi.org/10.1186/s12889-025-23880-0.
43. Halahleh K, Abu-Rmeileh NME, Abusrour MM. General oncology care in Palestine. In: Al- Shamsi HO, Abu-Gheida IH, Iqbal F, Al-Awadhi A, editors. Cancer in the Arab World. Singapore: Springer; 2022. https://doi.org/10.1007/978-981-16-7945-2_13.
44. Kun L, Gessl I, Filippou G, Ferrito M, Giacomelli R, Mandl P. Ultrasound in rheumatic and musculoskeletal diseases: from musculoskeletal to organ involvement. Joint Bone Spine. 2025;92(6):105920. https://doi.org/10.1016/j.jbspin.2025.105920.
45. Suji T, Sullivan R, Bowsher G. Radiology in conflict: scoping review. Confl Heal. 2024;18:8. https://doi.org/10.1186/s13031-023-00550-9.
46. Leung YY, Bird P, Haroon M, Kishimoto M, Shin K, Mathew AJ, et al. The APLAR recommendations for the management of psoriatic arthritis. Int J Rheum Dis. 2025;28(8):e70372. https://doi.org/10.1111/1756-185x.70372.
47. Sammaritano LR, Askanase A, Bermas BL, Dall'Era M, Duarte-García A, Hiraki LT, et al. 2025 American College of Rheumatology (ACR) guideline for the treatment of systemic lupus erythematosus. Arthritis Care Res (Hoboken). 2025; https://doi.org/10.1002/acr.25690.
48. Kerschbaumer A, Sepriano A, Bergstra SA, Smolen JS, van der Heijde D, Caporali R, et al. Efficacy of synthetic and biological DMARDs: a systematic literature review informing the 2022 update of the EULAR recommendations for the management of rheumatoid arthritis. Ann Rheum Dis. 2023;82(1):95–106. https://doi.org/10.1136/ard-2022-223365.
49. Alnaqbi KA, Aldabie G, Enizi AA, Abdulkarim S, Satti E, Lawati TA, et al. 2025 Consensus-based recommendations for the referral, diagnosis, monitoring, and management of axial spondyloarthritis in the Arabian Gulf countries. Semin Arthritis Rheum. 2025;75:152828. https://doi.org/10.1016/j.semarthrit.2025.152828.
50. Aljadeeah S, Satheesh G, Hafez S, Naguib M, Neilson A, Alaloul A, et al. Availability of essential medicines in 14 remaining health facilities in Gaza. Lancet. 2025;406(10511):1465–7. https://doi.org/10.1016/S0140-6736(25)01819-7.
51. World Health Organization. oPt emergency situation update 63 [Internet]. Cairo: WHO Regional Office for the Eastern Mediterranean; 2025. [cited 2026 Jun 15]. Available from: https://www.emro.who.int/images/stories/palestine/Sitrep_63.pdf.
52. Gaza Health Ministry warns of severe drug shortages as supplies run critically low. Anadolu Agency [Internet]. 2025. [cited 2026 Jun 15]. Available from: https://www.aa.com.tr/en/middle-east/gaza-health-ministry-warns-of-severe-drug-shortages-as-supplies-run-critically-low/3777129.

53. Akinci A, Kiliç G. Future of rehabilitation interventions for rheumatic patients in the Mediterranean region. Mediterr J Rheumatol. 2017;28(2):70–4. https://doi.org/10.31138/mjr.28.2.70.
54. World Health Organization.WHO rehabilitation need estimator [Internet]. 2021. [cited 2026 Jun 15]. Available from: https://vizhub.healthdata.org/rehabilitation/.
55. Palestinian Ministry of Health. Health annual report: Palestine 2020 [Internet]. 2021. [cited 2025 Nov 7]. Available from: https://www.moh.gov.ps/.
56. Physical and functional rehabilitation in the Occupied Palestinian Territory (West Bank and Gaza) [Internet]. Humanity & Inclusion; 2022. [cited 2026 Jun 15]. Available from: https://www.hi.org/sn_uploads/document/Factsheet_Rehabiliation_oPt_HI_March-2022.pdf.
57. Afana H, Dhair R. Total knee arthroplasty at Gaza Strip Palestine: compliance and retrospective comparative study. Int J Res Orthop. 2019;5(6):1044–9. https://doi.org/10.18203/issn.2455-4510.IntJResOrthop20194809.
58. World Health Organization. Gaza's many injured will need rehabilitation care and support for years to come, WHO report. [Internet]. Geneva: WHO; 2025. [cited 2026 Jun 15]. Available from: https://www.emro.who.int/opt/news/gazas-many-injured-will-need-rehabilitation-care-and-support-for-years-to-come-who-report.html.
59. Sebbag E, Felten R, Sagez F, Sibilia J, Devilliers H, Arnaud L. The worldwide burden of musculoskeletal diseases: a systematic analysis of the World Health Organization Burden of Diseases Database. Ann Rheum Dis. 2019;78(6):844–8. https://doi.org/10.1136/annrheumdis-2019-215142.
60. Al Meslamani AZ. Short and long-term economic implications of biosimilars. Expert Opin Biol Ther. 2024;24(7):567–70. https://doi.org/10.1080/14712598.2024.2307353.
61. World Health Organization. Right to health 2018: report on health access and barriers in the Occupied Palestinian Territory [internet]. Cairo: WHO Regional Office for the Eastern Mediterranean; 2019. [cited 2026 Jun 15]. Available from: https://www.emro.who.int/images/stories/palestine/documents/who_right_to_health_2018_web-final.pdf.
62. Miloslavsky EM, Marston B. The challenge of addressing the rheumatology workforce shortage. J Rheumatol. 2022;49(6):555–7. https://doi.org/10.3899/jrheum.220300.
63. McNeely CA, Barber BK, Giacaman R, Belli RF, Daher M. Long-term health consequences of movement restrictions for Palestinians, 1987–2011. Am J Public Health. 2018;108(1):77–83. https://doi.org/10.2105/AJPH.2017.304043.
64. World Health Organization. Monthly report on Health Access. Barriers for patients in the occupied Palestinian territory [Internet]. [cited 2026 Jun 15]. Available from: https://www.un.org/unispal/wp-content/uploads/2022/05/WHOAPRILMONTHLYRPT_260522.pdf.
65. National Resident Matching Program. results and data: specialties matching service 2019 appointment year. Washington, D.C: National Resident Matching Program; 2019.
66. Arab League of Associations for Rheumatology (ArLAR). [Internet]. [cited 2026 Jun 15]. Available from: https://www.arabrheumatology.org/aaaa-group.

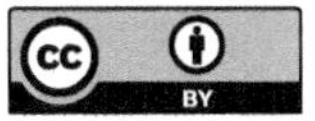

Chapter 13
Rheumatic Diseases in Qatar

Omar Alsaed, Mohamed Hammoudeh, and Samar Al Emadi

Abstract Qatar, a high gross domestic product (GDP) country, is located in the Arabian Gulf with an estimated population of 2.7 million, the majority being young individuals from different expatriates. Governmental health institutes mainly drive the primary, secondary, and tertiary healthcare systems: Hamad Medical Corporation (HMC), Sidra Medicine Hospital, and the Primary Health Care Corporation (PHCC).

The private health sector has developed significantly. As of September 2025, there were eight private hospitals, over 200 privately owned polyclinics, and various clinics, laboratories, pharmacies, and medical facilities. The rheumatology service in Qatar was founded in 1982 and has since expanded in different aspects, including the clinical care services, physician training, and education and research activities. There are 20 full-time adult rheumatology consultants and senior consultants, two pediatric rheumatology senior consultants distributed across all government facilities, and six rheumatologists in the private sector. Due to significant ethnicity variations in Qatar, various rheumatic diseases ranging from simple to complex illnesses are observed. The majority of these patients are managed at HMC. Osteoporosis care and fracture liaison services are led by a dedicated team of rheumatologists, part of the rheumatology division of HMC hospitals.

O. Alsaed · M. Hammoudeh · S. Al Emadi (✉)
Division of Rheumatology, Department of Medicine, Hamad Medical Corporation, Doha, Qatar
e-mail: oalsaed@hamad.qa; mhamoudeh@hamad.qa; salemadi@hamad.qa

K. A. Alnaqbi, G. Aldabie (eds.), *Rheumatic Diseases in the Arab World*,
https://doi.org/10.1007/978-981-92-0967-5_13

In this chapter, we will highlight the progression of rheumatology services in Qatar, starting with an introduction to the geographical and epidemiological data of Qatar's population, followed by rheumatic disease management and diagnostics. Furthermore, we will discuss the rheumatology fellowship training program and elaborate on the most essential studies initiated and published by the rheumatology division at HMC.

Keywords Qatar · Health system · Hamad medical corporation · Rheumatic diseases · Rheumatology services · Rheumatology workforce · Fracture liaison service · Biologic therapy · Biosimilars · Rheumatology Fellowship Training

13.1 Country Demographics

Qatar is one of the nations of the Gulf Cooperation Council. It is a peninsula in the Arabian Gulf that shares a southern border with Saudi Arabia. The approximate geographic surface area is 11,437 km^2. Doha, Al-Rayyan, Al-Khor, Al-Shamal, Al-Da'ayen, Al-Wakra, and Umm Salal are the seven municipalities of Qatar. Over the past 20 years, Qatar's population has significantly changed in size and composition. Approximately 668,629 people called Qatar home in 2005; by 2017, that number had risen to 2.7 million, with most of those residents being young foreigners from other nations. The report "*Qatar Population and Employment Projections 2017–2024: A Framework for National Planning*" provided this information. The two municipalities with the densest populations are Doha and Al-Rayyan. Based on the 2017 observed census, Fig. 13.1a depicts the age distribution of the people of Qatar and Fig. 13.1b shows how Qatar's population is distributed according to Qataris and non-Qataris based on the 2017 observed census [1].

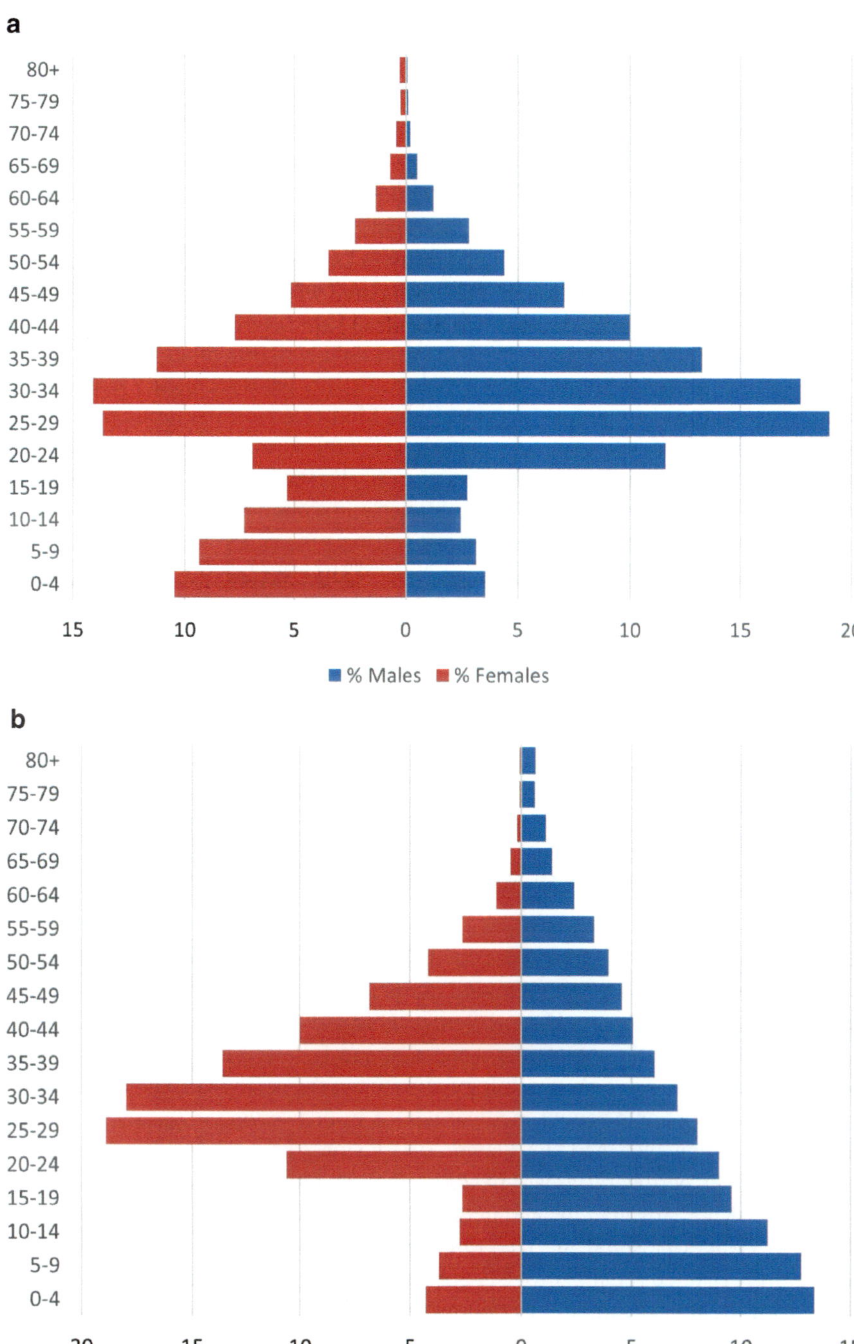

Fig. 13.1 (**a**) Qatar population age pyramid based on the 2017 observed census. (**b**) Qatar's population is distributed according to Qataris and non-Qataris based on the 2017 observed census. (This figure is reproduced from Alsaed et al. [1]. Licensed under CC BY 4.0.)

13.2 The Healthcare System in Qatar

Governmental healthcare institutes mainly handle the healthcare system in Qatar, including Hamad Medical Corporation (HMC), Sidra Medicine Hospital, and the Primary Health Care (PHC) Institute, and partially by the private health system. HMC has 14 Joint Commission International (JCI)-accredited facilities, including Hamad General Hospital, Al-Wakra Hospital, Al-Khor Hospital, the National Center for Cancer Care and Research, Women's Wellness and Research Center, Heart Hospital, Communicable Disease Center, Hazem Mebaireek General Hospital, Aisha Bint Hamad Al Attiyah Hospital, Ambulatory Care Center, Qatar Rehabilitation Institute, Hamad Dental Center, Cuban Hospital, and Rumailah Hospital. The PHCC has 31 centers across the country. HMC mainly leads secondary and tertiary care and the national ambulance service. Sidra Medicine Hospital provides secondary and tertiary healthcare for all pediatric specialties, while the PHCC provides primary public healthcare. Medical records from all HMC facilities, Sidra Hospital, and the 31 PHCC centers belong to the Ministry of Public Health. They are linked by a cloud-based electronic medical record software manager.

Healthcare in the private sector has grown recently over the last few years due to a rapid increase in the population. Eight leading hospitals (Al-Ahli Hospital, Doha Clinic, Al-Emadi Hospital, Turkish Hospital, Aster Hospital, the View Hospital, Aspetar, and Aman Hospital) provide inpatient and outpatient care. In addition to these eight private hospitals, many polyclinic centers across the country provide care for medically insured patients. None of these public or private hospitals offer medical tourism services.

13.3 Rheumatology Services in Qatar

Rheumatology service in Qatar was established in June 1982 after the first rheumatologist arrived to provide inpatient and outpatient rheumatology consultations for adult and pediatric patients at Hamad General Hospital in February 1982. Previously, patients with rheumatic complaints were seen and followed up by orthopedic surgeons. At that time, since rheumatology services in the nearby Gulf countries were limited, several patients sought medical advice in this service in Qatar. As part of HMC's expansion plan and the Qatar 2030 vision, rheumatology services have spread to cover peripheral areas. In 2005, rheumatology service care was established in Al-Khor Hospital, located in the northern region of Qatar. It was later initiated in Al-Wakra Hospital in 2012 to cover the southern geographical area. The number of registered rheumatologists gradually increased annually, especially after 2012, with the first rheumatology fellow graduating from the local rheumatology fellowship training program of Hamad General Hospital. Most rheumatologists and the rheumatology fellowship program faculty were qualified and trained in North

America and a few were from the United Kingdom. As of 2026, 15 consultants (5 females and 10 males) and 3 associate consultants (two females and one males) are affiliated with HMC.

These rheumatologists are distributed across the entire geographical area of Qatar: 11 in Hamad General Hospital, covering the capital and the central area; 2 in Al-Khor Hospital, covering the northern region; and 3 in Al-Wakra Hospital, covering the southern part. In addition, two pediatric rheumatology senior consultants are located in Sidra Medicine Hospital. Together with this highly qualified rheumatologists' staff, five dedicated rheumatology nurses have more than 10 years of experience. However, they are not formally certified in rheumatology nursing, as there is no formal training program in rheumatology for nursing in Qatar. The number of registered rheumatologists increased over the last four decades, and rapid growth in the population was reflected by an increased number of rheumatology clinics and patient visits to these clinics.

In 2004, the total number of outpatient clinic visits was 10,108. This number increased to 15,285 in 2011. There are 87 rheumatology clinics in HMC, and the average number of patient visits ranges from 2500 to 3000 outpatient visits per month. These figures were obtained from the annual reports of the rheumatology division in HMC. Electronic medical records (EMR) in all HMC facilities, Sidra Medicine Hospital, and the primary health care centers across Qatar are electronically linked by one cloud-based EMR software manager. This has significantly reduced the time to receive rheumatology care. The average waiting time to get an appointment with a rheumatologist ranges from 10 to 21 days. Non-obligatory medical insurance systems and the high costs of rheumatic disease medications and investigations make the private sector for rheumatology care services almost restricted to insured patients and patients able to afford the cost of care. Currently, there are six male rheumatologists in the private sector. However, we expect the private sector to develop further in the coming few years, as a medical insurance system will be obligatory in Qatar.

To build the links between rheumatologists in Qatar and rheumatologists in regional and international countries, Qatar Rheumatology Society (QRS) and Qatar Osteoporosis Society (QOS) were founded in 2019 under the umbrella of the Qatar Medical Association by a group of rheumatologists. Many local scientific activities were endorsed by the QRS and QOS, such as the annual rheumatology symposium, monthly rheumatology club meeting, and annual awareness day events (World Arthritis Day, World Lupus Day, and World Osteoporosis Day). The QRS is a member of the Arab League of Associations for Rheumatology (ArLAR) and the Asia Pacific League of Associations for Rheumatology (APLAR). QRS also supports patients by organizing educational activities and offering financial support to unprivileged patients with rheumatic disease who cannot afford the cost of expensive medications like biological drugs. This support is provided through many programs in collaboration between the QRS and the local charity institutes in Qatar. They aim to enable these patients to have healthy lives so they can maintain their work and income and simultaneously save their dignity. To date, the QRS's most notable accomplishment is providing biological disease-modifying anti-rheumatic medication (DMARD) therapy to around 500 patients.

The rheumatology division at HMC runs many specialized clinics in the rheumatology field. The Pregnancy and Rheumatic Disease Clinic is one of the distinguished specialized clinics in Qatar and the Middle East. It provides exceptional care to patients with rheumatic disease who are pregnant or planning to conceive. These patients have a unique structured care plan in collaboration with their obstetricians. Medical care at this clinic starts 6 months before pregnancy. It provides counseling for the proper time to have a new baby and medical advice on adjusting medications to be compatible with pregnancy. During pregnancy, the patient is followed closely in the specialized feto-maternal unit, which provides more frequent fetal ultrasound scanning and umbilical cord blood flow by doppler for antiphospholipid patients. Post-delivery, patients will receive counseling on the best contraceptive method for rheumatic disease and medication adjustment. All these measures were arranged to enable pregnant women with rheumatic disease to have healthy births and maintain their rheumatic disease in remission during pregnancy and post-delivery. Questionnaires, research templates, and patient-reported outcomes surveys were introduced recently to this clinic. The spondyloarthropathy and inflammatory bowel disease clinic and the psoriatic arthritis clinic are combined clinics run by a rheumatologist, dermatologist, and gastroenterologist. These clinics deal with complex and challenging cases.

Furthermore, there are five musculoskeletal (MSK) ultrasound clinics run by rheumatologists. Capillaroscopy and early arthritis clinics are the last two specialized clinics. Two fracture liaison service (FLS) clinics, run by rheumatologists utilizing the International Osteoporosis Foundation (IOF) standards, are dedicated to secondary osteoporotic fracture prevention. These FLS clinics operate at two facilities to ensure broad geographic coverage. The Osteoporosis and Organ Transplant Clinic offers specialized care for patients with osteoporosis who are planning or have undergone organ transplants, including those of the liver, kidney, lung, and bone marrow. Figure 13.2 shows the timeline for the progression milestones in rheumatology services in Qatar.

None of the hospitals providing rheumatology care or specialized rheumatology clinics is an accredited center of excellence. However, Hamad General Hospital has applied to IOF as an accredited center for Fracture Liaison Service (FLS).

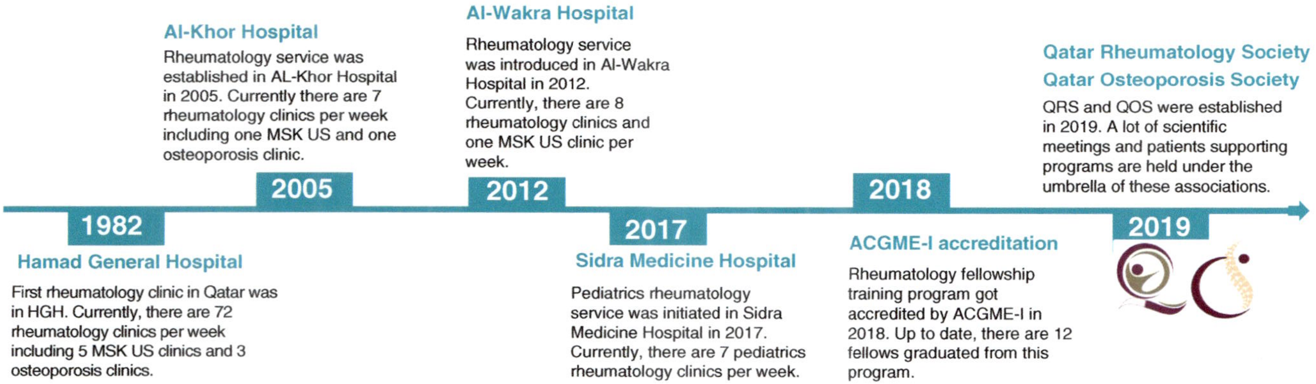

1982
Hamad General Hospital
First rheumatology clinic in Qatar was in HGH. Currently, there are 72 rheumatology clinics per week including 5 MSK US clinics and 3 osteoporosis clinics.

2005
Al-Khor Hospital
Rheumatology service was established in AL-Khor Hospital in 2005. Currently there are 7 rheumatology clinics per week including one MSK US and one osteoporosis clinic.

2012
Al-Wakra Hospital
Rheumatology service was introduced in Al-Wakra Hospital in 2012. Currently, there are 8 rheumatology clinics and one MSK US clinic per week.

2017
Sidra Medicine Hospital
Pediatrics rheumatology service was initiated in Sidra Medicine Hospital in 2017. Currently, there are 7 pediatrics rheumatology clinics per week.

2018
ACGME-I accreditation
Rheumatology fellowship training program got accredited by ACGME-I in 2018. Up to date, there are 12 fellows graduated from this program.

2019
Qatar Rheumatology Society
Qatar Osteoporosis Society
QRS and QOS were established in 2019. A lot of scientific meetings and patients supporting programs are held under the umbrella of these associations.

ACGME-I, Accreditation Council for Graduate Medical Education-international; QRS, Qatar Rheumatology Society; AOS, Qatar Osteoporosis Society; MSK US, musculoskeletal ultrasound; HGH, Hamad General Hospital.

Fig. 13.2 Timeline for the progression milestones in rheumatology services in Qatar. ACGME-I Accreditation Council for Graduate Medical Education-international, QRS Qatar Rheumatology Society, AOS Qatar Osteoporosis Society, MSK US musculoskeletal ultrasound, HGH Hamad General Hospital

13.4 Rheumatic Diseases in Qatar

13.4.1 Epidemiological Data

The population in Qatar has a unique structure; young expatriate males represent the population's main percentage of the population. This population category is dynamic; few stay in Qatar for more than 3–5 years. Therefore, we focused on the available data on rheumatic disease among Qatari citizens. Limited published studies demonstrate epidemiological data on certain rheumatic diseases and musculoskeletal (MSK) complaints in Qatar. In a community-oriented program for the Control of Rheumatic Diseases (COPCORD) survey, 1239 Qataris from randomly chosen homes in various towns participated. There were 563/1239 complaints with an MSK prevalence of 45.4%. The most typical locations for MSK pain complaints were the knee (24.5%) and back (23.3%). MSK abnormalities were present in 196 of 1239 people, or 15.8% of the population. Females (132/237; 55.6%) were slightly more likely than males (44.4%) to have MSK disorders. Most were noted to have degenerative etiology. The most prevalent illness was knee osteoarthritis (6.4%), followed by lumbar and cervical spondylosis (4%) and 2.3%, respectively. In this group, two women had rheumatoid arthritis (RA), one had connective tissue disease, and one had arthritis linked to inflammatory bowel illness. Qatar's overall MSK illness prevalence rate is comparable to regional and worldwide rates [2].

According to data from the HMC-owned RA registration, 23.6% of the participants were foreigners. Three-quarters of the patients—or around 76%—were seropositive. The most often prescribed synthetic DMARD was methotrexate (65.3%), followed by hydroxychloroquine (29.4%), sulfasalazine (21.2%), and leflunomide (13.7%), in that order. Biologic medications were administered to one-fourth of patients (26.4%) (etanercept, 9.3%; rituximab, 6%; tocilizumab, 5.6%; adalimumab, 4.4%; abatacept, 0.4%; certolizumab, 0.4%; infliximab, 0.2%) [3]. Hypertension (24.2%), diabetes mellitus (20.6%), dyslipidemia (10.9%), hypothyroidism (10.9%), and asthma and chronic obstructive pulmonary disease (1.4%) were the concomitant disorders that were most frequently present. Additionally, 37.6% had osteopenia, 11.6% had osteoporosis, and 48.6% had reduced bone density [4]. Numerous epidemiological studies on ankylosing spondylitis have been published in Qatar. Similar to global statistics, a higher percentage of men (70%) than women (2.3:1) are diagnosed with ankylosing spondylitis. The median age at diagnosis was 32, while the mean age was 41.5. 90% of individuals with sacroiliitis on magnetic resonance imaging (MRI) tested positive for HLA-B27, compared to 82% of patients from Qatar [5–7]. However, no prevalence studies on spondyloarthropathies are available yet in Qatar. Published data on rheumatic diseases in the pediatric age group in Qatar are minimal.

13.4.2 Risk Factors of Rheumatic Diseases

Hepatitis B incidence rates varied from 19.8 to 39.4 per 100,000 people annually in Qatar, according to epidemiological data on risk variables that worsened outcomes and increased the prevalence of rheumatic disease [8]. Between 0.3% and 11.2% of the general population had hepatitis C [9]. According to a recent survey, there are 25.2% reported to be active smokers in Qatar [10]. According to data from the Qatar National STEPwise Survey (2012), 43% of women and 40% of men in Qatar were considered obese (body mass index 30 kg/m^2) [11].

In Qatari households, the consanguinity percentage was calculated to be 66.2%, and 65% of Qataris are first cousins. This is based on a recent cross-sectional study [12].

Rheumatologists in Qatar provide osteoporosis treatment. According to estimates, 12.3% of postmenopausal women have osteoporosis [13]. Based on a single epidemiological investigation finished in 2007. The measured rate of low vitamin D status in Qatar was 90.4% (95% CI: 90.1–91.0; range 83–91%), according to a systematic evaluation of 16 papers [14]. For those over 50, the annual age-adjusted standardized incidence rate of osteoporotic hip fracture was 141.7 (141.1–142.2), 140.8 (140.2–141.3), and 162.7 (162.0–163.2) in 2017, 2018, and 2019 for the entire population of Qatar and 154.2 (153.6–154.7), 105.2 (104.7–105.7), and 176.6 (175.9–177.1) for Qataris, respectively [1].

13.4.3 Screening Programs for Rheumatic Diseases in Qatar

Currently, there is no national screening program for rheumatic diseases in Qatar; however, a dedicated clinic named the “early arthritis clinic” provides patients with inflammatory arthritis fast access to a rheumatologist assessment and management. Based on guidelines from the European Alliance of Associations for Rheumatology (EULAR) for immediate referral to specialized rheumatology services supporting early diagnosis and institution of therapy, this clinic was founded in 2017. Data on positive results for RA patients corroborate these recommendations [15]. Screenings for pulmonary hypertension by transthoracic echocardiography and interstitial lung disease by pulmonary function test in patients with autoimmune connective tissue disease are routine clinical practices in rheumatology clinics. Screening for osteoporosis by identifying high-risk patients for fracture using the Qatar Fracture Risk Assessment tool model (FRAX®) has been proposed to the Ministry of Public Health and approved. The lack of health economy experts in rheumatic diseases and osteoporosis and cost-effectiveness evidence is the most challenging part of initiating screening programs at the national level.

13.4.4 Laboratory Tests for Rheumatic Diseases

HMC has advanced diagnostic procedures in general, particularly in rheumatology. At the level of immunology testing, antinuclear antibody (ANA) test requests from all PHCs and HMC facilities are processed by a central HMC's immunology laboratory. Due to a large number of ANA requests from HMC and PHCs, estimated to be approximately 1300 tests per month, ANA testing is performed primarily by the enzyme-linked immunoassay (ELISA) technique (Phadia 250®). Furthermore, ANA testing can be achieved by the immunofluorescence technique if required. Other immunology tests include extractable nuclear antigens, antineutrophil cytoplasmic antibodies (ANCA), myeloperoxidase antibodies (MPO), proteinase three antibodies (PR3), C3, C4, beta 2-glycoprotein antibodies, anticardiolipin antibodies, rheumatoid factor, and anti-citrullinated peptide antibodies (ACPA), which are also available in HMC's immunology laboratory. Standard genetics tests, such as HLA B-27 and HLA B-51, are functional in HMC's molecular genetics lab. Other genetic and immunology tests related to the rheumatology field, such as Familial Mediterranean Fever gene mutations and other autoimmune biomarkers, are sent abroad through the referral laboratory.

13.4.5 Diagnostic Imaging for Rheumatic Diseases

Imaging scans are useful adjuvant diagnostic tools in challenging cases with suspected autoimmune rheumatic disease. Neuropsychiatric manifestations in autoimmune connective tissue disease are a dilemma that requires proper input from an expert neuroradiologist to reach the correct diagnosis. Enhanced MRI and computed tomography (CT) of the brain, together with specialized neuroradiologists and technicians, have been available in HMC since 1995. Large vessel vasculitis requires input from a specialized neuroradiologist. The Positron Emission Tomography (PET) scan center was established in 2013. A PET scan, an advanced imaging scan, is used to confirm the diagnosis of large vessel vasculitis in addition to other scans, such as magnetic resonance arteriography (MRA), CT angiography, and Doppler ultrasound. Diagnosis of axial spondyloarthropathy relies heavily on radiological findings, especially since the prevalence of HLA-B27 is low in Qatar [16]. MRIs of the sacroiliitis and spine are commonly requested imaging tests by rheumatologists. Thirteen certified MSK radiologists are working with the rheumatology team in HMC to interpret MRI findings within the correct clinical context, avoiding an improper diagnosis of axial SpA. Identifying inflammatory and structural changes of axial SpA is a cornerstone finding to confirm an axial SpA diagnosis. There are 11 MRI machines, and many CT scans and ultrasound machines are distributed at different HMC facilities. Monitoring inflammatory arthritis and large vessel vasculitis disease activity by bedside MSK ultrasound in a rheumatology clinic is evolving.

Within HMC's rheumatology team, six rheumatologists are trained to perform bedside MSK ultrasound diagnostic and therapeutic procedures. This has increased the diagnostic and management capabilities of complex joints, such as the shoulder joint, and deep-seated structures, such as the hip joint. Furthermore, using ultrasound for aspiration and steroid injection of the deep joints and soft tissues is becoming a common practice due to its favorable outcome and better patient satisfaction.

13.4.6 Management of Rheumatic Diseases in Qatar

Qualified rheumatologists initiate pharmacotherapy management in rheumatic disease in Qatar, as most medications used to treat rheumatic disease are immunosuppressive agents with potential adverse events. Conventional synthetic DMARDs (csDMARDs) and biological DMARDs (bDMARDs) are mainly available in tertiary hospitals (Hamad General Hospital, Al-Wakra Hospital, and Al-Khor Hospital). Prescribing these medications is strictly restricted to rheumatologists. All Cs-DMARDs and most bio-DMARDs are available to all patients. Etanercept, the first bDMARD, was introduced in HMC in 2000. Currently, five TNF inhibitors (etanercept, adalimumab, infliximab, certolizumab, and golimumab); seven non-anti-TNF bDMARDs (tocilizumab, secukinumab, ixekizumab, ustekinumab, risankizumab, guselkumab, and rituximab); and three JAK inhibitors (tofacitinib, baricitinib, and upadacitinib), as well as IVIG, anifrolumab, and belimumab, are available. In addition, several non-formulary biological medications can be requested for exceptional cases. All the csDMARDs and bDMARDs are provided to citizens free of charge and at an affordable supported price (20% of the market price) to patients with a Qatar residency number. Unprivileged patients who cannot afford the supported cost of the bDMARDs can get them through co-payment support programs, as mentioned earlier. These medications are also available in the private sector and are usually affordable for patients with medical insurance. To overcome the increasing cost of rheumatic disease medications, Qatar introduced biosimilars in 2023. By 2025, three biosimilar drugs—Amgevita, Erelzi, and Rixathon—are available for use in rheumatology.

Physiotherapy, occupational therapy, and rehabilitation programs work hand-in-hand with pharmacotherapy in treating patients with rheumatic disease. Qatar Rehabilitation Institute (QRI) is a facility that belongs to HMC. There are seven centers belonging to QRI and 11 physiotherapy centers belonging to PHCC distributed in different geographical areas. These centers are well-staffed with expert physiotherapists and equipped with the most modern machines. Hydrotherapy pools are also available in most centers.

13.4.7 Rheumatology Fellowship Training Program in Qatar

The rheumatology fellowship training program in Hamad General Hospital was established in 2008 under the umbrella of the medical education department of HMC. Eligible candidates must have graduated from an internal medicine residency training program and should be fully qualified with the Arab Board of Internal Medicine certification. The rheumatology fellowship training program is a three-year well-structured curriculum-based program. During these 3 years, the trainee should complete inpatient and outpatient general rheumatology training in Hamad General Hospital; 1-month rotations each in inpatient and outpatient pediatric rheumatology in Sidra Medicine Hospital; sports medicine clinics in Aspetar Hospital; a pregnancy and rheumatic disease clinic in HGH; a psoriatic arthritis combined clinic; and a musculoskeletal ultrasound clinic. Fellows interested in enhancing their knowledge in rheumatology-related immunology diagnostic tests, physical therapy, and rehabilitation medicine can join elective rotations in these specialties. Each trainee should complete the required number of procedures before graduation. These procedures should be performed under the direct supervision of training faculty. To assess and prove the trainee's proficiency development, each fellow is evaluated by the American College of Rheumatology Fellows-In-Training exam, a comprehensive exam that fellows must sit for every year throughout their fellowship. It is a full-day comprehensive test where their competency in different areas of rheumatology is assessed and compared with their peers in other rheumatology fellowship programs in the United States. They will receive a detailed report regarding their performance in different areas, which will be discussed in detail with their mentors. To build a trainee's competency in communication and professionalism skills, fellows have weekly clinics where they directly interact with patients from different backgrounds.

Furthermore, during the inpatient consult rotation, the trainee will be observed and evaluated for communication with other physicians and medical health professionals. Mastering the presentation skills and critically appraising the design, methodology, and findings of published rheumatology articles are priorities in the fellowship training program. It is attained during bi-weekly scientific rheumatology meetings. All fellows have the opportunity to contribute to research activities and are encouraged to publish a scientific paper before their graduation.

Hamad General Hospital's rheumatology fellowship training program is the only training program for adult rheumatology in Qatar. It is one of the 33 programs in HMC accredited by the Accreditation Council for Graduate Medical Education-International (ACGME-I). The original foundational accreditation date was January 2018, with several reaccreditation cycles completed since then, and the program maintains its current active ACGME-I accreditation status.

13.4.8 Rheumatology and Research in Qatar

Research activities in the rheumatology division of HMC started in 1992, with its first publication in a peer-reviewed journal [16]. Since then, several annual publications have been authored by rheumatologists affiliated with the rheumatology division of HMC. More than 300 publications (original articles, epidemiological papers, reviews, and book chapters) have been published in different peer-reviewed journals.

The two most important articles on genetics were the Genome-Wide Association Study (GWAS) on inflammatory arthritis among the Arab population and the incidence of HLA B-27 in ankylosing spondylitis in Arab countries [17, 18]. Three previously undiscovered gene locus variations (HLA region, intergenic 5q13, and 17p13 at SMTNL2/GGT6) were discovered due to a multinational investigation called GWAS in rheumatoid arthritis.

The study on the prevalence of HLA-B27 in ankylosing spondylitis also contributed important knowledge to the literature by demonstrating how much lower it was in the Arab population than in European and North American people. We anticipate that this discovery will affect local recommendations and clinical practice about whether to order HLA-B27 tests. In the field of osteoporosis, the prevalence of osteopenia and osteoporosis in postmenopausal Qatari women, epidemiological data on osteoporotic hip fracture, and the formulation of a Qatar Fracture Risk Assessment tool model (FRAX®) were the most eminent [1, 19, 20]. The Qatar FRAX model changed osteoporosis management practices in Qatar.

The rheumatology division has been granted funds for many research projects. Projects that were given funds of more than 100,000 Qatari Riyals are mentioned. GWAS in rheumatoid arthritis in the Arab population and pharmacogenomics of TNF-α inhibitors in autoimmune diseases were granted funds (900,000 USD and 445,900 USD, respectively) from the Qatar National Research Fund (QNRF). From the medical research center of HMC, the rheumatology division was granted funds to investigate seronegative antiphospholipid (600,000 Qatari Riyals) and corneal confocal microscopy studies in autoimmune diseases (350,000 Qatari Riyals).

Three worldwide clinical trials benefited from the HMC's rheumatology division's participation as a hub for recruiting:

1. Long-term remission in early rheumatoid arthritis after etanercept tapering [21].
2. An open-label phase 4 study in patients from the Middle East Investigating the safety, tolerability, and efficacy of tocilizumab in rheumatoid arthritis [22].
3. A randomized, double-blind trial comparing the clinical effectiveness and safety of etanercept versus sulfasalazine in individuals with ankylosing spondylitis [23].

The following regional and global studies are currently receiving its contributions:

1. A descriptive, prospective study to evaluate the clinical characteristics, pharmacology, biomarkers, demographics, and quality of life of patients with long-term organ damage and LUpus NEphritis (LUNELORD) [24].
2. Value of different REferral STrategies for axial spondylARThritis in the Arab countries (RESTART).
3. Toward developing a patient-reported outcome measure of glucocorticoid impact: glucocorticoid benefits and adverse events from the patient's and clinician's perspectives (OMERACT).
4. The APLAR spondyloarthropathy registry.
5. Opportunistic screening of bone fragility from X-ray and CT collaborative project scope.

As a result of all these research activities, the rheumatology division at HMC was awarded as the best research team in 2016 by the medical research center of HMC. Furthermore, in 2014, the Pfizer pharmaceutical company awarded the rheumatology division as the best research center for rheumatoid arthritis in the Gulf area and the best non-rheumatoid arthritis research center in the Middle East.

13.4.9 Rheumatology Scientific Meetings and Symposiums

The rheumatology division at HMC organized several rheumatology scientific meetings. The annual Qatar musculoskeletal ultrasound course (QMUSC), one of the unique courses in the Middle East, focuses on providing individualized training in small groups. This is guaranteed by the presence of internationally acclaimed trainers who will provide lectures, demos, and hands-on training. The instructors are world leaders in MSK ultrasound scanning, and most are from the EULAR faculty of the ultrasound certification program. The QMUSC is endorsed by EULAR for the basic and intermediate levels. Certifications from the QMUSC allow the trainees to attend the advanced-level course in recognized EULAR centers and sit for a final certification examination.

Furthermore, the QMUSC is endorsed by the European Federation of Societies for Ultrasound in Medicine and Biology (EFSUMB). Usually, in the days following the QMUSC, the organizing scientific committee will choose a particular track for rheumatologists, focusing on a specific rheumatology topic, such as crystal arthropathy, vasculitis, salivary glands, spondyloarthropathy, or ultrasound-guided procedures. In 2019, ultrasound-guided procedures training was performed on cadaveric models, followed by a sonoanatomy and dissection workshop for interested trainees. The next QMUSC will be held in December in December 2027 with its eleventh edition.

In addition, the rheumatology division organizes an annual rheumatology and osteoporosis symposium consisting of lectures and workshops in dual-energy X-ray absorptiometry (DXA) reading and interpretation and osteoporosis risk stratification and management using FRAX. Furthermore, the rheumatology division at HMC hosted the Pan Arab Rheumatology Conference in 2008, now called the ArLAR Congress.

13.5 Conclusion

Rheumatology care services in Qatar have improved dramatically in many aspects over the last four decades. The number of qualified rheumatologists and healthcare facilities providing specialized care in rheumatology and osteoporosis has increased to cope with a rapid increment in Qatar's population. This was associated with a significant improvement in the quality of rheumatology care provided to the public, which is currently up to international standards. The ACGME-I accredited rheumatology fellowship training program of Hamad General Hospital is a milestone in rheumatology service progression in Qatar. Due to its notable achievements in research activities, the rheumatology division at Hamad Medical Corporation has been granted many local and regional awards. Finally, the growing published data on rheumatic disease and osteoporosis in Qatar have paved the road for collaborative work with neighboring and Middle Eastern countries and the formulation of local and regional recommendations in rheumatic diseases and osteoporosis.

Authors' Conflict of Interest Declaration The authors have no conflicts of interest to declare.

Funding No third party financially supported this work.

References

1. Alsaed OS, Abdulla N, Lutf A, Abdulmomen I, Alam F, Alemadi SAR. The incidence rate of osteoporotic hip fracture in Qatar. Arch Osteoporos. 2021;16(1):150.
2. Aldeen Sarakbi H, Alsaed O, Hammoudeh M, Lutf A, Razzakh Poil A, Ziyada A, et al. Epidemiology of musculoskeletal complaints and diseases in Qatar: a cross-sectional study. Qatar Med J. 2020;2020(2):29.
3. Alam F, Hammoudeh M, Malallah Abdulaziz H, Sarakbi H, Mohammed Siam A, Mehdi S, et al. Disease activity and treatment patterns in rheumatoid arthritis in Qatar: data from the Qatar rheumatoid arthritis registry. Int J Clin Rheumatol. 2018;13(4)
4. Alam F, Hammoudeh M, Emadi SA. FRI0758-HPR Co-morbidity profile in patients with rheumatoid arthritis. Data from rheumatoid arthritis registry in Qatar. Ann Rheum Dis. 2017;76(Suppl 2):1504–5.
5. Abdelrahman MH, Mahdy S, Khanjar IA, Siam AM, Malallah HA, Al-Emadi SA, et al. Prevalence of HLA-B27 in patients with ankylosing spondylitis in Qatar. Int J Rheumatol. 2012;2012:860213.
6. Al-Allaf AW, Yahia YM. E092 a review of ankylosing spondylitis (AS) in Qatar: did it differ from the international figures? Rheumatology. 2019;58(Supplement_3)
7. Alam F, Lutf AQ, Abdulla N, Elsayed EHS, Hammoudeh M. Characteristics of ankylosing spondylitis patients living in Qatar. The Egyptian Rheumatologist. 2017;39(2):103–8.

8. Al Romaihi HE, Ganesan N, Farag EA, Smatti MK, Nasrallah GK, Hiatt SM, et al. Demographics and epidemiology of hepatitis B in the State of Qatar: a five-year surveillance-based incidence study. Pathogens. 2019;8(2)
9. Mohamoud YA, Riome S, Abu-Raddad LJ. Epidemiology of hepatitis C virus in the Arabian Gulf countries: systematic review and meta-analysis of prevalence. Int J Infect Dis. 2016;46:116–25.
10. AlMulla A, Mamtani R, Cheema S, Maisonneuve P, Abdullah BaSuhai J, Mahmoud G, et al. Epidemiology of tobacco use in Qatar: prevalence and its associated factors. PLoS One. 2021;16(4):e0250065.
11. Taheri S, Al-Thani M. Obesity in Qatar: current and future strategies. Lancet Diabetes Endocrinol. 2021;9(9):561–2.
12. Ben-Omran T, Al Ghanim K, Yavarna T, El Akoum M, Samara M, Chandra P, Al-Dewik N. Effects of consanguinity in a cohort of subjects with certain genetic disorders in Qatar. Mol Genet Genomic Med. 2020;8:e1051.
13. Bener A, Hammoudeh M, Zirie M. Prevalence and predictors of osteoporosis and the impact of lifestyle factors on bone mineral density. APLAR J Rheumatol. 2007;10(3):227–33.
14. Badawi A, Arora P, Sadoun E, Al-Thani AA, Thani MH. Prevalence of vitamin d insufficiency in Qatar: a systematic review. J Public Health Res. 2012;1(3):229–35.
15. Combe B, Landewe R, Daien CI, Hua C, Aletaha D, Alvaro-Gracia JM, et al. 2016 update of the EULAR recommendations for the management of early arthritis. Ann Rheum Dis. 2017;76(6):948–59.
16. Hammoudeh M, Siam AR. Salmonella peritonitis and splenic abscess in a patient with systemic lupus erythematosus. Ann Rheum Dis. 1992;51(1):140.
17. Saxena R, Plenge RM, Bjonnes AC, Dashti HS, Okada Y, Gad El Haq W, et al. A multinational Arab genome-wide association study identifies new genetic associations for rheumatoid arthritis. Arthritis Rheumatol. 2017;69(5):976–85.
18. Mustafa KN, Hammoudeh M, Khan MA. HLA-B27 prevalence in Arab populations and among patients with ankylosing spondylitis. J Rheumatol. 2012;39(8):1675–7.
19. Abdulla N, Alsaed OS, Lutf A, Alam F, Abdulmomen I, Al Emadi S, et al. Epidemiology of hip fracture in Qatar and development of a country-specific FRAX model. Arch Osteoporos. 2022;17(1):49.
20. Hammoudeh M, Al-Khayarin M, Zirie M, Bener A. Bone density measured by dual-energy X-ray absorptiometry in Qatari women. Maturitas. 2005;52(3–4):319–27.
21. Emery P, Hammoudeh M, FitzGerald O, Combe B, Martin-Mola E, Buch MH, et al. Sustained remission with etanercept tapering in early rheumatoid arthritis. N Engl J Med. 2014;371(19):1781–92.
22. Hammoudeh M, Al Awadhi A, Hasan EH, Akhlaghi M, Ahmadzadeh A, Sadeghi Abdollahi B. Safety, tolerability, and efficacy of Tocilizumab in rheumatoid arthritis: an open-label phase 4 study in patients from the Middle East. Int J Rheumatol. 2015;2015:975028.
23. Braun J, van der Horst-Bruinsma IE, Huang F, Burgos-Vargas R, Vlahos B, Koenig AS, et al. Clinical efficacy and safety of etanercept versus sulfasalazine in patients with ankylosing spondylitis: a randomized, double-blind trial. Arthritis Rheum. 2011;63(6):1543–51.
24. Al-Saleh J, Elbadawi F, Namas R, Elarabi M, Al-Emadi S, Gharib MH, et al. LUNELORD: A descriptive, prospective study on the demographics, disease characteristics and health-related quality of life of patients with LUpus NEphritis and long-term ORgan damage in rheumatology clinics in the Arabian Gulf. Lupus. 2026;35(7):653–66.

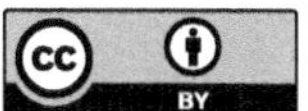
BY

Chapter 14
Rheumatic Diseases in the Kingdom of Saudi Arabia

Fahdah Al Okaily, Sami Bahlas, and Ibrahim Al-Homood

Abstract Millions of people throughout the world suffer from rheumatic illnesses and are affected by a wide range of inflammatory, autoimmune, and degenerative conditions. A significant global disparity between the frequency of rheumatic diseases and the availability of board-certified, highly qualified rheumatologists has been well-documented in research. Rheumatologists are in short supply in a number of nations, including the Kingdom of Saudi Arabia (KSA). The spectrum of rheumatic illnesses described in KSA appears to be similar to that seen in the West, albeit with some notable differences. Regarding the epidemiology of various rheumatic diseases reported, there are currently around 400 adult rheumatologists and around 80 pediatric rheumatologists (consultants, specialists, and fellows) working in different hospitals across KSA. The number of seats in rheumatology training programs in KSA is made public each year, as there is a shortage of rheumatologists, and there is no center for rheumatology research and development. Saudi rheumatology fellow trainees who enroll in the Saudi Commission for Health Specialties rheumatology programs go through a rigorous, 2-year, full-time training program during which they actively participate in patient care, with the scope of their responsibilities expanding as they gain more knowledge and experience. Specified research tasks must be finished within 2 years, and each fellow must also publish at least one peer-reviewed scientific paper. Researchers can share their research findings with the world's scientific community, meet their civic obligations, and advance their academic careers. To further strengthen rheumatology training and address the workforce shortage, scholarship programs can also play an important role.

F. Al Okaily (✉)
Prince Sultan Military Medical City, Riyadh, Kingdom of Saudi Arabia
e-mail: alokaily@yahoo.com

S. Bahlas
King Abdulaziz University Hospital, Jeddah, Kingdom of Saudi Arabia
e-mail: Lbahlas@kau.edu.sa

I. Al-Homood
King Fahad Medical City, Riyadh, Kingdom of Saudi Arabia
e-mail: iaalhomood@kfmc.med.sa

K. A. Alnaqbi, G. Aldabie (eds.), *Rheumatic Diseases in the Arab World*,
https://doi.org/10.1007/978-981-92-0967-5_14

Keywords Saudi Arabia · Rheumatic Diseases · Rheumatology Services · Rheumatology Workforce · Rheumatology · Capacity building · Rheumatology Fellowship · Pediatric Rheumatology · Biologic Therapy · Cost-Effective Care

14.1 Introduction

Although noteworthy distinctions have been identified, the range of rheumatic disorders seen in the Kingdom of Saudi Arabia (KSA) seems to be largely similar to that seen in the West [1]. Patients with rheumatic and musculoskeletal diseases can receive therapy using rheumatology's preventive, active, and rehabilitative methods [2]. Rheumatic illness disability has substantial social and health repercussions, including restrictions on patients' capacity for social and occupational functioning [3]. For instance, low back pain, which is estimated to affect over 60% of Saudis, accounts for a sizable portion of economic loss brought on by disability [3]. The need for rheumatology treatment has been rising rapidly in recent years, but there do not seem to be enough experts on this subject. Rheumatologists are in short supply in many nations, including KSA, which has a negative impact on many facets of rheumatic medical care [4]. Currently, approximately 400 adult and 80 pediatric rheumatologists (including consultants, specialists, and fellows) are practicing in various hospitals across the Kingdom. To increase the number of rheumatologists, certain measures should be taken to reduce the shortfall, such as encouraging specialization in rheumatology among medical students and internal medicine residents, ensuring adequate exposure to rheumatology, and having rheumatologists serve as mentors [4].

This chapter discusses the epidemiology and incidence of rheumatic diseases in KSA. It also emphasizes the value of rheumatologists and the future development of rheumatology training in KSA. A significant revamp of Saudi Arabia's health care system, including changes to the regulation of medical education, is anticipated as a result of Saudi Vision 2030.

14.2 Demography of the Kingdom of Saudi Arabia (KSA)

KSA, the largest country in the Arabian Peninsula, is located in Southwest Asia, on the Arabian Peninsula. The countries it borders include the United Arab Emirates (UAE), Oman, the Republic of Yemen, Iraq, Jordan, and Kuwait.

According to a 2024 survey, the population of Saudi Arabia is 35.3 million, of whom 55.6% are Saudi nationals and the remainder are non-Saudi immigrants. The average life expectancy at birth among Saudis is 78.0 years. The mean age of Saudi citizens is 26.6 years, and approximately 71% of the total population is under 35 years of age. About 22.5% are aged 0–14 years, 74.7% are between 15 and 64 years, and 2.8% are 65 years and above [5].

14.3 Country Health Care System

The KSA constitution establishes health care as a fundamental right to citizens and residents. To provide free health care to its residents, the public health system and the Ministry of Health (MoH) were founded in 1925 and 1949, respectively. Saudi Arabia's healthcare funding mainly comes from the government's budget [6], and its health spending as a percentage of GDP was 5.69% in 2023 [7].

Across the country, the MoH manages 17 regional directorates-general of health affairs [8]. Each regional health directorate oversees several hospitals and health sectors, each of which covers a number of primary health centers (PHC). The Kingdom's 2030 Vision established the Health Sector Transformation Program (scheduled to be implemented in 2022) which aims to ensure continuing development of health care services in the Kingdom and to focus efforts in this critical sector. This follows the success of the National Transformation Program and the completion of its strategic aims, which included updating the health sector to address issues within health services. This resulted in a boost of quality and efficiency, increased protection against health hazards, and emphasized the growth of the healthcare sector, in part due to privatization [9].

Furthermore, the government also plays an important role by providing various degrees of support to the healthcare sectors. Between 2007 and 2016, the Saudi government spent SR 484 billion on health care, establishing 2390 basic healthcare clinics and 284 hospitals [10], of which over 10 are considered tertiary referral hospitals. Patients are first seen in the primary care clinic for initial investigations and evaluation, after which a referral to the hospital rheumatologist will take place, according to their clinical condition. There is ongoing collaboration and communication between hospitals and primary health clinics in providing subspecialty care, such as rheumatology. Coordination between public health educational institutions and public health service organizations would aid the country in achieving its 2030 Vision which aims to build a sustainable public healthcare system.

14.4 Rheumatology Health Services

KSA aims to transform the health sector through Saudi Vision 2030, but there are still no specialized training programs for nurses in rheumatology. Moreover, there is a lack of data regarding certified rheumatology nurses, despite there being nurses who have worked across different rheumatology departments for significant periods of time. There is a need to establish a center of excellence specifically for rheumatology practice, research, and training, and one that encompasses both adult and pediatric rheumatology, as the number of pediatric rheumatologists in KSA is very limited. However, it should be noted there are many medical centers of excellence providing rheumatology care and training at a high standard.

The Charitable Association for Rheumatic Diseases (CARDS) provides social, psychological, and health-related services to improve the quality of life of patients living with rheumatic diseases. Medical services it provides include medication purchase and/or delivery, joint replacement, or bariatric surgeries and physiotherapies. CARDS also provide researchers access to its database to aid in recruiting patients for questionnaires, in accordance with high ethical standards [11].

14.5 Epidemiology of Rheumatic Diseases

Patients with joint, musculoskeletal (MSK), and connective tissue illnesses are treated with rheumatology in three ways: prevention, active therapy, and rehabilitative treatment [2]. Rheumatic disorders are chronic, persistent, and sometimes progressive diseases that can cause disabilities in affected patients. With some notable distinctions, the spectrum of rheumatic disorders reported in KSA is largely similar to that seen in the West. Different rheumatic diseases were reported, such as systemic lupus erythematosus (SLE), rheumatoid arthritis, spondyloarthritis (SpA), psoriatic arthritis (PsA), vasculitis, systemic sclerosis (SSc), idiopathic inflammatory myositis (IIM), Sjogren disease, osteoarthritis (OA), osteoporosis, gout, adult-onset Still's disease and fibromyalgia (FM) are described below.

14.5.1 Rheumatoid Arthritis (RA)

It is estimated that the prevalence of RA varies between Africa and the Middle East. Global and regional data from a Global Burden of Disease study suggests that the ratio is closer to 3:1 in Africa and the Middle East and that the incidence of RA in KSA is 0.06% [12]. Another study looked at the characteristics of RA patients who visited Riyadh's King Khalid University Hospital over 5 years. During this time, 195 patients with RA were examined, of which 155 were females and 40 were males. Within this group, 76.4% of patients reported a slow onset, and 45.1% used a form of regional medicine. Constitutional symptoms were noted in 40% of patients, and 79.5% had positive rheumatoid factors. Proximal interphalangeal (PIP), knee, and metacarpophalangeal (MCP) joints were the joints most frequently affected. Around 16% of patients had rheumatoid nodules and 14.4% had keratoconjunctivitis sicca [13]. In the Al Qassim Region, a house-to-house survey was conducted of 5890 Saudi adults aged 16 years or older. Using the standards established by the American College of Rheumatology for classifying RA, 13 cases of the disease were found. The prevalence of RA in this study was estimated to be 2.2 per 1000 people [14], and the prevalence in Taif was close to the global prevalence estimate [15]. In another study, the clinical, laboratory, and radiological characteristics, as well as the human leukocyte antigen (HLA)-DR phenotypes, were investigated in a group of 91 RA patients (72 females and 19 males). HLA-DR10 was identified as the most common HLA associated with RA in the studied group. When comparing patients with HLA-DR10 versus those without it, it was found that HLA-DR10 was associated with more progressive disease and lower hemoglobin and white blood cell count (WBC) [16].

Currently, epidemiological results found in the literature regarding RA in KSA are suboptimal. In fact, the exact prevalence of RA in the Saudi population remains uncertain. Therefore, conducting a nationwide study on the prevalence of RA in KSA is fundamentally important for developing effective management strategies for disease control.

To guide current practice, national registries are crucial. Middle Eastern and North African RA registries continue to be underrepresented, which also affects the ability to characterize a group of RA patients in KSA and assess the results against statistics from other countries. For the purpose of analyzing disease characteristics and remission rates in a tertiary care setting, the Rheumatoid Arthritis Saudi Database (RASD) was created [17]. In addition to this, the Saudi Arthritis Registry was established, with 2420 visits and 525 RA patients recruited from 10 sites across 4 provinces. Over 3 years, 30 centers plan to enroll over 4000 patients [18].

14.5.2 Systemic Lupus Erythematosus (SLE)

SLE is a chronic autoimmune disease of unknown etiology with growing incidence, predominantly affecting women. The prevalence of SLE in central KSA was studied in 2002: of the 10,372 studied, 2 cases of SLE were identified, and the prevalence of SLE was estimated to be 19.28 per 100,000 of the region's population. This result is comparable to that reported in Western countries [19].

Another study saw 624 SLE patients referred to King Khalid University Hospital, Riyadh. There were 566 females and 58 males (9.8:1) with a mean age of 34.3 (range 8–71) years and mean age at disease onset of 25.3 years (range 0.08–67). Hematological abnormalities were the most common manifestation (82.7%), followed by arthritis (80.4%) and mucocutaneous symptoms (64.3%). The prevalence of malar rash was 47.9%, discoid rash 17.6%, photosensitivity 30.6%, oral ulcers 39.1%, serositis 27.4%, nephritis 47.9%, and neuropsychiatric manifestations 27.6%. Lymphopenia (40.3%), anti-Ro (53.1%), anti-La (26.6%), anti-Sm (41.6%), anticardiolipin IgG (49.7%), and IgM (33.5%) antibodies were highly prevalent. Antinuclear antibodies were detected in 99.7% and anti-DNA in 80.1% patients. Low C3 and C4 were observed in 45.4% and 42.2%, respectively [20].

Lupus nephritis (LN) was found to be prevalent among Saudi patients and was typically associated with a worse prognosis. There were 299 (47.9%) cases of LN found in the 624 cases of SLE that were followed up at King Khalid University Hospital in Riyadh [20]. In addition, remission was seen in 226 (75.6%) patients, renal flares in 14 (4.7%), end-stage renal disease (ESRD) in 27 (9.0%), and 18 died (6.0%).

The majority of lupus patients are young women of child-bearing age. Researchers in KSA also took into account how lupus affects pregnant mothers. In a notable study, the pregnancy outcomes of 396 patients with SLE in KSA were examined. A retrospective analysis of all SLE patients' pregnancies between 1980 and 2006 was carried out. They found out that preterm deliveries were significantly more frequent in patients with lupus nephritis, as were anti-Ro/SSA antibodies, hypertension, history of intravenous cyclophosphamide treatment, and aPL, compared to those without these features. Moreover, high risk pregnancies were found to be associated with active lupus nephritis, anti-Ro/SSA antibodies, aPL, hypertension, Raynaud's phenomenon, and active disease at conception. SLE exacerbations also carry a higher risk of adverse pregnancy outcomes [21].

There has not been a prospective cohort study for SLE patients in Saudi Arabia until now. To recruit 1000 patients, Almaghlouth et al. from King Saud University established a countrywide SLE prospective research study. Physiological and molecular alterations linked to shifts in disease activity levels were found to be examples of secondary consequences. Results and analyses are currently being studied [22].

14.5.3 Axial Spondyloarthritis (AxSpA)

AxSpA is a chronic inflammatory disease that causes arthritis mainly in the axial skeleton but can also affect peripheral joints and internal organs. Unfortunately, there is a lack of information on the prevalence of axSpA in KSA. Some studies include reports of spondyloarthritis, including ankylosing spondylitis (AS) and psoriatic arthritis prevalence in adult patients in Riyadh and Jeddah. In one of the studies, they describe 15 patients with ankylosing spondylitis where they tested HLA-B27 on 12 out of 15 patients and 8 (out of 12) patients tested positive. All 15 patients had symmetrical radiographic sacroiliitis, 11 (73%) had radiographic (ankylosing) spondylitis, 9 (60%) had enthesitis, and 5 had peripheral joint disease (33%). There were two (13%) and one (7%) cases of conjunctivitis and uveitis, respectively [23]. Another study evaluated the prevalence of HLA-B27 in 134 patients with SpA recruited from five centers. HLA-B27 was positive in 60.4%, 69%, and 25.9% of patients with axSpA, AS, and nr-axSpA, respectively [24].

14.5.4 Psoriatic Arthritis (PsA)

PsA is a chronic inflammatory arthritis that predominantly affects patients with psoriasis and may also involve the spine and sacroiliac joints. A review of the literature identified several Saudi studies examining the prevalence of psoriasis and its associated comorbidities. In a retrospective cohort study conducted at King Abdulaziz Medical City in Riyadh, 49 out of 487 patients with psoriasis (10%) were diagnosed with PsA [25]. Similarly, a tertiary care center in the western region reported a PsA prevalence of 13% among 414 psoriasis patients [26]. Data from the Saudi Arabia Psoriasis Registry (PSORSA) indicated that 9.8% of enrolled psoriasis patients had comorbid PsA [27]. Furthermore, a study conducted in Riyadh on 141 patients with PsA found that the prevalence of hyperlipidemia was comparable to that of the general Saudi population [28].

14.5.5 Vasculitis

Vasculitis is a group of clinical diseases that causes chronic inflammation and destruction of blood vessel walls, leading to organ ischemia and damage. Due to the rarity of these illnesses and the lack of valid diagnostic criteria, an accurate estimate of the incidence and prevalence in KSA is limited.

Giant cell arteritis (GCA) was not previously documented in Saudi Arabia, either as individual cases or in epidemiological investigations, until 1997 [29]. GCA cases only make up four positive cases out of the 72 temporal artery biopsies performed over the last 15 years. In another retrospective study of 102 temporal artery biopsies, seven cases (6.8%) were found to be positive for GCA, indicating that the condition is uncommon in the Arab population [30].

The epidemiology of Behcet disease (BD) was studied in a tertiary hospital in Riyadh, involving 119 patients. The male to female ratio was 3.4:1. Disease manifestations showed a higher prevalence of CNS involvement. Of the 119 patients, 52 (44%) patients had central nervous system involvement (of which 12 had benign intracranial hypertension), 16% had pleuropulmonary involvement, 25% had deep venous thrombosis, 18% had arterial thrombosis and aneurysms, 4% had gastrointestinal manifestations, and 4% had epididymitis [31].

The male predominance of BD was also reported in a retrospective study conducted over a 25-year period in which the King Khaled Eye Specialist Hospital in Saudi Arabia examined 132 uveitis patients with BD. Male patients made up 77.3% of the total population. The most frequent diagnosis, panuveitis, affected 118 patients (89.4%). Bilateral episodes affected 75.8% of patients. At the time of presentation, 26.3% of the patients' eyes had retinal vasculitis, 25.4% had occlusive vasculitis, and 18.1% had macular edema [32].

HLA typing of BD among Saudis was reported in 60 patients. It revealed the frequencies of HLA-A*26, HLA-A*31, and HLA-B*51, which are significantly higher in patients with BD compared to controls [33].

Antineutrophil cytoplasmic antibodies (ANCA)-associated vasculitis (AAV) is a group of vasculitis disorders characterized by the presence of ANCA which comprises three diseases: granulomatosis with polyangiitis (GPA, previously known as Wegener's Granulomatosis [WG]), microscopic polyangiitis (MPA), and eosinophilic granulomatosis with polyangiitis (EGPA, previously known as Churg-Strauss syndrome). These disorders are uncommon in the Saudi population and are therefore not well studied. There is a study of 34 AAV patients (21 males: 13 females) comprising 23 GPA, 2 MPA, and 9 EGPA cases. The mean age of onset was 42.1 ± 17.6 years (range 11–75) and the mean duration of disease was 8.7 ± 5.1 years (range 1–20). The most frequently affected system was pulmonary in all the AAV patients (73.5%); especially with EGPA (100%) and GPA (65.2%), while renal involvement was 100% in MPA patients. Ophthalmological and upper airway involvement was higher in GPA cases. Neurological involvement was higher with EGPA. ANCA were detected in 79.4% of AAV patients; of them, c-ANCA and ANCA were confirmed in 77.8% and 22.2% of cases, respectively. ANCA was positive in 91.3% of GPA, 100% of MPA, and 44.4% of EGPA patients. In GPA, c-ANCA was detected in 80.9% and p-ANCA in 17.4% of cases. With MPA, c-ANCA was detected in 50% and p-ANCA in 50% of patients. In EGPA, c-ANCA was observed in 75% and p-ANCA in 25% of patients. All GPA patients had PR3. The 10-year survival in the AAV patients was 95%. The ANCA pattern was similar to Caucasian AAV patients but different from Japanese and Chinese AAV patients [34].

In another study, 52 patients with AAV were analyzed; of whom 62.5% had GPA, 25% had EGPA, and 12.5% had MPA. The relapse rate was 31.3%, while the remission rate was 68.8%. Additionally, 66.7% had lower respiratory involvement, and 43.8% had renal involvement. Birmingham Vasculitis Activity Score was not a potential predictor for relapse [35].

14.5.6 Systemic Sclerosis (SSc)

This rare chronic autoimmune connective tissue disease affects skin, blood vessels, and internal organs. The prevalence of this disease has not studied in KSA, and there are only a few reports. The prevalence of pulmonary arterial hypertension (PAH) in 57 Saudi patients with SSc was reviewed. PAH was confirmed by right heart catheter in 40 patients (87.5%, females). Their mean age was 45.43 ± 13.48 years. The mean pulmonary artery pressure was 42.9 ± 12.7 mmHg. Ten patients (25%) with SSc PAH died over a follow-up period of 37 ± 7 months. Saudi SSc-PAH patients have a younger disease onset and a lower mortality than described worldwide despite late presentation and requirement of combination therapy [36].

14.5.7 Idiopathic Inflammatory Muscle Diseases (IIM)

IIM are systemic diseases characterized by symmetrical proximal muscle weakness. These are uncommon medical conditions, with only a few reports found. They include three main types: adult dermatomyositis (DM), polymyositis (PM), and inclusion body myositis (IBM).

A study reported that 22 cases of dermatomyositis and polymyositis in Riyadh were associated with connective tissues, and malignancy and arthritis were more common in patients. Three patients died (14%) as a result of respiratory failure and underlying cancer [37]. There were 28 IIM patients, with a 3:1 ratio of female to male patients. Of the patients, 32.1% had pure polymyositis, 21.4% had pure dermatomyositis, 10.7% had juvenile dermatomyositis, and 35.7% had IIM combined with connective tissue diseases. Although the findings are similar to other global reviews, the association with malignancy was lower. Furthermore, a strong relation between comorbid illnesses and relapse was found [38].

Sixty patients with IIM were studied to evaluate the prevalence of malignancies among them. Four patients (6.7%) had neoplasms, including two males with lymphoma, a female with breast cancer, and a second with ovarian cancer. Cancer or its effects claimed the lives of two patients. Being over 40 years of age, dysphagia, necrotic rash, absence of interstitial lung disease (ILD), high ESR, and a negative anti-Jo-1 antibody were found to be possibly predictive risk factors for neoplasia [39].

14.5.8 Sjogren Disease (SjD)

Sjögren disease, formerly known as primary Sjögren's syndrome, is a chronic autoimmune disease characterized by diminished functionality of the exocrine glands due to lymphocytic infiltration and damage. To our knowledge, there are only a few studies in KSA on SjD. A cross-sectional study described 41 patients with SjD. The cohort had an average diagnosis delay of 2.2 ± 2.4 years, with a 1–11 year range. In 38 people (92.7%), a minor salivary gland biopsy was done. Extra-glandular manifestations were highly prevalent, with interstitial lung disease and arthritis accounting for 27 (65.9%) of the cases [40].

A retrospective study on the prevalence of interstitial lung disease (ILD) in SjD included 84 patients diagnosed with SjD-ILD, of which 40% had pulmonary hypertension (PH), 20% had severe PAH, and 50% exhibited negative autoimmune serology associated with SjD. Acute exacerbation was observed in 38% of the cohort during follow-up. For all patients, the 5-year survival rate was 56 [41].

14.5.9 Osteoarthritis (OA)

Osteoarthritis (OA) is the most common disease to cause joint pain around the world. In KSA, it was found to be common among the older female population. Few studies have been conducted on the prevalence of OA. One study utilized a house-to-house survey of randomly selected inhabitants of Al-Qaseem. A total of 10,406 persons were interviewed. Clinical OA of the knees was found to occur in 13% [42]. Another study looked at the radiographic evidence of osteoarthritis of the knee in 300 randomly chosen patients attending 14 primary care facilities for different medical conditions. Radiographic OA was seen in 89 males (53.3%) and 81 females (60.9%). The prevalence of osteoarthritis of the knee joint was 24.5% [43].

In another cross-sectional study of 200 primary health care center attendees in Makkah, a validated, reliable, self-administered, Arabic-based questionnaire was administered, and knee osteoarthritis was concluded to affect 41.5% [44] of attendees. The impact of knee OA was negative on Saudi elders' quality of life. The mental health component was more affected than the physical health component [45], along with increased functional and recreational difficulties. Physical activity was associated with lower knee OA severity, which implies a beneficial effect [46].

14.5.10 Osteoporosis

In KSA, the prevalence of osteoporosis and osteopenia among individuals aged 50 years and older is 37.8% and 28.2%, respectively [47]. In 2015, an estimated 7528 osteoporosis-related femoral fractures occurred nationwide among a population of 1,300,336 adults aged 55 years or above, as shown in Fig. 14.1 [48].

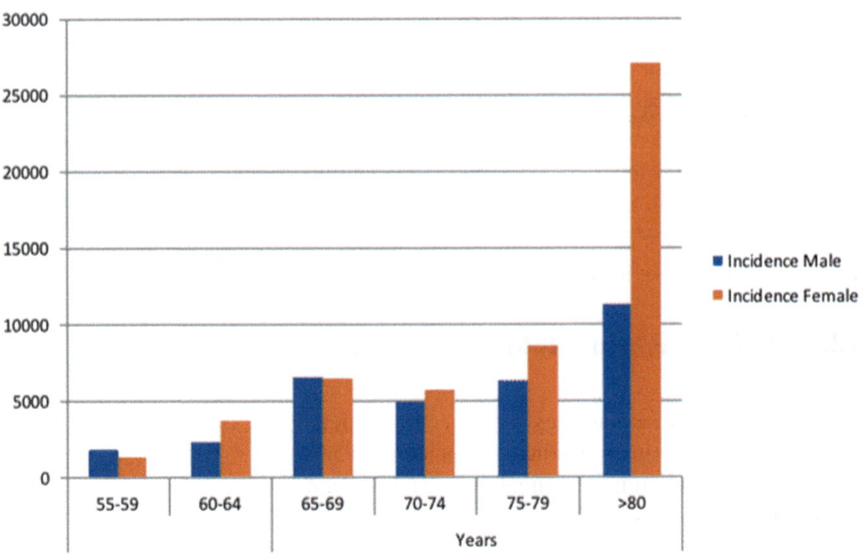

Fig. 14.1 Annual femur fracture rate in the KSA population, per 1000,000 person-years. (Data reproduced and adapted from Mir Sadat-Ali et al. [48]. Reproduced with permission from Springer Nature. © Springer Nature 2015)

14.5.11 Gout and Chondrocalcinosis

Globally, cases of hyperuricemia have increased significantly in recent decades. The prevalence of hyperuricemia in KSA was studied in a single center in Riyadh.

In total, 487 Saudis (250 men and 237 women) were questioned and examined. Of the 487 people, 41 (8.42%) had hyperuricemia (20 men and 21 women) [49]. Another study from Jeddah of 863 participants (586 male, 67.9%, and 277 female, 32.1%) detected hyperuricemia in 10.3% [50]. No data was found to study the epidemiology of gout.

Regarding chondrocalcinosis, a study was published on the prevalence of chondrocalcinosis in 150 subjects aged 50 years and above in a radiographic survey through 14 primary care clinics in North Riyadh, KSA. Six (3.9%) cases of chondrocalcinosis were identified in the whole age group (50–93). When the above 60 age group was considered, the prevalence rose to 6.7% [51].

14.5.12 Adult-Onset Still's Disease

Adult-Onset Still's disease is a rare systemic disease. Most of the reports are small series or case reports. The only large study included 14 Saudi patients diagnosed to have Adult-Onset Still's disease. The clinical and laboratory pattern of these patients are more or less similar to that in other reported series, apart from having lower cardiac and pulmonary involvement than the western series [52].

14.5.13 Fibromyalgia (FM)

FM is a chronic musculoskeletal pain with an unknown etiology. The prevalence of FM among medical students in KSA was analyzed, with a total of 450 participants. A total of 43 participants (9.6%) were found to have FM [53].

In a cross-sectional study, 183 physicians in training (PIT) completed a questionnaire. The prevalence of FM was (8.2%). Surgical residents had the highest prevalence (14.8%) followed by anesthetists (14.3%) and medical residents (13.4%) [54].

During the COVID-19 pandemic, a cross-sectional study among health workers in different health care settings in KSA was carried out. Of the 992 participants, the prevalence of Fibromyalgia using FiRST and LFESSQ was 12.6 and 19.8%, respectively. The prevalence was higher in females when compared to males [55].

14.6 Epidemiology of Pediatric Rheumatology Diseases in KSA

14.6.1 Juvenile Idiopathic Arthritis (JIA)

This is a group of diseases with arthritis as the main manifestation in patients aged <16 years.

Unfortunately, no proper epidemiological studies were conducted in KSA to evaluate the prevalence and incidence of each disease; however, there are many studies on the demographic and clinical characteristics of these disorders [56].

Almayouf et al. reported that the prevalence of JIA in Africa and the Middle East (including KSA) was found to be lower compared to global reports and commonly of the oligoarticular type. Moreover, ANA positivity and uveitis were found to be lower compared to other parts of the world [57].

14.6.2 Systemic Lupus Erythematosus (SLE)

A retrospective study of 152 patients (129 girls and 23 boys) was included. The mean age at onset of SLE was 8.8 ± 2.6 years, and permanent damage occurred in 52.6% of patients. Damage had affected the growth (26.8%), renal (17.1%), and neuropsychiatric (15.8%) domains, and 14 patients required dialysis for progressive renal disease; five of them underwent renal transplant. Infection was the main cause of death, and 8 out of 9 deaths were due to infection [58].

14.6.3 IgA Vasculitis

IgA vasculitis is the most common type of vasculitis in children. A retrospective study from the Aseer region included 89 children, of which 56.2% were boys and 43.8% were girls, with a male-to-female ratio of 1.28:1, and a mean age at diagnosis of 5.87 ± 2.81 years. Rash was present in 100%, arthritis in 72.2%, gastrointestinal tract involvement in 60.7%, and renal involvement in 23.5% of cases. Relapses occurred in 26% of cases [59].

14.7 Risk Factors of Rheumatic Diseases

A study conducted in Riyadh identified advanced age, female sex, low educational attainment, unemployment, smoking, obesity, and infrequent medical consultations (fewer than two visits within the previous 12 months) as significant risk factors for rheumatic diseases [60]. Another study reported hypertension (18.3%) and hypothyroidism (15%) as the most prevalent comorbidities among patients with rheumatic diseases, with a mean age of 47.87 ± 11.55 years and a female-to-male ratio of 6.5:1. Approximately 23.3% of patients with RA had a positive family history [61]. Furthermore, risk factors for progression to end-stage renal disease among patients with SLE included older age at disease onset and hypertension, as reported in a study from Riyadh [20].

14.8 Screening Programs for Rheumatic Diseases

General practitioners (GPs) are crucial in identifying rheumatic diseases such as RA in some health care systems, as they are sometimes the first point of contact for specialists, such as rheumatologists. In general practice, it can be challenging to recognize individuals who need to be referred to rheumatologists for suspected RA due to a variety of factors, including the fact that the disease frequently manifests slowly and that early-stage joint swelling may be asymmetric or monoarticular [62]. GPs have identified a number of obstacles to diagnosing RA, including a lack of knowledge of symptoms, the GP's gatekeeping role, poor communication with rheumatologists, and limits to laboratory testing. Future research in KSA should identify and address primary-care barriers to the early referral of suspected RA and strengthen bidirectional collaboration between general practice and rheumatology services.

The Saudi Society of Rheumatology (SSR) plays an important role in health education. It conducts awareness days for different rheumatology disorders, and these take place in malls and community centers. The health education departments of different hospitals also play similar roles within different regions in the kingdom. Early detection of rheumatology cases can also be accomplished during these events.

14.9 Diagnosis

Laboratory tests are available in KSA, and different tests used in the diagnosis of RA are accessible by patients. Almost all laboratory tests are available in tertiary hospitals, save for the few rare antibodies that are sent abroad. More advanced imaging, such as PET scans and angiography, is available in tertiary hospitals and large health facilities. In the diagnosis of rheumatic disease, radiologists play a very important role, particularly in MSK cases. In KSA, the exact number of MSK radiologists is unknown, although there is a good number of qualified radiologists working in the field of MSK radiology, of which many are graduates of the SCFHS fellowship program in MSK radiology. MSK ultrasound for the diagnosis and monitoring of rheumatic diseases is available in every hospital in KSA, and patients have easy access to such facilities:

14.10 Management

14.10.1 Medical

Early use of conventional synthetic disease-modifying antirheumatic medications (csDMARDs), which are regarded as the cornerstone of treatment for RA, is one way to implement the treat-to-target (T2T) strategy. Methotrexate (MTX), hydroxychloroquine (HCQ), sulfasalazine (SZZ), and leflunomide are examples of csDMARDs. Different types of biological or targeted synthetic DMARDs (tsDMARDs) are available in most hospitals. Other strategies, such as biosimilars, can also be used. Rehabilitation, physiotherapy, and occupational therapy are also available in KSA, as are orthopedic surgery facilities for all types of surgeries.

14.10.2 Cost-Effective Care for Rheumatic Diseases

In a study that involved 400 RA patients, with a mean age of 54, the disease lasted an average of 9 years. The anticipated average annual expense per patient was SAR 38,596. The price rose to SAR 75,097 for patients who underwent knee replacement surgery. With each additional comorbidity, the cost rose by a substantial SAR 3971. The cost of biologics was the main cost factor, followed by the price of lab and diagnostic tests and outpatient visits (84%, 5%, and 3%, respectively) [63]. However, in another study, it was shown that cost can be reduced by 27% (from SAR 62,193 to SAR 45,351) if patients switched from subcutaneous (SC) to oral tsDMARDs, and by 45% (from SAR 82,619 to SAR 45,351) if they switched from IV biologics. The average cost of oral tsDMARDs per patient was discovered to be 60% of the average cost of SC and IV biologics per patient [64]. The cost of medication for the treatment of RA is higher in a private clinic, and the best way to reduce the cost is the minimization of risk factors such as smoking, hypertension, and obesity.

14.11 Rheumatologists in KSA

There are an estimated 400 adult rheumatologists and around 80 pediatric rheumatologists. The rheumatology specialty appears to be favored by female doctors in KSA, reflected in the number of applicants to fellowship programs. The number of female rheumatologists is also increasing annually, of which the exact number cannot be determined, yet is still slightly less than the number of male rheumatologists.

We still have a shortage of rheumatologists and pediatric rheumatologists, especially in the peripheries. As a result, general pediatricians and adult rheumatologists manage child patients with JIA in some of the hospitals which are short on pediatric rheumatologists.

14.12 Rheumatology Fellowship Training

The first training program in KSA for adult rheumatology was established in the early 1990s at King Faisal Hospital, where a structured training program had a 2-year duration and accepted two candidates annually. This program was recognized by the Saudi Commission for Health Specialties (SCFHS) and was cancelled in 2009 after the establishment of the SCFHS Rheumatology fellowship training program. SCFHS is a health education and training regulatory body in charge of creating, approving, and overseeing professional health-related programs, as well as creating long-term medical education programs for health-related issues. It also establishes guidelines and standards for the practice of health professions in addition to monitoring and assessing training programs. SCFHS has a full set of "General Bylaws" and "Executive Policies" that regulate the process of training. The SCFHS fellowship program began with an annual intake of 10 candidates. Currently, the annual intake is 24 candidates distributed over 14 accredited training centers for a 2-year training period. With increased demand for training, another program was established at King Saud University in 2015, also recognized by SCFHS, with an intake of two to three candidates annually.

A pediatric fellowship program was established in 2004 at the King Faisal Hospital and Research Center, again with a 2-year training period. There are five accredited training centers for the pediatric rheumatology fellowship program.

Fellows who complete these training programs will be able to function as consultants with core competencies in rheumatology. The adult rheumatology training program curriculum ensures that "adult-learner" trainees must demonstrate full engagement with proactive roles through careful understanding of learning objectives, self-directed learning, openness to reflective feedback, and formative assessment. It also ensures conformance with the framework laid out by the Canadian Medical Education Directions for Specialists (CanMEDS). The training period of an adult rheumatology program is 2 years. The training covers general rheumatology inpatients, outpatient clinics, emergency, and referral services. Training also includes rotations in radiology, physiotherapy, immunology laboratory, pediatric rheumatology, research, and elective training in a specialized area of interest. Academic activities are also part of training. The Core Education Program (CEP) includes formal teaching and learning activities classified as universal topics, core specialty topics, and trainee-selected topics. At least 3 hours per week should be allocated to the CEP. This will be supplemented by practice-based learning activities such as morning reports or case presentations, morbidity and mortality reviews, journal clubs (including systematic reviews), hospital grand rounds, and other continuous medical education activities. Half-day educational activity (HDEA) is organized directly by the Rheumatology Scientific Committee. This activity is centered on topics and skills that are vital for training the fellows to master their basic and clinical knowledge.

During training, fellows will be assessed via periodical formative evaluations throughout the first and second years in order to ensure the CanMEDS competencies are met.

The assessment includes a promotional written examination at the end of the first year. At the end of the second year, fellows will be certified if they pass written and clinical examinations [65].

14.13 Research in Rheumatology

The amount of clinical research has grown in KSA ever since it became a mandatory requirement for doctor qualification and promotion. Research centers are established in many hospitals in KSA as well as institutional review boards (IRB). Clinical research studies may be used to promote or develop agents (drugs), equipment, techniques, and policies for prevention, diagnosis, treatment, and palliation. Researchers are typically advised to examine the literature and evaluate current data before planning a health research study to demonstrate the proposed study's feasibility and necessity. There are still unmet needs for epidemiological research within the kingdom.

14.14 Saudi Society of Rheumatology (SSR)

SSR was established in 2010, under the SCFHS [66]. The elected board works at different levels to promote rheumatology practice and training. The SSR advances the science of rheumatology, supports members in providing the best care possible for patients, and is a leading organization in the field of rheumatology with a significant positive impact on patient care. This will undoubtedly have an impact on children's and adults' lives who have rheumatic and musculoskeletal diseases in Saudi Arabia. There is also a group of rheumatologists who form the Arab Adult Arthritis Awareness Group, one of the Special Interest Groups established under the auspices of the Arab League of Association for Rheumatology. Working to reach all members of society in diverse Arabic-speaking nations and beyond, this group raises awareness of rheumatic and musculoskeletal disorders in Arabic as well as in English and French.

14.15 Conclusion

With an aging population, it is anticipated that the prevalence and burden of rheumatic illnesses will increase, placing further demand on the global rheumatology community and related healthcare resources. A significant global disparity between the incidence of rheumatic diseases and the availability of board-certified, highly qualified rheumatologists has been documented in research. Rheumatologists are in short supply in a number of nations, including KSA. Although there were some notable distinctions, the spectrum of rheumatic disorders reported in KSA looked to be largely similar to that seen in the West. Different rheumatic diseases have been reported and their epidemiology summarized. There are currently only around 400 adult rheumatologists and around 80 pediatric rheumatologists working in Saudi Arabia's hospitals. Each year, the number of seats in KSA's rheumatology training programs is released; these seats are distributed among reputable training facilities in the central, eastern, southern, and western regions of the Kingdom. Saudi doctors who join the SCFHS's Rheumatology Fellowship Program undergo a 2-year, full-time, tightly monitored training period during which they actively take part in patient treatment, with their duties increasing as they gain more experience and expertise. Each fellow has 2 years to complete the assigned research projects and submit at least one peer-reviewed scientific paper. Rheumatic diseases prevail, and sporadic cases have been reported from different areas of KSA. There is a lack of well-designed epidemiological studies of rheumatological diseases all over KSA; most of the available data are of small sample size and from single centers that may not reflect the real figures.

Conflict of Interest Declaration All authors agree that they have no conflict of interest.

References

1. Rajapakse CN. The spectrum of rheumatic diseases in Saudi Arabia. Br J Rheumatol. 1987;26(1):22–3.
2. Silva JAP, Woolf AD. Rheumatology in practice. The importance of rheumatic diseases. Springer; 2010. p. 1–13.
3. Aldera MA, Alexander CM, McGregor AH. Prevalence and incidence of low back pain in the Kingdom of Saudi Arabia: a systematic review. J Epidemiol Glob Health. 2020;10(4):269–75.
4. Al Maini M, Adelowo F, Al Saleh J, Al Weshahi Y, Burmester GR, Cutolo M, et al. The global challenges and opportunities in the practice of rheumatology: white paper by the world forum on rheumatic and musculoskeletal diseases. Clin Rheumatol. 2015;34(5):819–29.
5. General Authority for Statistics. Population estimates publication 2024. Riyadh: General Authority for Statistics; 2024 [cited 2026 Jun 15]. Available from: https://www.stats.gov.sa/documents/20117/2435273/Population+Estimates+Publication+2024+EN.pdf/7d123c57-1626-7d2f-ba7f-8a719f928f28.
6. Al-Yousuf M, Akerele TM, Al-Mazrou YY. Organization of the Saudi health system. East Mediterr Health J. 2002;8(4–5):645–53.

7. World Bank. Current health expenditure (% of GDP) - Saudi Arabia [Internet]. Washington (DC): World Bank; 2025 [cited 2026 Jun 15]. Available from: https://data.worldbank.org/indicator/SH.XPD.CHEX.GD.ZS?locations=SA.
8. Ministry of Health. Health Regions in Saudi Arabia [Internet]. [cited 2026 Jun 15]. Available from: https://samrindia.org/health-regions-in-saudi-arabia.
9. Rahman R. The privatization of health care system in Saudi Arabia. Health Services Insights. 2020;13:1178632920934497.
10. Ministry of Health (Saudi Arabia). Statistical yearbook 2021 [Internet]. Riyadh: Ministry of Health; 2021 [cited 2026 Jun 15]. Available from: https://www.moh.gov.sa/en/Ministry/Statistics/book/Documents/Statistical-Yearbook-2021.pdf.
11. Charitable Association for Rheumatic Diseases (CARD). [Internet] [cited 2026 Jun 15]. Available from: https://www.printo.it/pediatric-rheumatology/GB/family/9894/Charitable-Association-for-Rheumatic-diseases-(CARD).
12. Almoallim H, Al Saleh J, Badsha H, Ahmed HM, Habjoka S, Menassa JA, et al. A review of the prevalence and unmet needs in the management of rheumatoid arthritis in Africa and the Middle East. Rheumatol Ther. 2021;8(1):1–16.
13. Alballa SR. The expression of rheumatoid arthritis in Saudi Arabia. Clin Rheumatol. 1995;14(6):641–5.
14. Al-Dalaan A, Ballaa SA, Bahabri S, Biyari T, Sukait MA, Mousa M. The prevalence of rheumatoid arthritis in the Qassim region of Saudi Arabia. Ann Saudi Med. 1998;18(5):396–7.
15. Albishri J, Bukhari M, Alsabban A, Almalki FA, Altwairqi AS. Prevalence of RA and SLE in Saudi Arabia. Sch J Appl Med Sci. 2015;3(5D):2096–9.
16. Al-Arfaj AS. Characteristics of rheumatoid arthritis relative to HLA-DR in Saudi Arabia. Saudi Med J. 2001;22(7):595–8.
17. Almoallim H, Hassan R, Cheikh M, Faruqui H, Alquraa R, Eissa A, et al. Rheumatoid Arthritis Saudi Database (RASD): disease characteristics and remission rates in a tertiary care center. Open Access Rheumatol. 2020;12:139–45.
18. Al Rayes HM, Omair MA. Launching the Saudi arthritis registry. Clin Rheumatol. 2021;36(7):1537–43.
19. Al-Arfaj AS, Al-Balla SR, Al-Dalaan AN, Al-Saleh SS, Bahabri SA, Mousa MM, et al. Prevalence of systemic lupus erythematosus in Central Saudi Arabia. Saudi Med J. 2002;23(1):87–9.
20. Al Arfaj AS, Khalil N, Al Saleh S. Lupus nephritis among 624 cases of systemic lupus erythematosus in Riyadh, Saudi Arabia. Rheumatol Int. 2009;29(9):1057–67.
21. Al Arfaj AS, Khalil N. Pregnancy outcome in 396 pregnancies in patients with SLE in Saudi Arabia. Lupus. 2010;19(14):1665–73.
22. Almaghlouth IA, Hassen LM, Alahmari HS, Bedaiwi A, Albarrak R, Daghestani M, et al. National systemic lupus erythematosus prospective cohort in Saudi Arabia: a study protocol. Medicine (Baltimore). 2021;100(30):e26704.
23. Al-Arfaj A. Profile of ankylosing spondylitis in Saudi Arabia. Clin Rheumatol. 1996;15(3):287–9.
24. Omair MA, AlDuraibi FK, Bedaiwi MK, Abdulaziz S, Husain W, El Dessougi M, et al. Prevalence of HLA-B27 in the general population and in patients with axial spondyloarthritis in Saudi Arabia. Clin Rheumatol. 2017;36(7):1537–43.
25. Alrubaiaan MT, Alsulaiman SA, Alqahtani A, Altasan AN, Almehrij FO, Alrashid A, Mohamed OL. Prevalence and clinical predictors of psoriatic arthritis in Saudi patients with psoriasis: a single-center retrospective cohort study. Cureus. 2023;15(10):e46632. https://doi.org/10.7759/cureus.46632.
26. Alamri RA, Almahdi BH, Marghalani S. Prevalence of psoriatic arthritis and its risk factors among patients with psoriasis in a tertiary care center in Saudi Arabia. Cureus. 2025;17(4):e82782. https://doi.org/10.7759/cureus.82782.
27. Fatani MI, Binamer Y, Almudaiheem HY, Eshmawi MT, Aljehani FH, Alshammari S, et al. Demographics, clinical characteristics, and treatment patterns in patients with psoriasis:

insights from the Saudi Arabia psoriasis registry (PSORSA). Dermatol Ther (Heidelb). 2025;15(8):2031–45. https://doi.org/10.1007/s13555-025-01436-9.
28. Al Talhi K, Alotaiwi S, Alotaibi M, Alhamzi HA, Alrashedi S, Makkawy M, Alokaily F. Prevalence of hyperlipidemia in psoriatic arthritis patients in Riyadh, Saudi Arabia. Saudi Med J. 2024;45(12):1340–6. https://doi.org/10.15537/smj.2024.45.12.20240817.
29. Tahan AA, Rayess MA, Abduljabbar M, Moallem MA. Giant cell arteritis: report of two Saudi patients and review of the literature. Ann Saudi Med. 1997;17(2):237–9.
30. Chaudhry IA, Shamsi FA, Elzaridi E, Arat YO, Bosley TM, Riley FC. Epidemiology of giant-cell arteritis in an Arab population: a 22-year study. Br J Ophthalmol. 2007;91(6):715–8.
31. Al-Dalaan AN, Al Balaa SR, El Ramahi K, Al-Kawi Z, Bohlega S, Bahabri S, et al. Behçet's disease in Saudi Arabia. J Rheumatol. 1994;21(4):658–61.
32. Arevalo JF, Lasave AF, Al Jindan MY, Al Sabaani NA, Al-Mahmood AM, Al-Zahrani YA, et al. Uveitis in Behçet disease in a tertiary center over 25 years: the KKESH Uveitis Survey Study Group. Am J Ophthalmol. 2015;159(1):177–184.e1–2.
33. Al-Okaily F, Al-Rashidi S, Al-Balawi M, Mustafa M, Arfin M, Al-Asmari A. Genetic association of HLA-A26, -A31, and -B*51 with Behçet's disease in Saudi patients. Clin Med Insights Arthritis Musculoskelet Disord. 2016;9:167–73. https://doi.org/10.4137/CMAMD.S39879.
34. Al Arfaj AS, Khalil N. ANCA associated vasculitis in patients from Saudi Arabia. Pak J Med Sci. 2018;34(1):88–93.
35. Alahmari H, Daajani HA, Alsayed F, Alrashid A. ANCA-associated vasculitis clinical presentation and clinical predictors of relapse in Saudi Arabia. Open Access Rheumatol. 2021;13:213–20.
36. Al Otair HA, Idrees MM, Saleemi SA, Eltoukhy AM, Alhijji AA, Al Habeeb WA, et al. Pulmonary arterial hypertension in Saudi patients with systemic sclerosis: clinical and hemodynamic characteristics and mortality. Ann Thorac Med. 2019;14(1):83–9.
37. Al-Ballaa ST, Al-Dalaan AN, El-Ramahi KM, Al-Janadi MA, Al-Shaikh A, Bahabri S. Pattern of adult onset of polymyositis and dermatomyositis and association with malignancy. Ann Saudi Med. 1993;13(6):525–9.
38. Attar S, Babaeer E, Bagais M, Alrehaily W, Mozahim M. Inflammatory muscle disease, 15-year experience at tertiary centers. Intern Med. 2016;6(224):2.
39. Aljohani G, Awad EAB, Alshahrani K, Alsaqar MM, Albogami B, Almotywee SH, et al. The prevalence, clinical features, predictive factors and investigations to screen for cancer in patients with inflammatory myositis: a case series from two tertiary care centers in Riyadh, Saudi Arabia. Saudi Med J. 2021;42(1):100.
40. Omair MA, Al Qahtani BS, Al Hamad EH, Tashkandy YA, Othman NS, Al Shahrani KA, et al. Disease phenotype and diagnostic delay in Saudi patients with primary Sjögren's syndrome: an exploratory cross-sectional study. Saudi Med J. 2021;42(4):405.
41. Alhamad EH, Cal JG, Alrajhi NN, Paramasivam MP, Alharbi WM, AlEssa M, et al. Clinical characteristics and outcomes in patients with primary Sjogren's syndrome-associated interstitial lung disease. Ann Thorac Med. 2021;16(2):156–64.
42. Al-Arfaj AS, Alballa SR, Al-Saleh SS, Al-Dalaan AM, Bahabry SA, Mousa MA, et al. Knee osteoarthritis in Al-Qaseem, Saudi Arabia. Saudi Med J. 2003;24(3):291–3.
43. Al-Arfaj A, Al-Boukai A. Prevalence of radiographic knee osteoarthritis in Saudi Arabia. Clin Rheumatol. 2002;21(2):142–5.
44. Thigah AA, Khan AA. Prevalence of knee osteoarthritis among adult patients attending Al-iskan Primary Health Care Center, Makkah, Saudi Arabia. Ann Clin Anal Med. 2020;9(3):271–8.
45. Ateef M. Functional and higher level difficulties in knee osteoarthritis patients in Saudi Arabian populace. Saudi J Health Sci. 2018;7(1):49.
46. Aldosari AA, Majadah S, Amer KA, Alamri HH, Althomali RN, Alqahtani RF, et al. The association between physical activity level and severity of knee osteoarthritis: a Single Centre Study in Saudi Arabia. Cureus. 2022;14(4):e24377.

47. Saudi Ministry of Health. National Plan for osteoporosis prevention and management [Internet]. Riyadh: Ministry of Health; 2018 [cited 2026 Jun 15]. Available from: https://www.moh.gov.sa/en/Ministry/MediaCenter/Publications/Documents/NPOPM-2018.pdf.
48. Sadat-Ali M, Al-Dakheel DA, Azam MQ, Al-Bluwi MT, Al-Farhan MF, AlAmer HA, et al. Reassessment of osteoporosis-related femoral fractures and economic burden in Saudi Arabia. Arch Osteoporos. 2015;10:37.
49. Al-Arfaj AS. Hyperuricemia in Saudi Arabia. Rheumatol Int. 2001;20(2):61–4.
50. Abalkhail B, Milaat W, Kordy M. Prevalence of hyperuricemia in King Abdulaziz University. Jeddah Med Sci. 1998;6(1):31–8.
51. Al-Arfaj AS, Al-Boukai AA. Articular chondrocalcinosis in Saudi Arabia. Saudi Med J. 2002;23(5):577–9.
52. Al-Arfaj A, Al-Saleh S. Adult-onset still's disease in Saudi Arabia. Clin Rheumatol. 2001;20(3):197–200.
53. Samman AA, Bokhari RA, Idris S, Bantan R, Margushi RR, Lary S, et al. The prevalence of fibromyalgia among medical students at King Abdulaziz University: a cross-sectional study. Cureus. 2021;13(1):e12670.
54. Omair MA, Alobud S, Al-Bogami MH, Dabbagh R, Altaymani YK, Alsultan N, et al. Prevalence of fibromyalgia in physicians in training: a cross-sectional study. Clin Rheumatol. 2019;38(1):165–72.
55. AlEnzi F, Alhamal S, Alramadhan M, Altaroti A, Siddiqui I, Aljanobi G. Fibromyalgia in health care worker during COVID-19 outbreak in Saudi Arabia. Front Public Health. 2021;9:693159.
56. Bahabri S, Al-Sewairi W, Al-Mazyad A, Karrar A, Al-Ballaa S, El-Ramahai K, et al. Juvenile rheumatoid arthritis: the Saudi experience. Ann Saudi Med. 1997;17(4):417–8.
57. Al-Mayouf SM, Al Mutairi M, Bouayed K, Habjoka S, Hadef D, Lotfy HM, et al. Epidemiology and demographics of juvenile idiopathic arthritis in Africa and Middle East. Pediatr Rheumatol. 2021;19:166.
58. Al-Mayouf SM. Systemic lupus erythematosus in Saudi children: long term outcomes. Int J Rheum Dis. 2013;16(1):56–60.
59. Dawood SA, Abodiah AM, Alqahtani SM, Shati AA, Alqahtani YA, Alshehri MA, et al. Clinico-epidemiological profile and outcome of children with IgA vasculitis in Aseer region, Southwestern Saudi Arabia. Healthcare (Basel). 2021;9(12):1694.
60. Al-Ahmari AK. Prevalence of hypertension and its associated risk factors among patients with rheumatoid arthritis in the Kingdom of Saudi Arabia. Int J Gen Med. 2022;15:6507.
61. Alanazi F. Clinical profile and comorbidities associated with rheumatoid arthritis patients in Sudair, Saudi Arabia. J Pharm Bioallied Sci. 2021;13(Suppl 2):S1583.
62. Baymler Lundberg AS, Esbensen BA, Jensen MB, Hauge EM, Thurah A. Facilitators and barriers in diagnosing rheumatoid arthritis as described by general practitioners: a Danish study based on focus group interviews. Scand J Prim Health Care. 2021;39(2):222–9. https://doi.org/10.1080/02813432.2021.1913925.
63. Alghamdi A, Alsaif K, Alsahli M, Omair M, Almohammed O, Almalaq H, et al. PMS14 economic burden of rheumatoid arthritis in Saudi Arabia: a single-center cost of illness study. Value Health. 2020;23:S594.
64. Almudaiheem H, Mohamed O, Dawoud D, Alsuwayeh Y, Alenzi K, Mughari M, et al. PMS23-optimizing treatment for rheumatoid arthritis in the Kingdom of Saudi Arabia (OPTRA). Value Health. 2018;21:S291.
65. Saudi Commission for Health Specialties. Adult rheumatology fellowship [Internet]. [cited 2026 Jun 15]. Available from: https://scfhs.org.sa/en/training?title_op=contains&title_po_prog=Rheumatology+Fellowship.
66. Saudi Society for Rheumatology and Connective Tissue Diseases (SSRC) [Internet]. [cited 2026 Jun 15]. Available from: https://ssrc-sa.com/.

Chapter 15
Rheumatic Diseases in Somalia, Djibouti, and the Union of Comoros

Shamma Al Nokhatha and Khalid A. Alnaqbi

Abstract Healthcare systems in Africa are underdeveloped, particularly in low-income countries such as Somalia, Djibouti, and the Union of Comoros. As a result, the burden of musculoskeletal conditions is likely to be underestimated due to limited resources and inaccessible data. In this chapter, we provide an overview of the three countries (Somalia, Djibouti, and the Union of Comoros) and available data on musculoskeletal conditions.

Keywords Rheumatic diseases · Musculoskeletal diseases · Rheumatology workforce · Health services accessibility · Epidemiology · Africa · Somalia · Djibouti · Comoros

S. Al Nokhatha
Rheumatology Division, Sheikh Tahnoon bin Mohammed Medical City, SEHA/PureHealth, Al Ain, UAE
e-mail: Shamma.alnokhatha@gmail.com

K. A. Alnaqbi (✉)
Rheumatology Division, Sheikh Tahnoon bin Mohammed Medical City, SEHA/PureHealth, Al Ain, UAE

Internal Medicine Department, College of Medicine and Health Sciences, UAE University, Al Ain, UAE

College of Medicine, RAK Medical and Health Sciences, Ras Al Khaimah, UAE
e-mail: kalnaqbi@gmail.com; kalnaqbi@seha.ae

K. A. Alnaqbi, G. Aldabie (eds.), *Rheumatic Diseases in the Arab World*,
https://doi.org/10.1007/978-981-92-0967-5_15

15.1 Introduction

Somalia, Djibouti, and the Comoros Islands are among the low-income nations that experience difficulties in meeting their populations' healthcare needs [1]. Despite efforts to reach out to the respective health ministries, we were unable to establish contact. Consequently, our summary of information regarding rheumatic diseases in these regions is limited.

Due to limited resources and underdeveloped healthcare infrastructure in these countries, we could not identify formally established pediatric or adult rheumatology services in these countries. There is a scarcity of rheumatology care in Africa. As of October 2025, and based on available published sources and personal communications, we could not identify certified rheumatologists practicing in Somalia, Djibouti and the Comoros Islands. Additionally, a recent article did not identify any rheumatologists in these three countries [2]. It is highly likely that non-rheumatologists, such as internal medicine specialists or orthopedic surgeons, diagnose and treat rheumatic diseases in these countries. Moreover, no pediatric rheumatology centers were identified in these countries [3]. Little is known about the burden of rheumatic diseases in Africa, as there are limited epidemiological data. The morbidity and mortality associated with rheumatic diseases in Africa likely exceed those in other regions due to patients often presenting at advanced disease stages with limited treatment options [4].

15.2 Somalia

15.2.1 Country Demographics

The Federal Republic of Somalia, commonly known as Somalia, is located in the Horn of Africa. It is bordered by Djibouti, Kenya, and Ethiopia, with the Indian Ocean forming its eastern boundary. Mogadishu serves as the capital city. According to World Health Organization (WHO) data [5], in 2023, the total resident population was approximately 18,358,615. The official languages are Somali and Arabic, while Italian and English are also used in some contexts.

In 2021, the life expectancy at birth was about 54 years: 56.3 years for females and 51.7 years for males. In 2024, the fertility rate was estimated at 5.12 children per woman, with a birth rate of 37.4 births per 1000 population [6]. The maternal mortality ratio in 2023 was estimated at approximately 562.6 deaths per 100,000 live births [5], and the crude death rate at 11.2 deaths per 1000 population in 2024. The health expenditure was estimated at 2.5% of the national budget [6]. As of the most recent estimates, the literacy rate among individuals aged 15–19 years is approximately 62%, indicating moderate progress in youth education [7].

15.2.2 Healthcare System

Civil war since 1991, lack of financing of healthcare infrastructure, flooding, droughts, the 2010–2012 famine, malnutrition, and infections such as malaria, cholera, and locust plagues have significantly contributed to the low life expectancy in Somalia. These factors have also impeded the developmental progress of the health system [8, 9].

Furthermore, citizens commonly turn to traditional healers and community health workers for their healthcare needs. Unfortunately, there is no unified health system governance. Healthcare is primarily provided by the private sector due to limited government financial support, resulting in less than 30% of Somalis having access to essential health services [8, 9]. This dominance of private providers is evident in facility distribution data, with a 2017 density of 0.93 private facilities and 0.76 public facilities per 10,000 population [7].

Moreover, assistance from donors and development initiatives like the "Damal Caafimaad Project," funded by the World Bank, provides substantial aid to the Somali population. The unequal distribution of the workforce is evident, with a disproportionate concentration in urban areas compared to rural regions [9].

The Federal Ministry of Health partnered with the WHO regional office to formulate a comprehensive five-year strategic health plan spanning from 2021 to 2025. This plan addresses various health priorities, including communicable and non-communicable diseases, as well as maternal and child health [10].

Between 2016 and 2023, Somalia made notable advancements in the establishment of an integrated disease surveillance and response system (IDSRS). The factors contributing to this progress were categorized into 6 key areas: recognizing challenges with the existing surveillance system; utilizing the experience provided by the COVID-19 pandemic; integrating IDSRS into strategic planning documents; establishing a monitoring mechanism; implementing key activities gradually over an appropriate timeframe; and maintaining flexibility regarding predetermined deadlines [11].

There are approximately 846 healthcare facilities, including 7 reference hospitals, 27 district hospitals, 248 maternity and child health clinics, and 544 health posts. The public healthcare system is structured across four tiers, encompassing primary health units in rural regions, health centers at the sub-district level, referral health centers in districts, and regional hospitals situated in the regional capitals [8].

15.2.3 Physician Workforce in Somalia

WHO data indicate that Somalia continues to have one of the lowest physician densities globally, with only 0.48 physicians per 10,000 population in 2022, showing minimal improvement over previous years [12].

15.2.4 Health Risk Factors Associated with Rheumatic Diseases in Somalia

As of 2016, the prevalence of obesity in adults is estimated at 8.3% [6]. There is an association between obesity and increased tissue and plasma cytokines, which are also increased in certain rheumatic diseases, such as tumor necrosis factor and interleukin 6 [13].

According to the 2023 WHO country profile for Somalia, no recent nationally representative adult survey data on tobacco use are available. However, a subnational survey conducted in Somaliland among adolescents aged 13–15 reported a current tobacco use prevalence of 15.6% (14.3% among boys and 11.6% among girls) [14]. Interestingly, a survey and focus group conducted among Somali residents in London revealed a high prevalence of smoking (30%), with the majority (71%) also consuming qat. This behavior was predominantly observed among males (83%) aged 30–39 years [15].

According to the 2017 WHO report, the estimated prevalence of hepatitis B surface antigen (HBsAg) positivity in Somalia was 1.6% (95% CI 1.2–2.1) [16]. However, more recent analyses indicate substantially higher levels of hepatitis B virus (HBV) infection. For instance, a 2024 cross-sectional study conducted in Mogadishu reported an overall HBV seroprevalence of 13.3% among pregnant women [17], while a meta-analysis estimated a pooled HBV prevalence of 18.9% in the general population [18].

The 2017 WHO report also estimated the incidence of hepatitis C virus (HCV) infection at 62.5 (55.6–65.2) per 100,000 population [16], with a national prevalence of approximately 0.9% (95% CI 0.3–1.9%) [19]. In addition, the prevalence of hepatitis B and C among hemodialysis patients in Somalia was reported as 7.3% and 3.2%, respectively [20].

15.2.5 Burden and Characteristics of Rheumatic Diseases in Somalia

The age-standardized prevalence of musculoskeletal disorders for male and female sexes combined in 2020 is estimated to be between 1700 and less than 3100 [21]. In 2013, the point prevalence of neck pain exceeded 55 cases per 1000 individuals in Somalia. Additionally, the prevalence of osteoarthritis surpassed 46 cases per 1000 individuals. The age-standardized disability-adjusted life-year rate of musculoskeletal disorders in both sexes was 1998 per 100,000. Furthermore, the point prevalence of RA was documented to be over 3 cases per 1000 individuals [22].

A retrospective study conducted from 2010 to 2014, involving 100 patients of Somali origin receiving care at the rheumatology clinic in Minneapolis, USA, found that one-third had inflammatory rheumatic diseases, another third had osteoarthritis or myofascial pain, while the remaining third did not have any rheumatic diseases.

The study also noted a high rate of missed appointments for follow-up visits, with 50% of patients failing to attend [23].

In 2018, a study conducted among Somali residents in Minnesota, USA, identified 40 patients diagnosed with RA, comprising 10% of the sample. Among these patients, 98% were female, with only one male patient identified. The mean age at diagnosis was 54.6 years. Interestingly, seropositive patients were, on average, 12 years younger than seronegative patients, and the majority of seropositive cases were diagnosed before the age of 50. In terms of treatment received, the majority of patients did not use non-steroidal anti-inflammatory drugs, while most received prednisone. None of the patients received biologics. Additionally, the study observed a high rate of vitamin D deficiency and a low rate of missed appointments for follow-up visits [24].

15.2.6 Pediatric Rheumatology Education and Capacity Building in Somalia

The Pediatric Society of the African League Against Rheumatism (PAFLAR) has recently developed a virtual educational program aimed at providing physicians with essential insights into pediatric rheumatic diseases and their treatments. The educational content utilized during these sessions was derived from the Pediatric Musculoskeletal Matters online resource. The sessions covered a wide array of topics, including the pediatric musculoskeletal examination tool known as pediatric Gait, Arms, Legs, and Spine (pGALS), and discussions on the differential diagnoses and treatment strategies for various pediatric rheumatic conditions [25].

15.2.7 Availability of Rheumatology Medications in Somalia

Conventional disease-modifying anti-rheumatic agents (DMARDs) are available; however, to the best of our knowledge, there is no access to biological therapies or Janus kinase (JAK) inhibitors.

15.2.8 Research in Somalia

Clinical research remains limited in Somalia. In an effort to address this challenge, Somali universities took a significant step in 2021 by establishing the Somali Health Action Journal, an open-access medical journal. The Somali-Swedish Researchers' Association (SSRA) will initially host the journal for a few years [26].

In 2022, Somalia hosted its first National Institute of Health (NIH) Health Research Conference. The event was organized by the Somali NIH and the Federal Ministry of Health in collaboration with various partners, including WHO, the

Public Health Agency of Sweden, the Somali-Swedish Research Cooperation Initiative, the Somali-Swedish Researchers' Association, the Alliance for Health Policy and Systems Research, Somali universities, and the African Field Epidemiology Network. The conference concluded with the issuance of recommendations aimed at improving research efforts in Somalia [27].

15.2.9 Summary

In conclusion, political and economic stability in Somalia, sustaining financial support to the healthcare system in order to establish a strong infrastructure, and establishing reliable disease registries with manpower will advance healthcare delivery to citizens. Enhanced collaboration and communication among various tiers of government and stakeholders, including non-governmental organizations, United Nations agencies, and private providers, hold promise for overcoming challenges in implementing health policies and programs. Lastly, promoting research initiatives and fostering partnerships with academic institutions can further drive innovation and improve healthcare outcomes in Somalia.

15.3 Djibouti

15.3.1 Country Demographics

The Republic of Djibouti, or simply Djibouti, is located in the Horn of Africa, sharing borders with the Gulf of Aden and the Red Sea, positioned between Eritrea and Somalia. The capital is the city of Djibouti.

In 2024, the population was 994,974. Arabic and French are the official languages, but Somali and Afar are other major spoken languages. The birth rate is 21.8 births per 1000 population, with a total fertility rate of 2.11 children born per woman. The average life expectancy at birth is 65.9 years, with a median age of 26.3 and a mortality rate of 7 per 1000 people [28]. In 2023, the maternal mortality ratio was estimated at 162 deaths per 100,000 live births [29]. The literacy rate for people aged 15 and over was reported at 52.8% [30]. Health expenditure accounted for 2% of the gross domestic product (GDP) in 2020 [29].

15.3.2 Physician Workforce in Djibouti

According to WHO data, the physician density in Djibouti remains very low, at 2.11 physicians per 10,000 population in 2022, compared with 1.3 in 1999, showing only minimal improvement over the past two decades [12].

15.3.3 Health Risk Factors Associated with Rheumatic Diseases in Djibouti

Several population-level health risk factors relevant to rheumatic diseases have been reported in Djibouti. The prevalence of obesity among adults in Djibouti is estimated at 13.5% [28].

Tobacco use also appears to be more common among men than women. According to the 2012 Pan Arab Project for Family Health (PAPFAM) survey, tobacco use among adults in Djibouti was 18.0% in men and 2.0% in women (WHO, 2023) [31].

Infectious risk factors may also be relevant. According to a 2017 WHO report, the estimated prevalence of HBsAg positivity and the estimated incidence of HCV in Djibouti were comparable to those reported for Somalia [16]. A more recent study, however, found a prevalence of HCV infection of 0.3% among blood donors [19].

15.3.4 Burden and Characteristics of Rheumatic Diseases in Djibouti

In 2020, the age-standardized prevalence of musculoskeletal disorders for both males and females was estimated to be between 3900 and less than 4400 per 100,000. Similarly, the age-standardized prevalence of total osteoarthritis for both males and females was estimated to be between 5100 and less than 5800 per 100,000 [21]. In 2013, Djibouti exhibited comparable statistics to Somalia regarding the prevalence of neck pain and RA. Additionally, the age-standardized disability-adjusted life-year rate of musculoskeletal disorders in Djibouti was 2020 per 100,000 population for both sexes [22].

15.3.5 Access to Rheumatology Medications and Research Activity in Djibouti

There is no publicly documented data on the national availability of rheumatology-specific medications in Djibouti (such as DMARDs or biologics). Regional analyses of African essential medicines lists indicate that many countries list very few rheumatology drugs [32, 33]. Similarly, despite the increasing burden of musculoskeletal disorders in the region, locally driven rheumatology research appears to be virtually nonexistent, with studies noting that resources and literature remain extremely limited [34].

15.4 The Union of the Comoros

15.4.1 Country Demographics

The Union of the Comoros, or simply Comoros, lies in Southern Africa, comprising a cluster of islands situated at the northern entrance of the Mozambique Channel, approximately two-thirds of the distance from northern Madagascar to northern Mozambique. The capital is Moroni. The official languages are Arabic, French, and Shikomori.

In 2024, the estimated total population was 900,141, comprising 48.4% males and 51.6% females. In 2022, health expenditure accounted for 6.3% of the GDP [35]. As of 2024, the birth rate was 21.6 births per 1000 population, with a total fertility rate of 2.61 children per woman. The average life expectancy was 67.8 years, and the median age was 22.7 years. In 2023, the maternal mortality rate was estimated at 179 deaths per 100,000 live births [35]. In 2024, the crude death rate was estimated at 6.4 deaths per 1000 population [36].

In 2021, the literacy rate was 62% among individuals aged 15 years and older, underscoring the importance of investing in education to empower communities and improve health outcomes [36].

15.4.2 Physician Workforce in Comoros

The density of physicians improved by 2.3 per 10,000 population, increasing from 2.0 in 2004 to 4.2 in 2022 [12].

15.4.3 Risk Factors and Rheumatic Diseases in Comoros

In 2016, the prevalence of obesity among adults in Comoros was 7.8% [35]. In 2015, the overall prevalence of current cigarette smoking in the Comoros was 14.3%, with 18.5% among males and 9.9% among females. The use of non-cigarette tobacco products was less common, reported at 5.8% overall, including 6.7% among men and 4.9% among women [37]. According to the Global Smoking Tobacco and Health Resources (GSTHR) profile, in 2022, the prevalence of current tobacco smoking among adults aged 15 years and older was 11.9%, with 21.7% among males and 2.0% among females [38].

Like Somalia and Djibouti, the estimated prevalence of positive hepatitis B surface antigen is 1.6% (1.2–2.1%), and the estimated incidence of hepatitis C is 62.5 (55.6–65.2) per 100,000 [16].

Usenbo et al. conducted a systematic review in 2014 looking at the prevalence of six types of arthritis in Africa, namely rheumatoid arthritis, osteoarthritis, juvenile arthritis, psoriatic arthritis, gout, and ankylosing spondylitis. Unfortunately, there were no reported studies in Somalia, Djibouti, and Comoros [39].

The available arthritis reports are historical to reflect current disease trends. Collaborative research is a strategy to improve the health system in these nations despite their limited resources and unstructured healthcare systems.

15.5 Conclusion

Epidemiological studies on rheumatic diseases in Somalia, Djibouti, and Comoros are scarce. As of October 2025, we could not find certified rheumatologists in Somalia, Djibouti, or Comoros. There is an urgent need to train pediatricians and internists in these countries to specialize in rheumatology (pediatric or adult). Efforts should at least be focused on educating interested general pediatricians and internists in the recognition and treatment of various rheumatic diseases. International rheumatology organizations such as the Arab League of Associations for Rheumatology (ArLAR), the African League Against Rheumatism (AFLAR), and PAFLAR can offer educational courses to physicians in these countries. Local or regional cost-effective recommendations on the management of various rheumatic diseases are needed, considering socio-economic factors.

Authors' Conflict of Interest Declaration The authors declare that they have no conflicts of interest.

References

1. Al Maini M, Adelowo F, Al Saleh J, Al Weshahi Y, Burmester GR, Cutolo M, et al. The global challenges and opportunities in the practice of rheumatology: white paper by the World Forum on Rheumatic and Musculoskeletal Diseases. Clin Rheumatol. 2015;34(5):819–29.
2. Dey D, Paruk F, Mody GM, Kalla AA, Adebajo A, Akpabio A, et al. Women in rheumatology in Africa. Lancet Rheumatol. 2022;4(10):e657–e60.
3. Migowa AN, Hadef D, Hamdi W, Mwizerwa O, Ngandeu M, Taha Y, et al. Pediatric rheumatology in Africa: thriving amidst challenges. Pediatr Rheumatol Online J. 2021;19(1):69.
4. Adelowo O, Mody GM, Tikly M, Oyoo O, Slimani S. Rheumatic diseases in Africa. Nat Rev Rheumatol. 2021;17(6):363–74.
5. World Health Organization. Somalia [Country overview] [Internet]. [cited 2026 Jun 15]. Available from: https://data.who.int/countries/706.
6. Central Intelligence Agency. Somalia—The World Factbook [Internet]. [Last updated 2025 Sep 17, cited 2025 Oct 29]. Available from: https://www.cia.gov/the-world-factbook/countries/somalia/.
7. World Health Organization. Understanding the private health sector in Somalia. Cairo: WHO Regional Office for the Eastern Mediterranean; 2024. [Internet]. [cited 2026 Jun 15]. Available from: https://applications.emro.who.int/docs/9789292742041-eng.pdf.
8. Said AS, Kicha DI. Implementing health system and the new federalism in Somalia: challenges and opportunities. Front Public Health. 2024;12:1205327.

9. Gele A. Challenges facing the health system in Somalia and implications for achieving the SDGs. Eur J Public Health. 2020;30(Suppl 5):ckaa165.1147.
10. Morrison J, Malik S. Population health trends and disease profile in Somalia 1990–2019, and projection to 2030: will the country achieve sustainable development goals 2 and 3? BMC Public Health. 2023;23(1):66.
11. Ssendagire S, Karanja MJ, Abdi A, Lubogo M, Azad Al A, Mzava K, et al. Progress and experiences of implementing an integrated disease surveillance and response system in Somalia; 2016–2023. Front Public Health. 2023;11:1204165.
12. World Health Organization. Density of physicians (per 10 000 population) [Internet]. 2024 [updated 2025 Apr 30; cited 2026 Jun 15]. Available from: https://data.who.int/indicators/i/217795A.
13. Gremese E, Tolusso B, Gigante MR, Ferraccioli G. Obesity as a risk and severity factor in rheumatic diseases (autoimmune chronic inflammatory diseases). Front Immunol. 2014;5:576.
14. World Health Organization. Somalia: WHO report on the global tobacco epidemic, 2023—country profile [Internet]. Geneva: World Health Organization; 2023 [cited 2026 Jun 15]. Available from: https://cdn.who.int/media/docs/default-source/country-profiles/tobacco/gtcr-2023/tobacco-2023-som.pdf.
15. Straus L, McEwen A, Croker H. Smoking attitudes and prevalence of a Somali population in London. J Smoking Cessation. 2007;2(2):68–72. https://doi.org/10.1375/jsc.2.2.68.
16. World Health Organization. Global Hepatitis Report 2017. Geneva: World Health Organization; 2017. [cited 2026 Jun 15]. Available from: https://iris.who.int/bitstream/handle/10665/255016/9789241565455-eng.pdf?sequence=1.
17. Mohamud OM, Abdi AM, Osman WA, Ahmed AH, Osman NH, Tahlil AA. Sero-prevalence of hepatitis B virus and associated risk factors among pregnant women attending Demartino hospital, Mogadishu, Somalia. BMC Infect Dis. 2025;25(1):748.
18. Hassan-Kadle MA, Osman MS, Ogurtsov PP. Epidemiology of viral hepatitis in Somalia: systematic review and meta-analysis study. World J Gastroenterol. 2018;24(34):3927–57.
19. Chaabna K, Kouyoumjian SP, Abu-Raddad LJ. Hepatitis C virus epidemiology in Djibouti, Somalia, Sudan, and Yemen: systematic review and meta-analysis. PLoS One. 2016;11(2):e0149966.
20. Jeele MOO, Addow ROB, Adan FN, Jimale LH. Prevalence and risk factors associated with hepatitis B and hepatitis C infections among patients undergoing hemodialysis: a single-centre study in Somalia. Int J Nephrol. 2021;2021:1555775.
21. Collaborators GBDO. Global, regional, and national burden of osteoarthritis, 1990–2020 and projections to 2050: a systematic analysis for the Global Burden of Disease Study 2021. Lancet Rheumatol. 2023;5(9):e508–e22.
22. Moradi-Lakeh M, Forouzanfar MH, Vollset SE, El Bcheraoui C, Daoud F, Afshin A, et al. Burden of musculoskeletal disorders in the Eastern Mediterranean Region, 1990–2013: findings from the Global Burden of Disease Study 2013. Ann Rheum Dis. 2017;76(8):1365–73.
23. Miller E, Gertner E, Quirk R, McCarty M. Rheumatologic diagnoses, characteristics and needs of Somali patients referred to a rheumatology clinic serving the Somali population [abstract]. Arthritis Rheumatol [Internet]. 2015;67(suppl 10). [cited 2026 Jun 15]. Available from: https://acrabstracts.org/abstract/rheumatologic-diagnoses-characteristics-and-needs-of-somali-patients-referred-to-a-rheumatology-clinic-serving-the-somali-population/.
24. Waytz P, Forsberg A, Mahamed A. Is the care of rheumatoid arthritis in Somali patients associated with implicit bias? Minn Med. 2018;101:41–8.
25. Mahfud M, Jones M, Fader T, Hause E. A virtual pediatric rheumatology teaching initiative for physicians in Somaliland. Pediatr Rheumatol Online J. 2023;21(1):1.
26. Somali Health Action Journal (SHAJ). [Internet]. [cited 2026 Jun 15]. Available from: https://journals.ub.umu.se/index.php/shaj.
27. Bile K, Warsame M, Ahmed AD. Fragile states need essential national health research: the case of Somalia. Lancet Glob Health. 2022;10(5):e617–e8.
28. Central Intelligence Agency. Djibouti—The World Factbook [Internet]. [Last updated 2025 Oct 1, cited 2025 Oct 29]. Available from: https://www.cia.gov/the-world-factbook/countries/djibouti/.

29. Central Intelligence Agency. Djibouti—The World Factbook [Internet]. [Last updated 2023 Dec 6, cited 2025 Oct 30]. Available from: https://www.cia.gov/the-world-factbook/about/archives/2023/countries/djibouti/.
30. United Nations, Department of Economic and Social Affairs. Least developed country category: Djibouti Profile [Internet]. New York: United Nations; 2024 [cited 2026 Jun 15]. Available from: https://policy.desa.un.org/themes/least-developed-countries-category/least-developed-country-category-djibouti-profile.
31. World Health Organization. Djibouti: WHO report on the global tobacco epidemic, 2023—country profile [Internet]. Geneva: World Health Organization; 2023 [cited 2026 Jun 15]. Available from: https://cdn.who.int/media/docs/default-source/country-profiles/tobacco/gtcr-2023/tobacco-2023-dji.pdf.
32. Slamang W, Scott C, Foster HE. A quantitative comparison between the essential medicines for rheumatic diseases in children and young people in Africa and the WHO model list. Pediatr Rheumatol Online J. 2024;22(1):63.
33. Mody GM. Rheumatology in Africa-challenges and opportunities. Arthritis Res Ther. 2017;19(1):49.
34. Bayoumy K, MacDonald R, Dargham SR, Arayssi T. Bibliometric analysis of rheumatology research in the Arab countries. BMC Res Notes. 2016;9:393.
35. Central Intelligence Agency. Comoros—The World Factbook [Internet]. [Last updated 2025 Sept 17, cited 2025 Oct 30]. Available from: https://www.cia.gov/the-world-factbook/countries/comoros/.
36. Central Intelligence Agency. Comoros—The World Factbook [Internet]. [Last updated 2023 Dec 6, cited 2025 Oct 30]. Available from: https://www.cia.gov/the-world-factbook/about/archives/2023/countries/comoros/.
37. James PB, Kassim SA, Kabba JA, Kitchen C. Tobacco use among school-going adolescents in comoros: a secondary analysis of the 2015 comoros global youth tobacco survey. Biomed Res Int. 2022;2022:7134340.
38. Knowledge Action Change. Smoking, vaping, HTP, NRT and snus in Comoros [Internet]. Global Smoking Tobacco & Health Resources; 2025 [cited 2026 Jun 15]. Available from: https://gsthr.org/countries/profile/com/.
39. Usenbo A, Kramer V, Young T, Musekiwa A. Prevalence of Arthritis in Africa: a systematic review and meta-analysis. PLoS One. 2015;10(8):e0133858.

Chapter 16
Rheumatic Diseases in Sudan

Ziryab Imad Taha Mahmoud, Elnour Mohamed Elageb, and Wafaa Hassan Ahmed Albashir

Abstract Sudan is the third-largest African country and is characterized by rich multicultural and ecological diversity. The burden of rheumatic diseases in Sudan is substantial, although the exact number of cases remains undocumented due to the lack of a comprehensive database. However, the prevalence of these diseases is evident through the significant number of patients seeking admission to hospitals and receiving follow-up care in outpatient clinics.

In response to the growing need for specialized rheumatology care, the Rheumatology Fellowship Program was launched in 2018 after approval by the Sudanese Medical Specialization Board. Prior to this program, physicians had to travel abroad for additional training in rheumatology. As of January 2026, three batches have successfully completed the rheumatology fellowship training program, while a fourth batch comprising five trainees is currently undergoing training.

In recent years, Sudan's health system and infrastructure have been significantly challenged by prolonged sociopolitical instability. The civil war, known to be one of the longest in modern history, started in 1983 and remains prevalent in certain regions. Furthermore, the recent revolution against the military government in 2019 has had a substantial impact on the overall health sector, specifically affecting patients with rheumatic conditions due to the country's deteriorating economy. Unfortunately, access to healthcare is limited, with only about nine central public hospitals providing services, most of which are concentrated in the capital city of

Z. I. T. Mahmoud (✉)
Department of Internal Medicine, University of Bahri, Khartoum, Sudan

Merowe Medical City, Merowe, Sudan
e-mail: Ziryab2008@yahoo.com

E. M. Elageb
Military Teaching Hospital, Omdurman, Sudan
e-mail: Elagib62@hotmail.com

W. H. A. Albashir
Friendship Teaching Hospital, Omdurman and Aliaa Specialist Hospital, Omdurman, Sudan
e-mail: wafaa223@gmail.com

K. A. Alnaqbi, G. Aldabie (eds.), *Rheumatic Diseases in the Arab World*,
https://doi.org/10.1007/978-981-92-0967-5_16

Khartoum. Additionally, the cost structure of private hospitals may be perceived as high, potentially limiting affordability for a significant portion of the population.

Health insurance coverage is currently available to a restricted segment of the population. Unfortunately, there are certain medications and investigations that are not covered by existing insurance plans. The availability of advanced therapies remains constrained, with logistical and supply challenges affecting certain pharmaceutical companies and healthcare institutions.

The most prevalent rheumatic diseases in Sudan are rheumatoid arthritis, systemic lupus erythematosus, and gouty arthritis. Despite ongoing challenges, multiple initiatives are underway to strengthen rheumatology services, including the expansion of training opportunities and increased emphasis on research capacity building. Efforts to improve disease awareness and to enhance the collection of local epidemiological data remain key priorities for advancing rheumatologic care in Sudan.

Keywords Sudan · Health System · Rheumatic Diseases · Rheumatology Services · Rheumatology Workforce · Pediatric Rheumatology · Rheumatology Training · Health Services Accessibility · Armed Conflict

16.1 Introduction

Rheumatic and musculoskeletal diseases (RMDs) are a major cause of chronic morbidity and disability worldwide. In Sudan, their impact is compounded by limited healthcare resources, delayed diagnosis, and restricted access to specialist care.

Sudan is a geographically large and culturally diverse country with a young population and a healthcare system shaped by prolonged political instability, economic constraints, and workforce migration. These factors have important implications for the diagnosis and management of chronic conditions such as RMDs.

This chapter provides an overview of RMDs in Sudan, focusing on the healthcare system structure, availability of rheumatology services, disease patterns, risk factors, diagnostic and therapeutic challenges, and ongoing education and research initiatives. It aims to highlight current gaps in care and identify opportunities for strengthening rheumatology services in the country.

16.2 Country Demographics

Sudan (the land of the Blacks) has a long coastline along the Red Sea and shares boundaries with many countries. It is bordered by Egypt to the north, the Red Sea, Eritrea, and Ethiopia to the east, South Sudan to the south, the Central African

Republic and Chad to the west, and Libya to the northwest [1]. Following the secession of South Sudan in 2011, Sudan became the third largest country in Africa by land area [2].

Sudan is a crucial region of interaction between the cultural traditions of Africa and those of the Mediterranean world. Noticeably, Islam and Arabic are more prominent in the north, whereas indigenous African languages and cultural traditions are more prominent in the south [1].

Sudan comprises 18 states, each with its own council of ministers. Each state is further subdivided into localities (mudiriyat), which are in turn divided into villages (tazkiyat). Khartoum, the capital of Sudan, is situated roughly in the centre of the country, at the junction of the Blue Nile and White Nile rivers. It is part of the largest urban area in Sudan and is a center of commerce and government [3].

As of January 2026, Sudan's total population is approximately 48.9 million. Approximately 36.3% of the population resides in urban areas, with an estimated urbanization rate of 3.43% per year during the period 2020–2025 [3].

Sudan's population shows a near-equal distribution between males and females. The sex ratio at birth is estimated at 1.05 males per female. The population is young, with a median age of 19.5 years as of 2025. The median age is slightly lower among males (19.0 years) than among females (19.6 years). This is reflected in the age structure, with 40.1% of the population aged 0–14 years, 56.7% aged 15–64 years, and 3.2% aged 65 years or older (2024 estimate). The country also has a high birth rate of 32.95 births per 1000 population and a relatively low death rate of 6 deaths per 1000 population, based on 2025 estimates [3].

School life expectancy in Sudan was estimated at 7 years in 2015, indicating that children are expected, on average, to complete 7 years of formal education across primary to tertiary levels [3].

Sudan faces multiple development challenges, including high birth and mortality rates, relatively low life expectancy, limited educational attainment, and constrained healthcare resources. Health expenditure in Sudan remains limited, accounting for 2.8% of gross domestic product (GDP) in 2021 [3].

16.3 Health Sectors in Sudan

From a governance and administrative perspective, healthcare services in Sudan are managed across three levels: federal, state, and local. There is one main Federal Ministry of Health (FMOH) and 18 individual state ministries of health. The FMOH is responsible for developing national health policies, strategic planning, monitoring and coordination, training, and external relations. State ministries of health adapt these policies into state-level plans and oversee funding and implementation. At the local health levels, health authorities are primarily responsible for delivering healthcare services, in accordance with established plans and guidelines [4].

From a service delivery perspective, healthcare in Sudan is provided at three clinical levels: primary, secondary, and tertiary care. Primary health care (PHC) facilities consist of primary healthcare units, health centers, dressing stations, dispensaries, and rural hospitals [4]. At this level, care focuses on basic and preventive services, while secondary care provides specialist and referral services, and tertiary care delivers highly specialized treatment.

Within this health system context, providing high-quality healthcare is essential for disease prevention and for improving overall quality of life. As a lower-middle-income country, Sudan faces multiple public health challenges, including recurrent outbreaks of communicable diseases such as cholera, dengue fever, and Rift Valley fever [5]. Limited access to safe drinking water and sanitation continues to threaten public health in Sudan, with millions lacking basic water services and at risk of waterborne illnesses [6]. In parallel, the prevalence of non-communicable diseases, including obesity, type 2 diabetes, renal disease, and cancer, is increasing, resulting in a growing burden of multimorbidity [7]. Addressing these intersecting challenges and strengthening the healthcare system are essential to improving population health and quality of life.

Like many African countries, the healthcare sector in Sudan faces challenges related to insufficient funding and inadequate staffing, resulting in limited access to healthcare services [7]. Access to healthcare remains uneven in Sudan. In 2015, approximately 93% of the population had access to the basic PHC package, while only 60% had access to the full PHC package [8]. These gaps in comprehensive coverage are likely related, in part, to shortages of qualified healthcare professionals.

This workforce shortage is further illustrated by World Health Organization (WHO) data, which show that Sudan has a low physician density, with approximately 2.5 medical doctors per 10,000 population, corresponding to about 10,683 physicians nationwide based on the most recent available estimates from 2017 [9].

In addition to workforce constraints, the absence of a well-defined framework for implementing, monitoring, and evaluating healthcare policies and plans further adds to the difficulties faced by the health system. Moreover, the unequal distribution of healthcare facilities across regions continues to limit access to healthcare services, particularly in rural and underserved areas [8]. Addressing these issues is essential to improving the healthcare system and enhancing access to healthcare for all Sudanese citizens.

In response to these challenges, the Sudanese government is working in collaboration with the WHO to develop plans, policies, and strategies aimed at addressing deficiencies in the health sector. As part of these efforts, a novel interactive system is being developed to facilitate communication between different policy-making levels, thereby supporting decision-making, strategy implementation, and coordinated health sector processes.

Within this constrained health system environment, patients with RMDs face particular challenges in accessing adequate care. Due to Sudan's fragile health system and services, patients with RMDs are not adequately managed. Public hospitals do not provide full coverage for these patients, and most receive care in private hospitals. Likewise, health insurance companies offer only partial support. Unfortunately, coverage for expensive anti-rheumatic medications is limited, and the overall supply of these treatments remains insufficient to meet demand. National Medical Supplies attempts to subsidize some costs, but this remains inadequate, similar to other African countries [8, 10].

16.4 Rheumatology Services in Sudan

In Sudan, the development of rheumatology services has been comparatively slower than in many other African countries and globally. This can be attributed to a limited national budget and constrained resources across multiple sectors, including health, transport, water and sanitation, agriculture, housing, and education. Healthcare funding faces competing priorities, with greater emphasis placed on communicable diseases and the rising burden of non-communicable diseases [7, 11]. As a result, patients with RMDs often experience prolonged delays before receiving a timely diagnosis, which may lead to the development of complications and comorbidities.

The growing burden of RMDs in Sudan is partly driven by delayed diagnosis, influenced by limited access to education, sociocultural beliefs, and poverty. These challenges also reflect the maldistribution of limited national resources, with prolonged conflicts historically prioritized over investment in healthcare.

16.4.1 Referral Pathways

The absence of a well-defined and strictly implemented referral system between primary, secondary, and tertiary levels of healthcare services often leads to delays in diagnosing RMDs and initiating timely treatment, especially in rural areas. Similar challenges are observed within the public healthcare sector [12].

In the past, patients with RMDs in Sudan were predominantly assessed by orthopedic surgeons, largely due to limited disease awareness, a shortage of rheumatologists, and the small number of dedicated rheumatology outpatient clinics. In recent years, progress has been made with the establishment of rheumatology clinics in several hospitals, although some limitations remain, as these clinics are often integrated within general medicine departments. Examples include Academy Charity Teaching Hospital, Omdurman Teaching Hospital, and Ribat University Hospital. As awareness of RMDs increases, referrals to these centers have risen. However, these facilities receive patients from across Sudan, placing additional strain on their already limited resources.

To help meet the growing demand for rheumatology services, a more comprehensive rheumatology department was established at the Military Hospital in Khartoum. This department has been able to accommodate a larger number of patients.

16.4.2 Adult Rheumatology Clinics

The number of rheumatology outpatient clinics has increased over the past decade; however, services remain largely centralized in Khartoum. Rheumatology clinics are available at several tertiary hospitals, including Military Hospital, Khartoum Teaching Hospital, Omdurman Teaching Hospital, Friendship Teaching Hospital, Ribat University Hospital, Haj Elsafi Teaching Hospital, and Ibrahim Malik Teaching Hospital. Additional services are provided in Wad Madani (Gezira State) and El-Obayed (North Kordofan State), including a dedicated rheumatology center in Wad Madani and rheumatology services at El-Obayed International Hospital. These clinics receive referrals from all states in Sudan, from both public and private healthcare facilities, typically through direct referral letters.

While the private sector plays a significant role in providing rheumatology services in Sudan, its coverage is largely concentrated in urban areas. Consequently, the current centralization of rheumatology services may limit efforts to effectively reduce the burden of RMDs across the country. Following the recent war in Sudan, this already fragile system was severely disrupted, and patients experienced substantial difficulties in accessing care.

16.4.3 Pediatric Rheumatology Services

Before the onset of the armed conflict in 2023, pediatric rheumatology care in Sudan was primarily provided through a single dedicated department at Ahmed Gasim Teaching Hospital. At that time, the service operated with limited resources and staffing, comprising two pediatric rheumatologists, one immunologist, and three general pediatricians with a special interest in rheumatology. The service functioned with limited resources and relied on general pediatricians with an interest in rheumatology, supported intermittently by visiting specialists and collaborative efforts.

The average number of patients seen in each outpatient clinic was approximately 35. The majority of cases were related to juvenile idiopathic arthritis (JIA), juvenile systemic lupus erythematosus, juvenile dermatomyositis, juvenile systemic sclerosis, and autoinflammatory diseases, with a smaller proportion of patients diagnosed with chronic recurrent multifocal osteomyelitis and other less common conditions.

Clinical data from this center indicate that the majority of patients managed were female, and approximately half were referred from rural areas. This referral pattern was highlighted in a study of children with juvenile idiopathic arthritis

(JIA) attending the Ahmed Gasim clinic, underscoring the center's national referral role and the geographic disparities in access to pediatric rheumatology care in Sudan [13].

At present, there is no practicing pediatric rheumatologist in Sudan, and pediatric rheumatology services have been largely suspended since 2023 due to the armed conflict, staff displacement, and infrastructure damage.

16.4.4 Rheumatology Nurses/Nurse Practitioner

Sudan does not currently have dedicated rheumatology nurses or nurse practitioners. Currently, at Ahmed Gasim Teaching Hospital, the pediatric department lacks trained rheumatology nurses. As a result, medication administration and procedural support, including intra-articular injections and biologic infusions, are provided by trained nurses from other hospital units, such as intensive care or procedure rooms, due to the absence of specialized rheumatology nursing staff.

16.5 Electronic Medical Records (EMR)

Although comprehensive EMR systems are not yet widely implemented in Sudanese hospitals, digital health initiatives have gained increasing attention in recent years.

Sudan's national eHealth strategy outlines plans for the gradual development of centralized digital health records, aiming to improve data collection, continuity of care, and health system governance [14, 15]. Pilot EMR frameworks have been introduced in selected hospitals and health facilities, primarily supported by international organizations and humanitarian partners. In addition, recent initiatives to deploy digital health solutions across several hundred healthcare facilities reflect ongoing efforts to modernize patient data management, despite persistent challenges related to infrastructure limitations, electricity supply, internet connectivity, and healthcare workers' readiness for eHealth implementation [14, 15].

At present, most rheumatology services continue to rely on paper-based records, limiting longitudinal data tracking and research capacity.

16.6 Availability of Diagnostic Tests for Rheumatic Disease in Sudan

16.6.1 Laboratory Tests

Early diagnosis of RMDs is essential to achieve optimal clinical outcomes. Immunological laboratory tests are required to establish the diagnosis of many RMDs; however, these tests are largely unavailable outside the private sector and a limited number of governmental hospitals. In addition, access to genetic testing, such as HLA-B27 and HLA-B51, is highly restricted and currently limited to two private laboratories and two kidney transplant centers in Khartoum.

16.6.2 Imaging Tests

Advanced imaging facilities and modalities, including computed tomography (CT), CT angiography, magnetic resonance imaging (MRI) of the spine and sacroiliac joints, and MR angiography, are available in Sudan.

According to the latest available WHO data from 2013, Sudan has a CT scanner density of approximately 1.13 per million population and an MRI density of about 0.32 scanners per million population. Positron emission tomography (PET) scanning is not currently available [16], and patients who need it must seek services outside the country.

16.6.3 Availability of Musculoskeletal Radiologists

Due to the ongoing emigration of healthcare professionals, there is a severe shortage of musculoskeletal radiologists. To our knowledge, Sudan currently has only one musculoskeletal radiologist. In addition, the availability and quality of musculoskeletal ultrasonography remain limited, reducing its effectiveness in diagnosing and monitoring RMDs, despite its recognized importance and inclusion in the rheumatology fellowship training program.

16.7 Availability of Diagnostic Tests for Rheumatic Disease in Sudan

In Sudan, therapeutic regimens for RMDs are available in multiple centers; however, their availability is often limited by financial constraints and suboptimal distribution of medications by medical suppliers regulated by the National Medicines and Poisons Board.

In addition, some biologic therapies may be obtained through international medical supply channels. Surgical interventions are also available when clinically indicated.

Currently available biologic therapies in Sudan include golimumab, rituximab, and secukinumab. Other biologic agents, such as tocilizumab and anakinra, are in various stages of registration or accessed through limited international medical supply channels. Biosimilar medications are not yet widely available in Sudan, and their use remains limited due to regulatory delays, supply chain constraints, and cost considerations.

Multidisciplinary care involving rehabilitation services, physiotherapy, occupational therapy, and orthopedic departments is accessible in Sudan. However, stronger collaboration and the establishment of clear referral pathways are needed to optimize patient outcomes.

16.8 Accredited Rheumatology Centers in Sudan

Despite the presence of rheumatology services in several hospitals, there are currently no formally accredited rheumatology centers in Sudan.

16.9 Patient Support Groups

Formal patient support groups for RMDs are not yet established in Sudan.

16.10 Rheumatology Association in Sudan

The Sudanese Association of Rheumatology (SAR) is the leading professional body for rheumatology in Sudan. It aims to improve the care of patients with RMDs and to support the development of rheumatology subspecialties [17].

The association was established in 2011 under the umbrella of the Sudan Association of Physicians, at a time when only a small number of rheumatologists were actively involved. Over the following years, SAR became more active and increasingly engaged with the scientific and wider community, a development largely driven by the involvement of a new generation of rheumatologists. The association is now registered under the Sudan Doctors Union as an independent professional body, providing a platform for both adult and pediatric rheumatologists to collaborate and contribute to meaningful improvements in patient care.

As of January 2026, SAR has 49 members, including adult rheumatologists and physicians enrolled in the rheumatology fellowship. More than half of the members are female, reflecting the growing role of women in the specialty. The association is governed by a 10-member board, comprising six executive members and four advisory committee members.

16.11 Overview of Rheumatic Diseases in Sudan

16.11.1 Incidence and Prevalence of Rheumatic Diseases

Globally, RMDs are considered the second leading cause of disability [18]. However, data on the prevalence and incidence of RMDs in Sudan remain limited.

A study conducted at Omdurman Teaching Hospital (one of the rheumatology outpatient clinics in Khartoum State) revealed that the most common RMDs were rheumatoid arthritis (RA, 60.5%), followed by systemic lupus erythematosus (SLE, 12.9%), and gouty arthritis (8.9%). The study also showed rheumatoid arthritis (RA) was most prevalent in females, 76.6% versus 23.4% in males, while in SLE, 87.5% were females versus 12.5% in males. Gouty arthritis was more prevalent in males by 81.8% compared to 18.2% of females [19].

16.11.2 Clinical Characteristics and Disease Patterns

RA in Sudan tends to present at a younger age and with higher disease activity compared with high-income settings. A comparative study of Sudanese and Swedish patients demonstrated that individuals in Sudan developed RA at a younger age (43 vs. 56 years) and had a shorter disease duration at presentation (48 vs. 107 months), yet showed higher inflammatory markers and more active disease [20].

Female predominance was more marked in the Sudanese cohort, and a considerable proportion of patients were seronegative for rheumatoid factor. Access to advanced therapies differed substantially between the two settings, with Sudanese patients relying largely on conventional disease-modifying antirheumatic drugs and corticosteroids and no reported use of biologic agents, reflecting economic and healthcare system limitations. More recent data from Sudan further emphasize persistent challenges in RA management, including delayed diagnosis, limited access to specialist care, and restricted availability of biologic therapies, all of which contribute to ongoing disease burden and suboptimal outcomes [21].

Similar population-based differences have also been observed in SLE. Comparative analyses of Sudanese and Swedish SLE cohorts revealed distinct autoantibody profiles, with anti-histone and anti–double-stranded DNA antibodies more frequently detected in Swedish patients, while anti-Sm antibodies were significantly more common among Sudanese patients [22]. These findings underscore ethnic and population-related differences in disease expression.

Other connective tissue diseases have also been reported in Sudanese cohorts. A hospital-based study from Omdurman Military Hospital showed that mixed connective tissue disease (MCTD), although uncommon, predominantly affects women and often presents with non-specific musculoskeletal manifestations such as arthralgia, arthritis, and myositis [23]. Notably, only a minority of patients met diagnostic criteria at initial presentation, with many evolving from other rheumatic diagnoses, including RA and SLE, over time. This highlights the diagnostic complexity of connective tissue diseases in Sudan and the challenges of early recognition in resource-limited healthcare settings.

16.11.3 Risk Factors of Rheumatic Diseases in Sudan

RA, SLE, and gouty arthritis are the most common rheumatological diseases in Sudan [19]. However, there is limited data addressing the risk factors associated with the development of these diseases in Sudan.

Risk factors for RMDs can broadly be categorized into non-modifiable and modifiable factors, which may interact with one another. Non-modifiable risk factors include genetic background, sex, and race. Modifiable risk factors include diet, obesity, environmental exposures (such as infections), and lifestyle habits (such as smoking).

The development of RA is associated with genetic risk factors, such as HLA-DRB [11]. Consistent with the international studies, RA, SLE, and Sjogren disease are more frequently observed in females compared to males in Sudan [21]. Beyond RA, similar genetic susceptibility has been reported in other RMDs, particularly SLE. Genetic susceptibility to SLE involves multiple loci within the human leukocyte antigen (HLA) region, with HLA-DRB1 and HLA-DQB1 alleles consistently associated with increased disease risk across different populations, including Sudanese cohorts. Notably, the first genome-wide association study (GWAS) conducted in the Sudanese population confirmed the association of HLA-DRB1*03 with SLE and identified a novel suggestive signal within the ZNF236-DT gene, suggesting an additional genetic contributor to SLE susceptibility in this population [24].

A systematic review of tobacco use in Sudan examined published studies spanning more than a century and highlighted tobacco use as a persistent and significant public health concern [25]. The review showed wide variation in tobacco prevalence across different population groups, with higher rates consistently observed among males. Reported prevalence ranged from 1% to 25% among adolescents and from 10% to 47.5% among adults. Multiple forms of tobacco use were reported, including cigarette smoking, shisha, and the locally used smokeless tobacco "Toombak," often in combination. Tobacco use was common among adolescents, university students, and adults, with initiation frequently occurring at a young age. The authors emphasized the need for stronger prevention strategies, improved enforcement of tobacco control policies, and targeted public health interventions to reduce tobacco use in Sudan.

Furthermore, smoking has been identified as a significant risk factor for the development of many RMDs, such as RA, SLE, and Sjogren disease [26–28]. Despite that, Sudanese women do not often smoke. Therefore, it is hypothesized that the use of Dukhan, a traditional Sudanese adornment tool involving burning acacia wood, may serve as another environmental risk factor for RA, similar to cigarette smoking. It is noteworthy that Dukhan use is common among married Sudanese women [20]. Further research is necessary to examine the potential correlation between Dukhan use and the occurrence of RA in this population. These findings highlight tobacco exposure, including culturally specific practices, as a key modifiable environmental risk factor for RMDs in the Sudanese context.

In addition to environmental exposures, metabolic and inflammatory risk factors are increasingly relevant. Overall, obesity prevalence in Sudan is estimated at 21.2%, with women showing substantially higher rates than men (26.3% compared with 13.8%) [29]. In parallel, chronic inflammatory conditions such as periodontal disease have also been linked to RA in Sudan, further highlighting the role of systemic inflammation as a modifiable risk factor [30].

Chronic infections represent another important modifiable risk factor for RMDs, particularly in regions with high endemicity. Chronic viral infections such as hepatitis B virus (HBV) and hepatitis C virus (HCV) are known to be associated with inflammatory arthritis, mixed cryoglobulinemia, and other rheumatic manifestations [31, 32]. Studies conducted in high-risk groups have consistently shown elevated rates of HCV infection, with prevalence estimates ranging from 4.5% to 34.9%. Particularly high rates have been documented among patients undergoing hemodialysis, in whom prevalence varied between 8.5% and 34.9%, as well as among individuals with hemophilia, where rates of about 13% were reported. In contrast, most studies involving the general population have demonstrated much lower HCV prevalence, typically between 0% and 4%. The lowest reported rates were observed among blood donors, in whom no cases were detected, and among pregnant women, with a prevalence of approximately 0.6% [33].

Sudan is classified as a high-endemicity country for HBV infection, with hepatitis B surface antigen (HBsAg) prevalence reported in community and hospital populations ranging from approximately 6.8% to 26% across different regions [34–36]. General population estimates suggest an overall chronic HBV prevalence of around 9%, with higher rates documented in certain localities. These findings indicate substantial ongoing transmission and public health burden, underscoring the need for strengthened vaccination, screening, and prevention strategies.

Given that latent tuberculosis (TB) may pose a significant challenge during treatment with immunosuppressive medications commonly used in RMDs, understanding the burden of TB in Sudan is particularly important. TB remains a major communicable disease in the country, contributing substantially to morbidity and mortality. A systematic review estimated that TB prevalence across various clinical and community populations in Sudan is around 30.7%, with extrapulmonary TB also observed [37]. Regional data from River Nile State and Eastern Sudan confirm that pulmonary TB predominates, and male sex and lower educational status are associated with infection [38]. Recent evidence indicates that TB incidence increased during periods of armed conflict, and drug resistance among TB cases is a growing concern [39]. National health data suggest an incidence of approximately 50 cases per 100,000 population, underscoring the ongoing public health burden [40].

Gouty arthritis development is influenced by various risk factors, including urbanization, the adoption of a Western lifestyle, increased alcohol consumption, and the rising incidence of obesity, hypertension, diabetes, and renal disease [11].

Together, genetic susceptibility, environmental exposures, metabolic factors, chronic infections, and lifestyle changes interact within a resource-limited healthcare context to shape the risk and presentation of RMDs in Sudan.

16.12 Screening Programs for Rheumatic Diseases

There are no screening programs for RMDs in Sudan; if there are any, they are due to individual efforts and are usually inappropriately documented.

16.13 Research and Education

16.13.1 Education

The Rheumatology Fellowship Program in Sudan was established in 2018. As of January 2026, three batches have completed training, and a fourth batch consisting of five fellows is currently in training. The program has contributed significantly to expanding the national rheumatology workforce. Applicants are required to complete 4 years of training in general internal medicine before sitting for the mandatory rheumatology selection examination. The program consists of 2 years of structured training and concludes with the completion of a mandatory research publication.

At present, there is no dedicated rheumatology nursing training program in Sudan.

16.13.2 Research

Rheumatology Fellowship trainees are required to publish at least one research paper to complete their training program. This requirement encourages trainees to engage in research activities and contributes to improving the quality of publications and locally generated data within the rheumatology specialty.

The research office of the SAR is expanding and offers courses and training sessions aimed at enhancing research skills and understanding among its members. In addition, it supports young researchers by addressing common challenges encountered during research conduct and publication.

The Ziryab Research Group is one of the voluntary national research groups established in Sudan in May 2021 at Haj Elsafi Teaching Hospital in Khartoum. The group aims to promote physician engagement in research, facilitate documentation of rare cases, and support high-quality studies on the incidence and prevalence of RMDs in Sudan. It includes consultants and medical doctors from various regions of Sudan, as well as international collaborators from countries such as Ireland and the United Arab Emirates. The group has contributed to several peer-reviewed publications, such as SLE-related issues [41, 42] and connective tissue diseases in Sudanese populations, thereby strengthening locally generated evidence and international research collaboration.

16.14 Opportunities and Specific Challenges in Sudan

Rheumatology care in Sudan is delivered within a context of prolonged political instability, economic hardship, and healthcare workforce migration, all of which place sustained pressure on service delivery. The emigration of healthcare professionals has significantly reduced specialist capacity, particularly affecting patients with RMDs who require long-term, specialized care.

Within rheumatology, the limited number of specialists in Sudan, combined with the absence of subspecialization in complex diseases such as SLE and RA, poses a significant challenge to care delivery. Additionally, the lack of clinical nurse specialists further compromises long-term patient follow-up, placing additional strain on the already limited specialist workforce [18]. Key challenges and opportunities are summarized in Table 16.1.

In Sudan, many patients with RMDs manage much of their care on their own. Although the government provides some support through health insurance and medical supplies, this support is often limited. There is a clear need for stronger policies and better implementation to meet the growing demand for care and to support multidisciplinary management, which is important for these patients. At present, only patients who can afford to travel to neighboring countries are able to access more advanced care, particularly when specialized services or expensive treatments are required.

Table 16.1 Challenges and opportunities of rheumatology care in Sudan

Domain	Key challenges	Opportunities and future directions
Health system and governance	Political instability, armed conflict, weak infrastructure, and limited health expenditure	National health reform efforts; collaboration with the WHO and international partners
Policy and financing	Inadequate insurance coverage	Policy reform and cost-containment strategies
Workforce	Shortage of rheumatologists; emigration; no pediatric rheumatologists; no rheumatology nurses	Expansion of fellowship training; collaboration with international professional organizations to enhance diagnostic skills, and development of allied health roles
Geographic access	Services concentrated in Khartoum; limited rural access	Expansion to regional centers; decentralization strategies
Referral pathways	Poorly defined referral system; delayed diagnosis	Strengthening referral pathways; raising public awareness of RMDs, integration into primary care
Diagnostics	Limited immunological tests; restricted genetic testing; shortage of MSK radiologists	Investment in labs, MSK ultrasound training, diagnostic hubs
Imaging services	Low CT/MRI density; no PET availability	Gradual expansion of imaging capacity
Treatment availability	Limited medications; partial insurance; supply constraints	Registration of additional biologics; future biosimilar use
Multidisciplinary care	Lack of coordinated MDTs; no nurse specialists	Improved collaboration with rehabilitation and allied services
Pediatric rheumatology	No service since 2023	Rebuilding services through training and collaboration
Patient support and advocacy	No formal patient support groups	Potential SAR- and NGO-led initiatives
Research capacity	Limited epidemiological data	Mandatory trainee research; growing research groups
Digital health	Limited EMR implementation	Gradual implementation of the national eHealth strategy and pilot EMRs

Abbreviations: *CT* computed tomography, *EMR* electronic medical records, *MDT* multidisciplinary team, *MRI* magnetic resonance imaging, *MSK* musculoskeletal, *NGO* non-governmental organizations, *PET* positron emission tomography, *RMD* rheumatic and musculoskeletal diseases, *SAR* Sudanese Association of Rheumatology

16.15 Future of Rheumatic Disease Care in Sudan

Despite ongoing challenges, the future of rheumatology in Sudan holds promise. Recent national health reform efforts and growing engagement with international partners have highlighted opportunities to strengthen specialist training and improve healthcare delivery across the country. These broader initiatives create a supportive environment for advancing rheumatology services and training, with the potential to improve care for patients with RMDs nationwide [7, 12, 43]. Therefore, all healthcare stakeholders and non-governmental organizations (NGOs) are urged to develop coordinated plans and collaborate with the Ministry of Health in Sudan to advance RMD care nationwide.

16.16 Conclusion

Rheumatic diseases represent a significant and growing health burden in Sudan. Challenges related to limited epidemiological data, shortages of trained rheumatologists, delayed diagnosis, and restricted access to diagnostics and advanced therapies continue to affect patient outcomes, particularly in rural and underserved areas.

Despite these limitations, progress has been made through the development of local training programs, expanding research activity, and the growing role of professional organizations. Strengthening rheumatology care in Sudan will require coordinated efforts to improve early diagnosis, expand specialist and multidisciplinary services, enhance access to essential treatments, and support locally relevant research. With sustained national and international collaboration, meaningful improvements in the care of patients with rheumatic diseases in Sudan are achievable.

Conflict of Interest All the authors declare no conflict of interest.

References

1. Sabr ME, Britannica Editors. Sudan. Encyclopædia Britannica [Internet]. 2026. [cited 2026 Jun 15]. Available from: https://www.britannica.com/place/Sudan.
2. McKenna A. List of African countries by area. Encyclopædia Britannica [Internet]. 2025. [cited 2026 Jun 15]. Available from: https://www.britannica.com/topic/list-of-African-countries-by-area.
3. Central Intelligence Agency. Sudan [Internet]. The World Factbook. 2026. [cited 2026 Jan 17]. Available from: https://www.cia.gov/the-world-factbook/countries/sudan/.
4. RAD-Aid International. Republic of Sudan country report: health system overview [Internet]. 2019. [cited 2026 Jun 15]. Available from: https://rad-aid.org/wp-content/uploads/Sudan-CR.pdf.
5. World Health Organization. Public Health Situation Analysis: Sudan Conflict (10 March 2025). [Internet]. [cited 2026 Jun 15]. Available from: https://www.who.int/publications/m/item/public-health-situation-analysis-sudan-conflict-(10-march-2025).
6. UNICEF Sudan. Water, sanitation and hygiene [Internet]. UNICEF. 2022. [cited 2026 Jun 15]. Available from: https://www.unicef.org/sudan/water-sanitation-and-hygiene.
7. Charani E, Cunnington AJ, Yousif AHA, Seed Ahmed M, Ahmed AEM, Babiker S, et al. In transition: current health challenges and priorities in Sudan. BMJ Glob Health. 2019;4(4):e001723. https://doi.org/10.1136/bmjgh-2019-001723.
8. World Health Organization. Sudan national health care quality policy and strategy. 2017. [cited 2026 Jun 15]. Available from: https://platform.who.int/docs/default-source/mca-documents/policy-documents/policy/sdn-cc-31-01-policy-2017-eng-national-health-care-quality.pdf.
9. World Health Organization. Health workforce data and statistics [Internet]. 2026. [cited 2026 Jan 17]. Available from: https://www.who.int/data/gho/data/themes/topics/health-workforce.
10. Hitchon CA, Mody GM, Feldman CH, Lau Y, Shi S, Meltzer M, et al. Perceptions and challenges experienced by African physicians when prescribing methotrexate for rheumatic disease: an exploratory study. ACR Open Rheumatol. 2021;3(8):522–30. https://doi.org/10.1002/acr2.11290.
11. Adelowo O, Mody GM, Tikly M, Oyoo O, Slimani S. Rheumatic diseases in Africa. Nat Rev Rheumatol. 2021;17(6):363–74. https://doi.org/10.1038/s41584-021-00603-4.
12. Ebrahim MAE, Ghebrehiwot L, Abdalgfar T, Juni MH. Health care system in Sudan: review and analysis of strength, weakness, opportunity, and threats (SWOT analysis). Sudan J Med Sci. 2017;12(3):133–50. https://doi.org/10.18502/sjms.v12i3.924.

13. Salih O, Ali A, Elgadal A, Idris M, Taha Y. Juvenile idiopathic arthritis in Sudanese children: clinical characteristics and subtypes. Egypt Rheumatol. 2022;44(1):91–5. https://doi.org/10.1016/j.ejr.2021.10.002.
14. World Health Organization. Sudan eHealth Strategy [Internet]. 2005. [cited 2026 Jun 15]. Available from: https://cdn.who.int/media/docs/default-source/digital-health-documents/global-observatory-on-digital-health/sdn_ehealth.pdf.
15. UNICEF Sudan. Rebuilding Sudan's health system through digital innovations [Internet]. 2025 Sept 15. [cited 2026 Jun 15]. Available from: https://sudan.un.org/en/301575-rebuilding-sudan%E2%80%99s-health-system-through-digital-innovations.
16. World Health Organization. Medical devices [Internet]. Geneva: World Health Organization. [cited 2026 Jan 18]. Available from: https://www.who.int/data/gho/data/themes/topics/GHO/medical-devices.
17. Sudanese Association of Rheumatology (SAR) [Internet]. [cited 2026 Jan 23]. Available from: https://www.sudanar.org/.
18. Al Maini M, Adelowo F, Al Saleh J, Al Weshahi Y, Burmester GR, Cutolo M, et al. The global challenges and opportunities in the practice of rheumatology: white paper by the World Forum on Rheumatic and Musculoskeletal Diseases. Clin Rheumatol. 2015;34(5):819–29. https://doi.org/10.1007/s10067-014-2841-6.
19. Mirghani H, Suleiman A. Pattern of rheumatic disorders among Sudanese patients-Khartoum state. Int J Neurol Phys Ther. 2017;3(3):17–20. https://doi.org/10.11648/j.ijnpt.20170303.11.
20. Elshafie AI, Elkhalifa AD, Elbagir S, Aledrissy MI, Elagib EM, Nur MA, et al. Active rheumatoid arthritis in Central Africa: A comparative study between Sudan and Sweden. J Rheumatol. 2016;43(10):1777–86. https://doi.org/10.3899/jrheum.160303.
21. Ali ZAH, Abd El-Raheem GOH, Noma M. Status of rheumatoid arthritis practice and treatment in Sudan. Sci Afr. 2023:e01939. https://doi.org/10.1016/j.sciaf.2023.e01939.
22. Elbagir S, Elshafie AI, Elagib EM, Mohammed NA, Aledrissy MIE, Sohrabian A, et al. Sudanese and Swedish patients with systemic lupus erythematosus: immunological and clinical comparisons. Rheumatology (Oxford). 2020;59(5):968–78. https://doi.org/10.1093/rheumatology/kez323.
23. Abdelgalil Ali Ahmed S, Adam Essa ME, Ahmed AF, Elagib EM, Ahmed Eltahir NI, Awadallah H, et al. Incidence and clinical pattern of mixed connective tissue disease in Sudanese patients at Omdurman military hospital: hospital-based study. Open Access Rheumatol. 2021;13:333–41. https://doi.org/10.2147/OARRR.S335206.
24. Patasova K, Mohammed NA, Nur M, Elagib E, Elshafie A, Gunnarsson I, et al. Genetic associations with systemic lupus erythematosus in the Sudanese population. J Rheumatol. 2025;52(Suppl 1):138. https://doi.org/10.3899/jrheum.2025-0390.PV101.
25. Alzahrane A, West R, Ubhi HK, Brown J, Abdulqader N, Samarkandi O. Evaluations of clinical tobacco cessation interventions in Arab populations: a systematic review. Addict Behav. 2019;88:169–74. https://doi.org/10.1016/j.addbeh.2018.08.017.
26. Barbhaiya M, Tedeschi SK, Lu B, Malspeis S, Kreps D, Sparks JA, et al. Cigarette smoking and the risk of systemic lupus erythematosus, overall and by anti-double stranded DNA antibody subtype, in the Nurses' Health Study cohorts. Ann Rheum Dis. 2018;77(2):196–202. https://doi.org/10.1136/annrheumdis-2017-211675.
27. Costenbader KH, Feskanich D, Mandl LA, Karlson EW. Smoking intensity, duration, and cessation, and the risk of rheumatoid arthritis in women. Am J Med. 2006;119(6):503 e1–9. https://doi.org/10.1016/j.amjmed.2005.09.053.
28. Servioli L, Maciel G, Nannini C, Crowson CS, Matteson EL, Cornec D, et al. Association of Smoking and Obesity on the risk of developing primary Sjogren syndrome: a population-based cohort study. J Rheumatol. 2019;46(7):727–30. https://doi.org/10.3899/jrheum.180481.
29. Ahmed MH, Ali YA, Awadalla H, Elmadhoun WM, Noor SK, Almobarak AO. Prevalence and trends of obesity among adult Sudanese individuals: population based study. Diabetes Metab Syndr. 2017;11(Suppl 2):S963–S7. https://doi.org/10.1016/j.dsx.2017.07.023.
30. Buwembo W, Munabi IG, Kaddumukasa M, Kiryowa H, Nankya E, Johnson WE, et al. Periodontitis and Rheumatoid Arthritis in sub-Saharan Africa, gaps and way forward: a systematic review and meta-analysis. Open J Stomatol. 2019;9(10):215–26. https://doi.org/10.4236/ojst.2019.910023.

31. Cacoub P, Comarmond C, Domont F, Savey L, Desbois AC, Saadoun D. Extrahepatic manifestations of chronic hepatitis C virus infection. Ther Adv Infect Dis. 2016;3(1):3–14. https://doi.org/10.1177/2049936115585942.
32. Cacoub P, Terrier B. Hepatitis B-related autoimmune manifestations. Rheum Dis Clin N Am. 2009;35(1):125–37. https://doi.org/10.1016/j.rdc.2009.03.006.
33. Chaabna K, Kouyoumjian SP, Abu-Raddad LJ. Hepatitis C virus epidemiology in Djibouti, Somalia, Sudan, and Yemen: systematic review and meta-analysis. PLoS One. 2016;11(2):e0149966. https://doi.org/10.1371/journal.pone.0149966.
34. McCarthy MC, El-Tigani A, Khalid IO, Hyams KC. Hepatitis B and C in Juba, southern Sudan: results of a serosurvey. Trans R Soc Trop Med Hyg. 1994;88(5):534–6. https://doi.org/10.1016/0035-9203(94)90150-3.
35. Mudawi HM. Epidemiology of viral hepatitis in Sudan. Clin Exp Gastroenterol. 2008;1:9–13. https://doi.org/10.2147/ceg.s3887.
36. Mohamed YAG, Doutoum AA, Mahamat AB, Doungous DM, Gabbad AA, Osmab RM. Prevalence and risk factors of hepatitis B among the population at Algamosi locality, Gezira State, Sudan. Health. 2022;14. https://doi.org/10.4236/health.2022.1412084.
37. Badawi MM, SalahEldin MA, Idris AB, Idris EB, Mohamed SG. Tuberculosis in Sudan: systematic review and meta analysis. BMC Pulm Med. 2024;24(1):51. https://doi.org/10.1186/s12890-024-02865-6.
38. Elmadhoun WM, Noor SK, Bushara SO, Ahmed EO, Mustafa H, Sulaiman AA, et al. Epidemiology of tuberculosis and evaluation of treatment outcomes in the national tuberculosis control programme, River Nile state, Sudan, 2011–2013. East Mediterr Health J. 2016;22(2):95–102.
39. Mohammed AKY, Humida EHM, Ali AMO, Ahmed HG. Burden of tuberculosis in Western Sudan during The Sudan armed conflict. Cureus. 2025;17(1):e76944. https://doi.org/10.7759/cureus.76944.
40. World Health Organization. Sudan — tuberculosis country profile [Internet]. WHO Global Health Observatory. 2024. [cited 2026 Jun 15]. Available from: https://data.who.int/countries/729?utm_source=chatgpt.com.
41. Osman Ahmed Osman M, Imad Z, Abdalla Y, Hamza SB, Gafar M, Mohamed Ahmed Ali O. Calcinosis cutis in a patient with systemic lupus erythematosus: a case report. Cureus. 2025;17(12):e98457. https://doi.org/10.7759/cureus.98457.
42. Mahmoud Z, Osman M, Ahmed F, Mohammed S, Omer A. Quality of life in Sudanese systemic lupus erythematosus patients: A cross-sectional study. J Adv Res East Mediterr Reg. 2025;69:205–41. https://doi.org/10.5281/zenodo.17843636.
43. Wharton G, Ali OE, Khalil S, Yagoub H, Mossialos E. Rebuilding Sudan's health system: opportunities and challenges. Lancet. 2020;395(10219):171–3. https://doi.org/10.1016/S0140-6736(19)32974-5.

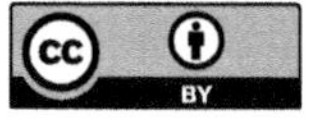

Chapter 17
Rheumatic Diseases in the Syrian Arab Republic

Salwa Al Cheikh, Mohammad Said Al Sawaf, Mohammed Alaswad, and Layla Kazkaz

Abstract The Syrian Arab Republic (or simply Syria) is located in western Asia; its capital is Damascus, the oldest continuously inhabited city in the world. It is a unitary republic with a population of 23,022,427, with a median age of 23.5 years for both sexes.

The Ministry of Health (MOH) is responsible for the management, planning, financing, and regulation of the health sectors, both public and private.

Syria's healthcare system comprises three primary services that collaborate seamlessly: rheumatology health services managed by the Military Medical Services Administration since 1979, those under the MOH since 1986, and services initiated by the Ministry of Higher Education in 1988. The Syrian Association for Rheumatology is the official association representing the country. It was established in 1995 and includes 66 members.

Under the MOH, Syrian patients with chronic rheumatic diseases receive all disease-modifying anti-rheumatic drugs (DMARDs), including biologics, free of charge. These medications are distributed to national hospitals and centers. The screening program of biologics adopted by the MOH is an international program. Furthermore, most immunological tests and various imaging modalities are available in the country.

The Syrian Board for Medical Specialties and the Medical Council for Rheumatic Diseases were established in 2013.

In 2017, the MOH established an unofficial registry and published the "Guide to Therapeutic Action for Patients with Arthritis and Immunological Diseases" in Arabic.

S. Al Cheikh
Faculty of Medicine, Damascus University, Damascus, Syria
e-mail: salwacheikh@gmail.com

M. S. Al Sawaf · L. Kazkaz (✉)
Syrian Association for Rheumatology, Damascus, Syria
e-mail: dr.swaf@gmail.com; dr.layla.kazkaz@gmail.com

M. Alaswad
Medical Centre Hospital, Hama, Syria
e-mail: dr.aswad97@gmail.com

K. A. Alnaqbi, G. Aldabie (eds.), *Rheumatic Diseases in the Arab World*,
https://doi.org/10.1007/978-981-92-0967-5_17

Keywords Rheumatic diseases · Rheumatology services · Syria · Syrian association for rheumatology · Rheumatology workforce · Biologic therapy · Rheumatology training · Medical education · Health services accessibility

17.1 Syria Demographics

Syria, officially known as the Syrian Arab Republic, is located in western Asia. It shares borders with the Mediterranean Sea to the west, Turkey to the north, Iraq to the east and southeast, Jordan to the south, and Palestine and Lebanon to the southwest. Cyprus lies to the west across the Mediterranean Sea. The capital city of Syria is Damascus, the oldest continuously inhabited city in the world [1].

Syria, known for its rich history, holds a pivotal place in human civilization. Its history spans thousands of years from the ancient city of Damascus to the ruins of Palmyra and the Crusader castles. It served as a crossroads of cultures, where the great civilizations of Mesopotamia, Egypt, Greece, and Rome intersected, leaving behind a legacy of architectural marvels and cultural exchange. Despite facing challenges today, Syria's historical significance endures as a testament to the resilience and endurance of its people and their enduring connection to the past.

Syria is divided into four traditional regions, including the coastal strip, the mountains, the cultivated steppe, and the desert steppe. It is a unitary republic administratively divided into 14 regional governorates, 107 districts, and 2480 subdistricts. The governorates of Syria include Damascus, Rural Damascus, Aleppo, Homs, Hama, Daraa, Deir ez-Zur, Al-Hasakah, Idlib, Latakia, Quneitra, Ar-Raqqah, As-Suwayda, and Tartus.

In 2023, the estimated population of Syria is 23,022,427, according to the latest United Nations data [1]. Sex distribution statistics indicate that approximately 49.99% of the population is female, while 50.01% is male [2]. As of 2018, approximately 54.2% of the population resides in urban areas. The median age in 2020 was 23 years for males and 24 years for females. The overall life expectancy in Syria is 75.2 years for both sexes, with females having a longer life expectancy at 77.8 years compared to males at 72.8 years [1].

17.2 Country Healthcare Sectors

The healthcare system in Syria is under the Ministry of Health's (MOH) jurisdiction. It is divided between public institutions complimented by the private healthcare sector. The system is relatively decentralized and focuses on offering primary healthcare at three levels: village, district, and provincial. Treatment courses are delivered per subdistrict. The MOH manages, plans, finances, and regulates the health sector.

The healthcare sector in Syria consists of entities that provide medical services, manufacture medical equipment and medications, administer medical insurance, and facilitate healthcare provision to patients.

17.3 Rheumatology Health Services

In the late 1980s, the majority of rheumatologists practicing in Syria had received their training overseas, primarily in European countries or the United States. However, after that period, training programs were initiated in hospitals under the Ministry of Defense, MOH, and later the Ministry of Higher Education in Syria.

1. *The Rheumatology Health Services Run by the Military Medical Services Administration*

   - In Damascus:
     The rheumatology unit at El-Tal Hospital was established in 1979. It was led by a female rheumatologist who had received sponsorship from Syrian authorities to specialize in rheumatology in London for 5 years. Subsequently, the unit received additional support from two consultant rheumatologists who joined the department after completing their training overseas. One consultant had received training in the United Kingdom (UK), while the other had trained in France. The department comprised a total of 20 beds.
     General Hospital, established in 1982, is the largest hospital in Syria and encompasses 10 floors and additional ancillary buildings. This modern hospital was designed by French architects and offers a comprehensive range of medical specialties, with a minimum of 1100 beds. With 38 departments, the hospital is staffed by highly qualified doctors sponsored by Syrian authorities to receive specialized training in various disciplines in countries such as the United States of America (USA), the UK, France, and other European nations. The nursing staff at General Hospital are also well-trained and proficient in their roles.
     Damascus Military Hospital (formerly known as Tishreen Hospital) is an important hospital in Syria that stays updated with the latest medical advancements. The military health services provide continuous support by inviting professors from the USA, UK, France, and other European countries to share their knowledge. The Rheumatology Department was established in 1982 by the same female rheumatologist previously at El-Tal Hospital, as she was

appointed the department head. Postgraduate doctors were trained in rheumatology, with 16 rotating house officers involved. The department had 14 nurses working in shifts. In 1989, two trainees passed their examination and became certified rheumatology specialists. The department has 36 beds, divided into female, VIP, and ordinary wings. It also includes an injection clinic and a preparatory room with a small pharmacy. The rheumatology clinics see around 70 patients per day, operating 5 days a week. Over time, the department expanded, and it now has two senior consultants (one male and one female), two male specialists, five registrars (one male and four females), and 16 senior house officers in training.

- In other cities:
  Lattakia, Tartous, and Homs each have one rheumatology unit.

2. *The Rheumatology Health Services Run by the MOH*

   In 1986, MOH employed a rheumatologist, who had already completed his specialty in rheumatology in England, to work in Damascus Hospital. Patients with rheumatic diseases at that time were managed by either an orthopedic surgeon, neurologist, internal medicine specialist, or cardiologist. There were officially 10 inpatient beds within the cardiology department (5 for males and 5 for females). However, there was a need to occupy 15 beds for males and the same for females most of the time.

   It is worth mentioning that almost all the immunological tests are available in Syria. Additionally, all DMARDs, including biologics, are provided free of charge by the MOH for patients with rheumatic diseases.

3. *The Rheumatology Health Services Run by the Ministry of Higher Education*

   Initially, rheumatology patients were admitted to the medical department and sometimes to neurology divisions at university hospitals, and training in rheumatology was basically for internal medicine residents.

   In 1991, an eight-bed rheumatology unit was established at Al-Mouwasat University Hospital, a 600-bed university hospital founded in 1943, later accompanied by a 20-bed rheumatology department at the National University Hospital (formerly known as Al Assad University Hospital), a 550-bed university hospital established in 1988. In each department, there are five rheumatologists and several internal medicine residents.

   A female rheumatologist who completed her specialized training in rheumatology in the USA was responsible for founding these two departments. While both departments were supported by advanced laboratory facilities and experienced radiology personnel, it was not until 2001 that the University of Damascus introduced a residency program in rheumatology.

Figure 17.1 depicts the timeline of major events related to rheumatology in Syria.

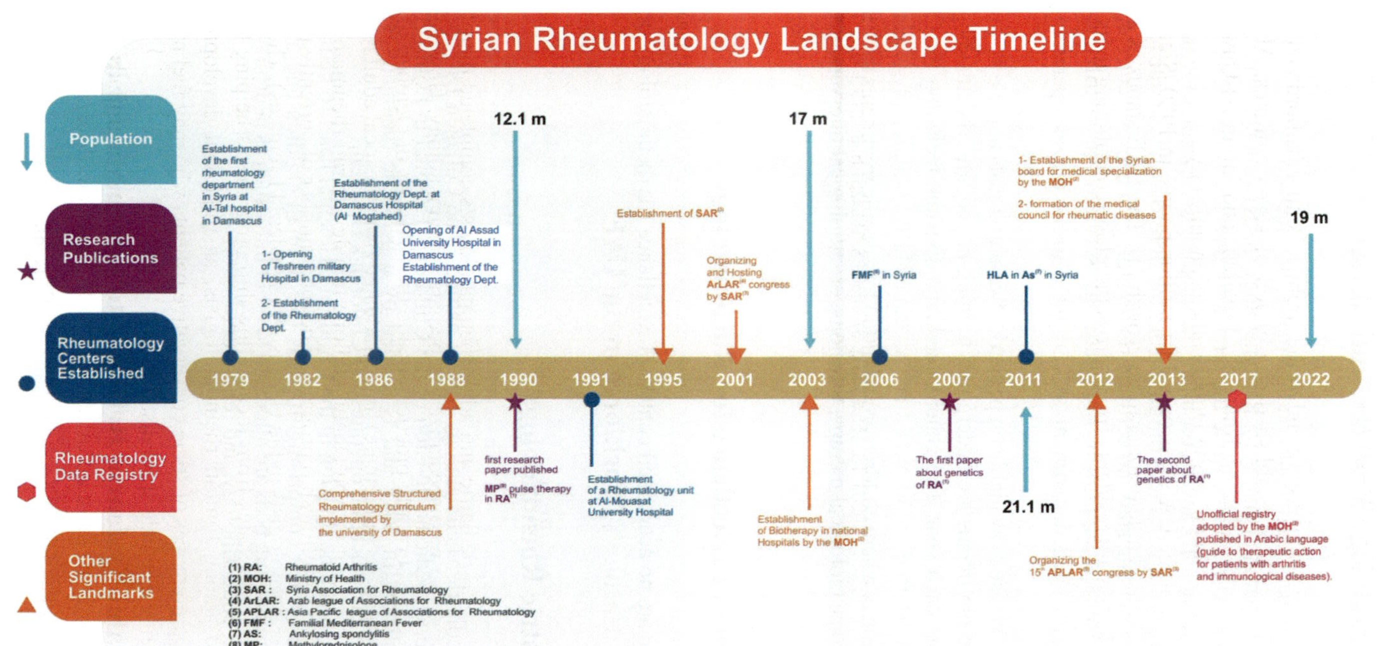

Fig. 17.1 Syrian rheumatology landscape timeline

17.4 Rheumatology Manpower: Registered Rheumatologists, Rheumatology Trainees, and Nurses

A total of 65 members (41 females and 24 males) are licensed by the MOH and are members of the Syrian Association for Rheumatology (SAR). Among them, 41 are consultants and senior consultants, while the remaining individuals consist of specialists and registrars. Additionally, seven consultant rheumatologists are not SAR members.

As for rheumatology trainees ranging from the first to fifth year, the total count is 84. Regarding nursing staff, no certified rheumatology nurses are currently available; however, nurses supporting rheumatology services are distributed across departments, with each department staffed by 6 to 14 nurses operating across three shifts.

There are no statistics available on pediatric rheumatologists at present. Currently, 34 postgraduate physicians are undergoing training in pediatric rheumatology, with varying numbers each year. The general medicine division, including the Collagen Diseases unit, is staffed by 30 nurses across three shifts. Additionally, a temporary residence division is where children are admitted for specific treatments such as intra-articular injections, biological therapy, infusions, or radiological interventions.

17.5 Centers of Excellence for Rheumatology

Currently, there are no accredited centers of excellence for rheumatology in Syria.

17.6 Pediatric Rheumatology

A dedicated pediatric rheumatology unit is named "The Collagen Diseases Unit" within the general medicine division of the Children's Hospital in Damascus. This unit was established in 2012 and is headed by a pediatric rheumatologist. The Ministry of Higher Education operates the Children's Hospital.

The general medicine division in the Children's Hospital has 116 beds, with the Collagen Diseases unit comprising 10 beds (5 for small children and 5 for older children). The remaining beds are allocated to other units such as neurology, pulmonary, metabolic, endocrinology, and renal units.

17.7 Available System of Referrals to Rheumatology in Syria

Referrals in healthcare can occur through various mechanisms. Public referrals involve patients from primary healthcare to higher-level healthcare facilities and back to primary healthcare as needed. This allows for comprehensive management of the patient's health needs using resources beyond what is available at their initial point of care, whether a community clinic, unit, dispensary, or health center. However, other referral mechanisms exist.

Self-referral is when patients bypass primary care facilities and directly seek care at higher-level centers, a common practice in Syria. Private referrals occur when patients request a personal referral from their general practitioner to an external private hospital or specialist. In these cases, the patient may receive a referral letter from the specialist to give to their general practitioner.

Some general practitioners may order tests, make a diagnosis, and then refer the patient to a specialist at a local hospital or a specialized hospital. Additionally, healthcare professionals may refer patients to rheumatologists for their expertise in diagnosis and treatment.

Referrals can also be made through charity organizations, which facilitate the referral process for patients in need. In emergencies, any doctor may refer a patient to a hospital's rheumatologist to promptly assess the patient's condition.

17.8 Syrian Association for Rheumatology (SAR)

The Syrian Association for Rheumatology (SAR) officially represents Syria. It is a non-profit association and includes 66 members [3]. It was established in 1995 under the umbrella of the Syrian Medical Association, which plays a significant role in creating, organizing, and supervising the associations of the different medical specialties.

SAR started with six rheumatologists and one consultant specializing in rehabilitation; therefore, it was named "The Syrian Association for Rheumatology and Rehabilitation." Subsequently, in 2001, the rehabilitation physicians formed their own association. Later, SAR established a committee focused on osteoporosis prevention, which later evolved into the Syrian Association for Osteoporosis Prevention in 2001. This new association included seven specialties: rheumatology, endocrinology, gynecology, orthopedic surgery, radiology, laboratory, and rehabilitation medicine.

SAR is currently a member of the Arab League of Associations for Rheumatology (ArLAR) and the Asia Pacific League of Associations for Rheumatology (APLAR).

- *SAR Objectives*
  SAR works nationally and locally to prevent and treat rheumatic diseases while raising awareness among the public and patients.
- *SAR Activities*
  SAR supports trainees in achieving high-quality standards of care for patients with rheumatic diseases, disseminates knowledge about new developments in rheumatology, strengthens collaboration between rheumatologists in Syria and other countries, and promotes research in the field.
  SAR organizes a variety of activities to disseminate knowledge and promote advancements in the field. This includes hosting two symposia each year, focus-

ing on specific topics in rheumatology, where experts provide the latest information on diagnosis and treatment. In addition, SAR conducts monthly clinical sessions in different national hospitals, facilitating collaborative discussions among colleagues to explore various diagnostic and therapeutic approaches. It also arranges an international congress every 2 years to promote international collaboration, featuring renowned speakers from esteemed universities.

SAR has successfully organized and hosted previous congresses, such as the ArLAR congress in 2001 and the 15th APLAR congress in 2012 (held in Jordan). It is also actively involved in teaching courses for trainees and young rheumatologists, publishing booklets for patient awareness, and contributing articles to international medical journals. The SAR council members meet monthly to ensure effective coordination of these activities and discussions.

- *Structure of the SAR*

  SAR has a well-structured organization that ensures effective leadership and representation. At its core is the executive committee, consisting of the president, vice president, secretary general, and treasurer. They are responsible for the overall management and decision-making within the association. The council members, including the chairs of Scientific Affairs, Social Affairs, and Public Relations, along with the immediate past president and honorary president nominated by the Syrian Medical Association and SAR's General Assembly, form an essential part of the organization. Representatives from various cities across Syria play a crucial role in connecting the council with members in different areas. SAR adheres to the internal discipline of the Syrian Medical Association, wherein the president and council members are elected by the general assembly for a three-year term. If they wish to continue, they can serve another term after one cycle has elapsed.

17.9 Overview of Rheumatic Diseases

17.9.1 Overview of Rheumatic Diseases in Syria

The prevalence of rheumatic diseases in Syria, as reported by unpublished data from the Ministry of Health, is shown in Table 17.1.

Some papers were published about the corticosteroids in rheumatoid arthritis (RA) [4], genetics of RA in Syria, including RA and genetic markers in Syrian and French populations [5], and the whole-exome sequencing for familial RA [6]. Furthermore, Syria participated in a large cohort of Arabic patients with RA to assess the epidemiology and treatment patterns [7].

A Syrian study found that the HLA-B27 allele was present in 1.4% of healthy individuals and in 60% of patients diagnosed with ankylosing spondylitis (AS), with HLA-B27*05 being the predominant variant [8].

Table 17.1 The prevalence of rheumatic diseases in Syria

	Disease	Prevalence	Male: Female	Mortality
1	Rheumatoid arthritis	0.16%	0.38:1	Overall mortality 1.6%
2	Ankylosing spondylitis	170/100,000	4.7:1	
3	Behcet's disease	160/100,000	2.13:1	
4	Systemic lupus erythematosus	15/100,000	0.24:1	
5	Familial Mediterranean fever	1/75,000	–	
6	Dermatomyositis / Polymyositis	5–20/(100,000)	–	
7	Sjogren Disease	40/(100,000)	33:67	
8	Vasculitis	3/100,000	3:5	
9	Giant cell arteritis	0.2/1000	2 males	
10	Psoriatic arthritis	150/100,000	115:129	
11	Rheumatic Fever	5/100,000	–	
12	Gout	1.40%	–	
13	Low back pain	800/100,000	–	
14	Neck Pain	3.30%	–	
15	Reactive arthritis	16/100,000	–	
16	Osteoarthritis	12.60%	–	

17.9.2 Common Risk Factors of Rheumatic Diseases in Syria

Lifestyle factors such as smoking and obesity are prominent contributors. Smoking, whether cigarettes or shisha, is widespread among young people of both sexes, often ranging from moderate to heavy use (1–3 packs daily). It is a known risk factor for developing rheumatic disease. The MOH keeps raising awareness about the hazards of smoking on health through social media, rallies, and campaigns.

Obesity is another major risk factor in all age groups in Syria. A study conducted in Aleppo revealed that obesity correlated with age, marital status, and consumption of certain food items, especially in women [9]. A high body mass index may also predispose individuals to certain rheumatic diseases [10].

Sociocultural practices, including consanguinity and endogamy, also contribute to rheumatic disease risk. Although these practices are less common than before in Syria due to increasing public awareness, they remain an issue, as seen in Syrian refugee children, particularly in familial Mediterranean fever (FMF) [11].

Finally, genetic factors have been explored in limited studies. Research on the frequency of MEFV gene mutations in Syrian patients with FMF and in the general population has provided important insights into the genetic underpinnings of this autoinflammatory disorder [12].

17.9.3 Screening Programs for Rheumatic Diseases

In 2017, the MOH established an unofficial registry in Arabic known as the "Guide to Therapeutic Action for Patients with Arthritis and Immunological Diseases." This comprehensive guide includes a summary of the international screening program for patients undergoing biological treatments for conditions such as juvenile idiopathic arthritis (JIA), RA, AS, psoriatic arthritis (PsA), Behcet's disease, and ANCA-associated vasculitis. The screening program involves several key steps:

(a) Screening for latent tuberculosis (TB) through a chest X-ray and a cutaneous tuberculin test. If the tuberculin test measures over 5 mm with a normal chest X-ray, prophylactic anti-TB treatment should be initiated.
(b) Screening for hepatitis B and C is also recommended.
(c) Specific tests are required to exclude active infection, demyelinating diseases, or congestive heart failure for each patient.
(d) Blood tests, including complete blood cell count, liver function tests, kidney function tests, acute phase reactants (erythrocyte sedimentation rate and C-reactive protein), rheumatoid factor (RF), and anti-cyclic citrullinated peptide (anti-CCP).

Moreover, all patients with autoimmune disease in Syria are screened for diabetes mellitus and hyperlipidemia.

17.10 Diagnosis of Rheumatic Diseases in Syria

17.10.1 Laboratory Tests

A range of laboratory tests is available, covering genetic, immunological, hypercoagulation, and therapeutic drug-level assessments.

Genetic testing encompasses HLA testing for HLA-B27, HLA-B5, HLA-B51, and HLA-DQ, as well as testing for FMF mutations within the MEFV gene, including specific mutations (M694V, M680I (G > C), M680I (G > A), V726A, M694I, E148Q, P369S, F479L, I692DEL, K695R, A744S, R761H, E148V, and E167D).

Immunological tests feature a comprehensive panel, including AMA M2 (antimitochondrial antibodies M2), cytoplasmic antineutrophil cytoplasmic antibody (cANCA), perinuclear antineutrophil cytoplasmic antibody (pANCA), anti-centromere, anti-Jo-1, anti-Sm, anti-U1 ribonucleoprotein (anti-URNP), anti-Scl-70, antinuclear antibodies (ANA), anti-double-stranded DNA, C3 and C4, RF, anti-CCP, smooth muscle antibodies, SS-A/Ro autoantibodies, and SS-B/La autoantibodies. Additionally, available hypercoagulation tests include anti-phospholipid antibodies (beta 2 glycoprotein, lupus anticoagulant, and anticardiolipin antibodies), protein C, protein S, anti-thrombin III, plasminogen, factor V Leiden, prothrombin, factor VIII, beta fibrinogen, plasminogen activator inhibitor, and human platelet antigen.

Furthermore, some tests, such as serum angiotensin-converting enzyme (ACE) and serum drug levels for tacrolimus and cyclosporin, can be ordered. The latter are used to monitor therapeutic drug levels, providing proper patient assessment for treatment guidance.

17.10.2 Imaging Services

Syria offers good accessibility to advanced imaging for both diagnosis and ongoing monitoring of medical conditions. These facilities, available in public and private sectors, encompass many modalities. This includes computed tomography (CT), high-resolution computed tomography (HRCT), CT angiography, and magnetic resonance imaging (MRI) for the spine and sacroiliac joints. Magnetic resonance angiography (MRA) and open MRI machines are available in various centers.

Other imaging modalities consist of bone scintigraphy, dual-energy X-ray absorptiometry (DXA), and positron emission tomography (PET) scans, which are accessible only in private centers, with three centers located in Damascus. Moreover, there is a notable number of musculoskeletal radiologists across different cities, and the availability of musculoskeletal ultrasound in both public hospitals and private centers further enhances the diagnosis of rheumatic diseases. For example, in Damascus, there are two centers in public hospitals and two centers in private hospitals.

17.11 Rheumatic Disease Management

17.11.1 Anti-rheumatic Medications

A variety of anti-rheumatic drugs are accessible for the treatment of different rheumatic diseases. Biologic DMARDs are available, including tumor necrosis factor inhibitors such as infliximab (Remicade), adalimumab (Humira), an adalimumab biosimilar (CinnoRa), golimumab (Simponi), and etanercept (Enbrel), as well as other biologics such as ustekinumab (Stelara) and rituximab. Conventional synthetic DMARDs, such as methotrexate, sulfasalazine, hydroxychloroquine, leflunomide, azathioprine, cyclophosphamide, cyclosporine, tacrolimus, and mycophenolate mofetil, are available, offering various treatment options for multiple rheumatic conditions. Table 17.2 presents the number of facilities (unpublished data from the Ministry of Health) that provide immunomodulatory and immunosuppressive treatments, as well as their geographical distribution.

Table 17.2 Geographical distribution of patients receiving immunomodulatory and immunosuppressive treatments in syria in 2022

Centers	Total	Males	Females
Damascus	2099	1000	1099
Al-Hasakah	17	9	8
Quneitra	120	31	89
As-Suwayda	489	180	309
Ar-Raqqah	41	16	25
Qamishli	22	6	16
Deir ez-Zur	90	34	56
Rif-Dimashq	331	167	164
Homs	361	122	239
Hama	697	202	495
Latakia	355	151	204
Tartus	263	124	139
Idlib	20	9	11
Aleppo	513	214	299
Daraa	143	75	68

17.11.2 Accessibility to Multi-disciplinary Specialties

17.11.2.1 Rehabilitation

Rehabilitation, specifically through physiotherapy and occupational therapy, plays a crucial role in managing rheumatic diseases, aiming to restore functionality [13]. Nearly all public hospitals in Syria have well-equipped physiotherapy departments typically overseen by specialized rehabilitation medicine physicians. Additionally, an important rehabilitation hospital, managed by military medical services, operates in Damascus, offering comprehensive facilities, including deep pool therapy and an artificial limbs unit. Moreover, prosthetic limb centers are also available in cities like Lattakia, Tartus, and Hama. These facilities provide a range of therapeutic options to patients, including exercises, ice, heat, and wax therapies, splints, and hydrotherapy, contributing to the comprehensive approach to rehabilitation.

17.11.2.2 Surgery

Orthopedic surgery is available in most public and private hospitals. This specialty is advanced in Syria and involves, for example, atlantoaxial subluxation, arthroplasties, tendon transfer and repair surgeries, scoliosis, kyphoplasty, vertebroplasty, etc.

17.12 Education and Research

17.12.1 Rheumatology Training Programs in Syria

17.12.1.1 Specialization Programs Run by the MOH

The rheumatology specialty training started in Damascus Hospital in 1987 by accepting two residents yearly, then two to three residents each year. The resident has to spend 2 years in the internal medicine department and 3 years in the rheumatology department. All residents follow training programs and duties designed by the Syrian Board for Medical Specialization and the Medical Council for Rheumatic Diseases.

In 2000, other training centers were started in Ibn Al-Nafees Hospital and the Red Crescent. Hospitals in addition to hospitals in Aleppo, Latakia, Tartus, and Suwayda.

17.12.1.2 Specialization Programs Run by the Ministry of Higher Education

In 2021, a comprehensive and well-structured rheumatology curriculum was introduced, consisting of 4 years in internal medicine followed by 2 years in rheumatology before residents could take the final written exam. Upon passing, residents could then proceed to the clinical exam. This curriculum and examination method were later adopted by other training programs in Syria and have since been regularly updated.

The Ministry of Higher Education program has another special requirement: residents are only qualified once they do clinical research, write their thesis, and defend it publicly. Regrettably, these research papers, authored in Arabic, were not well-known to the rheumatology societies that had studied the most in-depth rheumatic diseases in Syria. The thesis usually consists of around 60 pages of clinical research conducted by the resident under the close observation of department professors. After the agreement of the ethical research committee, the university sponsors the study, but the funding is usually limited. Examples of research outcomes include the prevalence of spondyloarthritis (SpA) in Syria, which is approximately 170 cases per 100,000 Syrians, and the prevalence of Behcet's disease in Syria, which is approximately 160 cases per 100,000 Syrians.

In 2008, the training programs in Syria changed their training requirement to 2 years in medicine and 3 years in rheumatology. In general, the two departments at Al-Mouwasat and the National University hospitals work together, and residents spend half of their 5 years in each hospital; professors and other qualified rheumatologists supervise the training.

Since establishing the Syrian Board for Medical Specialization and forming the Medical Council for Rheumatic Disease, candidates intending to train in rheumatology typically undergo a review process for their applications. Additionally, candidates often take written and clinical exams administered by the scientific committee. This process adds approximately 4–5 new rheumatologists to the rheumatology workforce each year. This number does not include physicians who leave Syria to work in other countries or get their qualifications abroad. This means that the number of rheumatologists in Syria is less than 0.5 for 100,000 inhabitants. It is important to note that the competency level of rheumatologists varies based on the quality of their training programs. This discrepancy significantly burdens the rheumatologists.

17.12.2 Availability of Formal Rheumatology Nursing Programs

There are two primary schools for nurses, one overseen by the MOH and the other by the Ministry of Higher Education. Approximately 200 nurses complete their training annually. Subsequently, they are assigned to various hospital or medical center departments to develop their skills further and gain experience. However, there are no formal training rheumatology programs for physician assistants or nurses in Syria.

17.12.3 Rheumatology Research in Syria

Rheumatology research in Syria has faced substantial barriers, including economic and administrative difficulties, the protracted crises since 2011, and the emigration of many researchers. Limited financial support and the lack of electronic medical records have further complicated data collection and verification, making research processes slow and often unreliable. As a result, most studies are conducted by master's and Ph.D. students or by professors fulfilling academic requirements for promotion.

Most rheumatology publications appear in journals affiliated with Damascus University and, more recently, other Syrian universities. However, these journals publish exclusively in Arabic and are not indexed in Index Medicus or PubMed, limiting the international visibility of Syrian research.

It is noteworthy that the fundamentals of medical research are typically taught in medical school and reinforced during postgraduate training. Nevertheless, some ambitious medical students and practitioners have taken the initiative to enhance their research skills by attending seminars and utilizing online resources, despite internet disruptions in Syria over the past 13 years [14]. Additionally, there is a growing need for medical secretaries and improved English proficiency to facilitate research endeavors.

Table 17.3 Key rheumatology research studies conducted in Syria

Title	Year of publication	Study type	Sample size	References
Familial Mediterranean fever in the Syrian population: gene mutation frequencies, carrier rates and phenotype-genotype correlation	2006	Case-control	325 (83 patients and 242 healthy controls)	[12]
Rheumatoid arthritis and genetic markers in Syrian and French populations: different effect of the shared epitope	2007	Comparative case-control	1259 (668 patients and 591 healthy controls in two distinct populations)	[5]
HLA-B27 and its subtypes in Syrian patients with ankylosing spondylitis	2011	Case-control	267 (50 patients and 217 healthy controls)	[8]
Assessing the Prevalence of disease-specific antinuclear antibodies and their detection in diagnosis of rheumatic disorders in Syria	2022	Cross-sectional	529	[16]
Cross-sectional study of COVID-19 infection in patients with rheumatic diseases in a sample of a Damascene population, Syria	2023	Cross-sectional	500	[17]
Analysis of septic arthritis in a sample of Syrian population: a retrospective study	2023	Retrospective cross-sectional	256	[18]
Clinical presentation and management of multisystem inflammatory syndrome in children associated with covid-19: a retrospective observational descriptive study in a pediatric hospital in Syria	2024	Retrospective observational	232	[19]
Rheumatic Diseases amidst conflict in northwest Syria: unveiling health challenges and implications	2024	Retrospective observational	488	[20]

Despite these challenges, a modest body of indexed literature has emerged, including original articles [5, 8, 12, 14–20] and case reports across different rheumatic diseases [21–26]. More recently, preprint studies have also started to appear [27–29]. Table 17.3 summarizes key rheumatology studies conducted in Syria.

17.13 Rheumatic Diseases and COVID-19: Clinical Outcomes and Insights from Syria

In Syrian patients with pre-existing rheumatic diseases who contracted COVID-19, poorer outcomes were attributed primarily to older age and comorbidities, rather than to the rheumatic disease itself or its treatment [17].

Complementing this adult-focused perspective, a 2024 retrospective observational study conducted at the Children's Hospital in Syria examined multisystem inflammatory syndrome in children (MIS-C) associated with COVID-19 infection. Among 232 pediatric COVID-19 cases, 11% (25 patients) were diagnosed with MIS-C, with a median age of 5.5 years and a predominance of males. The symptoms observed included fever, conjunctivitis, rash, and gastrointestinal features such as abdominal pain and diarrhea. Cardiac abnormalities noted were reduced left ventricular ejection fraction, coronary artery dilation and aneurysms, and pericardial effusion. Other findings included cavity changes, edema, cervical lymphadenopathy, neurological symptoms, and respiratory symptoms. Laboratory tests frequently showed leukocytosis, lymphopenia, and elevated levels of inflammatory markers (C-reactive protein, erythrocyte sedimentation rate, d-dimers, and ferritin), along with high serum creatinine and lactate dehydrogenase. Treatment for all patients included IVIG and aspirin, with most also receiving methylprednisolone. Remarkably, all patients fully recovered within 8 days of their hospital stay, with no reported mortality [19].

17.14 Cost-Effective Care for Rheumatic Diseases

In Syria, the MOH's Department of Infection and Chronic Diseases offers free-of-charge medications, including biologics, for treating chronic rheumatic conditions. Biologics are administered within the rheumatology departments and units at MOH hospitals. Table 17.4 below presents the drug list and associated expenses for 2021–2022.

Table 17.4 Cost of some disease-modifying anti-rheumatic drugs at the Ministry of Health (unpublished data)

Drugs	Pharmaceutical form	Dose	Unit price	Quantity in 2022	Total price 2022
Adalimumab	Vial	40 mg	360.0	6000	2,160,000
Azathioprine	Tablet	50 mg	0.08	1000	80,000
Cyclophosphamide	Vial	1000 mg	4.16	300	1248
Cyclophosphamide	Vial	200 mg	0.75	70	53
Cyclosporin	Tablet	100 mg	0.60	80,000	48,000
Cyclosporin	Tablet	25 mg	0.18	160,000	28,800
Cyclosporin	Tablet	50 mg	0.34	190,000	64,600
Etanercept	Vial	25 mg	51.15	9000	460,350
Golimumab	Vial	50 mg	800.00	8000	6,400,000
Hydroxychloroquine	Tablet	200 mg	0.80	300,000	240,000
Infliximab	Vial	100 mg	140.00	10,000	1,400,000
Methotrexate	Tablet	2.5 mg	0.08	350,000	28,000
Methylprednisolone	Vial	1000 mg	9.90	7000	69,300
Methylprednisolone	Vial	500 mg	5.00	2500	12,500
Rituximab	Vial	500 mg	517.00	4000	2,068,000
Teriparatide	pen	20μg/80μl	217.55	900	195,795
Tocilizumab	Vial	200 mg	311.00	3000	933,000
Tocilizumab	Vial	400 mg	623.00	3000	1,869,000
Tocilizumab	Vial	80 mg	123.00	3000	369,000
Ustekinumab	Vial	45 mg	2,000	700	14,000,000
					Total: **US $ 25,549,756**

17.15 Implications of the Syrian Crisis

Syria historically developed a relatively strong rheumatology service infrastructure, but the crisis since 2011 has profoundly disrupted these systems, leading to marked regional disparities in clinical service availability, education, and training [30, 31]. Moreover, a significant increase in healthcare professionals' migration has led to a shortage in medical service availability, placing additional strain on an already overburdened system [32].

Remaining healthcare professionals are frequently required to work extended shifts, often exceeding 16 h a day, and manage over 40 patients per shift, which significantly restricts opportunities for comprehensive training and skill development [33].

While there is no specific updated data about the implications of the Syrian crisis on the status of rheumatology across all the different regions of Syria, one recent retrospective study conducted in northwest Syria [20] specifically documented a severe shortage of rheumatologists (with only three specialists serving a population of 5.5 million); disrupted provision and reduced accessibility of rheumatology diagnostic tests due to damaged infrastructure and import restrictions; a significant lack of available and affordable medications, exacerbated by the destruction of pharmaceutical factories; a critical shortage of human resources and trainers in the field; and the high cost and unavailability of many essential rheumatic investigations.

Regarding residency training, a study by Soqia et al. evaluating the impact of war on medical residents' specialty choices found that economic pressures and security concerns have driven many residents to prioritize specialties that facilitate migration [32]. This can suggest that many residents who initially had an interest in internal medicine and rheumatology training may have shifted toward other specialties that better align with their migration goals. For instance, some may opt for fields with fewer shifts and lighter workloads (compared to internal medicine), such as pathology or radiology, to allocate more time for foreign language proficiency and residency examination requirements abroad.

17.16 Challenges and Opportunities

We present here some challenges in the care of patients with rheumatic diseases in Syria.

1. Shortages of Rheumatologists: Syria faces a significant shortage of rheumatologists, limiting access to specialized care for patients with rheumatic diseases.
2. Lack of Specialized Clinics/Programs: There is a notable absence of specialized clinics or programs dedicated to specific rheumatic diseases, impeding comprehensive and tailored care for patients.
3. Insufficient Training for Healthcare Professionals: Currently, there are no formal training programs for nurses or physician assistants specializing in rheumatology, leading to a shortage of skilled healthcare providers in this field.
4. Absence of Accredited Centers of Excellence: Syria lacks accredited centers of excellence for rheumatology, which could serve as hubs for specialized care, research, and education.
5. Limited Research: The country faces challenges in conducting rheumatology research, with limited resources and infrastructure for research initiatives. Additionally, economic challenges since 2011 have further delayed research efforts and medical tourism [34].

Furthermore, there are opportunities for improving the care of patients with rheumatic diseases, such as:

1. Expertise in Specific Diseases: While shortages exist, some rheumatologists in Syria possess expertise in specific rheumatic diseases based on their training and experience. This includes conditions such as systemic lupus erythematosus, SpA, pediatric rheumatology, and more, offering specialized care within the constraints of available resources.
2. Government Support for Medication Access: The MOH plays a pivotal role in providing all DMARDs, including biologics, free of charge for patients in public

hospitals. Additionally, patients in the private sector may receive coverage through insurance companies or other organizations, ensuring access to necessary treatments.

Despite the challenges faced, opportunities exist to improve rheumatic disease care in Syria through strategic investments in training, infrastructure development, and research initiatives. Collaboration between healthcare stakeholders, government agencies, and international partners can help address these challenges and enhance the quality of care for patients with rheumatic diseases.

17.17 The Future of Rheumatic Diseases Care in Syria

Despite the significant strides we have made in recent years, including the establishment of rheumatology as an independent specialty, the implementation of a robust competence-based rheumatology curriculum, and the training of eager and knowledgeable residents, we remain unsatisfied with our achievements. This is because of the limited number of research publications from our region.

While we are unaware of any official plans to enhance rheumatology services in Syria, we believe the path to improving these services for our patients is clear. To achieve this, the following steps must be undertaken promptly.

17.17.1 Improvement of the Education and Training of New Rheumatologists

To ensure that physicians are well-prepared to address the multi-systemic manifestations of rheumatic diseases, we propose that a foundation in internal medicine be a prerequisite for beginning a residency in rheumatology. Trainees should rotate through a reputable university department with a regularly updated curriculum, offering exposure to various educators with different approaches, different patient settings, and rheumatic conditions. Additionally, the importance of accreditation, quality control, and periodic evaluations (every 3–5 years) of educational rheumatology units should be recognized. Furthermore, developing a nationally standardized academic curriculum for all rheumatology training centers is essential.

17.17.2 Training General Practitioners

We share the global concern regarding the shortage of rheumatologists, particularly given the unique challenges faced by rheumatologists, many of whom are females responsible for caring for their families. As a result, a significant number of rheumatic patients are managed by general practitioners whose knowledge of rheumatology may require updating.

To address this issue, it is imperative for the MOH and the Syrian Medical Association to ensure adequate training in rheumatology and provide ongoing medical education for internists and general practitioners. While steps have been taken by the Syrian Medical Association to address this need across all specialties, further efforts are needed to ensure that all healthcare providers are equipped to effectively manage rheumatic conditions.

17.17.3 Patient-Centered Rheumatology Services

Syria stands out as one of the few countries that offer high-quality medical care free of charge to all its citizens, including essential medications for chronic diseases such as biologics. Despite facing significant challenges over the past 13 years, this commitment to accessible healthcare has endured. With improved administrative processes, Syria has the potential to emerge as a leading example in providing comprehensive healthcare to its population.

17.17.4 Research

A more realistic approach to supporting research is necessary, particularly for rheumatologists in public health sectors and universities who serve as the driving force for research. Financial support is essential to enable them to dedicate adequate time to research. Additionally, implementing electronic medical records is crucial for data collection, streamlining appropriate data gathering, and serving as valuable tools for ongoing quality enhancement. Training medical secretaries and nurses in research will significantly contribute to this effort. Regrettably, the absence of dedicated rheumatology nurses in these centers raises concerns about potential burnout among rheumatologists. Despite these challenges, we believe that with genuine efforts, our already active health institutions in Syria have the potential to transform the quality of our healthcare system positively. We hope that rheumatologists in Syria will be integral to driving this reform forward.

17.18 Conclusion

Syria, a small country abundant in resources, practices medicine and rheumatology according to the latest recommendations. While clinical rheumatology is advancing, research progress remains limited due to economic and administrative challenges.

Notably, Syria is one of the rare nations offering quality medical care to all its citizens free of charge, including biologics for chronic diseases, under the Ministry of Health.

With the establishment of the Syrian Board for Medical Specialties, aspiring rheumatologists undergo rigorous evaluation through written and clinical exams administered by the scientific committee. Approximately 4–5 new rheumatologists are inducted into the field of rheumatology annually. It is worth mentioning that pediatric rheumatology is still in its early developmental stages.

Improving the education and training of new rheumatologists and general practitioners and fostering research are essential for shaping the hopeful future of rheumatic disease care and perspectives in Syria despite the numerous challenges in providing proper rheumatology services.

Conflict of Interest Declaration The authors declare they have no conflicts of interest.

References

1. Wikipedia. Demographics in Syria [Internet]. Last Updated 2026 Jun 7 [cited 2026 Jun 15]. Available from: https://en.wikipedia.org/wiki/Demographics_of_Syria#cite_note-41.
2. Wikipedia. Women in Syria [Internet]. Last Updated 2026 Jun 12 [cited 2026 Jun 15]. Available from: https://en.wikipedia.org/wiki/Women_in_Syria#cite_note-6.
3. The Syrian Association for Rheumatology [Internet]. [cited 2026 Jun 15]. Available from: www.rheumatology-syria.com.
4. Kazkaz L. Methylprednisolone pulse therapy in the symptomatic relief of rheumatoid disease. Acta Ther. 1990;16(4):329–35.
5. Kazkaz L, Marotte H, Hamwi M, Angélique Cazalis M, Roy P, Mougin B, Miossec P. Rheumatoid arthritis and genetic markers in Syrian and French populations: different effect of the shared epitope. Ann Rheum Dis. 2007;66(2):195–201. https://doi.org/10.1136/ard.2004.033829. Epub 2006 Oct 26. PMID: 17068065; PMCID: PMC1798494.
6. Okada Y, Diogo D, Greenberg JD, Mouassess F, Achkar WA, Fulton RS, et al. Integration of sequence data from a Consanguineous family with genetic data from an outbred population identifies PLB1 as a candidate rheumatoid arthritis risk gene. PLoS One. 2014;9(2):e87645. https://doi.org/10.1371/journal.pone.0087645. PMID: 24520335; PMCID: PMC3919745.
7. Dargham SR, Zahirovic S, Hammoudeh M, Al Emadi S, Masri BK, Halabi H. Epidemiology and treatment patterns of rheumatoid arthritis in a large cohort of Arab patients. PLoS One. 2018;13(12):e0208240. https://doi.org/10.1371/journal.pone.0208240. Erratum in: PLoS One. 2019; 14(3): e0214258.
8. Harfouch EI, Al-Cheikh SA. HLA-B27 and its subtypes in Syrian patients with ankylosing spondylitis. Saudi Med J. 2011;32(4):364–8.
9. Fouad M, Rastam S, Ward K, Maziak W. Prevalence of obesity and its associated factors in Aleppo, Syria. Prev Control. 2006;2(2):85–94. https://doi.org/10.1016/j.precon.2006.09.001.
10. Valero-Jaimes JA, López-González R, Martín-Martínez MA, García-Gómez C, Sánchez-Alonso F, Sánchez-Costa JT, et al. Body mass index and disease activity in chronic inflammatory rheumatic diseases: results of the cardiovascular in rheumatology (Carma) project. J Clin Med. 2021;10(3):382. https://doi.org/10.3390/jcm10030382.
11. Karadağ ŞG, Sönmez HE, Demir F, Çakan M, Öztürk K, Tanatar A, et al. Rheumatic diseases in Syrian refugee children: a retrospective multicentric study in Turkey. Rheumatol Int. 2020;40(4):583–9. https://doi.org/10.1007/s00296-020-04534-3.

12. Khouri H, Joma M, Al-Cheikh S, et al. Familial Mediterranean fever in the Syrian population: gene mutation frequencies, carrier rates and Mattit phenotype-genotype correlation. Eur J Med Genet. 2006;49(6):481–6. https://doi.org/10.1016/j.ejmg.2006.03.002.
13. Fedorchenko Y, Mahmudov K, Abenov Z, Zimba O, Yessirkepov M. Rehabilitation of patients with inflammatory rheumatic diseases and comorbidities: unmet needs. Rheumatol Int. 2024;44(4):583–91. https://doi.org/10.1007/s00296-023-05529-6.
14. Al Saadi T, Abbas F, Turk T, Alkhatib M, Hanafi I, Alahdab F. Medical research in war-torn Syria: medical students' perspective. Lancet. 2018;391(10139):2497–8. https://doi.org/10.1016/S0140-6736(18)31207-8.
15. Wakitani S, Murata N, Toda Y, Ogawa R, Kaneshige T, et al. The relationship between HLA-DRB1 alleles and disease subsets of rheumatoid arthritis in Japanese. Br J Rheumatol. 1997;36:630–6.
16. Babelly W, Ghrewaty AJ, Dababo MK. Assessing the prevalence of disease-specific antinuclear antibodies and their detection in the diagnosis of rheumatic disorders in Syria. Int J Pharm Sci Nutr. 2022;15(2):5855–62.
17. Khalayli N, Kudsi M. Cross-sectional study of COVID-19 infection in patients with rheumatic diseases in a sample of a Damascene population, Syria. Ann Med Surg (Lond). 2023;85(4):689–93. https://doi.org/10.1097/MS9.0000000000000274.
18. Khalayli N, Shahada Z, Kudsi M, Alcheikh S. Analysis of septic arthritis in a sample of the Syrian population: a retrospective study. Int J Surg Glob Health. 2023;6(5):e 0330. https://doi.org/10.1097/GH9.0000000000000330.
19. Shhada E, Hamdar H, Nahle AA, Mourad D, Khalil B, Ali S. Clinical presentation and management of multisystem inflammatory syndrome in children associated with covid-19: a retrospective observational descriptive study in a pediatric hospital in Syria. BMC Infect Dis. 2024;24(1):322. https://doi.org/10.1186/s12879-024-09197-0.
20. Zakaria W, Ibrahim Y. Rheumatic diseases amidst conflict in northwest Syria: unveiling health challenges and implications. Avicenna J Med. 2024;14(2):115–22. https://doi.org/10.1055/s-0044-1786826.
21. Abir K, Yousser M, Omar D, Alcheikh S. Unusual pulmonary masses in beta thalassemia major. EC Pulmonol Respiratory Med. 2016;2(5):181–6.
22. Hamsho S, Alannouf I, Ashour AA. Rapidly progressive felty syndrome after sudden discontinuation of methotrexate: a case report and review of literature. Int Med Case Rep J. 2022;15:473–7. https://doi.org/10.2147/IMCRJ.S365004.
23. Hamsho S, Alaswad M, Alsmodi H, Sleiay M, Hoha G, Alcheikh S. Idiopathic granulomatous mastitis with extramammary manifestations: a case report. Ann Med Surg (Lond). 2023;85(12):6192–5. https://doi.org/10.1097/MS9.0000000000001397.
24. Kudsi M, Hodaifa Y, Tarcha R, Almajzoub R, Hamsho S, Ghazal A. Glomerulonephritis as a renal manifestation in a patient with systemic sclerosis overlapped with anti-neutrophil cytoplasmic antibody-associated vasculitis. Int J Surg Glob Health. 2024;7(2):e0418. https://doi.org/10.1097/GH9.0000000000000418.
25. Hamsho S, Alaswad M, Makhlouf Z, Alcheikh S. Septal atrial thrombosis as a primary presentation of antiphospholipid syndrome in a patient with ANA-negative systemic lupus erythematosus: a case report. Ann Med Surg (Lond). 2024;86(4):2189–93. https://doi.org/10.1097/MS9.0000000000001668.
26. Alaswad M, Hamsho S, Sultan E, Al-Ibrahim M, Merza A, Al-Baroudi Y. Sulfasalazine's potential in managing rheumatoid nodules: insights from a case report. Medicine (Baltimore). 2024;103(31):e39209. https://doi.org/10.1097/MD.0000000000039209.
27. Assaad N, Khayali N, Kudsi M. Rheumatoid arthritis in Syria: knowledge and awareness among the general population. Res Square. 2022; https://doi.org/10.21203/rs.3.rs-2194091/v2.
28. Hamsho S, Almasri IA, Alaswad M, Sleiay M, Alabdullah H, Aboud M. The association between smoking and clinical and radiological severity in patients with primary knee osteoarthritis: the first cross-sectional study in Syria. Res Square. 2023; https://doi.org/10.21203/rs.3.rs-3515256/v1.

29. Haj Ali D, Kudsi M. Awareness about rheumatic diseases: a survey from a Syrian population. Res Square. 2023; https://doi.org/10.21203/rs.3.rs-2515336/v1.
30. Alhaffar MHDBA, Janos S. Public health consequences after ten years of the Syrian crisis: a literature review. Glob Health. 2021;17:1–11. https://doi.org/10.1186/s12992-021-00762-9.
31. Jabbour S, Leaning J, Nuwayhid I, Ager A, Cammett M, Dewachi O, et al. 10 years of the Syrian conflict: a time to act and not merely to remember. Lancet. 2021;397:1245–8. https://doi.org/10.1016/S0140-6736(21)00623-1.
32. Soqia J, Yakoub-Agha L, Mohamad L, Alhomsi R, Shamaa MA, Yazbek A, et al. Syrian crisis' effect on specialty choice and the decision to work in the country among residents of six major hospitals in Damascus. PLoS One. 2024;19:e0295310. https://doi.org/10.1371/journal.pone.0295310.
33. Abdelrahman S, Haar R. The effect of conflict on healthcare workers in Syria: results of a qualitative survey. Berkeley Sci J. 2021;26(1):79–84. https://doi.org/10.5070/BS326157104.
34. Alnaser H. The challenges facing Syrians and the effects of medical tourism on global economic growth. E3S Web Conf. 2023;420:05007. https://doi.org/10.1051/e3sconf/202342005007.

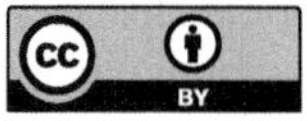

Chapter 18
Rheumatic Diseases in Tunisia

Hiba Boussaa, Hanene Lassoued Ferjani, Saoussen Miladi, Nejla El Amri, Kawther Ben Abdelghani, and Elyes Bouajina

Abstract Rheumatology in Tunisia has expanded in the last decades, with more than 220 specialists, including 142 females, practicing in the private and public sectors. The geographic distribution of rheumatologists needs to be more balanced in favor of coastal cities. More than ten hospital-university rheumatology departments provide practical training to students, residents, and paramedical staff in addition to health care activities. There are three centers of reference dedicated to pediatric rheumatology in our country. Our official rheumatology association is the Tunisian League Against Rheumatism (LITAR), established in 1975. Each year, the LITAR organizes the Tunisian Rheumatology Congress and the National Day of Rheumatology. Tunisians and foreign speakers, especially French and Maghrebians, present high-level scientific conferences, workshops, and updates.

The first Biologic National Registry (BINAR), subsidized by the LITAR, was launched in 2018 and includes more than 500 patients treated with biological disease-modifying anti-rheumatic drugs (DMARDs) for rheumatoid arthritis and spondyloarthritis.

Rheumatic and musculoskeletal disorders (RMDs) are prevalent in Tunisia, and their prevalence can reach one-third of the population. Extensive studies estimating the incidence and prevalence of chronic inflammatory rheumatism in our country still need to be conducted. Osteoarthritis is the most frequent disease. Post-menopausal osteoporosis is a widespread disease in Tunisia, as at least 16% of women over 50

H. Boussaa · S. Miladi · K. Ben Abdelghani (✉)
Faculty of Medicine of Tunis, University of Tunis El Manar, Tunis, Tunisia

Department of Rheumatology, Mongi Slim University Hospital, Tunis, Tunisia
e-mail: hibaboussaa@gmail.com; saoussenmiladi@gmail.com; kawther_ba@yahoo.fr

H. Lassoued Ferjani
Department of Rheumatology, Mohamed Kassab Institute of Orthopedics, La Manouba, and Faculty of Medicine of Tunis, University of Tunis El Manar, Tunis, Tunisia
e-mail: lassouedferjanihanene@gmail.com

N. El Amri · E. Bouajina
University of Sousse, Faculty of Medicine of Sousse, Department of Rheumatology, Farhat Hached University Hospital, Sousse, Tunisia
e-mail: elamri_nejla@yahoo.fr; elyes.bouajina@rns.tn

K. A. Alnaqbi, G. Aldabie (eds.), *Rheumatic Diseases in the Arab World*,
https://doi.org/10.1007/978-981-92-0967-5_18

have experienced one or more fractures. A strong partnership exists between rheumatologists, immunologists, genetic specialists, physical and rehabilitation physicians, orthopedists, internists, ophthalmologists, dermatologists, and gastroenterologists. The availability of musculoskeletal radiologists is limited, primarily due to their significant immigration to other countries. Thankfully, musculoskeletal ultrasonography is available in all rheumatology departments. Synthetic, biological, and targeted DMARDs are available in our country. Access to specific treatments requires enrollment in the national health insurance fund or an access program. Our four faculties of medicine provide 20 training programs related to rheumatology. The first postgraduate training program in pediatric rheumatology in Tunisia and the first Francophone program in Africa have been recently established. Furthermore, a master's degree program has been introduced to provide training in ultrasonography.

Keywords Tunisia · Rheumatic diseases · Rheumatology · Arthritis · Biological Therapy · Antirheumatic Agents · Health Services Accessibility · Health Workforce · Medical Education

18.1 Country Demographics

18.1.1 Geographic Data

Tunisia is located in North Africa and covers an area of 63,170 square miles (163,610 km^2) [1]. Its Western border begins in Algeria (965 km), and its southeastern border is in Libya (459 km). Tunisia is also divided into six geographical regions. These regions are Northeast Tunisia, Greater Tunisia, Northwest Tunisia, Central-West Tunisia, Central-East Tunisia, and South Tunisia. The southern part of Tunisia is semi-arid, changing to an arid desert near the Sahara Desert. Tunisia also has a fertile coastal plain, the Sahel, along the eastern Mediterranean coast. The urban network is between the capital, Tunis, and the Sahel on the eastern coastal strip. Tunisia is divided into 24 governorates, the governorates being the highest administrative unit. The governorates are subdivided into 264 districts. Among the districts, there are municipalities.

18.1.2 Demographic Data

Tunisia's population was 12,048,847 in 2024, divided into 49.6% men and 50.4% women [2]. The northern and central cities, where the most significant economic hub is based, account for 61% of the total population. In contrast, only 14.5% of Tunisians are in the south.

18.2 Country Healthcare Sectors

The Tunisian health system consists of two main sectors: the public and private sectors, both of which have experienced significant growth since the 1990s. The public system is structured into three levels to provide comprehensive healthcare services. At the first level, primary health care is delivered through basic health centers, district hospitals, and maternity wards. This level has been instrumental in improving access to primary healthcare in underserved areas. However, the potential of district hospitals is limited by the need for additional technical capacity [3]. The second level consists of regional hospitals, which face challenges in terms of productivity due to a shortage of specialist physicians. The third level encompasses universities, 24 teaching hospitals, centers, and specialized institutes, which provide advanced medical education and specialized care.

The private health system consists of 3101 general practitioners and 3614 specialists (49% of doctors in Tunisia) working in private clinics and medical centers (unpublished data from the Ministry of Health). The private sector benefits from Tunisia's high-quality medical resources and uses health tourism as a new source of income for the country.

18.3 Rheumatology Health Sectors

The number of rheumatologists in Tunisia has steadily increased (Fig. 18.1). Currently, there are more than 200 specialists in rheumatology practice in our country.

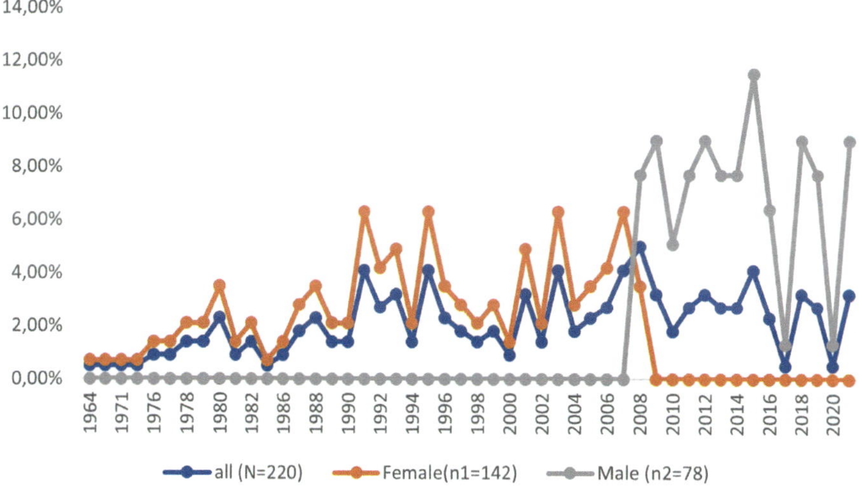

Fig. 18.1 Rheumatologist's number per year. (Unpublished data from the Ministry of Health)

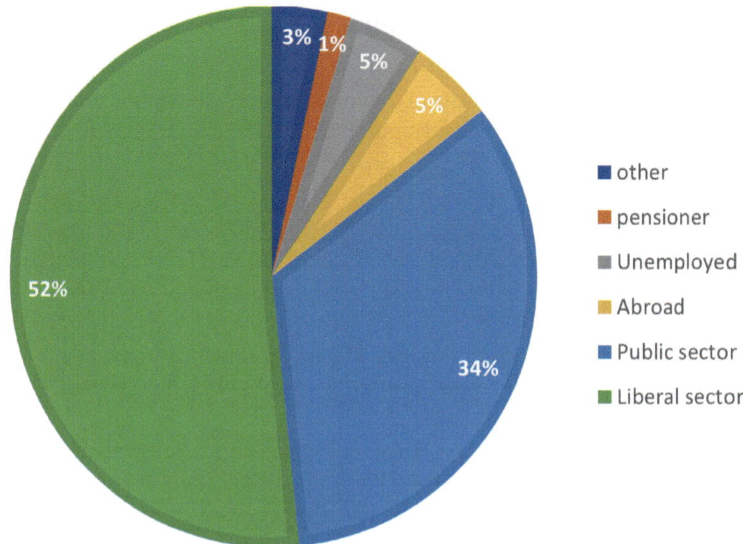

Fig. 18.2 Distribution of the rheumatologists according to the work sector. (Unpublished data from the Ministry of Health)

As shown in Fig. 18.2, the distribution of rheumatologists is divided into four sectors: the public sector, the private or liberal sector, retired rheumatologists (pensioners), and those currently unemployed. More than half of the rheumatologists work in the private sector. Additionally, females predominate the rheumatology specialty, accounting for approximately 65% of rheumatologists.

The geographic distribution of rheumatologists is highly imbalanced in favor of coastal cities (Fig. 18.3). According to unpublished data from the Ministry of Health, the governorate of Greater Tunis accounts for the highest number of rheumatologists distributed as follows: 54.2% work in free practice, 16.2% in university hospitals, and 8.5% in public hospitals. Sousse and Monastir, the greatest governorates of the Sahel, account for a quarter of the rheumatologists with the same sector distribution (17 in public hospitals and 24 in private clinics).

18.3.1 Rheumatology Centers Distribution

The rheumatology departments of hospital universities are based in the major cities of the capital and the Sahel. In Tunis, five rheumatology departments serve patients from the north and the northwest. At the levels of Sahel's significant cities, represented by Sousse, Monastir, Mahdia, and Sfax, rheumatology departments are located near the corresponding faculty of medicine and welcome patients from central and southern Tunisia.

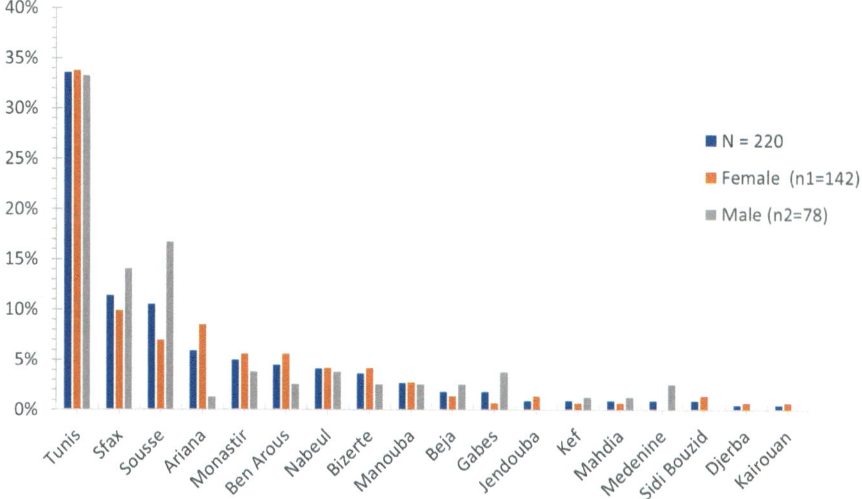

Fig. 18.3 Rheumatologist density in Tunisia's governorate. (Unpublished data from the Ministry of Health)

18.3.2 Rheumatology Center Activities

Education:
University hospital departments are mandatory in the practical training of students, residents, and paramedical staff. Indeed, bedside teaching is a vital component of medical education and one of the most effective ways to learn clinical and communication skills. Moreover, interdepartmental and interdisciplinary staff provide opportunities for mutual exchange of experience and improvement of knowledge [4, 5].

Healthcare:
University hospital departments, in addition to their academic pursuits, offer a range of medical services to patients daily. These services include consultations, short- and long-term hospitalizations, and a variety of medical procedures. Among these procedures are intra-articular injections, musculoskeletal ultrasound (MSUS), acupuncture, mesotherapy, and therapeutic education.

Research activities:
Research units within university hospital departments conduct extensive experimental, longitudinal, and epidemiological studies, which are reimbursed by the Ministry of Health.

Pediatric rheumatology in Tunisia:
Pediatric rheumatology has been introduced recently in Tunisia. Currently, there are three centers of referrals dedicated to pediatric rheumatology. They are located in the capital and receive patients from the center and the south of the country. The first two centers specialize in rheumatic diseases of pediatric and adult patients.

Additionally, they offer outpatient consultations, day clinics, and hospitalization, especially for children with rheumatic, autoinflammatory, and bone diseases. Conventional DMARDs (cDMARDs) are available in these centers. However, only three biologics are approved for children (tocilizumab, etanercept, and adalimumab), and a coordinated response from the National Health Insurance Fund (CNAM) is required. The third center, Bechir Hamza Hospital, specializes in pediatric diseases.

Through the collaborative efforts of rheumatologists and pediatricians, the Faculty of Medicine of Tunis created the first postgraduate training program in pediatric rheumatology in Tunisia and the first Francophone training in Africa in 2021. The first class consisted of 30 learners (Tunisians and Africans) working as pediatricians, rheumatologists, and orthopedic surgeons in the public and private sectors. This theoretical and practical training, taught exclusively online, will undoubtedly be essential in developing pediatric rheumatology in Tunisia and Africa.

Pediatric rheumatology is actively expanding its presence in Africa. The first initiative began in 2019 with the establishment of the Pediatric Society of the African League Against Rheumatism (PAFLAR) [6]. Members of this African society, including Tunisian rheumatologists, are actively involved in academic training. To promote research activities and to determine clinical characteristics of pediatric rheumatology, the PAFLAR working group established the first African registry for patients with juvenile idiopathic arthritis in December 2021. Tunisia has a notable presence in this group through its rheumatologists.

The Juvenile Inflammatory Rheumatism (JIR) Cohort, established in 2013, is an international network that facilitates collaboration between rheumatology departments in European countries and two Tunisian centers. This network comprises physicians from 11 Francophone countries, offering participating centers academic learning and research opportunities. In October 2019, collaboration between the JIR centers and Tunisian departments began, and they are currently working on publishing their first paper [7].

Tunisian pediatric rheumatologists are also participating in the second edition of the Sister Hospital Initiative organized by the Pediatric Rheumatology European Society (PRES). This initiative aligns with PReS's mission to advance care and enhance the health and well-being of children and young people with rheumatic conditions. Furthermore, it embodies the ethos of the Global Musculoskeletal Task Force, which emphasizes the importance of collaboration and learning from one another.

This proposal brought together a Tunisian pediatric rheumatology center to share its expertise and experience with the European center. It was an excellent opportunity to explore the differences between the health systems of the involved hospitals, learn about organizational aspects of managing children with rheumatic diseases, and facilitate knowledge exchange to explore the possibilities for more comprehensive and concrete treatments [8].

18.4 Official Rheumatology Association

The Tunisian League Against Rheumatism (LITAR), founded in 1975, is a not-for-profit professional association committed to advancing the rheumatology specialty. The LITAR aims to promote knowledge concerning rheumatic and musculoskeletal disorders (RMDs) and study general interest problems relating to epidemiology, prevention, and education for patients with RMDs.

The LITAR has gradually organized and structured itself to empower the development and progress of the specialty. With 220 members, the LITAR intends to be a place of gathering and exchanging information. Administrators, universities, hospitals, or liberal rheumatologists rely on a board of nine members to make strategic and administrative decisions.

The communication of high-level scientific information emerging from Tunisian research and the collaboration of our French-speaking guests mainly pass through the Tunisian Congress of Rheumatology and the National Day of Rheumatology. Achievement of quality continuing education is also supported by regular participation in international congresses organized by the French Society of Rheumatology (SFR), the European Alliance of Associations for Rheumatology (EULAR), and the American College of Rheumatology (ACR).

The Tunisian Congress of Rheumatology annually hosts over 100 participants for scientific sessions, including plenary presentations and e-poster presentations, as well as practical workshops and symposiums organized in collaboration with pharmaceutical industry partners. The LITAR provides registration and accommodation support for rheumatology residents.

The National Day of Rheumatology takes place annually in one of our coastal towns to attract a growing number of young rheumatologists. The event offers interactive training sessions and scientific presentations highlighting the latest advances in rheumatic diseases. The aim is to actively engage participants and provide them with valuable knowledge and insights, fostering their interest and passion for rheumatology.

The LITAR also organizes open days to facilitate meetings between rheumatologists and patients and raise awareness about the most common types of RMDs, such as osteoarthritis, chronic inflammatory diseases, osteoporosis, and gout. Illustrations, quizzes, and role-playing games are used to facilitate the transmission of critical messages.

One notable accomplishment of the LITAR was the creation of the Biologic National Registry (BINAR) in 2018, which served as the first Tunisian registry. It encompasses patients with rheumatoid arthritis (RA) or spondyloarthritis (SpA) who have received their initial biologic disease-modifying anti-rheumatic drug (bDMARD) within the last 2 years. The registry includes 500 patients who have been assessed for disease activity parameters, maintenance of therapy, and any adverse events over 2 years.

The official website of the LITAR offers access to the latest national conferences and supports continuing medical training through clinical and radiological quizzes.

The website also provides an agenda of national and international events and current master's degrees in rheumatology. Awareness videos and practical information about RMDs are also available [9].

In the coming years, LITAR will encounter several challenges, one of which involves optimizing the use of modern communication tools like social media. This effort aims to strengthen the reputation and significance of rheumatology while improving patient care. Another challenge is keeping pace with scientific advancements, which will require significant investment in top-notch research, particularly to support young rheumatologists.

18.5 Overview of Rheumatic Diseases in Tunisia

18.5.1 Musculoskeletal Manifestations

A prospective cross-sectional survey of a Tunisian population was conducted in 2005 in collaboration with the National Institute of Public Health, encompassing all Tunisian regions. The Community Oriented Program for Control of Rheumatic Diseases (COPCORD) Stage I was implemented in households across urban and rural areas. Primary healthcare workers administered the World Health Organization and the International League of Associations for Rheumatology (WHO-ILAR) core questionnaire during the final home visit of the survey. Overall, 1582 subjects were included. The mean age was 36.7 years. There was a positive correlation between age and musculoskeletal manifestations. The prevalence of musculoskeletal pain was 31.1% in the studied sample and 38.7% among the 1280 persons over 15 years old. Women were significantly affected more frequently (43.2%) than men (29.1%). There was no significant difference between urban and rural populations. The most symptomatic sites were the knees (19.3%), lumbar spine (15.9%), and shoulders (8.7%). About 60% of symptomatic subjects had a functional disability, and 16.2% stopped working [10].

18.5.2 Rheumatoid Arthritis (RA)

RA is a chronic inflammatory disease with widespread synovial joint involvement that predominantly affects peripheral joints. The most recent data show that the global RA prevalence estimate was 0.46% [11].

In 2001, a prospective survey was conducted in the northern region of Tunisia to determine the prevalence of RA [12]. The survey involved 18,000 individuals aged 15 years and above residing in the Tebourba district. Out of the 13,102 respondents, 200 were identified as potential cases of RA and were subsequently referred to two rheumatologists for further evaluation. Among these individuals, 26 were diagnosed with RA based on the revised 1987 ACR, resulting in a prevalence rate of 0.18% [0.16–0.2]. The average age of the diagnosed patients was 58.6 years, ranging from 24 to 80 years. The mean age at disease onset was 51.4 years, ranging from 18 to 72 years. Of the 26 patients, 77% had received a diagnosis of RA and were receiving DMARDs as part of their treatment. The prevalence of RA was significantly higher among women (0.35% vs. 0.01% in men, $p < 0.001$) and individuals residing in urban areas (0.35% vs. 0.01% in rural areas, $p < 0.001$). However, it is essential to acknowledge some limitations of this survey. The screening process for suspected RA patients involved only hand X-rays and rheumatoid factor, without evaluating the more specific anti-citrullinated protein antibodies (ACPA). The 2010 ACR/EULAR criteria had not yet been established at the time of the survey. These limitations may have led to an underestimation of the prevalence of RA in Tunisia.

18.5.3 Spondyloarthritis (SpA)

Despite the lack of epidemiologic studies estimating the incidence and prevalence of SpA disease in Tunisia, it is commonly considered a public health problem due to its apparent frequency and severity. Indeed, a study conducted in the Public Health Service of Monastir, including 50 patients with SpA, showed a major socioeconomic burden and significant impact on patients' quality of life [13].

An interesting and recent study was conducted in a single rheumatology center in Tunisia. It included 200 patients with axial SpA, fulfilling the 2009 Assessment of SpondyloArthritis International Society (ASAS) criteria to determine their clinical and radiological characteristics in Tunisian patients. One hundred and sixty (80%) patients had ankylosing spondylitis (AS), and 40 (20%) patients had non-radiographic axial SpA (nr-axSpA). Patients with nr-axSpA were significantly younger, with a mean age of 39.4 years compared to 44.3 years in the ankylosing spondylitis (AS) group ($p = 0.03$). Male gender was less frequent in nr-axSpA patients (52.5% versus 73.1%; $p = 0.01$). A family history of SpA was reported more frequently in patients with nr-axSpA compared to patients with AS (20% versus 6.2%; $p = 0.007$). The frequency of HLA-B27 positivity was similar between the nr-axSpA and AS groups. The symptom duration was significantly shorter in the nr-axSpA group (10.1 versus 17.5 years; $p < 0.0001$). Patients with nr-axSpA had a higher prevalence of enthesitis than AS patients (45% vs. 15.6%; $p < 0.0001$). There was no significant difference between the two groups in peripheral arthritis, dactylitis, and uveitis. However, coxitis was more frequently complicated in AS patients than in nr-axSpA patients (40.6% vs. 19.3%; $p = 0.02$) [14].

In another study, which included 165 Tunisian patients with SpA, hip involvement was noted in 36.4% of cases and bilateral in 27.3% of cases. The following parameters were associated with coxitis: age over 40 (OR = 2.688 [1.020–7.083],

$p = 0.045$), radiographic sacroiliitis (OR = 5.656 [1.007–31.769], $p = 0.049$), and very high disease activity (OR = 5.328 [1.774–16.002], $p = 0.003$) [15].

18.5.4 Osteoarthritis (OA)

In 2019, the WHO estimated that around 528 million people worldwide live with osteoarthritis. Those over 55 years old account for 73% of those with the condition, and females make up 60%. OA can affect any joint but is most common in the hips, knees, hands, feet, and spine [16].

A prospective survey on a representative sample of the national population was conducted in 2001 in the north of Tunisia to determine the prevalence of knee and hip OA [17, 18]. A random selection was made from the population over 40 years living in the district of Tebourba. One thousand participants were evaluated for hip OA, and 300 for knee OA. In the second step, patients suspected of OA were referred for clinical and X-ray examinations. The prevalence of knee OA was about 25%. Women were more frequently affected (30.6% vs. 21.9%), but the difference was insignificant. The prevalence of knee OA increased significantly with age ($p < 0.0001$). People between 70 and 79 were the most affected (55.2%). It was more frequent among the rural population, but the difference was not statistically significant. Knee OA was unilateral in 78% of cases. It involved most frequently the medial femorotibial compartment (75%). The prevalence of radiographic knee OA was 32%. The prevalence of hip OA was 6.3%. Men were more frequently affected than women (8.9% vs. 5.3%), but the difference was insignificant. The prevalence of hip OA was higher in people aged between 60 and 69 years (7.3%). It was more frequent among the urban population, but the difference was not statistically significant. Hip OA was unilateral in 68% of cases. The prevalence of radiographic hip OA was 24.4%.

18.5.5 Osteoporosis

Osteoporosis is a condition marked by reduced bone density and the deterioration of bone tissue structure, leading to greater vulnerability to fractures and weakened bones. Hip fracture is the most detrimental event, associated with 20% mortality and 50% permanent loss of function. In Tunisia, a cross-sectional survey was conducted between 2001 and 2003, and it included 1123 women ages more than 45 years, randomly selected from Ariana and Manouba governorates. Participants underwent a bone mineral density (BMD) test using dual-energy X-ray absorptiometry (DEXA). The mean age was 59.3 years. Ninety-six women reported fractures after low-energy trauma. The most frequent sites of fractures were the wrist (85%), the hip (6%), the humerus (6%), and the vertebrae (2%). The mean BMD was

0.903 g/cm^2 in the lumbar spine and 0.912 g/cm^2 in the femoral neck. The prevalence of osteoporosis was 24%. The mean age among osteoporotic women was 67.2 years. The history of fractures was significantly higher in women with osteoporosis compared to women with a normal BMD (24% vs. 12.9%, $p < 0.001$) [19]. It is essential to mention that this study was based on a Tunisian BMD reference curve established in 2001 following a national survey that included 1033 healthy women over 20 years old. This has prevented misdiagnosis of osteoporosis in 2.1% with the Middle Eastern curve and overestimates in 8.2–12% with the Western curve [20].

A prospective study was conducted to determine the prevalence of osteoporotic fractures in the country and better understand the extent of this problem. The study randomly selected a sample of women over 50 from the population of Manouba. Fractures occurring after low-energy trauma in the femoral neck, wrist, or proximal humerus were recorded, while vertebral fractures were identified through lateral X-rays of the thoracolumbar spine. The study included 1311 women with an average age of 64.07 years, and the average age at menopause was 48.29 years. Among these women, 212 (16.2%) had experienced a fracture in one of the specified locations. Vertebral fractures accounted for approximately 60% of all fractures, while wrist fractures comprised 32%, proximal femoral fractures 4.5%, and proximal humeral fractures 3.7% [21].

A more recent study was conducted to assess the prevalence of asymptomatic vertebral fracture (VF) among high-risk Tunisian postmenopausal women. Participants were referred for BMD assessment and a vertebral fracture assessment scan using DEXA. Two hundred and ten postmenopausal women were included. The overall prevalence of VF was 26.2%, and approximately 10% had multiple VFs. The prevalence of VF was significantly higher in older participants, those having a history of prior severe fragility fracture or at least one intrinsic fall [22].

The incidence of fractures of the upper extremity of the femur in Tunisia was also estimated in 2001 through a prospective multicenter study [23]. The overall incidence rate was 74.4 per 100,000 inhabitants per year, with rates of 80.4 for women and 68.4 for men. When considering the fractures of low-energy trauma occurring in people over 50 years old, which reflect osteoporotic fractures, the incidence was 213.5 per 100,000 per year. However, this data had only been evaluated at one center in the capital.

The risk of mortality after fractures is strongly associated with factors such as advanced age (over 90 years), the presence of other medical conditions, and the instability of the fracture. In a study that examined 100 consecutive trochanteric fractures in patients aged 60–96 years, it was found that the estimated mortality rate after 2 years was 28%. The study also observed several complications, including 4 cases of thromboembolism, 14 complications related to immobility, 2 infections, 6 secondary displacements resulting in loss of fixation, four non-unions, and 9 unions. Secondary and late complications significantly impacted functional outcomes ($p = 0.046$) [24].

18.6 Risk Factors for Rheumatic Diseases in Tunisia

18.6.1 Rheumatoid Arthritis (RA)

RA is well known to be influenced by environmental and genetic factors, particularly the human leucocyte antigen (HLA) system. In 2016, a study investigated the association of HLA class II DRB1 and DQB1 alleles and DRB1-DQB1 haplotypes with RA susceptibility in Tunisian subjects. One hundred and ten RA patients and 116 controls were included. The study confirmed the association of HLA-DRB1*04, specifically the HLA-DRB1*04:05 subtype, and DRB1*04-DQB1*03 haplotype with RA susceptibility in Tunisians [25].

A previous study also showed a positive association of HLA-DRB1*04 and HLA-DRB1*10 with RA and significant associations with the disease severity in the south Tunisian population [26].

Moreover, another study showed that the shared epitope (SE) QRRAA expressed in DRBI*04 alleles is related to the susceptibility to RA in Tunisia (OR = 2.03, $p = 0.039$). However, it was not found to be involved in the severity of RA [27].

18.6.2 Spondyloarthritis (SpA)

In 2009, a case-control study that included 100 consecutive Tunisian patients (85 males and 15 females with a mean age of 38.4 years) with AS according to the modified New York criteria and 100 control individuals revealed the presence of HLA-B27 in 62% of patients against 3% in controls ($p = 0.0000$, OR = 52.6, $15.6 < CI < 166.7$) [28].

Clinical, radiographic, and biologic characteristics of AS patients were also assessed. A comparison of the HLA-B27-positive and HLA-B27-negative patients revealed that HLA-B27 was correlated with age, male sex, family history of SpA, age at disease onset, acute onset, spinal involvement at presentation, uveitis, bilateral and destructive hip arthritis, and high modified Sharp/van der Heijde scoring system (modified Stoke Ankylosing Spondylitis Spine Score, mSASSS), which is a radiographic scoring method used to assess the progression of structural damage in AS [29].

Similar results were found in Sfax, the second largest city of Tunisia, located in the southwest, with a population of nearly 900,000. Eighty-five patients diagnosed with AS ($n = 68$) and reactive arthritis ($n = 17$) were selected and compared with 100 healthy controls. A significantly increased frequency of HLA-B27 in 62.4% of SpA patients was noted (OR = 53.55). The most frequent association was observed for HLA-B27 in AS (OR = 52.23). All patients' mean age at symptom onset was 30 years, revealing a slightly younger mean age (28 years) for HLA-B27-positive patients (33 years). HLA-B27 was significantly higher in men than women (85% vs. 15%, $p = 0.03$) [30].

18.6.3 Osteoarthritis (OA)

In the Tunisian population, the prevalence of knee OA increased with age ($p < 0.0001$), body mass index ($p = 0.048$), and a history of trauma ($p = 0.03$). Smokers suffered more from knee OA (29.2% vs. 27.8%), but the difference was insignificant [17].

The prevalence of hip OA was significantly higher among older men ($p < 0.0001$). Body mass index, smoking, and trauma were not associated with hip OA [18].

18.6.4 Osteoporosis

A Tunisian cross-sectional study enrolled 134 osteoporotic menopausal women aged 50 years or more to evaluate the frequency of hypovitaminosis D. The latter was found in 45.2% of all women and was significantly more frequent among women with fractures (51% vs. 25%, $p < 0.01$). BMD in femoral and lumbar sites was statistically lower in women with fractures ($p < 0.001$) [31].

Genetic factors play a role in determining BMD, a surrogate osteoporosis measure. The vitamin D receptor (VDR) was the initial gene investigated as a potential candidate linked to BMD in adult individuals and those experiencing bone loss after menopause. VDR polymorphisms ApaI and TaqI were analyzed in 566 postmenopausal Tunisian women. The GG ApaI genotype ($p = 0.02$; OR = 1.86) and the TT TaqI polymorphism ($p = 0.02$; OR = 1.53) were associated with osteopenia development but not osteoporosis. The GG ApaI genotype was associated with a 3-fold higher risk of vertebral fractures [32].

The receptor activator of nuclear factor kappa B ligand (RANK-L) stimulates bone resorption by activating RANK signaling. Therefore, it is considered a candidate gene regulating susceptibility to osteoporosis. Polymorphic sites in the RANK-L gene (rs9533155 -693G > C and rs9533156 -643C > T polymorphisms) were determined in 566 postmenopausal Tunisian women. This study demonstrated the association of the -643C > T polymorphism with BMD variation and osteoporosis risk ($p = 0.01$; OR = 2.15) in postmenopausal Tunisian women [33].

18.7 Screening Programs for Rheumatic Diseases

Rheumatic diseases are responsible for increased morbidity with severe socioeconomic consequences. In Tunisia, national efforts are being made to promote the dissemination of information and raise awareness about RMDs.

Training courses on the most common RMDs are regularly offered to general practitioners working at primary health centers to help them recognize these conditions. Round table discussions are organized with related specialists such as orthopedic surgeons, dermatologists, ophthalmologists, and gastroenterologists to increase their awareness about the appropriate timing to refer patients to rheumatologists. In order to bring consistency to the identification process, Tunisian guidelines have been introduced to determine the specific circumstances under which a patient should be considered a possible case of SpA [34]. Consequently, the patient must be referred to a rheumatologist for further assessment. Similarly, an update of the recommendations for rheumatoid arthritis is currently being elaborated.

Furthermore, health caravans are organized nationwide, particularly in underserved villages, to reach individuals who may be suffering from RMDs but lack access to medical care. These caravans are often covered by the media to enhance their effectiveness. Young rheumatologists actively participate in these events, where people undergo screening through interviews and clinical examinations. They are referred to the nearest rheumatology department in case of need for additional investigations. As a result of these medical caravans, many patients are now being accurately diagnosed and receiving consistent follow-up care for their RMDs.

However, specific and standardized screening programs for rheumatic diseases do not exist in Tunisia. This is probably due to the heterogeneity of clinical presentations and the diversity of the affected sites. Moreover, such programs need financial support, which allows the prescription of immunological and imaging tests on a larger scale.

18.8 Diagnostic Services for Rheumatic Diseases in Tunisia

18.8.1 Laboratory Services

In Tunisia, the public health sector comprises eight immunology departments (four in Tunis, one each in Ariana, Sousse, Monastir, and Sfax) and three genetic departments (two in Tunis and one in Sfax). Collaboration with these specialties is essential in daily practice. Routine rheumatology tests, such as HLA typing, autoantibody testing, hepatitis, human immunodeficiency virus (HIV) serology, and MEFV mutations, are commonly performed. However, certain tests may be unavailable, particularly for rare bone diseases. In such cases, samples are sent to France through a collaborative framework between the two countries.

18.8.2 Imaging Services

In recent decades, musculoskeletal ultrasound (MSUS) has attracted significant interest among rheumatologists. Indeed, MSUS emerged as a helpful tool in diagnosing and monitoring rheumatic diseases, with the advantage of being accessible, reproducible, and well-accepted by patients. In Tunisia, MSUS is available in all rheumatology departments. Rheumatologists and residents have been gradually trained since the introduction of a master's degree called "Ultrasonography in Rheumatology" in 2018 at the Faculty of Medicine of Tunis. This training program also introduces learners to ultrasound-guided interventions.

According to the latest data published by the Tunisian Ministry of Health in 2021, the country accounts for 198 computed tomography (CT) scans and 66 magnetic resonance imaging (MRI) devices. Seventy-four percent of both examinations are located in the private sector [35].

The total number of positron emission tomography (PET) scans in Tunisia is four. The first one was introduced in 2016 in a private clinic in the capital. Then, three public hospitals in Tunis, Sousse, and Sfax were equipped with PET scans. This acquisition offers optimal medical care for cancer and vasculitis patients.

Musculoskeletal radiology is quite limited in Tunisia. Only two centers specialized in osteoarticular diseases: the Mohamed Kassab National Institute of Orthopedics in Manouba and the Center for Traumatology and Major Burns in Ben Arous. These centers employ eight radiologists. There are approximately 10 musculoskeletal radiologists in the private sector.

18.9 Management of Rheumatic Diseases in Tunisia

18.9.1 Availability of Antirheumatic Medications

cDMARDs such as methotrexate (oral route) and sulfasalazine are usually available at hospitals and primary health centers. Antimalarial drugs and azathioprine are also available in these structures. These medications are only delivered on medical prescriptions.

Methotrexate (injection route), leflunomide, bDMARDs, and targeted synthetic DMARDs require a request for reimbursement from CNAM. The CNAM accounts for 54 regional and local centers distributed across all the governorates of Tunisia. Processing of patients' files takes 2–3 weeks. When the response is favorable, patients can withdraw their treatment from the polyclinics of the National Social Security Fund (CNSS). There are six polyclinics in Tunis: Bizerte, Sousse, Sfax, and Gafsa. This procedure needs to be renewed every 6 months.

In 2018, an access program was established with the pharmaceutical industry partners to provide biologics to patients who require this treatment but are not affiliated with the CNAM.

18.9.2 Access to Multidisciplinary Specialties

All rheumatology departments have rehabilitation centers, including physiotherapy, exercise training, and occupational therapy. Patients can also be referred to one of the five physical and rehabilitation medicine departments in Tunis: Sousse, Monastir, and Sfax.

There are two pediatric orthopedic departments at the Bechir Hamza Children's Hospital and the Mohamed Kassab National Institute of Orthopedics, both in Tunis. Orthopedic departments are also available in all the university hospitals in Tunisia. A strong partnership exists between rheumatologists, internists, ophthalmologists, dermatologists, and gastroenterologists.

A total of 10 occupational departments are available in Tunisia and distributed as follows: five in Tunis, two in Sousse, one in Monastir, one in Mahdia, and one in Sfax.

18.10 Education and Research

18.10.1 Education

There are four faculties of medicine in Tunisia. The oldest is the Faculty of Medicine of Tunis, founded in 1964. Each faculty offers training to approximately 2000 students annually. After 5 years of medicine, students sit for a national specialty contest called "residency in medicine" to choose a medical, surgical, or fundamental specialty. Four rheumatology positions were open per year. Since 2017, the number of positions has increased threefold, and the number of rheumatologists per promotion has increased 12-fold annually.

The faculties offer specialized training for rheumatology residents through college courses, post-university training, and postgraduate certifications throughout their academic journey. Postgraduate training programs enhance professional skills, lead to better patient outcomes, and promote the application of evidence-based procedures. The faculties provide 20 training programs, as highlighted in Table 18.1. Candidates must choose only one program per year.

Apart from postgraduate rheumatology training, other training programs are available for hospital-university doctors, including pedagogy, biostatistics, artificial intelligence, simulation, therapeutic education, telemedicine, and medical English.

18.10.2 Research

In recent years, there has been a remarkable surge in medical research in Tunisia. This growth can be attributed to the increased accessibility of resources, which has facilitated a revolution in research and made it possible to publish articles in international journals since 2000.

According to ShanghaiRanking 2021, the University of Tunis El Manar ranked among the top 900-1000 universities globally for the fourth consecutive year [36]. It also achieved a subject ranking of 401–500 in Clinical Medicine. The university is the top-ranked institution in Tunisia [37].

Table 18.1 Rheumatology training programs in Tunisia

	Faculty of Medicine of Sfax	Faculty of Medicine of Monastir	Faculty of Medicine of Sousse	Faculty of Medicine of Tunis
Training Programs	Podiatry Musculoskeletal Tumors Immunotherapy (Biotherapy) in Auto-immune and Inflammatory Diseases Imaging in Musculoskeletal Diseases Musculoskeletal Ultrasonography Chronic Pain and Palliative Care	Podiatry Spine Pathology Immunotherapy in Tumoral and Inflammatory Diseases Geriatrics	Management of Systemic Diseases and Auto-immunes Geriatrics Musculoskeletal Anatomy Assessment and Treatment of Pain	Podiatry Musculoskeletal Diseases in Children and Adolescent Geriatrics Imaging in Musculoskeletal Diseases Ultrasonography in Rheumatology Management of Chronic Pain

Notably, the University of Tunis El Manar is the sole representative of the Maghreb region among the 18 African universities and the 15 universities from Arab countries listed in the ranking. Additionally, the University of Tunis El Manar is ranked number one in Tunisia and the Maghreb region. In terms of specific disciplines, the university has achieved commendable rankings of 401–500 in clinical medicine and 301–400 in public health [36].

The number of articles published in the field of rheumatology is steadily growing. As of September 2025, a PubMed search yielded over 294 papers (171 related to RA, 88 focusing on SpA, and 35 on osteoporosis). The manuscripts are published in indexed journals such as "Rheumatology," "Joint Bone Spine," "Clinical Experimental Rheumatology," and "Clinical Rheumatology." Original articles on inflammatory rheumatic disease accounted for over half of the publications.

As of 17 September 2025, we identified 583 studies involving Tunisia published on the trials' website www.clinicaltrials.gov, with 10 related to rheumatology.

18.10.3 Rheumatology Nursing Programs

In Tunisia, there is no formal nursing program to certify nurses in rheumatology. However, a nursing training program was conducted in the rheumatology department of Mongi Slim University Hospital between November 2021 and June 2022, with the participation of the rheumatology department of Strasbourg University Hospital via video conference. The program included five modules on inflammatory rheumatic disease care and daily management, improvement of nurses' skills, educational therapy, rehabilitation, psychotherapy, and nutrition. Quizzes and questions were shared with the French speakers. A final evaluation of the 22 participants was performed at the end of each session.

18.11 Economic Challenges and Cost-Containment Strategies for Advanced Therapies

Healthcare costs remain a real challenge in low-income countries. In the last few decades, advances in biological therapy have changed the outcomes and prognosis of rheumatic diseases, offering patients a better quality of life and autonomy. However, this led to significant financial costs and negatively impacted the economic system. Since 2011, Tunisia has had indecisive public policymaking and growing protectionism. The political instability and the COVID-19 pandemic have contributed to the economy's decline, with slow growth and rising debt levels. To address this financial problem, the CNAM proposed austerity measures to narrow fiscal deficits. This approach is based on eliminating expensive medications and reducing the duration of treatment with other medications (such as anti-osteoporotic agents). The therapeutic arsenal is limited to tumor necrosis factor inhibitors, anti-interleukin (IL) 6 receptors, anti-IL-17, anti-CD20, and Janus kinase (JAK) inhibitors (tofacitinib). In inflammatory rheumatic diseases, such as RA and SpA, bDMARDs are not allowed as first-line therapies. The CNAM requires a non-response and/or a contraindication to cDAMRDs before switching to bDMARDs. To reduce expenditures, the CNAM's strategy is also based on rapid tapering of bDMARDs as soon as remission is obtained.

In addition to the efforts made by pharmaceutical industries to lower the prices of biologics, biosimilars were introduced in Tunisia. Biosimilars have demonstrated efficacy, tolerability, and safety comparable to the original biologics in treating rheumatic diseases. Moreover, they offer a more cost-effective alternative, substantially reducing the economic burden on patients and the country [37, 38].

18.12 Challenges and Emerging Opportunities

18.12.1 Health Workforce Challenges

Like many Arab countries, Tunisia experiences a significant brain drain, with nearly half of its scientific emigrants comprising health professionals. Factors such as higher standards of living, higher salaries, access to advanced technology, and more stable political conditions in developed nations attract young Tunisian physicians seeking opportunities abroad. This trend has had a detrimental effect on Tunisia's health systems, resulting in a loss of investment in health professional education and a decline in contributions to the healthcare system. Consequently, certain governorates in Tunisia face shortages of specialist physicians and nurses.

In addition to emigration to other countries, Tunisia also faces an internal brain drain within its healthcare system, characterized by migration from rural to urban areas and from the public to private sectors. This phenomenon exacerbates the unequal distribution of healthcare resources across Tunisia's governorates. To address the internal medical brain drain, the Ministry of Health has implemented measures to incentivize doctors to work in rural and disadvantaged areas by offering more privileges, such as salary increases and on-call bonuses. Furthermore, a quota system has been introduced for residency positions in these regions.

18.12.2 Medical Tourism

Worldwide, individuals seek private medical care by traveling to hospitals that serve international patients. In Tunisia, medical tourism is scarce. It is rare for Tunisians to leave the local healthcare system and pay privately to access care abroad. However, Tunisia seems an essential destination for wellness tourists from nearby countries (Libya and Algeria) and Europe. The main tourists' motivations are highly competent medical staff and the low cost of medical procedures.

Patients suffering from rheumatic disease are among the many Libyans traveling to seek care in our country. The Global Wellness Institute has shown that Tunisia was visited by 577,300 wellness tourists in 2017 [39]. Seawater-based thalassotherapy is a tourist destination, followed by esthetic and orthopedic surgery.

18.13 The Future of Rheumatic Disease Care in Tunisia

In discussing the prospects and shortcomings of rheumatology in your country, it is important to focus on specific areas of improvement within the field rather than the broader context of health system modernization. This approach allows for a more targeted assessment of the challenges and opportunities within rheumatology practice. First, there is an absolute need to increase the number of trained rheumatologists to achieve a higher ratio of specialists per citizen. Additionally, improving academic conditions for teaching the specialty and upgrading and enhancing rheumatology departments within hospitals is essential. Improving access to expensive medications like biologics, ensuring the availability of generalized ultrasound machines, and improving access to MRI scans are crucial. Lastly, allocating more significant budgets to the research field is essential for further advancement in rheumatology.

18.14 Conclusion

The field of rheumatology in Tunisia is witnessing remarkable growth and development with a continuous increase in the number of rheumatologists and the availability of diverse postgraduate training programs. Our population faces persistent musculoskeletal disorders, and it is important to highlight certain local specificities, such as the prevalence of severe SpA and a high frequency of fractures. Despite having skilled practitioners, there are challenges related to timely access to healthcare due to regional disparities in the distribution of rheumatologists. Financial constraints faced by insurance funds contribute to difficulties in accessing expensive treatments. However, health authorities are trying to improve access to new and effective medications. Tunisia has a wealth of well-trained and qualified researchers; however, there is a need to allocate increased research budgets to support their work further.

Conflict of Interest The authors declare they have no conflicts of interest.

References

1. Tunisia [internet]. [cited 2026 Jun 15]. Available from: https://www.nationsonline.org/oneworld/tunisia.htm.
2. Central Intelligence Agency. Tunisia—The World Factbook [Internet]. Last updated: 2025 Sept 8. [cited 2025 Sept 17]. Available from: https://www.cia.gov/the-world-factbook/countries/tunisia/#people-and-society.
3. Jdidi J, Mejdoub Y, Yaich S, Ben Ayed H, Kassis M, Fki H, et al. Private-public partnership: a solution for the development of health system in Tunisia. Tunis Med. 2017;95(3):160–7.
4. Adelowo O, Mody GM, Tikly M, Oyoo O, Slimani S. Rheumatic diseases in Africa. Nat Rev Rheumatol. 2021;17(6):363–74. https://doi.org/10.1038/s41584-021-00603-4.
5. Dey D, Paruk F, Mody GM, Kalla AA, Adebajo A, Akpabio A, Abu-Zaid MH, du Toit R, Ngandeu-Singwe M, Courage UU, Koussougbo OD, Migowa A, Moosajee F, Nomena RH, Olaosebikan HB, Palalane E, Lebughe PL, Sahli H, Cames LM, Mohamed D, Ndongo S, Idrissa C, Hmamouchi I. Women in rheumatology in Africa. Lancet Rheumatol. 2022;4(10):e657–60. https://doi.org/10.1016/S2665-9913(22)00255-7.
6. Paediatric Society of the African League Against Rheumatology (PAFLAR). [Internet]. [cited 2026 May 19]. https://paflar.org.
7. Hamdi W, Ferjani H, Carlomagno R, Dusser P, Echaubard S, Belot A, et al. Factors associated with poor prognosis of hip arthritis in juvenile idiopathic arthritis: data from the JIR cohort. Musculoskeletal Care. 2023;21(3):806–14. https://doi.org/10.1002/msc.1755.
8. Migowa AN, Hadef D, Hamdi W, Mwizerwa O, Ngandeu M, Taha Y, et al. Pediatric rheumatology in Africa: thriving amidst challenges. Pediatr Rheumatol Online J. 2021;19(1):69. https://doi.org/10.1186/s12969-021-00557-7.
9. Ligue Tunisienne Anti Rhumatismale [Internet]. [cited 2026 May 19]. Available from: https://litar.org.tn/.
10. Laatar A, Hajem S, Kerkeni S, Chekili S, Belhassine B, Hajri R, et al. Prevalence of musculoskeletal complaints and disability in Tunisia: a WHO-ILAR COPCORD study. Ann Rheum Dis. 2005;64(Suppl 3):1791.

11. Almutairi K, Nossent J, Preen D, Keen H, Inderjeeth C. The global prevalence of rheumatoid arthritis: a meta-analysis based on a systematic review. Rheumatol Int. 2021;41(5):863–77.
12. Hajri R, Ben Hamida A, Laatar A, Bahri M, Saadallaoui K, Moalla M, et al. Epidemiological study to assess prevalence of rheumatoid arthritis in Tunisian population. Ann Rheum Dis. 2003;62(5):533.
13. Younes M, Jalled A, Aydi Z, Zrour S, Korbaa W, Ben Salah Z, et al. Socioeconomic impact of ankylosing spondylitis in Tunisia. Joint Bone Spine. 2010;77(1):41–6.
14. Ben Abdelghani K, Gzam Y, Fazaa A, Miladi S, Sellami M, Souabni L, et al. Non-radiographic axial spondyloarthritis in Tunisia: main characteristics and detailed comparison with ankylosing spondylitis. Clin Rheumatol. 2021;40(4):1361–7.
15. Tbini H. Hip involvement in spondyloarthritis: frequency and risk factors [Medicine thesis]. Tunis: University of Tunis El Manar; 2022. p. 59p.
16. Osteoarthritis [Internet]. Last updated on 14 July 2023. [cited 2026 May 19]. Available from https://www.who.int/news-room/fact-sheets/detail/osteoarthritis.
17. Hajri R, Ben Hamida A, Bahri M, Laatar A, Zakraoui L, Moalla M, et al. The prevalence of osteoarthritis of the knee in Tunisian population. Ann Rheum Dis. 2002;61(Suppl):472.
18. Hajri R, Ben Hamida A, Laatar A, Bahri M, Zakraoui L, Moalla M, et al. Epidemiological study to assess prevalence of osteoarthritis of the hip in Tunisian population. Ann Rheum Dis. 2002;61(Suppl):472.
19. Kerkeni S. Prevalence of densitometric osteoporosis in Tunisian women: an epidemiological study [Medicine thesis]. Tunis: University of Tunis El Manar; 2005. p. 108.
20. Nasraoui R. Determination of the osteodensitometric reference values of the average Tunisian population [Medicine thesis]. Tunis: University of Tunis El Manar; 2006. p. 59.
21. Sellami S, Sahli H, Meddeb N, Hamza S, Chahed M, Ben M'Barek R, et al. Prevalence of osteoporotic fractures in Tunisian women. Rev Chir Orthop Reparatrice Appar Mot. 2006;92(5):490–4.
22. El Amri N, Daldoul C, Lataoui S, Baccouche K, Belghali S, Zeglaoui H, et al. Asymptomatic vertebral fracture in Tunisian post-menopausal women at risk: prevalence and risk factors. Arch Osteoporos. 2021;16(1):139.
23. Zakraoui L, Laatar A, Labidi R, Zouari B. Incidence de la fracture de l'extrémité supérieure du fémur (FESF) en Tunisie: étude épidémiologique nationale. Rev Rhumatisme Ed Fr. 2002;69:1042.
24. Mnif H, Koubaa M, Zrig M, Trabelsi R, Abid A. Elderly patient's mortality and morbidity following trochanteric fracture. A prospective study of 100 cases. Orthop Traumatol Surg Res OTSR. 2009;95(7):505–10.
25. Lagha A, Messadi A, Boussaidi S, Kochbati S, Tazeghdenti A, Ghazouani E, et al. HLA DRB1/DQB1 alleles and DRB1-DQB1 haplotypes and the risk of rheumatoid arthritis in Tunisians: a population-based case-control study. HLA. 2016;88(3):100–9.
26. Ben Hamad M, Mahfoudh N, Marzouk S, Kammoun A, Gaddour L, Hakim F, et al. Association study of human leukocyte antigen-DRB1 alleles with rheumatoid arthritis in south Tunisian patients. Clin Rheumatol. 2012;31(6):937–42.
27. Dhaouadi T, Sfar I, Abdelmoula L, Bardi R, Jendoubi-Ayed S, Makhlouf M, et al. Association of specific amino acid sequence (QRRAA) of HLA-DRB1*0405 with rheumatoid arthritis in a Tunisian population. Arch Inst Pasteur Tunis. 2010;87(1–2):53–9.
28. Kchir MM, Hamdi W, Laadhar L, Kochbati S, Kaffel D, Saadellaoui K, et al. HLA-B, DR and DQ antigens polymorphism in Tunisian patients with ankylosing spondylitis (a case-control study). Rheumatol Int. 2010;30(7):933–9.
29. Hamdi W, Kaffel D, Ghannouchi MM, Laadhar L, Makni S, Kchir MM. Clinical, radiographic and biologic particularities of ankylosing spondylitis in Tunisian patients according to the presence or the absence of the HLA B27 and its sub-types. Rev Med Liege. 2012;67(7–8):430–6.
30. Mahfoudh N, Siala M, Rihl M, Kammoun A, Frikha F, Fourati H, et al. Association and frequency of HLA-A, B and HLA-DR genes in south Tunisian spondyloarthritis (SpA) patients. Clin Rheumatol. 2011;30(8):1069–73.

31. Bahlous A, Farjallah N, Bouzid K, Klouz A, Mohsni A, Sahli H, et al. Hypovitaminosis D in Tunisian osteoporotic postmenopausal women and the relationship with bone fractures. Tunis Med. 2009;87(3):188–90.
32. Sassi R, Sahli H, Souissi C, Sellami S, Ben Ammar El Gaaied A. Polymorphisms in VDR gene in Tunisian postmenopausal women are associated with osteopenia phenotype. Climacteric. 2015;18(4):624–30.
33. Sassi R, Sahli H, Cheour E, Sellami S, El Gaaied ABA. −643C>T RANKL gene polymorphism is associated with osteoporosis in Tunisian postmenopausal women. Climacteric. 2017;20(4):374–8.
34. La prise en charge diagnostique et thérapeutique des spondyloarthrites | INEAS [Internet]. Last updated: April 2021. [cited 2026 Jun 14]. Available from: https://www.litar.org.tn/public/uploads/files/pdf_guide_poche/Guide-pratique-de-prise-en-charge-des-spondyloarthrites-660e90087ac28.pdf.
35. Ministère de la Santé, République Tunisienne. Carte sanitaire 2021 Tunisie [Internet]. Scribd; 2021 [cited 2026 Jun 15]. Available from: https://www.scribd.com/document/850366609/carte-sanitaire-2021-Tunisie.
36. ShanghaiRanking's Academic Ranking of World Universities 2021 Press Release [Internet]. [cited 2026 Jun 15]. Available from: https://www.shanghairanking.com/rankings/arwu/2021.
37. Phisalprapa P, Kositamongkol C, Limsrivilai J, Aniwan S, Charatcharoenwitthaya P, Pisespongsa P, et al. Cost-effectiveness and budget impact analysis of infliximab and its biosimilar in patients with refractory moderate-to-severe Crohn's disease using real-world evidence in Thailand. J Med Econ. 2020;23(11):1302–10.
38. Atzeni F, Gerratana E, Bongiovanni S, Talotta R, Miceli G, Salafi F, et al. Efficacy and safety of biosimilar and originator etanercept in rheumatoid arthritis patients: real-life data. Isr Med Assoc J. 2021;23(6):344–9.
39. Global Wellness Institute – Global Wellness Tourism Economy: Middle East & North Africa [Internet]. [cited 2026 May 19]. Last updated: November 2018. Available from: https://globalwellnessinstitute.org/wp-content/uploads/2019/04/MiddleEastNAfrica_TourismEconomyMonitor2018revweb.pdf.

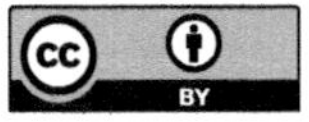

Chapter 19
Rheumatic Diseases in the United Arab Emirates

Suad Hannawi, Amna Almheiri, Mohamed Almarzooqi, and Khalid A. Alnaqbi

Abstract Rheumatic diseases represent a growing global health concern due to their increasing prevalence and substantial impact on health and economic systems. Easy access to rheumatology care can expedite the diagnosis and treatment of these conditions and help reduce disparities. In the United Arab Emirates (UAE), there has been sustained investment in health infrastructure to meet the population's healthcare needs. However, policy development, workforce planning, and service delivery are often hampered by many challenges, such as shortages of physicians and nurses, skill imbalances, maldistribution, limited budget, and gaps in education and research.

This chapter presents a narrative review supported by data collected from multiple sources that sheds light on the rheumatology landscape in the UAE. We

S. Hannawi (✉)
Alkuwait Hospital, Emirates Health Services, Dubai, UAE
e-mail: soad.hanawi@ehs.gov.ae

A. Almheiri
Research and Innovation, PureHealth, Abu Dhabi, UAE

Rheumatology Division, Sheikh Shakhbout Medical City, PureHealth, Abu Dhabi, UAE
e-mail: dramnaa@gmail.com

M. Almarzooqi
Sheikh Khalifa Medical City, SEHA/PureHealth, Abu Dhabi, UAE
e-mail: dralmarzouqi@live.com

K. A. Alnaqbi
Division of Rheumatology, Sheikh Tahnoon bin Mohammed Medical City, SEHA/PureHealth, Al Ain, UAE

Internal Medicine Department, College of Medicine & Health Sciences, UAE University, Al Ain, UAE

College of Medicine, RAK Medical and Health Sciences University, Ras Al Khaimah, UAE
e-mail: kalnaqbi@gmail.com

K. A. Alnaqbi, G. Aldabie (eds.), *Rheumatic Diseases in the Arab World*,
https://doi.org/10.1007/978-981-92-0967-5_19

describe the disease burden, service availability, education and training pathways, research activity, and key opportunities and challenges. Recent policy initiatives signal a strong governmental commitment to strengthening subspecialty capacity and improving the organization and quality of rheumatology care.

Keywords United Arab Emirates · Rheumatic Diseases · Rheumatology Services · Rheumatology Workforce · Health System · Biologic Therapy · Biosimilars · Rheumatology Training · Pediatric Rheumatology · Electronic Medical Records

19.1 Introduction

The United Arab Emirates (UAE) is a relatively young country that has accomplished notable milestones both locally and globally in recent years. Achievements in healthcare were made possible by its high-caliber healthcare professionals.

Expedited and consistent access to rheumatologists improves early diagnosis and management, uses disease-modifying anti-rheumatic drugs (DMARDs) judiciously, controls disease activity, and improves the overall quality of patients with rheumatic disease.

Any attempt to improve health services requires analyzing the currently available resources and understanding the opportunities and challenges. Yet, data on rheumatological diseases from the UAE are limited [1].

Moreover, the UAE health system is presently working in an environment of rapid social and economic changes. The health system is also under continuous analysis and development by health providers and healthcare receivers [2]. The expectations of our patients have grown consistently with the population's rising knowledge, potential, and wealth, resulting in strong pressure on the health system to satisfy patients' expectations [2]. Hence, medical and public health measures are vital for enhancing the treatment of patients with rheumatic conditions. These interventions are as equally important as economic and social interventions [3].

This chapter will discuss the rheumatology workforce in the UAE and present our vision to further enhance the service.

19.2 Country Demographics

The UAE is situated at the eastern end of the Arabian Peninsula, bordered by Oman and Saudi Arabia. It was established as a union of seven emirates: Abu Dhabi, Dubai, Ajman, Sharjah, Ras Al Khaimah, Fujairah, and Umm-Al-Quwain. Abu Dhabi is the nation's capital, while Dubai is the economic city.

The population of the UAE was only 1.01 million people in 1980. Since then, it has experienced remarkable demographic growth [4]. The UAE stands as a beacon of multiculturalism, with residents from across the globe contributing to its diverse social and cultural fabric.

As of June 2025, the estimated population of the UAE was 11.35 million, comprising approximately 63.8% males and 36.2% females. Emirati citizens account for about 11.5% of the population, while expatriates make up 88.5%. The median age of the UAE population is 31.6 years. The population is predominantly within the working-age group (25–54 years), which represents 64.1% of the total. Those aged 0–14 years constitute 15.98%, 15–24 years make up 12.71%, 55–64 years represent 5.40%, and 65 years and above account for 1.79% [4]. The population is heavily concentrated in its three most populous emirates, Abu Dhabi, Dubai, and Sharjah, which together account for approximately 85% of the population [4].

19.3 The UAE Health Sectors

The UAE health system consists of an intricate network of regulatory, operational, and payer entities. Together, these entities support the delivery of world-class healthcare to the people living in the country. The three main regulators are the Ministry of Health and Prevention (MOHAP)/Emirates Health Service (EHS), the Department of Health—Abu Dhabi (DOH) [previously known as Health Authority Abu Dhabi (HAAD)], and the Dubai Health Authority (DHA). These health entities have expanded in recent years and were subjected to major restructuring to improve the quality of public health in parallel with a rapidly growing population. Regulatory bodies are aiming for higher standards of care and delivering various new cutting-edge medical advances. In some areas, regulatory bodies have a dual role as operators as well. For example, MOHAP serves as the nation's major healthcare policy maker, as well as serving as an operator for healthcare services for the Northern Emirates, alongside the emirate-level regulatory bodies and operators in Sharjah, Fujairah, Ras Al Khaimah, Umm Al Quwain, and Ajman.

19.3.1 Health Organization

Table 19.1 provides an overview of the main healthcare regulators, operators, and payers within the UAE health system.

19.3.1.1 Ministry of Health and Prevention (MOHAP)

MOHAP is the main federal authority that reports directly to the Prime Minister's Office. It is responsible for unifying the UAE's health policies, developing comprehensive, nationwide health services, and ensuring accessibility of healthcare remains consistent across the country. It is also the primary healthcare regulator in the northern emirates and a partial health regulator in Dubai [5]. The Federal Health Authority handles the supervisory responsibilities for MOHAP, focusing on increasing the productivity and competitiveness of the UAE health system.

Table 19.1 Regulators, operators, and payers in the UAE

Entity	Category	Coverage	Role/Function
Ministry of Health and Prevention (MOHAP)	Regulator	Five emirates (Sharjah, Fujairah, Ajman, Ras Al Khaimah, and Umm Al Quwain) and partially in Dubai	The federal health authority is responsible for national health policies, public health legislation, licensing of professionals and facilities, and regulation of healthcare services across the UAE. Oversees service provision in the Northern Emirates and supervises Emirates Health Services (EHS)
Emirates Health Services (EHS)	Operator	Five emirates (Sharjah, Fujairah, Ajman, Ras Al Khaimah, and Umm Al Quwain) and partially in Dubai	Executes healthcare delivery on behalf of MOHAP across the Northern Emirates. Operates hospitals, primary care, and specialty centers. Implements national programs and manages electronic medical records (Wareed)
Ministry of Finance (MoF)	Payer	MOHAP and the EHS	Provides federal healthcare funding, especially to MOHAP and EHS facilities. Oversees financial allocations for national health programs and supports federal-level health initiatives
Department of Health (DOH)—Abu Dhabi	Regulator	Emirate of Abu Dhabi	Regulates healthcare in Abu Dhabi, sets clinical and insurance standards, accredits facilities, monitors outcomes, and implements population health initiatives. Ensures high-quality care through compliance inspections
PureHealth Group (e.g., Abu Dhabi SEHA healthcare facilities, SEHA Clinics, Sheikh Shakhbout Medical City, Yas Clinic, PureLab, Daman insurance)	Operator	Emirate of Abu Dhabi Some services (e.g., insurance and laboratories) extend across the UAE	The UAE's largest integrated healthcare network managing Abu Dhabi's public hospitals and clinics. Provides tertiary care and digital health integration
Daman Insurance Company	Payer	Emirate of Abu Dhabi; network and plans extend across the UAE	The UAE's largest health insurer (part of PureHealth). Provides medical insurance to over three million people. Manages reimbursement systems across public and private sectors

(continued)

Table 19.1 (continued)

Entity	Category	Coverage	Role/Function
Dubai Health Authority (DHA)	Regulator	Emirate of Dubai	Governs healthcare services in Dubai, including private and public sectors. Regulates medical licensing, insurance coverage, and quality standards. Promotes health tourism and oversees clinical education and research
Dubai Health (DHA Corporation)	Operator	Emirate of Dubai	Manages Dubai's network of public hospitals (e.g., Dubai Hospital, Rashid Hospital, Latifa Hospital, Hatta Hospital). Implements the DHA's clinical and academic directives through the Dubai Academic Health Institution
Private Insurance Companies	Payer	Across the UAE	Offer supplementary or employer-based health insurance plans. Operate under regulatory frameworks of DOH, DHA, and MOHAP to ensure coverage compliance and access to healthcare services

On 26 September 2016, Federal Law No. 16 was issued to separate planning and regulatory responsibilities from healthcare service provision. As a result, MOHAP became the regulatory authority, while the Emirates Health Services (EHS) was designated as the executive and healthcare delivery body. The law was implemented in 2021. EHS is responsible for providing healthcare across five emirates—Sharjah, Fujairah, Ajman, Ras Al Khaimah, and Umm Al Quwain—and partially in Dubai. EHS, as a federal health institute, provides free health services to all UAE citizens and Gulf Cooperation Council (GCC) residents in the UAE. Additionally, EHS provides emergency health services to all GCC visitors in the UAE and private insurance to all EHS employees and UAE residents with special needs [6].

19.3.1.2 Abu Dhabi: Department of Health (DOH) and Healthcare Providers

DOH is the regulator of healthcare in Abu Dhabi. It shapes and maintains the regulations of the health system, and it ensures a high standard of healthcare for the community by monitoring and analyzing the health status of the population, enforcing the adoption of best medical practices, setting performance targets, inspecting healthcare facilities, promoting public health programs, and engaging the community in disaster response. Additionally, DOH sets the guidelines for service range, insurance premiums, and reimbursement rates [7].

The main healthcare operator in Abu Dhabi is PureHealth, which encompasses the Abu Dhabi Health Services Company (SEHA), Sheikh Shakhbout Medical City (SSMC), and Yas Clinic, in addition to various private hospitals and clinics. Established by Emiri Decree No. 10 of 2007, SEHA initially functioned as the primary public healthcare provider across the Abu Dhabi, Al Dhafra, and Al Ain regions, and included the Ambulatory Health Services (AHS) network [8].

In 2020, all services at Al Mafraq Hospital in Abu Dhabi, which was owned by SEHA and included both pediatric and adult rheumatology, were relocated to the newly opened SSMC, a joint venture comanaged with the Mayo Clinic from 2019 to 2023 [8].

In January 2022, PureHealth formally consolidated several major healthcare entities—including SEHA, Daman, The Life Corner, and AHS—under its umbrella, becoming the largest integrated healthcare group in the Middle East [9]. Subsequently, in March 2024, PureHealth integrated SSMC [10], and in February 2025, it rebranded AHS as SEHA Clinics.

SEHA Company owns and operates more than 14 hospitals with a combined capacity of over 3000 beds and employs more than 2300 physicians. SEHA's network covers all three regions of Abu Dhabi: Abu Dhabi City (including Sheikh Khalifa Medical City and SEHA Kidney Care), Al Dhafra (Al Dhafra Hospitals), and Al Ain (including Sheikh Tahnoon bin Mohammed Medical City, Tawam Hospital, and Al Ain Hospital) [11].

19.3.1.3 Dubai Health Authority (DHA) and Healthcare Providers

The DHA was formed in 2007 to look after the health service in the emirate of Dubai. DHA is the regulator of Dubai's healthcare sector, including all public and private healthcare facilities, hospitals, clinics, and services in Dubai and its free trade zones [12]. In addition to its regulatory role, the DHA develops health policies and standards for service delivery, health insurance, and medical tourism. It also implements public health and preventive programs, oversees occupational health and safety, and guides medical education and clinical research within the emirate [13].

In line with its vision to integrate healthcare and education, the Dubai Academic Health Institution (DAHI) was established under Law No. 13 of 2021 as Dubai's first integrated academic health system, aimed at elevating the standard of care and advancing health for humanity. The following entities are affiliated with DAHI: Dubai Healthcare Corporation of the DHA and its hospitals and organizational units (such as Dubai Hospital, Latifa Hospital, Hatta Hospital, and Rashid Hospital), Mohammed bin Rashid University of Medicine and Health Sciences, Al Jalila Medical Education and Research Support Foundation, and Al Jalila Children's Specialty Hospital [14]. In 2023, Dubai Health was introduced as the public-facing brand of the corporation [12].

Rheumatology services under DHA are currently provided at Dubai Hospital and Hatta Hospital.

19.3.1.4 Ministry of Defense and Medical Services

The Ministry of Defense provides medical services for military personnel and their families and also for Emiratis who are enrolled in the mandatory national service.

19.3.1.5 Abu Dhabi Police and Medical Services

Abu Dhabi Police provides medical services, including rheumatology, for prisoners.

19.4 Payers of the UAE Health System

There are different paying entities providing the required financial support for healthcare services within the UAE. Some are government-owned, and some are privately owned. There are two major payers: Daman Insurance Company and the Ministry of Finance (MoF).

19.4.1 Ministry of Finance (MoF)

The federal authority is responsible for providing finance for the UAE healthcare sector, including MOHAP and the EHS.

19.4.2 Dubai Health Authority (DHA)

In November 2013, Dubai Health Insurance Law No. 11 of 2013 was passed, mandating health insurance for every resident in Dubai. The UAE nationals who register with DHA are covered by the Dubai government [15].

19.4.3 Private Insurance Companies

There are numerous health insurance companies across the UAE. Daman was established in 2006 in the emirate of Abu Dhabi, and it is the leading health insurer in the UAE. It is currently part of PureHealth, the UAE's largest integrated healthcare platform. It provides insurance to more than three million people and covers over 3000 medical facilities within the UAE and worldwide [16].

19.5 Rheumatology Workforce in the UAE

19.5.1 Rheumatologists

A total of 18 Emirati pediatric and adult rheumatologists completed their training abroad, including five who specialized in pediatric rheumatology. However, some have since retired or currently practice outside the UAE. As of October 2025, five Emirati rheumatologists (all female) have graduated from the local adult rheumatology fellowship program in Abu Dhabi, and one female Emirati rheumatologist has completed the Dubai fellowship program. The total number of currently practicing Emirati adult rheumatologists in the UAE is 19 (8 males, 11 females). The growing number of female graduates from local fellowship programs is helping to narrow the gender gap among Emirati rheumatologists, an important development that aligns with the preferences of some conservative patients who may feel more comfortable consulting a female specialist.

Furthermore, non-Emirati rheumatologists with diverse backgrounds and expertise are contributing to the care of patients with rheumatic diseases in the UAE, practicing across different types of healthcare institutions.

19.5.2 Emirates Health Services (EHS) Rheumatology Services

EHS oversees a network of 120 healthcare facilities, including 17 hospitals (with a total of 1649 beds), 103 health centers, 10 public health centers, 61 primary healthcare centers, and 20 fitness centers for rehabilitation [17]. Despite the remarkable increase in the number of healthcare workers in the UAE, there remains an opportunity to strengthen the availability of trained physicians and nurses, particularly among Emirati professionals. Physicians currently represent about 20% of the total health workforce at EHS. Among them, 82% are non-Emiratis, while Emiratis account for only 10% of physicians and 3% of nurses [18, 19].

Rheumatology services are available in six major tertiary hospitals. No rheumatology service is available in any primary or secondary hospitals. The rheumatology services are available in:

1. Al Kuwait Hospital—Dubai, the only federal EHS hospital in Dubai.
2. Al Qassimi Hospital—one of the three main hospitals in Sharjah.
3. The Women and Children Hospital, where only the pediatric rheumatology service is available (in Sharjah).
4. Obaidullah Hospital—one of the two hospitals in Ras Al Khaimah.
5. Al Fujairah Hospital—the main EHS hospital in Fujairah.
6. Umm Al Quwain—where two clinics of rheumatology are conducted.

Rheumatologists working in the private sector in all the emirates (except for Dubai and Abu Dhabi) are licensed by the MOHAP.

19.5.3 Abu Dhabi Rheumatology Services

The number of facilities that are licensed for rheumatology services within Abu Dhabi as of May 2022 was as follows: 70 hospitals (22 public and 48 private) and 25 centers (19 public and 6 private) [unpublished data].

Rheumatology services under SEHA cover the three main regions of Abu Dhabi: Abu Dhabi City, Al Dhafra, and Al Ain. As of October 2025, the only hospital in Abu Dhabi city providing pediatric and adult rheumatology services is SSMC. Al Dhafra Hospitals offer adult rheumatology services within their network. In Al Ain, rheumatology care is available at the new Sheikh Tahnoon bin Mohammed Medical City (STMC), as well as Tawam Hospital and Al Ain Hospital. Additionally, several SEHA Clinics (i.e., primary healthcare centers) in Abu Dhabi and Al Ain have in-house rheumatologists.

Mubadala Health was established in 2021 to provide patients with access to specialized medical care within the UAE. It has partnered with many internationally recognized specialized centers to enhance regional healthcare capacity, address the UAE's most pressing healthcare needs, and reduce the need for patients to travel abroad for specialized treatment. The organization operated, managed, and developed a portfolio of advanced medical facilities, including Cleveland Clinic Abu Dhabi (CCAD), Healthpoint, and the National Reference Laboratory, among others [20]. In 2023, Mubadala Health joined forces with G42 Healthcare, part of the Abu Dhabi-based artificial intelligence group G42, to establish M42—a technology-enabled, integrated healthcare company that combines clinical excellence with data-driven innovation [21]. Both CCAD and Healthpoint provide adult rheumatology services but do not currently offer pediatric rheumatology care.

19.5.4 Dubai Health Authority (DHA) Rheumatology Services

The Rheumatology Unit at Dubai Hospital offers specialized clinics, including general rheumatology, early arthritis, antenatal rheumatology, combined rheumatology–nephrology, and musculoskeletal ultrasound clinics [22]. Rheumatology services at Hatta Hospital are covered by a consultant rheumatologist.

19.5.5 Ministry of Defense Rheumatology Services

Rheumatology services include general rheumatology clinics, infusion day care, and inpatient consultations.

19.5.6 Abu Dhabi Police Rheumatology Services

Abu Dhabi Police provides medical services for prisoners. Rheumatology services include only general rheumatology clinics.

19.5.7 Pediatric Rheumatology in the UAE

There are currently six practicing pediatric rheumatologists in the UAE, mostly in the Emirate of Abu Dhabi. The EHS initiated a specialized Al Qassimi Women's and Children's Hospital in Sharjah (AQWCH), with one rheumatologist covering the pediatric rheumatology service. Al-Jalila Specialty Children's Hospital (AJCH) in Dubai offers pediatric rheumatology services covering the Emirate of Dubai, while both AQWCH and AJCH provide the pediatric rheumatology services to the Northern Emirates. AQWCH and AJCH assess children up to the age of 18 years. The service is run by a consultant pediatric rheumatologist who covers outpatient clinics, inpatient consultations, and day care infusions.

Currently, PureHealth group—which oversees SSMC and SEHA hospitals—exclusively provides the main pediatric rheumatology services in the Emirate of Abu Dhabi. At SSMC, there is a dedicated pediatric rheumatology division. In Al Ain, pediatric rheumatology care is provided at Tawam Hospital, supported by one full-time and one part-time consultant from the College of Medicine and Health Sciences, UAE University.

Due to the rarity of pediatric rheumatology services in the UAE, they are primarily located within tertiary hospitals. Referrals to the pediatric rheumatology clinic come from various sources, including general pediatrics, adult rheumatologists, and orthopedic surgeons. Additionally, the clinics welcome walk-in patients and self-referrals. Beyond outpatient consultations, inpatient consultations are provided across a wide range of hospitals, both governmental and private. Procedures such as intra-articular injections and infusions such as intravenous (IV) biologics and IVIG are carried out as day-case treatments. Pharmacies at these tertiary hospitals offer a comprehensive range of DMARD medications, encompassing both synthetics and biologics.

The pediatric services cover a diverse spectrum of pediatric diseases, including JIA, systemic SLE, scleroderma, juvenile dermatomyositis, and other connective tissue diseases. Most supporting specialties are located within the same hospitals, including orthopedic surgery, physiotherapy, occupational therapy, ophthalmology, genetics, dietary services, and gastroenterology, among others.

19.6 Rheumatology Nurses/Nurse Practitioner/ Physician Assistant

With the increasing demand for rheumatology services, the role of rheumatology nurses has expanded in Western countries. The European Alliance of Associations for Rheumatology (EULAR) has updated its recommendations defining nurses' roles in managing chronic inflammatory arthritis. Nurse-led clinics have also proven effective in monitoring such patients, allowing rheumatologists to focus on complex cases and advanced treatments [23].

Unfortunately, there are no certified nurses in rheumatology, rheumatology nurse practitioners, or physician assistants in the UAE. However, educational sessions and workshops have also been held at local rheumatology meetings and conferences in the UAE to enhance the knowledge of nurses who work with rheumatologists. For example, the Rheumatology department at Al Ain Hospital conducted a series of educational sessions (face-to-face and virtual) from 2018 to 2020 for nurses working at rheumatology clinics, presented by rheumatologists and nurses. In October 2017, the Emirates Society for Rheumatology (ESR) nominated a nurse from Al Ain Hospital who presented on the need for having rheumatology nurses in Arabia at the 19th annual meeting of the Asia Pacific League of Associations of Rheumatology (APLAR) held in Dubai. In November 2018, the ESR sponsored some nurses from the UAE to attend a rheumatology nursing preceptorship at St. Vincent's Hospital in Ireland. To the best of our knowledge, the first hands-on rheumatology nursing preceptorship in the Arabian Gulf region was held at Al Ain Hospital in December 2019 [8]. It was a one-day program that provided theoretical and practical sessions to nurses who work with rheumatologists in the UAE. It focused on dealing with rheumatic patients and their caregivers (e.g., education, pediatric and adult patients, challenging patients) and calculating scores of commonly used patient-reported outcomes (e.g., spondylitis scores and Health Assessment Questionnaire score). The program was primarily conducted by nurses from Al Ain Hospital experienced in rheumatology, utilizing their knowledge and skills acquired during the American accreditation of rheumatology programs at Al Ain Hospital in April 2019.

Over time, some nurses have obtained certificates in Musculoskeletal Imaging Techniques Ongoing Sonography (MITOS).

19.7 Diagnosis of Rheumatology Patients

19.7.1 Emirates Health Services (EHS)

The EHS in all the northern emirates and partially Dubai provides the needed laboratory and radiological diagnostic tools to help diagnose and manage rheumatology patients. All tertiary hospitals within the EHS have the capability to conduct genetic testing for HLA-B27. Other genetic tests (e.g., HLA-B51, MEFV M694V mutation) are performed in a private laboratory with the EHS covering its expenses. Furthermore, each tertiary hospital has computed tomography (CT), CT angiography, magnetic resonance imaging (MRI) (e.g., spinal, sacroiliac joints, and peripheral joints), magnetic resonance angiography (MRA), and dual-energy X-ray absorptiometry (DEXA). Musculoskeletal ultrasound examination is performed, although mainly by general radiologists or sonographers. Nevertheless, many rheumatologists in the UAE can perform ultrasound examinations in their clinics. A Positron Emission Tomography (PET) scan is not available at EHS. Although we do not know the exact number of musculoskeletal radiologists in the UAE, the number seems to be small.

19.7.2 Dubai Health and Mubadala Healthcare Facilities

Similar to EHS, numerous tests (routine blood and urine, genetic tests, imaging) are available to support the care of patients with rheumatic disease. Certain tests can be sent abroad. A PET scan is available at CCAD [24].

19.7.3 PureHealth Healthcare Facilities

Most of the common tests are available at PureLab (owned by PureHealth). Routine blood tests (infectious, inflammatory markers, and autoimmune serology) can be ordered. Examples include rheumatoid factor, anti-CCP, antinuclear antibodies, extractable nuclear antigens, dsDNA IgG, anti-neutrophilic cytoplasmic antibody (ANCA) and its subtypes, complement levels, and various urine tests. Genetic markers, such as HLA-B27 and HLA-B51, are available. Some tests are sent abroad, such as the MEFV M694V mutation and the TPMT enzyme genetic mutation. Similar to EHS, almost all imaging modalities are available at PureHealth healthcare facilities in addition to bone scans.

PET scan is available at SSMC in Abu Dhabi and at Tawam Molecular Imaging Centre (operated by M42) in Al Ain city [25, 26].

19.7.4 Private Hospitals

Similar to other government-owned facilities, a wide range of laboratory tests are available in private hospitals, with certain specialized tests referred to outsourced laboratories. Imaging modalities such as CT, CTA, MRI, MRA, bone densitometry (DEXA), and musculoskeletal ultrasound are routinely accessible across private hospitals. PET scans and bone scans are also available in select private facilities in Abu Dhabi and Dubai [27–32].

19.8 Availability and Accessibility of Rheumatic Drugs in the UAE

Most pharmaceutical companies register rheumatic drugs in the UAE as soon as international regulatory bodies approve them, such as the US Food and Drugs Administration (FDA) and the European Medicines Agency (EMA). In fact, the UAE is among the first countries in the region to use cutting-edge medications once they are approved by the FDA or EMA. All conventional DMARDs are available in the UAE, while almost all targeted DMARDs and biologic DMARDs are available, Table 19.2.

Table 19.2 Availability of various rheumatic and musculoskeletal medications in the UAE

Conventional synthetic DMARDs: methotrexate, hydroxychloroquine, sulfasalazine, leflunomide, azathioprine, mycophenolate mofetil, mycophenolic acid, cyclophosphamide, tacrolimus, cyclosporine
Targeted synthetic DMARD
Apremilast
Tofacitinib
Baricitinib
Upadacitinib
Biologics DMARDs
A. *TNF inhibitors*:
Originators:
Etanercept (Enbrel), adalimumab (Humira), infliximab (Remicade, IV), certolizumab (Cimzia), golimumab (Simponi SC)
TNF inhibitors Biosimilars
Etanercept biosimilars (Elrezi, Brenzys), adalimumab biosimilars (Amgevita, Hyrimoz), infliximab biosimilar (Ixifi, Remsima IV and SC)
B. *IL-1 inhibitors*: anakinra, canakinumab
C. *IL-12/23 inhibitor*: ustekinumab and its biosimilar (Wezlana)
D. *IL-17 inhibitors*: secukinumab, ixekizumab, bimekizumab
E. *IL-23 inhibitors*: guselkumab, risankizumab
F. *CTLA4-IgG*: Abatacept (IV and SC)
G. *IL-6 inhibitors*: Tocilizumab (IV and SC)
H. *CD20 inhibitor*: rituximab originator (MabThera), rituximab biosimilars (Rixathon, Ruxience, Truxima), obinutuzumab
I. *Biologic drugs for systemic lupus erythematosus*: belimumab (IV and SC), anifrolumab, obinutuzumab
Anti-osteoporosis drugs: Bisphosphonates (e.g. alendronate, risedronate, ibandronate, zoledronate, pamidronate); teriparatide; abaloparatide; denosumab; romosozumab
Others: inebilizumab, avacopan, nintadenib, cevimeline, pilocarpine, allopurinol, febuxostat, pegloticase

Abbreviations: *DMARDs* disease-modifying anti-rheumatic drugs, *TNF* tumor necrosis factor, *IL* interleukin, *IV* intravenous, *SC* subcutaneous, *CTLA4-IgG* cytotoxic T-lymphocyte-associated antigen 4 immunoglobulin G

Pharmaceutical companies marketing voclosporin, intravenous golimumab, rilonacept, filgotinib, and sarilumab have not registered their medications in the country yet. To address the high costs of medications, the EHS, DHA, DOH, and SEHA of Abu Dhabi have each developed their own biosimilar guidelines. Notably, the UAE has led the Gulf consensus recommendations on the use of biosimilars in inflammatory arthritis [33]. Furthermore, in a recently published paper on international comparative analysis and a roadmap to sustainable biosimilar markets, the UAE contributed to proposing a set of elements that should form the foundation for sustainable biosimilar policy development over time [34].

Furthermore, if a non-formulary medication is needed by a rheumatologist at any healthcare facility, it can be requested after providing a medical report and a non-formulary medication request. Afterward, the healthcare facility will purchase the medication on a case-by-case basis.

19.9 Accredited Rheumatology Centers in the UAE

The Joint Commission International (JCI) is an independent nonprofit organization that accredits and certifies healthcare organizations and programs across the globe. The JCI has accredited all the EHS hospitals. Apart from the general accreditation, no specific accreditation for subspecialties has been received in the EHS.

In April 2019, Al Ain Hospital in Al Ain city received American accreditation for its rheumatology programs, namely, Ankylosing spondylitis, SLE, RA, and JIA programs. This was the first and only rheumatology center outside the United States to receive such prestigious accreditation [8]. Further details on this accreditation are discussed in the chapter "Accreditation of Rheumatology Programs in the Arab World" in this book.

19.10 Electronic Medical Records (EMR)

19.10.1 Emirates Health Services (EHS)

The electronic medical record, EMR (Cerner), is connected throughout all the EHS medical services centers. The name of the EMR is Wareed. Each file (patient) has a unique Medical Record Number (MRN) in each hospital throughout the EHS. All the MRN numbers for the same patient are connected by another unified number, the CMRN (Central Medical Record Number). The CMRN is connected to the national identification number of the patient. Therefore, all hospital visits, investigations, and past medical histories of the patients can be viewed by any physician in any EHS-owned hospital/clinic [35–37]. This well-connected electronic file system facilitates the referral system that can take place from all other non-rheumatology clinics across EHS-owned hospitals and clinics by inserting an order of referral in the system. Afterward, the referred patient can call the rheumatology clinic or call center to book an appointment at the rheumatology clinic (based on the referral order). Alternatively, the physician can log into the rheumatology clinics' system and book an appointment electronically. On the other hand, rheumatology associations/societies have no role in the referral of rheumatology patients, as their role is limited to public awareness and physician education. Also, some charitable societies have a role in financial support of patients to cover the costs of medications, especially for patients who do not have insurance coverage.

19.10.2 SEHA Abu Dhabi Health Services Company and Sheikh Shakhbout Medical City

SEHA utilizes an EMR system from Cerner™ called Salamtak, where any patient record from all SEHA facilities is available under one MRN. SEHA is also part of the Health Information Exchange (HIE) program named Malaffi, where patient records from most healthcare providers are shared across facilities within the Abu Dhabi region, making it effortless for physicians to have access to patients' records at any facility within the Abu Dhabi region [8]. The use of HIF drastically reduces the cost of care and duplicate investigations, as any results and documents within Abu Dhabi are available to most of the facilities.

Rheumatologists have a special platform on the Salamtak system, with numerous electronic patient-reported outcome measures (ePROMs) related to rheumatology incorporated into the EMR to be used in daily clinical practice and research [8].

19.10.3 Dubai Hospital

Dubai Hospital uses Epic™ as the EMR.

19.10.4 Mubadala Health

Cleveland Clinic Abu Dhabi (CCAD) uses Epic™ as the EMR, while Healthpoint uses Cerner™.

19.10.5 Private Hospitals

Almost all private hospitals in the UAE use different EMRs.

19.11 Emirates Society for Rheumatology (ESR)

The UAE's official society representing rheumatologists is the Emirates Society for Rheumatology (ESR), a nonprofit organization that was established in 2008 under the Emirates Medical Association (EMA) that reports to the Ministry of Social Affairs. As per the EMA bylaws, nurses cannot be members of the ESR and can only be members of the Emirates Nursing Association, which is similar to but independent from the EMA and also reports to the Ministry of Social Affairs. With that in mind, the ESR organizes an annual meeting and periodical workshops aimed at enhancing the expertise of nurses across the UAE in the field of rheumatic diseases [38].

The society has a role in establishing rheumatology guidelines for the UAE, such as the Dubai Standard of Care for RA, and consensus-based recommendations for the evaluation and non-pharmacological and pharmacological management of psoriatic arthritis (PsA) in the UAE [39, 40].

19.12 Patient Support Groups

In April 2006, the Emirates Arthritis Foundation was launched to help patients who could not afford their treatment. Registration faced some challenges, requiring it to be renamed the Middle East Arthritis Foundation, which was launched in 2007 under the Fujairah Free Zone but not as a nonprofit organization. Its mandate is to increase awareness and education about arthritis in the region. Its goal is to improve the quality of life for people with arthritis through leadership training and in the prevention, control, and cure of the disease. The two main activities are patients' support events on World Arthritis Day and the Walkathon for Arthritis. Other events have been occurring sporadically [41].

Friends of Arthritis Patients' Society was a public benefit society registered by the Ministry of Community Development under Ministerial Resolution No. 52 for the year 2021. It was originally established in October 2008 by a decree of the Sharjah Government within the umbrella of the Health Education Department of the Supreme Council for Family Affairs in Sharjah. Its activities included walkathons and educational events for the public, either in-person at various cities or via virtual platforms [42, 43]. The focus was on disease education, screening, and prevention of different rheumatic diseases such as osteoporosis. Many educational activities were conducted by healthcare professionals (such as rheumatologists and dietitians) and personal trainers. These activities were held in collaboration with different entities such clubs (e.g., Sharjah Self-defence Sports Club, Al Dhaid Club, and Dibba Al-Hisn Sports Club), the Emirates Red Crescent, and Zayed Search and Rescue Volunteers Team. The society was formally dissolved in July 2025.

19.13 Overview of Rheumatic Diseases in the UAE

Data on rheumatological diseases in the UAE are scarce. Yet, a few publications have tackled some of the common rheumatological diseases.

Unpublished data obtained from the DOH (Table 19.3) revealed the top five most common reasons for a rheumatology encounter in 2019 (in order from most common to least common) were (1) osteoarthritis (OA), (2) spondyloarthropathies, (3) gout, (4) rheumatoid arthritis, and (5) osteoporosis. Other common reasons for seeking rheumatology services were lupus, Sjogren disease, JIA, scleroderma, polymyalgia rheumatica (PMR), and vasculitis, respectively.

Based on the DOH data from 2019, the female-to-male ratio of specific rheumatic disorders was analyzed using visit counts. The female-to-male ratios were as follows: 0.17:1 for gout, 1.09:1 for OA, 7.03:1 for SLE, 1.09:1 for scleroderma, 1.81:1 for RA, 1.12:1 for vasculitis, 2.14:1 for JIA, 1.35:1 for Sjogren disease, 2.40:1 for PMR, 0.83:1 for spondyloarthropathy, and 4.41:1 for osteoporosis. Additionally, a total of 237,379 rheumatology encounters were recorded in Abu Dhabi. The distribution of these encounters based on the patient's nationality was as follows: 57.6% for expatriates, 38.2% for UAE nationals, and 4.2% for patients of unrecorded nationality.

19.13.1 Rheumatoid Arthritis (RA)

RA is mostly studied in the UAE, particularly regarding its comorbidities. RA has an estimated prevalence rate of 2.72%. The prevalence is higher in females (3.73%) compared to males (1.28%) [1]. Subclinical atherosclerosis is more predominant among RA patients in the UAE than among the control participants [44, 45]. In addition to the traditional and nontraditional cardiovascular disease (CVD) risk factors [46], uric acid and subclinical kidney function were found to contribute to accelerating atherosclerosis in the UAE-RA population [47]. UAE-RA patients also have more vitamin D deficiency than their age-sex-matched controls [48].

Table 19.3 Rheumatology visits from 2019 in the Emirate of Abu Dhabi

2019	Gout	OA	SLE	Scl	RA	Vasculitis	JIA	Sjogren Disease	PMR	SpA	OP
0–14	55	272	117	21	796	–	643	168	6	143	129
15–29	3364	3205	1015	62	1977	18	181	294	17	6325	350
30–44	16,547	20,790	2137	181	6826	53	28	508	72	27,779	1321
45–59	9200	41,505	975	92	5249	35	15	340	81	20,562	4491
60+	2592	33,510	201	35	2201	11	6	157	136	11,249	9336

OA osteoarthritis, *SLE* systemic lupus erythematosus, *Scl* scleroderma, *RA* rheumatoid arthritis, *JIA* Juvenile idiopathic arthritis, *PMR* polymyalgia rheumatica, *SpA* spondyloarthritis, *OP* osteoporosis

19.13.2 Vitamin D Deficiency

Vitamin D deficiency is a prevalent health issue in the UAE, with an overall occurrence of 29.5% in Dubai [49]. In the UAE, RA patients have more vitamin D deficiency than age-sex-matched controls [48]. This deficiency is reported as an outcome and a cause of subclinical renal impairment [50]. Therefore, screening for 25-vitamin D deficiency might be important to improve bone health in the UAE.

19.13.3 Systemic Lupus Erythematosus (SLE)

In the UAE, the female:male ratio in SLE is markedly high: 27:1 for the whole population and 21:1 among Arabs. Local patients (Emiratis) develop the disease at an earlier age than expatriates [51]. This finding was also similar to another study that showed a female:male ratio of 20.5:1, with a mean age at disease onset of 28.9 years [52]. Also, Al Dhanhani et al. found that the prevalence of SLE in the UAE is much higher than in other countries of the GCC [53].

In another study conducted in Dubai, the clinical presentations of the lupus cohort were as follows: arthritis (88%), hematological abnormalities (62%), malar rash (60%), leukopenia (54%), hair loss (58%), fever (51%), proteinuria (50%), photosensitive rash (43%), anemia (44%), serositis (31%), mouth ulcers (27%), vasculitis (19%), discoid lupus (13%), brain infarcts (13.2%), neuropsychiatric symptoms (10%), and hemolytic anemia (10%). The 5-year survival rate was 94% [52].

19.13.4 Psoriatic Arthritis

A cross-sectional population-based study of 3985 patients attending primary healthcare clinics in the UAE estimated the prevalence of PsA to be 0.3%. Yet, the study was not focused on PsA per se [54]. Apart from this, no other study has looked at or studied PsA in the UAE.

The ESR published two papers on non-pharmacological and pharmacological recommendations on the management of PsA [39, 40].

19.13.5 Scleroderma

The Emirates Systemic Sclerosis (SSc) Registry, a multicenter initiative, was established, and its first research article was released in 2023. In the UAE, the prevalence of systemic sclerosis was 7.78 per 100,000 patients. Diffuse cutaneous SSc showed a higher association with anti-Scl-70 antibodies, while limited cutaneous SSc had a stronger link to anti-centromere antibodies. The diffuse cutaneous type frequently presented with sclerodactyly, breathing difficulties, interstitial lung disease, and digital ulcers compared to the limited type. However, telangiectasia and pulmonary arterial hypertension were predominantly observed in the limited cutaneous [55].

19.13.6 Osteoarthritis

A recent study conducted on the incidence and prevalence of OA cases as well as patients with OA of the hip and/or knees during the period from January 1, 2014, to May 31, 2020, revealed rates of 1.7% and 2%, respectively. Furthermore, the study gathered OA-related data from the Dubai Real-World Claims Database and highlighted the significant financial impact of osteoarthritis in the UAE [56].

19.13.7 Osteoporosis

Considering that 7% of the UAE population is above 50 years of age, this might indicate a small number of people suffering from osteoporosis. On the other hand, there is data showing osteoporosis prevalence of around 2.5% at an average age of 42 years (based on screening of 1825 asymptomatic individuals). Moreover, 2.25 osteoporotic hip fractures per 100 individuals were recorded at a major hospital in Abu Dhabi [57]. This report emphasizes the need to consider osteoporosis and hypovitaminosis D as major health challenges that require preventive and curative actions. The prevalence of osteoporosis in the UAE reflects its distinct population makeup, with Emirati nationals making up just 20% (having a female-to-male ratio of 1:1.1) and expatriates comprising 80% (with a female-to-male ratio of 1:4). In short, accurate epidemiological prevalence figures for osteoporosis are not available in the UAE [58].

A consensus statement of the GCC countries' osteoporosis societies regarding the diagnosis and management of postmenopausal women with osteoporosis was published in 2020 [59]. The Emirates Osteoporosis Society participated in this consensus. In addition, the first UAE recommendations on managing osteoporosis were published recently [60].

19.14 Rheumatological Diseases Risk Factors in the UAE

19.14.1 Environmental Pollution

Environmental pollution remains a significant yet often under-recognized public health challenge in the UAE. A national modeling study estimated that in 2008, approximately 651 deaths (around 7% of all deaths) were attributable to outdoor air pollution alone, with additional impacts from indoor air pollution and occupational exposures [61]. Although precise data on Disability-Adjusted Life Years (DALYs) are limited, these findings indicate that environmental factors contribute substantially to the national disease burden [62]. According to the UAE's Long-Term Strategy for Net Zero by 2050 (published in 2023), the government's decarbonization roadmap targets multiple sector—including transport, industry, and waste management—while advancing clean energy, sustainable infrastructure, and circular economy principles [63]. Consistent with this strategy, the UAE has integrated environmental health into its national health policies by investing in clean energy infrastructure, banning leaded gasoline, and expanding public transportation to reduce emissions and waste-related exposures.

19.14.2 Smoking

Smoking has been proven as a risk factor for RA [64, 65], SLE [64], psoriasis and PsA [66], osteoporosis [67], and primary vasculitis [68].

In the UAE, an overall prevalence of tobacco smoking of 21.6% among men and 1.9% among women was reported in a national review of studies [69]. In a separate cohort of applicants to the Abu Dhabi Premarital Screening Program in 2011, 3.5% of women and 19.2% of men reported being current cigarette smokers. Among that cohort, Arab expatriate men had the highest cigarette-smoking prevalence (31.4%), and Emirati women the lowest (0.7%) [70]. While the highest prevalence in men was among those aged 20–39 years, the mean age of female smokers in the national review was reported as 32.8 ± 11.1 years [69].

The most common forms of tobacco use include cigarette smoking (77.4%), followed by 15.0% midwakh use (a special pipe for smoking), 6.8% water pipe use, and 0.66% cigar use [71].

Approximately 11% of RA patients in the UAE were found to be smokers [1]. The number of cigarettes/day also showed a significant association with the carotid intima-media thickness (cIMT) of UAE-RA patients [48]. In short, avoiding smoking is a feasible primary prevention strategy for RA, PsA, psoriasis, SLE, osteoporosis, and vasculitis.

19.14.3 Sunlight

In the UAE, the average annual number of sun hours is 3580. Exposure to sunlight enhances disease flare-up of SLE skin manifestations and, most probably, lupus development [72].

19.14.4 Obesity

Despite inconsistent results about the relationship between increased body mass index (BMI) and rheumatological diseases, some research suggests an association between increased BMI and RA [73], SLE [74], knee OA [75], and PsA [76].

In the UAE, not much data is known about the relation of BMI with rheumatological diseases. Still, among RA patients, a statistically significant difference was observed in BMI at the time of diagnosis between females and males, with a higher BMI in females (31.4 ± 6.61) compared to males (28.8 ± 6.03) [1].

19.14.5 Vitamin D Deficiency

Given that vitamin D synthesis and its production in humans depend on sun exposure, vitamin D deficiency is supposed to be an unnoticeable clinical problem in a sunny area like the UAE. Yet, it has been proven to be a major health issue. Al-Anouti et al. examined vitamin D levels in a random sample of university students in Al Ain city. Interestingly, the average vitamin D level during summer was 20.9 ± 14.9 and 27.3 ± 15.7 ng/mL in females and males, respectively [77].

Similarly, a study from Dubai showed that the prevalence of vitamin D levels <30 ng/ml (deficiency and insufficiency) is 81% based on a sample of 2836 individuals who attended the biggest government hospital in Dubai [49]. Most researchers attributed this to the avoidance of sun exposure in addition to inappropriate dietary habits.

19.14.6 Hypertension

The pooled prevalence of hypertension in the UAE was found to be 31%, with a higher prevalence observed in Dubai (37%) than in the Abu Dhabi region (29%). The level of awareness was only 29% [78]. A retrospective study in Abu Dhabi among Emirati participants of a national cardiovascular screening program (2011–2013) reported an approximately 10% increase in hypertension prevalence over the past decade. In multivariable analysis, age, systolic and diastolic blood pressure, HbA1c, and HDL-cholesterol levels were significantly associated with hypertension [79].

The most frequent comorbidity associated with RA in the UAE is dyslipidemia (43.5%), followed by hypertension (37.9%) and diabetes mellitus (34.5%) [1]. Additionally, systolic and diastolic blood pressure were found to be associated with the thickness of the cIMT (a surrogate marker for CVD) in UAE-RA patients [46, 47].

19.14.7 Diabetes Mellitus

The prevalence of diabetes among adult citizens in the Northern Emirates of the UAE was reported to be 25.1% [80]. It increased with age, lower education, obesity, positive family history, hypertension, dyslipidemia, snoring, and low high-density lipoprotein (HDL) levels. According to some studies, the highest prevalence rates are observed among Asians (16.4%) and non-Emirati Arabs (15.2%), while the lowest rates are found in Africans and Europeans (11.9%). The research underscores the pressing need for diabetes prevention and control programs across the entire UAE population, given that 64% of diabetes cases among migrants in the UAE go undiagnosed [81].

The only data available about diabetes in rheumatological diseases revealed a diabetes prevalence of 34.5% in UAE-RA patients [1]. In both diabetic and nondiabetic UAE-RA patients, a high fasting blood glucose level was identified as a key contributor to atherosclerotic risk [46].

19.14.8 Dyslipidemia

The overall prevalence of dyslipidemia was found to be 72.5%. Specifically, 42.8% of individuals exhibited elevated total cholesterol levels, while 29% had elevated triglyceride levels. Moreover, 38.6% demonstrated high levels of low-density lipoprotein (LDL) cholesterol, and 42.5% exhibited low levels of high-density lipoprotein (HDL) cholesterol. Additionally, a high cholesterol ratio was observed in 72.3% of the population. The study also revealed that risk factors for dyslipidemia were male gender, middle-aged individuals (30–59 years old), diabetes mellitus, central obesity, and smoking [82].

Others investigated the overall prevalence of metabolic syndrome in the UAE, which was 37.4%.

Metabolic syndrome had varying prevalence rates among different populations: 34% in Emiratis, 35% in Arab non-Emiratis, and 41% in Asians. Factors such as age, gender, ethnicity, marital status, education level, and BMI showed a positive correlation with the occurrence of metabolic syndrome [83].

Dyslipidemia was reported in 43.5% of UAE-RA patients [1], and others found that 16% of UAE-RA patients were confirmed to have dyslipidemia and are on anti-lipid medications. High LDL and triglycerides proved to be CVD risk factors in UAE-RA patients [46, 47].

19.14.9 Consanguinity

The consanguinity rate in the UAE is high, and it has increased from 39% to 50.5% in one generation. Generally, an increase in consanguinity had been reported in Dubai, but it was higher in Al Ain (54.2%) than in Dubai (40%) [84]. The most common type of consanguineous marriage was between first cousins, ranging from 20.7% to 29.7% [85]. Double first-cousin marriages are more common in the UAE (3.5%) compared to other populations [84]. Unfortunately, the effect of consanguinity on rheumatological diseases in the UAE has not been studied.

19.15 Screening Programs for Rheumatic Diseases

Prevention is better than treatment. Therefore, the WHO established recommendations for disease screening and prevention. Generally, the recommendations state that screening and prevention should be devoted to diseases that have a significant effect on health, and a recognizable asymptomatic period during which screening can be conducted on individuals at high risk can be accurately identified [86, 87].

Prevention strategies are typically divided into primary, secondary, and tertiary interventions [86]. Primary prevention involves efforts to prevent the onset of diseases by either eliminating associated risk factors or boosting an individual's resistance to the disease in question. Secondary prevention aims to halt the progression of a disease from an asymptomatic phase to a symptomatic one. Tertiary prevention focuses on delaying or mitigating the effects of an already established disease [86].

While most rheumatic diseases are addressed with tertiary prevention, the rising global prevalence underscores the importance of introducing primary prevention strategies for these diseases. However, in the UAE, screening programs for rheumatic diseases are currently limited and would greatly benefit from more structured organization and broader outreach. Many of the existing initiatives have originated from the individual efforts of motivated rheumatologists rather than coordinated national strategies. Establishing and managing screening programs for rheumatic diseases, however, present numerous logistical and operational challenges. The following sections highlight the key obstacles and opportunities related to implementing such programs.

19.15.1 Challenges at the Health Institutional Level

Health institutions, whether governmental or private, often rely on pharmaceutical companies to sponsor screening or educational initiative. However, the approach to pharmaceutical companies lacks a clear institutional pathway; instead, it usually stems from individual rheumatologists' efforts. These rheumatologists independently propose and approach pharmaceutical companies for financial support related to any rheumatology-associated screening or educational project.

Furthermore, the limited involvement of stakeholders or their representatives poses an additional challenge in implementing screening programs. An opportunity for improvement lies in increasing stakeholder engagement and involving their representatives in screening programs. This collaboration is essential to ensure that the benefits of the screening programs at the healthcare facilities (hospitals and primary care centers) and that the potential consequences of late diagnosis of rheumatic diseases are recognized. Directives for screening programs for rheumatic diseases should be integrated into healthcare policies.

19.15.2 Challenges at the Public Level

At the public level, there is a need to prioritize efforts to enhance awareness of rheumatic diseases. Furthermore, certain educational meetings have witnessed low attendance. It is crucial to understand the diverse cultural landscape and varying socioeconomic status within the UAE to plan effective educational approaches for the public. Additionally, due to the intricate demographics of the UAE, effective screening initiatives should cater to multiple languages and accessible communication channels.

19.15.3 Challenges at Other Specialties Level

Collaborating within a multidisciplinary rheumatology team delivers more holistic care and is associated with improved clinical outcomes and higher patient satisfaction [88, 89]. Thus, establishing collaborative teamwork necessitates the engagement of specialists from every relevant field, such as dermatology, gastroenterology, and orthopedic surgery. Improving knowledge and communication about extra-musculoskeletal involvement and co-managing any comorbidity will achieve multidisciplinary collaboration and enhance screening initiatives. Furthermore, building a culture of teamwork and organizing combined activities requires participation from every specialty and level of the organization and recognizing each team member for their efforts.

19.16 Education in Rheumatology

19.16.1 Continuous Medical Education (CME)

Across MOHAP, the Ministry of Presidential Affairs (MOPA), and DHA, approximately 26 million (2019) and 22 million (2020) were invested to improve health workforce training and continuing professional development. These investments ensure that health workers continuously upgrade their skills, ultimately leading to better confidence, output, and career satisfaction. Also, there are mandatory existing national and/or subnational systems for continuing professional development (CPD) linked to relicensing. The CPD system is integrated into national education plans for the health workforce [90].

Moving forward, there is an opportunity for health institutes to allocate budgets for specialties and establish a clear framework for rheumatology education. Rheumatologists attend scientific educational activities face-to-face and virtually as part of periodic meetings in rheumatology entities such as the annual meetings of EULAR or the American College of Rheumatology, ESR, and the Arab League of Associations for Rheumatology (ArLAR), and as part of pharmaceutical company-sponsored meetings.

19.16.2 Rheumatology Fellowship Training Programs

All the currently 19 practicing Emirati rheumatologists graduated from Canada, the United States, Germany, Australia, Ireland, the United Kingdom, France, KSA, and the UAE. Among these Emirati rheumatologists are only four female pediatric rheumatologists.

In October 2019, the first adult rheumatology fellowship program was launched at SSMC in Abu Dhabi, with the pediatric rheumatology fellowship following in September 2022. The duration of each program is 3 years. Both programs have been accredited by the Accreditation Council for Graduate Medical Education International (ACGME-I). Two seats are offered to new applicants to the adult program annually, and a total of six fellows for the whole program can exist at all times. To be eligible for the program, the candidate's prerequisite is to be board-certified in Internal Medicine Specialty. As of October 2025, the 3-year adult program has four fellows, and the pediatric program is currently training one fellow. Eight fellows have graduated from the adult program.

The National Institute of Health Specialty (NIHS) was established by Cabinet Decree No. 28 of 2014 as a national institution responsible for regulating and organizing professional development for the health workforce with a particular emphasis on specialty training. In October 2021, a scientific rheumatology committee was established to develop Emirati curricula for pediatric and adult rheumatology fellowship programs. The curricula are based on ACGME and the Royal College of Physicians and Surgeons of Canada standards, with some modifications to reflect the UAE culture. The pediatric and adult programs are of 3-year duration each. The graduating fellows are expected to take the Emirati certification (board) examination at the end of the third year. Both programs at SSMC have received NIHS accreditation, with the pediatric rheumatologist program achieving accreditation in 2023, followed by the adult program in January 2024 [8]. The first batch of candidates passed the adult exit examinations in 2025 and received the Emirati Board of Rheumatology certification.

In 2023, the second rheumatology fellowship program was established in Dubai with a 2-year training period. It is accredited by the Saudi Central Board for Accreditation of Healthcare Institutions (CBAHI) [8]. It currently trains two fellows (a male and a female). Furthermore, one female Emirati fellow graduated from the Dubai Adult Rheumatology Fellowship Program in 2025.

19.16.3 Rheumatology Nurses/Nurse Practitioner/ Physician Assistant

Unfortunately, there is no rheumatology nursing program offered by any academic institute in the UAE.

19.17 Rheumatology Research in the UAE

The UAE has made commendable strides in rheumatology research, with several noteworthy publications originating from dedicated personal efforts. However, there is a vast opportunity to expand research, especially concerning the prevalence, incidence, distribution, and characteristics of common rheumatological diseases and their effects on the population. While there have been complexities in navigating the health system in the UAE, this underscores the potential for fostering stronger institutional and administrative support for research at various levels. As health entities in the UAE primarily focus on service provision, there is an opportunity to emphasize and prioritize research within these institutions [91]. Providing protected time for researchers at healthcare facilities, boosting financial resources for studies, establishing specialized rheumatology research centers, and expanding research training can be key areas of growth. Additionally, increasing public awareness about the significance of clinical research can further propel the field forward [8, 91].

Furthermore, many steps in the last few years have paved the road for establishing an acceptable framework and requirements that can support rheumatology researchers. For example, MOHAP, DHA, and DOH have developed guidelines for conducting clinical trials (the guidelines are made accessible on the official websites of all health entities), and research ethics committees and institutional review boards have been structured across the health entities [92–97]. Such changes have facilitated the approval and conduction of different clinical trial phases (phases I, II, III, and IV).

Although most of the published research is observational, the latest changes in the infrastructure of the UAE research environment are promising for future interventional trials in rheumatology. By establishing appropriate infrastructure, allocating resources, providing guidelines and regulations, allowing researchers ample time to conduct their studies, granting due recognition, and securing necessary funds, rheumatologists can independently sustain their research efforts, ultimately enhancing the quality of rheumatology care services. To sustain conducting research on rheumatic diseases, support needs to be at the macro-level (e.g., government), meso-level (e.g., regional health authorities, hospitals), and micro-level (e.g., clinical programs).

19.18 Opportunities for Enhancing Rheumatology Care

The WHO recommended some opportunities for improving the UAE's health [98]. Some of the recommendations that can be applied specifically to rheumatology services are as follows:

1. Improving coordination between health authorities
2. Improving quality of care
3. Working on the accreditation of all health facilities
4. Setting appropriate standards and guidelines
5. Increasing and encouraging social participation in the health sector decision-making process
6. Improving governance function in health with a focus on evidence-based policy
7. Improving health planning formulation, regulation, and legislation
8. Promoting health in all policies tactics to address inequities in health
9. Developing human resources with an emphasis on local health workforce production
10. Expanding surveillance and prevention of noncommunicable diseases

The following sections highlight several opportunities to advance and optimize rheumatology care delivery in the UAE.

19.18.1 Promoting Subspecialty Training in Rheumatology

To the best of our knowledge, among all the practicing rheumatologists in the UAE, four of them (Emiratis) have undergone further formal subspecialty training at accredited programs in Canada and Ireland. One rheumatologist has undertaken a Spondyloarthritis Clinical Research Fellowship at the University of Toronto as part of the Clinician Investigation Program, which is accredited by the Royal College of Physicians and Surgeons of Canada. Two rheumatologists have undertaken a Lupus Clinical Research Fellowship at the same university. The fourth rheumatologist has undertaken a Musculoskeletal Ultrasound Fellowship in Ireland.

A structured clinic is a dedicated, protocol-driven service for a defined patient group, delivered by a coordinated multidisciplinary team using standardized care pathways, scheduled assessments, and routine outcome tracking [99]. Five subspecialty clinics in Tawam Hospital and Sheikh Tahnoon bin Mohammed Medical City (STMC) have been established, including Spondyloarthritis (SpA), Lupus, Procedure Clinics, Interstitial Lung Disease (combining Rheumatology and Respirology services), and Sjogren Clinic. A structured SpA Clinic was launched in 2014 at Al Ain Hospital, the first of its kind in the Arabian Gulf region. The SpA Clinic moved to Tawam Hospital in September 2020 during the COVID-19 crisis. A Musculoskeletal Ultrasound Clinic at Tawam Hospital was launched in early 2022, and a second clinic was opened at STMC in 2024. Additionally, a structured Sjogren Clinic was launched at STMC in February 2024.

More subspecialized rheumatologists are needed to help establish structured subspecialty clinics in the UAE. This will also aid in establishing Clinical Rheumatology subspecialty Fellowship training programs similar to those found in developed countries.

19.18.2 Promoting Rheumatology Nursing to Improve Quality of Care

Having structured specialty programs for rheumatology nursing in the region will significantly improve the quality of care for patients with rheumatic diseases. Offering incentives or higher salaries to specialized rheumatology nurses can play a crucial role in attracting and retaining experienced professionals in this complex rheumatology field.

19.18.3 Cultivating Collaboration Among Health Authorities

Health authorities such as MOHAP, DHA, and DOH play a vital role in health strategic planning and policy development. At the same time, there is room to enhance coordination among these health authorities and establish a mechanism for managing various diseases, including rheumatic conditions.

19.18.4 Embracing a Multidisciplinary Approach

Rheumatic diseases are primarily systemic, impacting various body systems and necessitating cross-specialty collaboration for effective comanagement. Additionally, the creation of integrated clinical practice guidelines encompassing prevention, treatment, and rehabilitation is imperative for advancing rheumatology services.

19.18.5 Education and Knowledge Enhancement

The UAE has a promising opportunity to foster collaboration between academic institutes, health authorities and healthcare providers, enabling the seamless exchange of knowledge. Strengthening these partnerships would significantly boost research advancements.

19.19 Summary and Conclusion

Over the past decades, the UAE has demonstrated significant advancements in healthcare infrastructure and specialized services, positioning rheumatology among the most well-developed disciplines in the region. Rheumatology care is considered among the best in the Arab world, partly due to the presence of rheumatologists trained in diverse international programs who bring varied expertise. Numerous public and private health institutions offer state-of-the-art imaging and laboratory services essential for the evaluation of rheumatic diseases. Most of the advanced therapies for rheumatic diseases are available in the UAE, making it one of the first countries globally to register several new medications. There are numerous opportunities for rheumatologists to attend and participate in educational activities in the UAE and abroad. Emirati curricula and certifications for pediatric and adult rheumatology fellowships have been established, which will help improve the shortage of rheumatologists in the country, especially among Emirati physicians. There are some opportunities to expand the care spectrum to medical tourism, and to study various rheumatic diseases that are being diagnosed and treated in the country using proper research designs. As in any country, ongoing challenges include workforce shortages and the need to strengthen research efforts, particularly through the establishment of disease registries.

Acknowledgments We would like to thank Dr. Elsadeg Sharif (consultant pediatric rheumatologist at Al Jalila Children's Specialty Hospital in Dubai) and Dr. Khulood Khawaja (consultant and former Chair of the Pediatric Rheumatology division at Sheikh Shakhbout Medical City in Abu Dhabi) for providing their perspectives on pediatric rheumatology in the UAE. We also appreciate Dr. Humeira Badsha, consultant rheumatologist at Mubadala Health Dubai and Co-founder of the Middle East Arthritis Foundation, for sharing her insights on the Foundation.

Conflict of Interest The authors have no conflicts of interest to declare.

Disclaimer The views and opinions expressed in this chapter are those of the authors and do not necessarily reflect the official policy or position of their affiliated institutions or organizations.

References

1. Namas R, Joshi A, Ali Z, Al Saleh J, Abuzakouk M. Demographic and clinical patterns of rheumatoid arthritis in an Emirati cohort from United Arab Emirates. Int J Rheumatol. 2019;2019:3057578.
2. Hannawi S, Al Salmi I. Health workforce in the United Arab Emirates: analytic point of view. Int J Health Plann Manag. 2014;29(4):332–41.
3. Hannawi S, AlSalmi I. The world health report 2000-health system improving performance. Indian J Soc Dev 2015;15(2).
4. Global Media Insight. UAE population statistics [Internet]. 2026. [cited 2026 Jun 17]. Available from: https://www.globalmediainsight.com/blog/uae-population-statistics/#UAE_Population_2025_Key_Statistics.

5. Emirates Health Services. Home. United Arab Emirates: Emirates Health Services; 2026. [cited 2026 Jun 17]. Available from: https://www.ehs.gov.ae/en/home.
6. Emirates Health Services. Health legislation. United Arab Emirates: Emirates Health Services; 2026. [cited 2026 Jun 17]. Available from: https://www.ehs.gov.ae/en/about-us/health-legislation.
7. Department of Health – Abu Dhabi (DoH). About us. Abu Dhabi (UAE): Department of Health – Abu Dhabi; 2026. [cited 2026 Jun 17]. Available from: https://www.doh.gov.ae/en/about.
8. Alnaqbi KA, Fazal F, Namas R. From sand to excellence: a deep dive into Abu Dhabi's rheumatology landscape. Mediterr J Rheumatol. 2024;35(1):73–82. https://doi.org/10.31138/mjr.011123.fst.
9. PureHealth. Home. Abu Dhabi (UAE): PureHealth Holding PJSC; 2026. [cited 2026 Jun 17]. Available from: https://purehealth.ae/.
10. Abu Dhabi Media Office. PureHealth completes integration of Sheikh Shakhbout Medical City. Abu Dhabi (UAE): Abu Dhabi Media Office; 2024. [cited 2026 Jun 17]. Available from: https://www.mediaoffice.abudhabi/en/health/purehealth-completes-integration-of-sheikh-shakhbout-medical-city/.
11. Abu Dhabi Health Services Company (SEHA). About us. Abu Dhabi (UAE): SEHA; 2026. [cited 2026 Jun 17]. Available from: https://www.seha.ae/about-us.
12. Dubai Health. Inaugural report 2023. Dubai (UAE): Dubai Health; 2023. [cited 2026 Jun 17]. Available from: https://dubaihealth.ae/documents/d/dubai-health/dubai-health-inaugural-report-2023.
13. Dubai Health Authority (DHA). About us [Internet]. Dubai (UAE): DHA; [cited 2026 Jun 17]. Available from: https://www.dha.gov.ae/en/AboutUs.
14. Government of Dubai. Law No. (13) of 2021 Establishing the Dubai Academic Health Institution. Dubai (UAE): Dubai Legislation Portal; 2021. [cited 2026 Jun 17]. Available from: https://dlp.dubai.gov.ae/Legislation%20Reference/2021/Law%20No.%20(13)%20of%202021%20Establishing%20the%20Dubai%20Academic%20Health%20Institution.html.
15. Government of Dubai. Law No. (11) of 2013 Concerning Health Insurance in the Emirate of Dubai [Internet]. Dubai (UAE): Dubai Legislation Portal; 2013 [cited 2026 Jun 17]. Available from: https://dlp.dubai.gov.ae/Legislation%20Reference/2013/Law%20No.%20(11)%20of%202013.pdf.
16. The National Health Insurance Company – Daman. About us [Internet]. Abu Dhabi (UAE): Daman; 2026. [cited 2026 Jun 17]. Available from: https://www.damanhealth.ae/about-us/.
17. Emirates Health Services. EHS in numbers [Internet]. UAE: EHS; 2026. [cited 2026 Jun 17]. Available from: https://www.ehs.gov.ae/en/open-data/ehs-in-numbers.
18. Kronfol NM. Perspectives on the health care system of the United Arab Emirates. East Mediterr Health J. 1999;5(1):149–67.
19. El-Haddad M. Nursing in the United Arab Emirates: an historical background. Int Nurs Rev. 2006;53(4):284–9.
20. Mubadala. Mubadala inaugurates fully integrated health network [Internet]. Abu Dhabi (UAE): Mubadala; 2021. [cited 2026 Jun 17]. Available from: https://www.mubadala.com/en/news/mubadala-inaugurates-fully-integrated-health-network.
21. M42. Who we are [Internet]. Abu Dhabi: M42 Health; 2026. [cited 2026 Jun 17]. Available from: https://m42.ae/who-we-are/about-m42/.
22. Dubai Health Authority. Dubai hospital—rheumatology services [Internet]. Dubai: DHA; 2026. [cited 2026 Jun 17]. Available from: https://dha.gov.ae/uploads/122021/fb431907-99dd-4912-8db0-47a6aa474e05.pdf.
23. Bech B, Primdahl J, van Tubergen A, Voshaar M, Zangi HA, Barbosa L, et al. 2018 update of the EULAR recommendations for the role of the nurse in the management of chronic inflammatory arthritis. Ann Rheum Dis. 2020;79(1):61–8.

24. Cleveland CliSnic Abu Dhabi. PET Scan [Internet]. Abu Dhabi (UAE): Cleveland Clinic Abu Dhabi; [cited 2026 Jun 17]. Available from: https://www.clevelandclinicabudhabi.ae/en/health-library/health-resources/diagnostics-and-testing/pet-scan.
25. Sheikh Shakhbout Medical City. Positron Emission Tomography (PET) scan [Internet]. Abu Dhabi: SSMC; 2026. [cited 2026 Jun 17]. Available from: https://ssmc.ae/doctors-specialities/positron-emission-tomography-pet-scan/.
26. M42. Tawam Molecular Imaging Centre (TMIC), Al Ain—PET/CT molecular imaging [Internet]. Abu Dhabi: M42; 2026. [cited 2026 Jun 17]. Available from: https://m42.ae/tmic/.
27. Burjeel Medical City. Nuclear Medicine [Internet]. Abu Dhabi (UAE): Burjeel Medical City; [cited 2026 Jun 17]. Available from: >https://burjeelmedicalcity.com/specialities/nuclear-medicine/.
28. Mediclinic Airport Road Hospital. Diagnostic nuclear medicine & molecular imaging. Abu Dhabi: Mediclinic Airport Road Hospital; 2026. [cited 2026 Jun 17]. Available from: https://www.mediclinic.ae/en/airport-road-hospital/services-and-specialities/nuclear-medicine/our-services.html.
29. Gulf International Cancer Center. [Internet]. Abu Dhabi (UAE): Gulf International Cancer Center; [cited 2026 Jun 17]. Available from: https://gulficc.com/.
30. American Hospital Dubai. Advanced Radiology Services [Internet]. Dubai (UAE): American Hospital Dubai [cited 2026 Jun 17]. Available from: https://www.ahdubai.com/services/medical-imaging-and-nuclear-medicine-center.
31. Clemenceau Medical Center – Dubai (CMC). PET-CT Scan [Internet]. Dubai (UAE): CMC; [cited 2026 Jun 17]. Available from: https://cmcdubai.ae/solution/pet-ct-scan/.
32. Mediclinic City Hospital – Comprehensive Cancer Centre. Nuclear Medicine (including PET/CT) [Internet]. Dubai (UAE): Mediclinic City Hospital; [cited 2026 Jun 17]. Available from: https://www.mediclinic.ae/en/City-Hospital-Comprehensive-Cancer-Centre/services-and-specialities/nuclear-medicine.html.
33. Alnaqbi KA, Al Adhoubi N, Al Dallal S, Al Emadi S, Al Herz A, El Shamy A, et al. Consensus-based overarching principles and recommendations on the use of biosimilars in the treatment of inflammatory arthritis in the Gulf region. BioDrugs. 2024;38(3):449–63. https://doi.org/10.1007/s40259-023-00642-1.
34. Alnaqbi KA, Bellanger A, Brill A, Castañeda-Hernández G, Clopés Estela A, Delgado Sánchez O, et al. An international comparative analysis and roadmap to sustainable biosimilar markets. Front Pharmacol. 2023;14:1188368. https://doi.org/10.3389/fphar.2023.1188368.
35. Cerner Corporation. UAE Ministry of Health and Prevention renews relationship with Cerner to provide electronic health record [Internet]. GlobeNewswire; 2016 Nov 21 [cited 2026 Jun 17]. Available from: https://www.globenewswire.com/news-release/2016/11/21/891682/0/en/UAE-Ministry-of-Health-and-Prevention-Renews-Relationship-with-Cerner-to-Provide-Electronic-Health-Record.html.
36. Emirates Health Services [Internet]. United Arab Emirates [updated 2026 Apr 29; cited 2026 Jun 17]. Available from: https://patient.ehs.gov.ae/FE/Login.aspx.
37. Alshamsi AI, Abuquta A, Ibrahim A, AlSaadi A, Altaee E, AlAli N. Leaving against medical advice: a mixed method study to explore the prevalence, causes, and challenges in the Emirates Health Services' hospitals. Front Disaster Emerg Med. 2024;2:1474687. https://doi.org/10.3389/femer.2024.1474687.
38. Emirates Society for Rheumatology [Internet]. [cited 2026 Jun 17]. Available from: https://www.esr.ae.
39. Alnaqbi KA, Hannawi S, Namas R, Alshehhi W, Badsha H, Al-Saleh J. Consensus statements for evaluation and nonpharmacological management of psoriatic arthritis in UAE. Int J Rheum Dis. 2022;25(7):725–32. https://doi.org/10.1111/1756-185X.14357.
40. Alnaqbi KA, Hannawi S, Namas R, Alshehhi W, Badsha H, Al-Saleh J. Consensus statements for pharmacological management, monitoring of therapies, and comorbidity management of psoriatic arthritis in the United Arab Emirates. Int J Rheum Dis. 2022;25(10):1107–22. https://doi.org/10.1111/1756-185X.14406.

41. Middle East Arthritis Foundation [internet]. 2026. [cited 2026 Jun 17]. Available from: https://arthritis.ae/.
42. Sharjah Events. Friends-of-Arthritis-Patients (9th Charitable Marathon) – Event Archive. [Internet]. Sharjah (UAE): SharjahEvents.ae; 2022 Mar 16 [cited 2026 Jun 17]. Available from: https://cms.sharjahevents.ae/en/organizer/friends-of-arthritis-patients/.
43. Emirates News Agency (WAM). Friends of arthritis patients to launch 11th marathon on February 25. Abu Dhabi: WAM; 2024. [cited 2026 Jun 17]. Available from: https://www.wam.ae/en/article/b1pkkp7-friends-arthritis-patients-launch-11th-marathon.
44. Hannawi S, Hannawi H, Alokaily F, Naredo E, Moller I, Al Salmi I. Recent-onset of rheumatoid arthritis leads to increase in wall thickness of left anterior descending coronary artery. An evidence of subclinical coronary artery disease. Saudi Med J. 2018;39(12):1213–7.
45. Hannawi SM, Hannawi H, Alokaily F, Al Salmi I. Subclinical atherosclerosis in rheumatoid arthritis patients of the Gulf Cooperated Council. Saudi Med J. 2020;41(9):1022–5.
46. Hannawi S, Hannawi H, Alokaily F, Al Salmi I. Variables associated with subclinical atherosclerosis among rheumatoid arthritis patients of Gulf Cooperative Council countries. Saudi Med J. 2020;41(2):128–37.
47. Hannawi S, AlSalmi I, Moller I, Naredo E. Uric acid is independent cardiovascular risk factor, as manifested by increased carotid intima-media thickness in rheumatoid arthritis patients. Clin Rheumatol. 2017;36(8):1897–902.
48. Hannawi S, Hannawi H, Salmi IA. Rheumatoid arthritis patients have vitamin D deficiency compared to age sex matched control. What contribute to this. Ann Rheum Dis. 2019;78:1622–3.
49. Abdelgadir EIE, Rashid F, Basheir AMK, Alawadi F, Al Suwidi H, Eltinay A. Vitamin D deficiency, the volume of the problem in the United Arab Emirates. A cohort from the Middle East. Middle East J Endocrinol Diab. 2016;3(2):1–5.
50. Hannawi S, Al Salmi I. In Rheumatoid Arthritis: Vitamin-D Deficiency Is an Outcome and a Cause of Subclinical Renal Impairment [abstract]. Arthritis Rheumatol. 2017;69(suppl 10). [cited 2026 Jun 17]. Available from: https://acrabstracts.org/abstract/in-rheumatoid-arthritis-vitamin-d-deficiency-is-an-outcome-and-a-cause-of-subclinical-renal-impairment/.
51. Al-Attia HM, George S. Characterization of systemic lupus erythematosus in patients in U.A.E. Clin Rheumatol. 1995;14(2):171–5.
52. AlSaleh J, Jassim V, ElSayed M, Saleh N, Harb D. Clinical and immunological manifestations in 151 SLE patients living in Dubai. Lupus. 2008;17(1):62–6.
53. Al Dhanhani AM, Agarwal M, Othman YS, Bakoush O. Incidence and prevalence of systemic lupus erythematosus among the native Arab population in UAE. Lupus. 2017;26(6):664–9.
54. Al Saleh J, Sayed ME, Monsef N, Darwish E. The prevalence and the determinants of musculoskeletal diseases in Emiratis attending primary health care clinics in Dubai. Oman Med J. 2016;31(2):117–23.
55. Namas R, Elarabi M, Khan S, Mubashir A, Memisoglu E, El-Kaissi M, et al. Comprehensive description of the prevalence, serological and clinical characteristics, and visceral involvement of systemic sclerosis (scleroderma) in a large cohort from the United Arab Emirates Systemic Sclerosis Registry. J Scleroderma Relat Disord. 2023;8(2):137–50.
56. Al-Saleh JA, Albelooshi AA, Salti AA, Farghaly M, Ghorab AM, Linga S, et al. Burden, treatment patterns and unmet needs of osteoarthritis in Dubai: a retrospective analysis of the Dubai real-world claims database. Rheumatol Ther. 2022;9(1):151–74.
57. Al Taie WAM, Rasheed AM. The correlation of body mass index, age, gender with bone mineral density in osteopenia and osteoporosis: a study in the United Arab Emirates. Clin Med Diagn. 2014;4(3):42–54.
58. Al Anouti F, Taha Z, Shamim S, Khalaf K, Al Kaabi L, Alsafar H. An insight into the paradigms of osteoporosis: from genetics to biomechanics. Bone Rep. 2019;11:100216.
59. Al-Saleh Y, Al-Daghri NM, Sabico S, Alessa T, Al Emadi S, Alawadi F, et al. Diagnosis and management of osteoporosis in postmenopausal women in Gulf Cooperation Council (GCC) countries: consensus statement of the GCC countries' osteoporosis societies under the auspices

of the European Society for Clinical and Economic Aspects of Osteoporosis and Osteoarthritis (ESCEO). Arch Osteoporos. 2020;15(1):109.
60. Al Izzi M, Al Suhaili A, El Serafi A, Abogamal A, Tapponi L, Brodzinski Z. Launching the Emirates Osteoporosis Society (EOS) Guidelines 2022 in the United Arab Emirates. New Emirates Med J. 2023;4(1):e260123213159.
61. MacDonald Gibson J, Thomsen J, Launay F, Harder E, DeFelice N. Deaths and medical visits attributable to environmental pollution in the United Arab Emirates. PLoS One. 2013;8(3):e57536. https://doi.org/10.1371/journal.pone.0057536.
62. Gibson JM, Farah ZS. Environmental risks to public health in the United Arab Emirates: a quantitative assessment and strategic plan. Environ Health Perspect. 2012;120(5):681–6.
63. United Arab Emirates. UAE Long-Term Low-Emission Development Strategy: Net Zero by 2050 [Internet]. UAE: Ministry of Climate Change & Environment; 2023 [cited 2026 May 9]. Available from: https://unfccc.int/sites/default/files/resource/UAE_LTLEDS.pdf?n=1673557627.
64. Majka DS, Holers VM. Cigarette smoking and the risk of systemic lupus erythematosus and rheumatoid arthritis. Ann Rheum Dis. 2006;65(5):561–3.
65. Hannawi SM, Hannawi H, Al Salmi I. Cardiovascular risk in rheumatoid arthritis: literature review. Oman Med J. 2021;36(3):e262.
66. Pezzolo E, Naldi L. The relationship between smoking, psoriasis and psoriatic arthritis. Expert Rev Clin Immunol. 2019;15(1):41–8.
67. Al-Bashaireh AM, Haddad LG, Weaver M, Chengguo X, Kelly DL, Yoon S. The effect of tobacco smoking on bone mass: an overview of pathophysiologic mechanisms. J Osteoporos. 2018;2018:1206235.
68. Khabbazi A, Alinejati B, Hajialilo M, Ghojazadeh M, Malek MA. Cigarette smoking and risk of primary systemic vasculitis: a propensity score matching analysis. Sarcoidosis Vasc Diffuse Lung Dis. 2019;36(3):243–50.
69. Razzak HA, Harbi A, Ahli S. Tobacco smoking prevalence, health risk, and cessation in the UAE. Oman Med J. 2020;35(4):e165.
70. Aden B, Karrar S, Shafey O, Al Hosni F. Cigarette, water-pipe, and Medwakh smoking prevalence among applicants to Abu Dhabi's Pre-marital Screening Program, 2011. Int J Prev Med. 2013;4(11):1290–5.
71. Al-Houqani M, Ali R, Hajat C. Tobacco smoking using Midwakh is an emerging health problem—evidence from a large cross-sectional survey in the United Arab Emirates. PLoS One. 2012;7(6):e39189.
72. Klareskog L, Gregersen PK, Huizinga TW. Prevention of autoimmune rheumatic disease: state of the art and future perspectives. Ann Rheum Dis. 2010;69(12):2062–6.
73. Feng X, Xu X, Shi Y, Liu X, Liu H, Hou H, et al. Body mass index and the risk of rheumatoid arthritis: an updated dose-response meta-analysis. Biomed Res Int. 2019;2019:3579081.
74. Cozier YC, Barbhaiya M, Castro-Webb N, Conte C, Tedeschi S, Leatherwood C, et al. A prospective study of obesity and risk of systemic lupus erythematosus (SLE) among Black women. Semin Arthritis Rheum. 2019;48(6):1030–4.
75. Zhou ZY, Liu YK, Chen HL, Liu F. Body mass index and knee osteoarthritis risk: a dose-response meta-analysis. Obesity (Silver Spring). 2014;22(10):2180–5.
76. Love TJ, Zhu Y, Zhang Y, Wall-Burns L, Ogdie A, Gelfand JM, et al. Obesity and the risk of psoriatic arthritis: a population-based study. Ann Rheum Dis. 2012;71(8):1273–7.
77. Al Anouti F, Thomas J, Abdel-Wareth L, Rajah J, Grant WB, Haq A. Vitamin D deficiency and sun avoidance among university students at Abu Dhabi, United Arab Emirates. Dermatoendocrinol. 2011;3(4):235–9.
78. Bhagavathula AS, Shah SM, Aburawi EH. Prevalence, awareness, treatment, and control of hypertension in The United Arab Emirates: a systematic review and meta-analysis. Int J Environ Res Public Health. 2021;18(23):12693.

79. Alketbi LB, Al Hashaikeh B, Fahmawee T, Sahalu Y, Alkuwaiti MHH, Nagelkerke N, et al. Hypertension and its determinants in Abu Dhabi population: a retrospective cohort study. J Hypertens. 2025;43(2):308–17. https://doi.org/10.1097/HJH.0000000000003907.
80. Sulaiman N, Mahmoud I, Hussein A, Elbadawi S, Abusnana S, Zimmet P, et al. Diabetes risk score in the United Arab Emirates: a screening tool for the early detection of type 2 diabetes mellitus. BMJ Open Diabetes Res Care. 2018;6(1):e000489.
81. Sulaiman N, Albadawi S, Abusnana S, Mairghani M, Hussein A, Al Awadi F, et al. High prevalence of diabetes among migrants in the United Arab Emirates using a cross-sectional survey. Sci Rep. 2018;8(1):6862.
82. Mahmoud I, Sulaiman N. Dyslipidaemia prevalence and associated risk factors in the United Arab Emirates: a population-based study. BMJ Open. 2019;9(11):e031969.
83. Mahmoud I, Sulaiman N. Prevalence of metabolic syndrome and associated risk factors in the United Arab Emirates: a cross-sectional population-based study. Front Public Health. 2021;9:811006.
84. al-Gazali LI, Bener A, Abdulrazzaq YM, Micallef R, al-Khayat AI, Gaber T. Consanguineous marriages in the United Arab Emirates. J Biosoc Sci. 1997;29(4):491–7.
85. Al-Gazali L, Hamamy H. Consanguinity and dysmorphology in Arabs. Hum Hered. 2014;77(1–4):93–107.
86. Finckh A, Deane KD. Prevention of rheumatic diseases: strategies, caveats, and future directions. Rheum Dis Clin N Am. 2014;40(4):771–85.
87. World Health Organization. Screening programmes: a short guide [Internet]. Geneva: WHO. [cited 2026 Jun 17]. Available from: https://www.who.int/europe/teams/ncd-management/screening.
88. Sayers S, Lam D, Shah Q, Evans J, Parkes M, Stober C, et al. Impact on patient outcomes of spondyloarthritis-inflammatory bowel disease multi-disciplinary meetings. Rheumatology (Oxford). 2025;64(2):815–20. https://doi.org/10.1093/rheumatology/keae116.
89. Ndosi M, Lewis M, Hale C, Quinn H, Ryan S, Emery P, et al. The outcome and cost-effectiveness of nurse-led care in people with rheumatoid arthritis: a multicentre randomised controlled trial. Ann Rheum Dis. 2014;73(11):1975–82. https://doi.org/10.1136/annrheumdis-2013-203403.
90. MOHAP. United Arab Emirates Ministry of Health and Prevention (MOHAP). In: National Health Workforce Account (NHWA) report 2019–2020 [Internet]. Dubai (UAE): MOHAP; 2020. [cited 2026 Jun 17]. Available from: https://mohap.gov.ae/documents/20117/1212145/NHWA+UAE+Report+2019-2020-472.pdf.
91. Hannawi S, Hannawi H. Rheumatology research setting in the United Arab Emirates. Saudi Med J. 2022;43(6):637–55.
92. Ministry of Health and Prevention. Ministerial Decree No. (730) of the year 2018 approving the guidelines for conducting clinical trials [Internet]. United Arab Emirates: Ministry of Health and Prevention; 2018 [cited 2026 Jun 17]. Available from: https://mohap.gov.ae/en/w/ministerial-decree-no.-730-of-the-year-2018-approving-the-guidelines-for-conducting-clinical-trials.
93. Ministry of Health (UAE), Drug Control Department. Guidance for conducting clinical trials based on drugs/medical products & good clinical practice. 2006. [cited 2026 Jun 17]. Available from: https://mohap.gov.ae/documents/20117/454960/2c69fad1-9af2-4113-9147-1d8d25da1fdd.pdf.
94. Dubai Health Authority. Submissions of new applications and opinions to DSREC [Internet]. 2019. [cited 2026 Jun 17]. Available from: https://dha.gov.ae/uploads/122021/045bbafa-9072-4624-a1d8-83b2abe0d55b.pdf.
95. Department of Health – Abu Dhabi. Guidelines for conducting clinical trials with investigational products and medical devices. 2020. [cited 2026 Jun 17]. Available from: https://www.doh.gov.ae/-/media/Feature/Resources/Guidelines/Guidelines-for-Conducting-Clinical-Trials-with-Investigational-Product.ashx.

96. Department of Health – Abu Dhabi. Standard on human subject research. 2020. [cited 2026 Jun 17]. Available from: https://www.doh.gov.ae/-/media/C07A10ADB6504312A601E3A514D43084.ashx.
97. Department of Health – Abu Dhabi (DoH). Research and Innovation – Research Governance and Forms [Internet]. Abu Dhabi (UAE): DoH; [cited 2026 Jun 17]. Available from: https://www.doh.gov.ae/en/research/landing-page.
98. World Health Organization. Regional Office for the Eastern Mediterranean. United Arab Emirates: health systems profile – key country indicators and strategic priorities [Internet]. Cairo: WHO-EMRO; 2013. [cited 2026 Jun 17]. Available from: https://applications.emro.who.int/docs/Country_profile_2013_EN_15403.pdf.
99. Rotter T, de Jong RB, Lacko SE, Ronellenfitsch U, Kinsman L. Clinical pathways as a quality strategy. In: Busse R, Klazinga N, Panteli D, Quentin W, editors. Improving healthcare quality in Europe: characteristics, effectiveness and implementation of different strategies [Internet]. Copenhagen (Denmark): European Observatory on Health Systems and Policies; 2019. (Health Policy Series, No. 53). Chapter 12. Available from: https://www.ncbi.nlm.nih.gov/books/NBK549262/.

Chapter 20
Rheumatic Diseases in Yemen

Arwa Aljohi, Nabil Al-Ashmory, Thekra Alabsi, and Abdulrahman Jamel

Abstract Rheumatic diseases represent a growing global health challenge, yet data from conflict-affected countries such as Yemen remain extremely limited. This chapter provides the most comprehensive overview to date of the rheumatology landscape in Yemen, drawing on available literature, unpublished clinical data, and expert insights. Yemen's prolonged conflict has severely weakened the health system, resulting in critical shortages of rheumatologists, limited diagnostic capacity, inadequate access to essential medications, and the absence of national registries or coordinated care pathways. Pediatric and adult rheumatic disease patterns from existing clinical reports highlight a predominance of rheumatoid arthritis and systemic lupus erythematosus, high rates of misdiagnosis, and delays in referral, particularly in rural regions. Diagnostic services remain constrained by limited autoantibody testing, imaging capacity, biopsies, and a reliance on paper-based records. Additional country-specific risk factors, including widespread consanguinity, smoking, khat chewing, infections, and low socioeconomic status, likely exacerbate disease burden. The chapter concludes by outlining key opportunities for strengthening rheumatology services through workforce development, improved diagnostics, tele-rheumatology, national registry establishment, and regional collaboration. Together, these actions are essential to improving outcomes and reducing disability among Yemenis living with rheumatic diseases.

A. Aljohi (✉)
Rheumatology and Rehabilitation, Alsheikh Othman polyclinic, Aden, Yemen
e-mail: aljohiarwa@gmail.com

N. Al-Ashmory
Rheumatology and Rehabilitation, University of 21 September, Sanaa, Yemen
e-mail: nabilalashmory@gmail.com

T. Alabsi
Internal Medicine and Rheumatology, Kuwait University Hospital, Sanaa University, Sanaa, Yemen
e-mail: Thekrasaif@gmail.com

A. Jamel
Rheumatology and Rehabilitation at Taiz University, Taiz, Yemen
e-mail: dr.abdulrahman.a.jamel@gmail.com

K. A. Alnaqbi, G. Aldabie (eds.), *Rheumatic Diseases in the Arab World*,
https://doi.org/10.1007/978-981-92-0967-5_20

Keywords Yemen · Healthcare · Conflict · Rheumatic disease · Rheumatology

20.1 Yemen Demographics

The Republic of Yemen, or simply Yemen, is in the Middle East, at the southwestern end of the Arabian Peninsula. It is the second-largest country on the Peninsula, occupying 527,968 km^2, and has a coastline of 1906 km along the Arabian Sea, the Gulf of Aden, and the Red Sea [1]. The Bab el-Mandeb Strait, which connects the Red Sea and the Gulf of Aden, is one of the busiest shipping lanes in the world. Yemen's name, "Arabia Felix," was inspired by the concepts of prosperity and blessings. This fertile and commercially prosperous region, known by the ancient Romans as such, was once the residence of many ancient kingdoms. Sana'a is the country's largest city and national capital, while Aden is the country's economic center [2]. Yemen is divided into 22 governorates.

As of 2024, Yemen has a population of approximately 32.14 million, with a median age of about 22 years, reflecting a young demographic structure. The sex ratio shows slight variation across age groups, with roughly 1.04 males for every female in the 0–14-year group, 1.03 males per female among those aged 15–64 years, and 0.78 males per female in the population aged 65 years and older. The birth rate is approximately 23.4 births per 1000 people, while the death rate is approximately 5.5 per 1000 people. The total fertility rate stands at 2.82 children per woman, and life expectancy at birth is estimated at 68.2 years. A substantial share of the population resides in rural and tribal areas, consistent with its predominantly agrarian and communal social structure. Additionally, the country faces significant limitations in its healthcare workforce, with a physician density of only 0.1 per 1000 population reported in 2023 [1].

Historically, Yemen was known to the Romans as *Arabia Felix* ("Fortunate Arabia") for its prosperity, fertile lands, and flourishing incense trade, supported by remarkable engineering feats such as the ancient Marib Dam. The region was home to influential civilizations, including the Sabaean, Himyarite, and Hadrami kingdoms, that shaped its political, cultural, and commercial identity [2, 3]. Yemen's strategic position along major trade routes further enriched its heritage, contributing to the development of distinctive architectural, linguistic, and cultural traditions that continue to characterize the country today.

In contrast, modern Yemen has faced prolonged political instability, with the conflict that escalated in 2015 leading to widespread destruction, displacement, and one of the world's most severe humanitarian crises. The ongoing war has devastated infrastructure and significantly weakened the country's health, economic, and social systems [4].

20.2 Healthcare System in Yemen

Healthcare in Yemen is centrally administered by the Ministry of Public Health and Population (MoPHP), with governance extending to the Governorate Health Offices (GHOs) at the governorate level and the District Health Offices (DHOs) at the district level [4].

However, years of armed conflict have severely weakened the health system, contributing to the deterioration of healthcare facilities and a decline in health expenditure, which represented only 2.5% of the national budget in 2022. The physician density also remains critically low, estimated at 0.1 physicians per 1000 population in 2023 [1, 4, 5]. According to the World Health Organization Eastern Mediterranean Regional Office (WHO EMRO), only 45% of Yemen's health facilities remain fully functional, with widespread shortages of essential medicines, equipment, and staff, and a heavy dependence on out-of-pocket payments for most services and medications [6].

The prolonged conflict has pushed Yemen into one of the world's worst humanitarian crises, leaving nearly 21 million people in need of assistance and more than 80% of the population living below the poverty line [4]. It has disrupted essential health programs and supply chains, contributing to high rates of child malnutrition, low immunization coverage, and recurrent outbreaks of infectious diseases. As a result, healthcare delivery now relies heavily on international humanitarian and development organizations [4, 7].

Significant disparities in healthcare access persist between urban and rural areas, and the ongoing conflict has further worsened health outcomes.

Yemen's digital health infrastructure remains limited, with most hospitals relying on fragmented, paper-based systems and only a few public health programs supported by electronic platforms such as the district health information software 2 (DHIS2) and the electronic Disease Early Warning System (eDEWS) [8, 9]. In this context, rheumatology services face similar challenges: most clinics operate without structured clinical databases or formal disease registries, resulting in inconsistent and incomplete patient documentation. Establishing a standardized, nationwide rheumatic disease registry is therefore urgently needed to support epidemiological research, monitor disease burden, and improve clinical decision-making within the constraints of Yemen's current health system.

20.3 Rheumatology Services in Yemen

The demand for specialized rheumatology care in Yemen is significant, driven by a rising prevalence of rheumatic diseases.

20.3.1 Rheumatology Workforce

In Yemen, there is a severe shortage of rheumatologists. As of 2023, only seven adult specialists (two females and four males) are available, along with one pediatric rheumatologist. These clinicians provide care for patients with musculoskeletal diseases across seven outpatient clinics nationwide: three in Sanaa, one in Ibb, one in Aden, and three in Hadramout.

A notable development in pediatric care is the establishment of a pediatric rheumatology clinic at Al-Mukalla Hospital in Hadramout in January 2010, which began registering pediatric rheumatic disease cases and increasing awareness among physicians and families.

Given Yemen's population size, this number is markedly insufficient, and public awareness of rheumatology as a specialty remains limited, partly because rheumatology is not well integrated into medical school training. Most of the available rheumatologists received their postgraduate training abroad.

Due to the shortage of specialists, orthopedic surgeons and internists often serve as the first point of contact for patients with rheumatic symptoms. As a result, misdiagnosis and underdiagnosis are common, especially at the primary healthcare level. Furthermore, Yemen lacks formally trained rheumatology nurses, which further constrains service delivery.

20.3.2 Access to Rheumatology Services in Yemen

Effective management of rheumatic diseases requires coordinated, multidisciplinary care that includes rheumatologists, specialized nursing, physiotherapy, and occupational therapy. In Yemen, however, access to such comprehensive services remains limited [4]. Most patients rely initially on primary care or general medical services, as rheumatology expertise is scarce and specialized centers are not widely available. This overall lack of specialized rheumatology access has negatively affected outcomes across a wide range of rheumatic diseases, leading to delayed diagnosis, suboptimal treatment, and preventable disease progression.

Rehabilitation services in the country are predominantly oriented toward war-related injuries. Many rehabilitation centers focus primarily on supporting people wounded in the conflict and therefore have limited capacity or experience in managing chronic rheumatic and musculoskeletal conditions. This creates important gaps in non-trauma rehabilitation, including the long-term functional and mobility needs of patients with rheumatic diseases.

According to the International Committee of the Red Cross (ICRC) Semi-Annual Activity Report for 2025, physical rehabilitation services were provided through five ICRC-supported rehabilitation centers and two wheelchair-service structures across five governorates, demonstrating that rehabilitation services exist but remain constrained and insufficiently aligned with the needs of rheumatology patients [7]. In addition, King Salman Relief Center (KSRC) supports four additional physical rehabilitation centers as part of the health sector program [10], demonstrating that rehabilitation services exist but remain constrained and insufficiently aligned with the needs of rheumatology patients.

20.4 Availability of Diagnostic Tests for Rheumatic Diseases in Yemen

20.4.1 Laboratory Tests

In Yemen, the available diagnostic investigations for patients with rheumatic disease are limited and considered preliminary. Not all autoantibodies are available, and immunofluorescent tests are limited to private labs and scarce in public laboratories. The synovial analysis is available in most health laboratories. However, the quality of trained technicians could be improved. Polarized microscopy or capillaroscopy is not available. Fortunately, the HLA-B27 test is available, but its cost remains a barrier for many patients, limiting their ability to afford it.

20.4.2 Imaging Tests

Imaging plays a crucial role in diagnosing, monitoring, and predicting the outcome of rheumatic diseases. Conventional radiological imaging is available in most public and private health facilities across Yemen.

Military hospitals in Aden and Sanaa offer magnetic resonance imaging (MRI), and several private hospitals and imaging centers also provide MRI services. According to the latest available WHO data (2013), Yemen has a computed tomography (CT) scanner density of approximately 3.61 per million population and an MRI density of about 1.15 scanners per million population; positron emission tomography (PET) scanning is not available [11].

Musculoskeletal ultrasonography (MSUS) is widely accepted in the rheumatology community for detecting synovitis and tenosynovitis in inflammatory joint diseases [12]. However, access to trained MSUS operators remains limited in Yemen, restricting its routine use in rheumatology clinics.

20.4.3 Biopsy

A biopsy is a valuable diagnostic tool in many rheumatic diseases, helping confirm diagnoses, assess disease severity, and guide prognosis, particularly in conditions with organ involvement such as lupus nephritis. However, in Yemen, kidney biopsy and other important tissue biopsies (including muscle, nerve, vessel, salivary gland,

and synovial biopsies) are hardly available due to limited technical capacity and the shortage of trained interventional radiologists and pathologists.

20.5 Availability of Treatment in Yemen

20.5.1 *Disease-Modifying Anti-Rheumatic Drugs (DMARD)*

Conventional DMARDs are available in the major cities of most governorates. However, biological DMARDs and targeted synthetic DMARDs are limited in availability across the country. The only options for the few patients who can afford them are to travel abroad (Egypt, Jordan, or India) or make a special request to larger pharmacies.

20.5.2 *Plasma Exchange*

Immune dysregulation and autoantibody production drive many rheumatic diseases, making antibody removal a useful therapeutic strategy. Therapeutic plasma exchange is a safe and minimally invasive option that can benefit selected rheumatic conditions [13]. Unfortunately, this service is available only in one private hospital in Yemen.

20.6 Overview of Rheumatic Diseases in Yemen

In 2021, non-communicable diseases accounted for 41.5% of total deaths. The leading causes of death per 100,000 population were ischemic heart disease (78.4), collective violence and legal intervention (54.9), COVID-19 (48.1), stroke (47.3), preterm birth complications (33.7), lower respiratory infections (33.5), road injuries (29.9), birth asphyxia and trauma (19.6), hypertensive heart disease (17.7), and diarrheal diseases (13.8) [14]. Against this broader national health backdrop, rheumatic diseases represent an under-recognized yet significant burden, with patterns that differ between children and adults.

20.6.1 *Pediatric Rheumatology Services and Rheumatic Disease Patterns in Yemen*

A recent observational study at the pediatric rheumatology clinic in Al-Mukalla Hospital, Hadramout province, assessed pediatric rheumatic disease (PRD) cases from January 2010 to December 2016, diagnosed using validated criteria [15]. Out of 26 patients with PRD (70.3%) referred, 16 were sent by pediatricians (43.2%), two by either an orthopedic surgeon or a dermatologist (5.4%), six were transferred from peripheral hospitals (16.2%), and two were identified during admission to the pediatric ward (5.4%). The remaining 11 patients (29.7%) presented to the clinic for the first time after prolonged evaluations in multiple private clinics.

A total of 37 PRD cases were documented. Juvenile idiopathic arthritis was the most frequent diagnosis (24.3%), followed by systemic lupus erythematosus (SLE, 13.5%). Autoinflammatory syndromes and non-inflammatory musculoskeletal pain each accounted for 10.8% of cases. Scleroderma and vasculitis represented 8.1% each. Less common conditions, including enthesitis-related arthritis, juvenile polymyositis, sarcoidosis, septic arthritis, and osteomyelitis, each occurred in 2.7% of patients. Post-streptococcal reactive arthritis and rheumatic fever were each reported in 5.4% of cases [15].

Among the referred cases, 70.3% were initially misdiagnosed, and 48.8% had received an incorrect diagnosis before presentation. The reported mortality rate was 5.4%, attributed to severe disease complications or poor treatment adherence. Overall, PRDs constituted 86% (37/43) of evaluated cases, with 83.8% (31/37) originating from the Hadhramout province. The female-to-male ratio was 1:0.9, and the mean age at presentation was 8.86 ± 4.11 years [15].

20.6.2 Adult Rheumatology Patient Characteristics and Disease Distribution

In contrast to pediatric patterns, adult rheumatic diseases in Yemen show a different epidemiological profile. In an unpublished study involving patients attending rheumatology clinics in Aden and Sanaa from January to May 2022, the mean age of patients was 41 years (±12.43), and 82% were female (Fig. 20.1). Rheumatoid arthritis (RA) was the most common rheumatic disease, accounting for 62.5% of all cases (Fig. 20.2). The female-to-male ratio among RA patients was 8:1, and 89% of all patients with SLE were female. SLE represented the second most frequent condition, followed by spondyloarthropathies (SpA).

The study also reported a rise in the diagnosis of fibromyalgia (5%) and reactive arthritis (1.2%). This pattern is likely influenced by the ongoing conflict, which has disrupted healthcare services and increased exposure to physical and psychological stressors (Table 20.1). The collapse of the healthcare system and inadequate water and sanitation have contributed to higher rates of communicable diseases, some of which can trigger or mimic rheumatic conditions. Additionally, the prolonged conflict may exacerbate underlying genetic susceptibility, acting as a precipitating factor for rheumatic disease onset or flares.

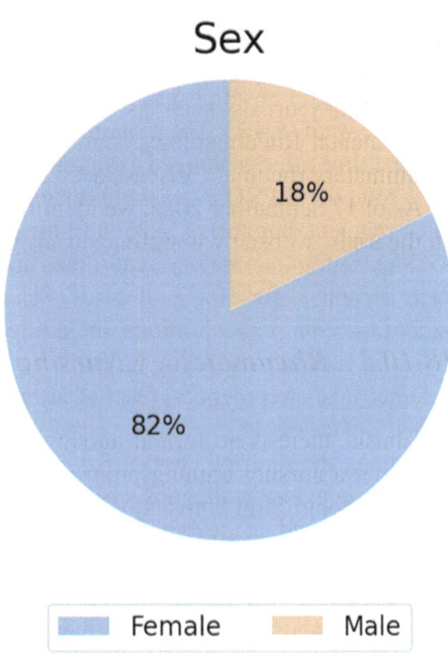

Fig. 20.1 Sex Presentation of Rheumatic Disease in Rheumatology Clinics at Aden and Sanaa (unpublished data)

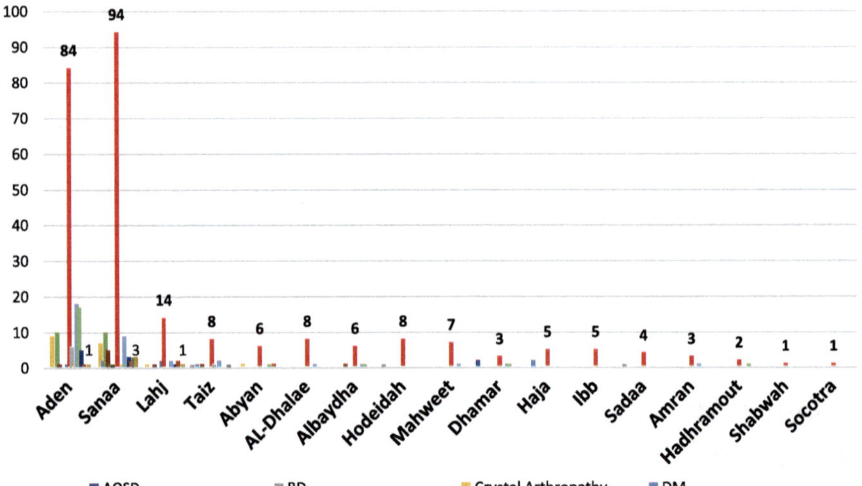

Fig. 20.2 Distribution of rheumatic diseases by governorates (unpublished data)
Abbreviations: *AOSD* adult-onset Still's disease; *FM* fibromyalgia; *PsA* psoriatic arthritis; *SLE* systemic lupus erythematosus; *BD* Behçet disease; *MCTD* mixed connective tissue disease; *RA* rheumatoid arthritis; *SpA* spondyloarthritis; *SS* Sjögren syndrome; *DM* dermatomyositis; *PM* polymyositis; *SSC* systemic sclerosis

Table 20.1 Rheumatic disease presentation in Aden and Sanaa Clinics (unpublished data)

Disease	Frequency	Percentage
RA	259	62.5%
SLE	36	9%
SpA	23	6%
FM	20	5%
Crystal arthropathies	18	4.3%
MCTD	9	2.2%
SS	9	2.2%
SSc	6	1.4%
Reactive arthritis	7	1.2%
DM	5	0.9%
Vasculitis	6	1.7%
Undifferented CTD	4	1%
BD	3	0.7%
PsA	3	0.7%
Sarcoidosis	2	0.5%
AOSD	2	0.5%
Overlap CTD	1	0.2%
PM	1	0.2%
Total	414	100

RA rheumatoid arthritis, *SpA* spondyloarthropathy, *SLE* systemic lupus erythematosus, *FM* fibromyalgia, *MCTD* mixed connective tissue disease, *JIA* juvenile idiopathic arthritis, *SS* Sjögren syndrome, *SSc* systemic sclerosis, *PsA* psoriatic arthritis, *AOSD* adult-onset Still disease, *PM* polymyositis, *RF* rheumatic fever, *CTD* connective tissue disease, *BD* Behçet disease

20.6.3 Patterns of Autoimmune and Rheumatic Diseases in Hospital-Based Studies

Beyond clinic observations, broader epidemiological analyses provide additional insight. The first comprehensive assessment of autoimmune and rheumatic diseases in Yemen was conducted across six major health facilities in Sana'a between 2014 and 2017 [16]. RA (39.2%) and SLE (36.9%) were the most common systemic autoimmune conditions, with a marked predominance among women. Antiphospholipid syndrome accounted for 16.4% of cases, while Sjögren's syndrome (2.6%), mixed connective tissue disease (1.8%), systemic sclerosis (1.6%), vasculitis (0.9%), and polymyositis (0.5%) were observed less frequently. The study also highlighted that autoimmune hepatitis, Graves' disease, Hashimoto's disease, and celiac disease were the leading organ-specific autoimmune disorders. Overall, autoimmune diseases primarily affected young adults and showed a steady increase in frequency over the study period.

These findings underscore the strong female predominance, the rising burden of autoimmune diseases in Yemen, and the urgent need for population-level studies to better define incidence, risk factors, and regional patterns.

20.6.4 Clinical and Laboratory Characteristics of SLE in Yemen

A hospital-based study from Al-Thawra Hospital in Sana'a analyzed 149 Yemeni patients with SLE to describe their clinical and laboratory features [17]. Most patients were young adults, with women representing three-quarters of all cases. Fatigue, fever, joint pain, photosensitivity, renal involvement, and malar rash were the most frequently reported manifestations. Serologically, antinuclear antibodies (ANA) were positive in more than 95% of patients and were significantly associated with most clinical symptoms. Anti-dsDNA antibodies were found in nearly 60% and correlated particularly with fever and fatigue. Anti-Sm antibodies were detected in about one-quarter of patients but showed no strong relationship with clinical features. The study also identified sunlight exposure and psychosocial stress as risk factors for triggering SLE.

Overall, the findings highlight the predominance of SLE among young women in Yemen, the high frequency of systemic involvement, and the reliance on limited but essential immunological tests for diagnosis.

20.7 Risk Factors for Rheumatic Diseases

Understanding country-specific risk factors is essential for developing appropriate educational strategies, strengthening healthcare services, and tailoring public health interventions related to rheumatic diseases in Yemen.

20.7.1 Genetic Factor

RA appears to have a hereditary component, according to family studies. Both candidate genes and whole-genome screening have been used extensively to investigate genetic factors linked to RA [18]. The risk of developing RA is 3 to 5 times higher in individuals with first-degree relatives who have the condition [19]. Yemen has one of the highest consanguinity rates in the region, with more than 40% of marriages occurring between blood relatives and the majority between first cousins

[20]. Recent studies confirm this trend: Khayat et al. and Al-Asfar et al. both reported persistently high consanguinity levels across Yemeni communities. These patterns increase the likelihood of clustering hereditary and autoimmune conditions within families, thereby raising the genetic susceptibility to rheumatic diseases.

20.7.2 Socioeconomic Status

Socioeconomic disadvantage is consistently associated with poorer functional outcomes, higher disease activity, and reduced access to advanced therapies in RA [21]. Yemen, one of the world's poorest nations, faces extreme resource constraints, low health literacy, and fragmented specialist services, all of which increase the likelihood that patients with rheumatic diseases will experience delayed diagnosis, suboptimal treatment, and worse long-term outcomes. Together, these factors suggest that low socioeconomic status in Yemen is a major, and often under-recognized, risk determinant for adverse outcomes in rheumatic diseases.

20.7.3 Environmental Causes

Environmental exposures are a significant concern in Yemen. Khat leaves often contain pesticide residues (i.e., organophosphates and organochlorines) and heavy metals (e.g., lead, cadmium, and iron) at levels that pose health risks [22]. A growing body of evidence demonstrates that many of these pesticides possess immunotoxic, genotoxic, and endocrine-disrupting properties. Pesticide exposure can impair lymphocyte function, alter cytokine profiles, disrupt immune regulation, and contribute to autoimmunity, allergy, cardiac disease, infection susceptibility, and malignancy [23].

Experimental work further demonstrates that exposure to organochlorine pesticides, such as hexachlorocyclohexane (HCH) isomers and dichlorodiphenyltrichloroethane (DDT) derivatives, can increase disease activity in systemic sclerosis, reducing lymphoproliferative responses and promoting IL-4 production, a profibrotic cytokine, in patient-derived immune cells [24]. In the Agricultural Health Study, lifetime use of several pesticides, including methyl bromide and cyclodiene organochlorines, was associated with a higher prevalence of antinuclear antibodies and other autoantibodies [25]. Consistent with these findings, a study among pesticide sprayers found a higher frequency of rheumatoid arthritis and allergic rhinitis [26].

20.7.4 Smoking

Current smoking is a well-established, modifiable risk factor in inflammatory rheumatic diseases and is linked with increased disease activity, functional disability, and radiographic progression in conditions such as RA and axial spondyloarthritis [27–29].

In Yemen, smoking remains an important public health concern. The 2013 Demographic and Health Survey conducted among adults aged 15 years and older reported a current smoking prevalence of 20.7% in males and 6.0% in females. More recent WHO age-standardized estimates from 2019 indicate that tobacco use continues to be widespread, with 35.3% of men and 8.9% of women using tobacco (smoked or smokeless), and 21.4% of men compared to 3.7% of women classified as current cigarette smokers [30].

20.7.5 Khat (Catha edulis)

Khat chewing, a psychostimulant, is highly prevalent in Yemen, particularly among men, and is deeply rooted in social and cultural practices [31, 32]. Evidence shows that khat chewing is frequently accompanied by the use of other substances such as cigarettes, reflecting a pattern of clustered risk behaviors among regular khat users [33]. Long sessions of khat chewing often involve prolonged sitting in flexed-knee postures, which may contribute to mechanical stress on the knee joints; frequent knee-bending activities have been associated with focal knee lesions and increased osteoarthritis risk [34]. Chronic khat chewing is also implicated in several oral and dental disorders, including periodontal disease and changes in subgingival microbiota [35, 36].

Furthermore, studies from Yemen indicate that khat users report significantly more joint pain and higher uric acid levels than non-chewers, suggesting a potential link to arthritic conditions [37]. Khat chewing is also associated with poorer health-related quality of life and lower socioeconomic status, which may further compound rheumatic disease outcomes. Taken together, these findings indicate that khat chewing may act as an under-recognized lifestyle risk factor in rheumatic disease development and progression in Yemen.

20.7.6 Infections

Yemen faces a substantial burden of communicable diseases, many of which have intensified due to the ongoing conflict and collapse of essential public health services. Recurrent outbreaks of cholera, diphtheria, tuberculosis, dengue, and chikungunya have been widely documented, reflecting the breakdown of water and sanitation systems, declining vaccination coverage, and disruptions in disease control programs [38–42]. Some of these infections, particularly chikungunya and dengue, are well known for causing acute febrile polyarthritis that can mimic or trigger inflammatory rheumatic diseases [41].

The COVID-19 pandemic further strained the already fragile healthcare system, worsening access to routine care and complicating the management of chronic diseases, including rheumatic conditions [40]. Collectively, these infectious disease pressures create diagnostic challenges, contribute to delays in appropriate rheumatologic evaluation, and may precipitate or exacerbate musculoskeletal symptoms in susceptible individuals.

In 2020, the prevalence of hepatitis B surface antigen (HBsAg) among children under five was 1.76% [43]. In 2024, the estimated incidence rate of tuberculosis is 39.7 cases per 100,000 population [44, 45]. Pooled HCV antibody prevalence in the general population in Yemen was 1.9%, and the prevalence among hemodialysis patients ranged between 40% and 62.7% [46].

20.7.7 Obesity

Obesity is strongly associated with many rheumatic diseases, with epidemiological studies showing that overweight or obese individuals face a higher risk of developing rheumatic conditions as well as experiencing greater disease severity [47]. In Yemen, recent population-based data indicate that 20.3% of adults are overweight and 10.3% are obese, highlighting a growing burden that may worsen rheumatic disease outcomes [48].

20.8 Screening Programs for Rheumatic Diseases

In Yemen, most health screening initiatives have been severely disrupted by the ongoing conflict. While international non-governmental organizations (NGOs) primarily support communicable disease screening and vaccination programs, these remain the most consistently implemented nationwide. However, no established screening or vaccination programs exist specifically for rheumatic diseases. As a result, early detection of rheumatic conditions remains largely dependent on clinical presentation rather than organized screening efforts.

20.9 Economic Burden of Rheumatic Diseases

Yemen has one of the highest musculoskeletal disease burdens in the Eastern Mediterranean Region, with an age-standardized disability-adjusted life-year (DALY) rate of 2125 per 100,000 population in 2013, disproportionately affecting women (2362) more than men (1864), reflecting a female-to-male ratio of 1.27 [49].

Musculoskeletal and rheumatic diseases impose a significant and rising economic burden worldwide, particularly in low-income countries where disability, reduced productivity, and impaired quality of life are major contributors to societal cost [47, 50]. As these diseases frequently affect individuals during their most productive years, initiatives that support patients to remain employed or return to work after disease flares are essential.

Recent analyses have demonstrated substantial global spending on rheumatic disease treatments, largely driven by the introduction and widespread use of costly biologic and targeted synthetic DMARDs. This expansion has emphasized the importance of cost-effectiveness evaluations to guide resource allocation and ensure equitable access to high-value therapies [51–53]. Studies in the Middle East and North Africa (MENA) region have shown that using biosimilar biologics can reduce treatment costs by 17–21%, highlighting the potential economic impact in low-resource settings [54].

In Yemen, however, conducting such evaluations is extremely challenging due to the country's weakened health system, severe shortages of essential medicines, fragmented services, and reliance on out-of-pocket payments for nearly all medications [5, 6]. Access to conventional DMARDs is inconsistent, and biologic therapies are generally unavailable or unaffordable for the vast majority of patients. As a result, oral corticosteroids remain widely used because they are inexpensive and readily accessible, leading to their well-recognized and frequently observed complications.

20.10 Education and Research

Yemen is currently experiencing a severe collapse in both the healthcare and education sectors due to the ongoing armed conflict [55]. The primary focus of intervention efforts is on emergency response and acute health crises, but the education sector has also been critically impacted [56, 57]. Research capacity is similarly weakened, as Yemen's health system has been fragmented and under-resourced, limiting opportunities for specialty training and academic inquiry [56].

Conducting clinical research in Yemen is particularly challenging due to limited infrastructure, resource constraints, and political instability. Additionally, there is a marked shortage of rheumatologists, and few academic institutions provide structured support for training or advancing specialization in rheumatology. Furthermore, many Yemeni clinicians face significant clinical workloads that limit their ability to engage in research activities, resulting in minimal local data and limited capacity for evidence-based decision-making [4, 5, 55].

20.11 Specific Challenges

20.11.1 Limited Availability of Rheumatology Care

Rheumatology services in Yemen remain severely underdeveloped. The very limited number of specialists, along with the country's economic constraints, restricts patient access to proper evaluation and long-term follow-up. The low socioeconomic status also affects patients' ability to adhere to prescribed DMARDs, resulting in undertreatment and preventable complications.

20.11.2 Limited Access to Health Services

Access to rheumatology care in Yemen is hampered by a shortage of specialists, their concentration in urban centers, and limited services in rural areas. Many patients cannot afford DMARDs or advanced therapies, further restricting their treatment options.

20.11.3 Absence of National Rheumatology Association

Yemen currently lacks an official national rheumatology association. The absence of such a body limits opportunities for coordinated professional development, standardized training, national guidelines, and advocacy for improved rheumatology services.

20.12 Future Directions for Improving Rheumatology Care in Yemen

Clinical rheumatology research remains limited in Yemen, largely due to resource constraints, the shortage of specialists, and the ongoing conflict. Strengthening rheumatology education and research will require coordinated long-term planning, policy support, and external collaboration.

Key opportunities for Yemen include the following:

1. Capacity building in rheumatology workforce
   The MoPHP, together with universities and emerging professional societies, could support residency programs, fund subspecialty fellowships abroad, and incentivize the return of trained specialists.
2. Integrating tele-rheumatology as a national strategy
   A practical opportunity for Yemen is the adoption of tele-rheumatology, modeled after successful implementations in Syria, Gaza, and South Sudan, where remote consultations improved continuity of care despite mobility restrictions and health system fragmentation [58, 59]. Telehealth platforms, supported by NGOs or academic partnerships, can provide virtual specialist reviews, follow-up visits, medication monitoring, and physician-to-physician consultations.
3. Establishing a national rheumatic disease registry
   Establishing a national rheumatic disease registry would also enable multi-center research, help quantify disease burden, and support analyses of genetic, environmental, cultural, and socioeconomic determinants of rheumatic diseases in Yemen.
4. Improving access to essential medications
   MoPHP, NGOs, and donors could create procurement partnerships for affordable DMARDs and explore the adoption of biosimilars, which have successfully reduced treatment costs in several MENA countries.
5. Expanding public and professional awareness
   Nationwide campaigns, through radio, community leaders, schools, and NGOs, can promote early recognition of musculoskeletal symptoms. Training primary care physicians to recognize inflammatory arthritis would improve timely referrals.
6. Creating the Yemen Rheumatology Association
   Establishing such a body would be an important step toward improving rheumatic disease care. A national association could organize scientific meetings, continuing medical education, and collaborative activities with regional and international societies, such as the Arab League of Associations for Rheumatology (ArLAR) or the Asia Pacific League of Associations for Rheumatology (APLAR). It would also play a central role in developing structured training programs for medical students, general practitioners, and future rheumatology trainees, thereby strengthening the subspecialty workforce in the country.
7. Strengthening academic and research collaborations
   Given Yemen's limited research infrastructure, collaborations with regional universities could facilitate data-sharing, joint publications, structured training programs, and research mentorship. This is similar to successful academic partnerships formed during periods of conflict in other countries.

20.13 Conclusion

Yemen faces a substantial burden of rheumatic diseases, yet decades of conflict, economic hardship, and a fragile health system have limited the country's ability to provide timely and effective care. The severe shortage of rheumatologists, restricted diagnostic capacity, and limited availability of essential medications contribute to delayed diagnosis, mismanagement, and preventable complications. Pediatric and adult data consistently highlight the predominance of rheumatoid arthritis and systemic lupus erythematosus, along with high rates of misdiagnosis and under-referral.

Improving rheumatology services in Yemen will require expanding specialist training, strengthening diagnostic services, ensuring reliable access to DMARDs, and developing national registries to track disease burden. Tele-rheumatology and regional partnerships offer practical, cost-effective support in the current crisis. Coordinated efforts between the Ministry of Public Health and Population, academic institutions, and international partners are essential to advancing care, research, and long-term outcomes for Yemenis living with rheumatic diseases.

Conflict of Interest The authors declare no conflicts of interest.

References

1. Central Intelligence Agency. Yemen – The World Factbook [Internet]. Washington, DC: Central Intelligence Agency; 2025. [cited 2025. Nov 21]. Available from: https://www.cia.gov/the-world-factbook/countries/yemen/.
2. Encyclopaedia Britannica. Yemen [Internet]. London: Encyclopaedia Britannica; 2025. [cited 2026 Jun 15]. Available from: https://www.britannica.com/place/Yemen.
3. UNESCO World Heritage Centre. World heritage list [Internet]. Paris: UNESCO; 2025. [cited 2026 Jun 15]. Available from: https://whc.unesco.org/en/list/.
4. Al Waziza R, Sheikh R, Ahmed I, Al-Masbhi G, Dureab F. Analyzing Yemen's health system at the governorate level amid the ongoing conflict: a case of Al Hodeida governorate. Discov Health Syst. 2023;2(1):15. https://doi.org/10.1007/s44250-023-00026-w.
5. Qirbi N, Ismail SA. Health system functionality in a low-income country in the midst of conflict: the case of Yemen. Health Policy Plan. 2017;32(6):911–22. https://doi.org/10.1093/heapol/czx031.
6. World Health Organization. Understanding the private health sector in Yemen [Internet]. Cairo: WHO Regional Office for the Eastern Mediterranean; 2019. [cited 2026 Jun 15]. Available from: https://applications.emro.who.int/docs/9789292742546-eng.pdf.
7. International Committee of the Red Cross (ICRC). Yemen | International Committee of the Red Cross [Internet]. 2025. [cited 2026 Jun 15]. Available from: https://www.icrc.org/en/where-we-work/yemen.
8. World Health Organization, Regional Office for the Eastern Mediterranean (WHO EMRO). Strengthening Yemen's disease early warning system during the COVID-19 pandemic [Internet]. Cairo: WHO EMRO; 2025. [cited 2026 Jun 15]. Available from: https://www.emro.who.int/pandemic-epidemic-diseases/news/strengthening-yemens-disease-early-warning-system-during-the-covid-19-pandemic.html.

9. United Nations Yemen. UNICEF Yemen National Health Information System – DHIS2 Platform [Internet]. 2025. [cited 2026 Jun 15]. Available from: https://yemen.un.org/en/298266-unicef-yemen-national-health-information-system-dhis2-platform.
10. KSRelief-supported artificial limbs centers in Yemen have provided services to 25,000 patients [Internet]. ReliefWeb. 2019. [cited 2026 Jun 15]. Available from: https://reliefweb.int/report/yemen/ksrelief-supported-artificial-limbs-centers-yemen-have-provided-services-25000-patients.
11. World Health Organization. Medical devices [Internet]. Geneva: World Health Organization; 2025. [cited 2025 Nov 25]. Available from: https://www.who.int/data/gho/data/themes/topics/GHO/medical-devices.
12. Sapundzhieva T, Sapundzhiev L, Batalov A. Practical use of ultrasound in modern rheumatology-from A to Z. Life (Basel). 2024;14(9):1208. https://doi.org/10.3390/life14091208.
13. Bai Z, Chen Y, Dong L. Experience of therapeutic plasma exchange in rheumatic diseases: albumin may be a suitable substitute for plasma. Arch Rheumatol. 2021;36(3):398–408. https://doi.org/10.46497/ArchRheumatol.2021.8447.
14. World Health Organization. Yemen | Country overview [Internet]. 2025. [cited 2026 Jun 15]. Available from: https://data.who.int/countries/887.
15. Dahman HAB. Challenges in the diagnosis and management of pediatric rheumatology in the developing world: lessons from a newly established clinic in Yemen. Sudan J Paediatr. 2017;17(2):21–9. https://doi.org/10.24911/SJP.2017.2.2.
16. Al-Haimi RM, Othman AM, Al-Shamahy HA, Al-Moyed KA, Al-Selwi AHA. Common autoimmune diseases among Yemeni patients in Sana'a City, Yemen. Yemeni J Med Sci. 2020;14(1):22–7. https://doi.org/10.20428/yjms.v14i1.1722.
17. Al-Shamahy HA, Dhaifallah NH, Al-Ezzy YM. Clinical and laboratory manifestations of yemeni patients with systemic lupus erythematosus. Sultan Qaboos Univ Med J. 2014;14(1):e80–7. https://doi.org/10.12816/0003340.
18. Oliver JE, Silman AJ. What epidemiology has told us about risk factors and aetiopathogenesis in rheumatic diseases. Arthritis Res Ther. 2009;11(3):223. https://doi.org/10.1186/ar2585.
19. Frisell T, Holmqvist M, Kallberg H, Klareskog L, Alfredsson L, Askling J. Familial risks and heritability of rheumatoid arthritis: role of rheumatoid factor/anti-citrullinated protein antibody status, number and type of affected relatives, sex, and age. Arthritis Rheum. 2013;65(11):2773–82. https://doi.org/10.1002/art.38097.
20. Jurdi R, Saxena PC. The prevalence and correlates of consanguineous marriages in Yemen: similarities and contrasts with other Arab countries. J Biosoc Sci. 2003;35(1):1–13. https://doi.org/10.1017/s0021932003000014.
21. Izadi Z, Li J, Evans M, Hammam N, Katz P, Ogdie A, et al. Socioeconomic disparities in functional status in a national sample of patients with rheumatoid arthritis. JAMA Netw Open. 2021;4(8):e2119400. https://doi.org/10.1001/jamanetworkopen.2021.19400.
22. Oyugi AM, Kibet JK, Adongo JO. A review of the health implications of heavy metals and pesticide residues on khat users. Bull Natl Res Cent. 2021;45(1):158. https://doi.org/10.1186/s42269-021-00613-y.
23. Mokarizadeh A, Faryabi MR, Rezvanfar MA, Abdollahi M. A comprehensive review of pesticides and the immune dysregulation: mechanisms, evidence and consequences. Toxicol Mech Methods. 2015;25(4):258–78. https://doi.org/10.3109/15376516.2015.1020182.
24. Alsulimani A, Das S, Akhter N, Ahmad A, Jawed A, Beigh S, et al. Pesticide exposure promotes disease activity by decreasing lymphoproliferative activity and increasing IL-4 production in systemic sclerosis patients. Immunopharmacol Immunotoxicol. 2025;47(1):112–9. https://doi.org/10.1080/08923973.2024.2445731.
25. Parks CG, Santos ASE, Lerro CC, DellaValle CT, Ward MH, Alavanja MC, et al. Lifetime pesticide use and antinuclear antibodies in male farmers from the agricultural health study. Front Immunol. 2019;10:1476. https://doi.org/10.3389/fimmu.2019.01476.

26. Koureas M, Rachiotis G, Tsakalof A, Hadjichristodoulou C. Increased frequency of rheumatoid arthritis and allergic rhinitis among pesticide sprayers and associations with pesticide use. Int J Environ Res Public Health. 2017;14(8):865. https://doi.org/10.3390/ijerph14080865.
27. Di Giuseppe D, Discacciati A, Orsini N, Wolk A. Cigarette smoking and risk of rheumatoid arthritis: a dose-response meta-analysis. Arthritis Res Ther. 2014;16(2):R61. https://doi.org/10.1186/ar4498.
28. Nam B, Koo BS, Choi N, Shin JH, Lee S, Joo KB, et al. The impact of smoking status on radiographic progression in patients with ankylosing spondylitis on anti-tumor necrosis factor treatment. Front Med (Lausanne). 2022;9:994797. https://doi.org/10.3389/fmed.2022.994797.
29. Akar S, Kaplan YC, Ecemis S, Keskin-Arslan E, Gercik O, Gucenmez S, et al. The role of smoking in the development and progression of structural damage in axial SpA patients: a systematic review and meta-analysis. Eur J Rheumatol. 2019;6(4):184–92. https://doi.org/10.5152/eurjrheum.2019.19073.
30. World Health Organization. WHO report on the global tobacco epidemic, 2021: Yemen country profile [Internet]. Geneva: WHO; 2021. [cited 2026 Jun 15]. Available from: https://cdn.who.int/media/docs/default-source/country-profiles/tobacco/who_rgte_2021_yemen.pdf.
31. Manghi RA, Broers B, Khan R, Benguettat D, Khazaal Y, Zullino DF. Khat use: lifestyle or addiction? J Psychoactive Drugs. 2009;41(1):1–10. https://doi.org/10.1080/02791072.2009.10400669.
32. Wedegaertner F, Al-Warith H, Hillemacher T, te Wildt B, Schneider U, Bleich S, et al. Motives for khat use and abstinence in Yemen—a gender perspective. BMC Public Health. 2010;10:735. https://doi.org/10.1186/1471-2458-10-735.
33. Lemma AF, Robert U, Lajtai L. Khat use and users' readiness to quit khat: qualitative research in the case of street people in Addis Ababa. J Addict Ther Res. 2022;6:001–6. https://doi.org/10.29328/journal.jatr.1001020.
34. Virayavanich W, Alizai H, Baum T, Nardo L, Nevitt MC, Lynch JA, et al. Association of frequent knee bending activity with focal knee lesions detected with 3T magnetic resonance imaging: data from the osteoarthritis initiative. Arthritis Care Res (Hoboken). 2013;65(9):1441–8. https://doi.org/10.1002/acr.22017.
35. Al-Hebshi NN, Al-Sharabi AK, Shuga-Aldin HM, Al-Haroni M, Ghandour I. Effect of khat chewing on periodontal pathogens in subgingival biofilm from chronic periodontitis patients. J Ethnopharmacol. 2010;132(3):564–9. https://doi.org/10.1016/j.jep.2010.08.051.
36. Al-Sharabi AK, Shuga-Aldin H, Ghandour I, Al-Hebshi NN. Qat chewing as an independent risk factor for periodontitis: a cross-sectional study. Int J Dent. 2013;2013:317640. https://doi.org/10.1155/2013/317640.
37. Ahmed KA-A, Abdoh TH, Farah HS, Al-Qaisi TS, Qaisi KMA, Alhmoud JF. Adverse effects of Khat (Catha edulis) chewing in Yemeni adults: a case-control study. Medico-legal Update. 2021;21(3):331–6. https://doi.org/10.37506/mlu.v21i3.3010.
38. Ng QX, De Deyn M, Loke W, Yeo WS. Yemen's cholera epidemic is a one health issue. J Prev Med Public Health. 2020;53(4):289–92. https://doi.org/10.3961/jpmph.20.154.
39. Badell E, Alharazi A, Criscuolo A, Almoayed KAA, Lefrancq N, Bouchez V, et al. Ongoing diphtheria outbreak in Yemen: a cross-sectional and genomic epidemiology study. Lancet Microbe. 2021;2(8):e386–e96. https://doi.org/10.1016/S2666-5247(21)00094-X.
40. Alsabri M, Alhadheri A, Alsakkaf LM, Cole J. Conflict and COVID-19 in Yemen: beyond the humanitarian crisis. Glob Health. 2021;17(1):83. https://doi.org/10.1186/s12992-021-00732-1.
41. Furuya-Kanamori L, Liang S, Milinovich G, Soares Magalhaes RJ, Clements AC, Hu W, et al. Co-distribution and co-infection of chikungunya and dengue viruses. BMC Infect Dis. 2016;16:84. https://doi.org/10.1186/s12879-016-1417-2.
42. World Health Organization. Global Tuberculosis Programme – data [Internet]. 2025. [cited 2026 Jun 15]. Available from: https://www.who.int/teams/global-programme-on-tuberculosis-and-lung-health/data.

43. World Health Organization. Hepatitis B surface antigen (HBsAg) prevalence among children under 5 years (%): Yemen [Internet]. Geneva: WHO; 2025. [cited 2026 Jun 15]. Available from: https://data.who.int/indicators/i/62D8ABE/F513188.
44. World Health Organization. Tuberculosis profile – Yemen [Internet]. Geneva: WHO; 2025. [cited 2025 Nov 25]. Available from: https://worldhealthorg.shinyapps.io/tb_profiles/?_inputs_&tab=%22charts%22&lan=%22EN%22&iso3=%22YEM%22&entity_type=%22country%22.
45. World Health Organization. Global tuberculosis report 2025 [Internet]. Geneva: WHO; 2025. [cited 2026 Jun 15]. Available from: https://iris.who.int/server/api/core/bitstreams/e97dd6f4-b567-4396-8680-717bac6869a9/content.
46. Chaabna K, Kouyoumjian SP, Abu-Raddad LJ. Hepatitis C virus epidemiology in Djibouti, Somalia, Sudan, and Yemen: systematic review and meta-analysis. PLoS One. 2016;11(2):e0149966. https://doi.org/10.1371/journal.pone.0149966.
47. Gremese E, Tolusso B, Gigante MR, Ferraccioli G. Obesity as a risk and severity factor in rheumatic diseases (autoimmune chronic inflammatory diseases). Front Immunol. 2014;5:576. https://doi.org/10.3389/fimmu.2014.00576.
48. Ibrahim AIM Sr, Bourkhime H, Benmaamar S, El Harch I, Otmani N, Mohammed S, et al. The double burden of obesity and underweight in Yemeni adults. Cureus. 2023;15(12):e50829. https://doi.org/10.7759/cureus.50829.
49. Moradi-Lakeh M, Forouzanfar MH, Vollset SE, El Bcheraoui C, Daoud F, Afshin A, et al. Burden of musculoskeletal disorders in the Eastern Mediterranean Region, 1990-2013: findings from the Global Burden of Disease Study 2013. Ann Rheum Dis. 2017;76(8):1365–73. https://doi.org/10.1136/annrheumdis-2016-210146.
50. Woolf AD, Pfleger B. Burden of major musculoskeletal conditions. Bull World Health Organ. 2003;81(9):646–56.
51. Westhovens R, Annemans L. Costs of drugs for treatment of rheumatic diseases. RMD Open. 2016;2(2):e000259. https://doi.org/10.1136/rmdopen-2016-000259.
52. Donges E, Staatz CE, Benham H, Kubler P, Hollingworth SA. Patterns in use and costs of conventional and biologic disease-modifying anti-rheumatic drugs in Australia. Clin Exp Rheumatol. 2017;35(6):907–12.
53. Huang Y, Li J, Agarwal SK. Economic and humanistic burden of rheumatoid arthritis: results from the US National Survey Data 2018–2020. ACR Open Rheumatol. 2024;6(11):746–54. https://doi.org/10.1002/acr2.11728.
54. Almaaytah A, Elhajji FD. Comparative cost efficiency of the originator drug infliximab and its biosimilar for the treatment of rheumatoid arthritis in the MENA region. Int J Pharm Investig. 2019;9(1):12–5.
55. Zakham F, Vapalahti O, Lashuel HA. Education and research are essential for lasting peace in Yemen. Lancet. 2020;395(10230):1114. https://doi.org/10.1016/S0140-6736(20)30162-8.
56. Al-Awlaqi S, Dureab F, Tambor M. The National Health Cluster in Yemen: assessing the coordination of health response during humanitarian crises. J Int Humanit Action. 2022;7(1):9. https://doi.org/10.1186/s41018-022-00117-y.
57. Khaled F. A war of attrition: higher education in Yemen. Sana'a Center for Strategic Studies; 2024. [cited 2026 Jun 15]. Available from: https://sanaacenter.org/files/A_War_of_Attrition_Higher_Education_in_Yemen_en.pdf.
58. Parkes P, Pillay TD, Bdaiwi Y, Simpson R, Almoshmosh N, Murad L, et al. Telemedicine interventions in six conflict-affected countries in the WHO Eastern Mediterranean region: a systematic review. Confl Heal. 2022;16(1):64. https://doi.org/10.1186/s13031-022-00493-7.
59. Ziade N, Hmamouchi I, El Kibbi L, Daou M, Abdulateef N, Abutiban F, et al. Telehealth in rheumatology: the 2021 Arab League of Rheumatology Best Practice Guidelines. Rheumatol Int. 2022;42(3):379–90. https://doi.org/10.1007/s00296-021-05078-w.

Chapter 21
Arab League of Associations for Rheumatology (ArLAR)

Fatemah Abutiban, Hebah AlHajeri, Amjad Alkadi, and Fatemah Baroun

Abstract The Arab League of Associations for Rheumatology (ArLAR) was established in 1995 to strengthen the relations between rheumatologists in the Arab countries. The main aims of this league were to keep abreast of global medical developments, promote health awareness among Arabs, and play a significant role in the global scientific movement.

It was necessary to establish such a regional Arab league for many reasons, such as geographic proximity, ease of travel, proximity of time zones, convenient calendar arrangements, and shared sponsoring pharmaceutical companies.

Over the years, and since its establishment, ArLAR has conducted 14 biannual congresses, with the last one being held in Kuwait in March 2023. The ArLAR activities are organized and managed by dedicated scientific and media committees.

The vision of ArLAR is to be an internationally recognized professional league for rheumatology. One of its main missions is to enhance education and research among Arab countries and to build formal bridges between Arab rheumatologists and international rheumatology communities.

ArLAR comprises a board of directors, an executive committee, a scientific committee, a general assembly, a media committee, and eight special interest groups. The board aims to maintain continuous collaboration among the committees and

F. Abutiban (✉) · F. Baroun
Jaber AlAhmad Hospital, Department of Medicine, Ministry of Health,
Kuwait City, State of Kuwait
e-mail: ffbaroun@gmail.com; fbaroun@gmail.com; amjad.alqadi@hotmail.com

H. AlHajeri
Mubarak Al Kabeer Hospital, Department of Medicine, Ministry of Health,
Kuwait City, State of Kuwait
e-mail: hebah.Alhajeri@gmail.com

A. Alkadi
Al-Sabah Hospital, Department of Medicine, Ministry of Health,
Kuwait City, State of Kuwait
e-mail: amjad.alqadi@hotmail.com

K. A. Alnaqbi, G. Aldabie (eds.), *Rheumatic Diseases in the Arab World*,
https://doi.org/10.1007/978-981-92-0967-5_21

offer opportunities to engage medical staff and the public in ArLAR activities. The league has well-constructed bylaws, formed in 2019 and written in Arabic, the official language of the league. The bylaws were updated again in 2023.

Keywords Arab League of Associations for Rheumatology · ArLAR · Rheumatology · Rheumatology Societies · Arab World · Rheumatology Education · Rheumatology Research · Special Interest Groups · Rheumatology Congress · Arab Journal of Rheumatology

21.1 History of the ArLAR

The Arab League of Associations for Rheumatology (ArLAR) is a nonprofit professional society committed to advancing the rheumatology specialty. ArLAR was founded on March 29, 1995, originally known as the Pan Arab Society of Rheumatic Diseases [1].

The idea started with the first successful congress for Arab rheumatologists in Rabat, Morocco, in 1981, before the establishment of the society [2, 3]. During the second meeting of the Arab rheumatologists in Cairo on 28–31 March 1995, the Pan Arab Society of Rheumatic Diseases was established. Since then, regular biannual congresses have been held in different Arab countries, and several publications and scientific materials have been published. In 1999, the first bylaws were written in English.

During the 11th Pan Arab Rheumatology Congress, held in Dubai, the United Arab Emirates, in January 2014, the society's name was changed to the "Arab League of Associations of Rheumatology – ArLAR" to keep up with the elevated corresponding international leagues [2, 3]. The Emirates Society for Rheumatology proposed this step for rheumatology. Since then, five congresses have taken place; the first being in Dubai (UAE) in January 2014, followed by Marrakech (Morocco) in March 2016, then in Muscat (Oman) in February 2018 [1–3], and the ArLAR21 Jordan e-Congress, which was conducted virtually in March 2021 during the COVID-19 pandemic. The ArLAR23 congress was held in Kuwait (Kuwait City) in March 2023, and it was hosted in a hybrid format with predominantly on-site presentations. The most recent ArLAR congress was held in Algeria in April 2025. (Table 21.1).

Since the official establishment of ArLAR, there has been an expanded number of memberships, from seven founding rheumatology national societies to 16 as of January 2025. The Jordanian Society wrote the first constructed bylaws in Arabic for the rheumatology initiative in 2018, when more special interest groups (SIGs) were formed, covering the most important topics needed to run a rheumatology

Table 21.1 History of ArLAR congresses

Number of the meeting	Place of the meeting	Date of the meeting	Status of the league
First Arab Congress of rheumatology	Rabat, Morocco	June 1981	Before ArLAR establishment
Second meeting	Cairo, Egypt	March 1995	Establishment of pan Arab Society of Rheumatic diseases
Third meeting	Riyadh, KSA	October 1997	Pan Arab Society of Rheumatic diseases
Fourth meeting	Amman, Jourdan	September 1999	Pan Arab Society of Rheumatic diseases
Fifth meeting	Damascus,Syria	September 2001	Pan Arab Society of Rheumatic diseases
Sixth meeting	Beirut, Lebanon	September 2003	Pan Arab Society of Rheumatic diseases
Seventh meeting	October 6 city, Egypt	February 2006	Pan Arab Society of Rheumatic diseases
Eighth meeting	Doha, Qatar	January 2008	Pan Arab Society of Rheumatic diseases
Ninth meeting	Dead Sea, Jordan	April 2010	Pan Arab Society of Rheumatic diseases
Tenth meeting	Jeddah, KSA	January 2012	Pan Arab Society of Rheumatic diseases
Eleventh meeting	Dubai, UAE	January 2014	Establishment of ArLAR
Twelfth ArLAR meeting	Marrakesh, Morocco	March 2016	ArLAR
Thirteenth ArLAR meeting	Muscat, Oman	February 2018	ArLAR
Fourteenth ArLAR meeting	Jordan, Amman	March 2021	ArLAR
Fifteenth ArLAR meeting	Kuwait City, Kuwait	March 2023	ArLAR
Sixteenth ArLAR meeting	Alger, Algeria	April 2025	ArLAR

league successfully [2]. The scientific activities have also evolved since then, and there have been more contributions from all the members. By creating the ArLAR College, a continuous medical education platform was formed to provide regular educational webinars and workshops to rheumatologists around the time of the main scientific activity of the league, the biannual ArLAR Congress.

21.2 Councils and Committees of ArLAR

21.2.1 Board of Directors

The board of directors is the highest authority of ArLAR. It consists of the presidents of the national Arab societies' members or deputies. Its mission includes setting or modifying the bylaws, approving new applications for membership, initiating new special SIGs, and electing the members of the executive council [2].

21.2.2 The Executive Council

The executive council is responsible for implementing and monitoring the execution of all the recommendations and plans of the board of directors. The members are the current ArLAR president, the immediate past president, the president-elect, the secretary-general, the treasurer, and the president of the scientific committee [2].

21.2.3 The Scientific Committee

The scientific committee members are representatives of the national societies, with the president being an elected member of the board of directors. The mission of the committee includes organizing and monitoring the continuous medical education of the members, organizing scientific webinars, monitoring the activities of the SIGs, and helping organize and plan the annual ArLAR Congress [2].

21.2.4 The General Assembly

The ArLAR General Assembly consists of all representatives of the full-member National Societies or other organizations and chairpersons of SIGs. The role of the General Assembly is advisory, where all its members can propose awareness programs and scientific research on rheumatic and musculoskeletal diseases, as well as projects related to improving the performance of ArLAR [2].

21.2.5 *The Media Committee*

In 2021, ArLAR formed an official media committee responsible for managing the multimedia communication channels for ArLAR. It is chaired by a member of Arab society, where the next ArLAR congress will be held, and includes members from other Arab societies with experience in media and networking. Furthermore, the committee manages different social media platforms of ArLAR, for example, Facebook, Instagram, Twitter, and LinkedIn accounts. It also manages the ArLAR official website, establishes and manages an E-bulletin, and produces and handles any multimedia videos for ArLAR [1].

21.3 ArLAR Membership

ArLAR is composed of "National Scientific Medical Societies" specialized in the management of rheumatic and musculoskeletal diseases, which are officially recognized by the authorities of their respective countries, such as the ministries of health or medical associations [2].

A national Arab rheumatology society shall be admitted as a member after obtaining the majority of the board of directors' votes. Other organizations may be admitted as supporting members or observers in ArLAR's General Assembly if they agree and commit to ArLAR's objectives and Articles of Association and upon the approval of the majority of the Board of Directors. These organizations may include:

- Nongovernmental health bodies, including but not limited to patient support societies and associations
- Groups conducting and interested in scientific research on rheumatic and musculoskeletal diseases
- National and regional organizations concerned with health awareness and prevention of rheumatic and musculoskeletal diseases
- Bodies, groups, and societies specialized in some rheumatic and musculoskeletal diseases
- Health care companies and health insurance companies
- Manufacturers and distributors of pharmaceuticals and medical devices

ArLAR membership shall entitle members to the following rights and privileges:

- Benefit from participation in the scientific and social activities organized by ArLAR
- Free subscription to periodic and nonperiodic publications as well as the scientific journal of ArLAR
- Submission of proposals and opinions to support, improve, or modify ArLAR's activities

- Be nominated for positions in ArLAR's various institutions and committees according to the type of membership in ArLAR
- Attendance at meetings of ArLAR's General Assembly and Board of Directors according to the type of membership

21.4 ArLAR Educational Activity

One of the main goals of establishing ArLAR is to engage rheumatologists in various educational activities provided by expert Arab rheumatologists. This goal has been achieved through the annual ArLAR Congress and the ArLAR College. ArLAR scientific activities are organized and run by the scientific committee.

21.4.1 ArLAR Congress

The ArLAR biannual scientific congress is one of the most important events and activities of ArLAR. This congress is a four-day scientific program held every 2 years in an Arab country with a full member state through its national society. The ArLAR Congress is chaired by the ArLAR President, who is also the chairperson of the national society elected to hold the ArLAR Congress. The congress targets academics, physicians, researchers, and others interested in adult and pediatric rheumatology, where distinguished and renowned regional and international speakers deliver remarkable presentations, workshops, and poster sessions.

The official language of the congress is English. The program usually comprises parallel sessions for adult and pediatric Rheumatology and different workshops. The ArLAR SIGs also contribute to the congress with workshops and sessions organized by the SIG committees.

In March 2020, the 14th ArLAR congress was supposed to be held in Amman, Jordan. However, due to the COVID-19 pandemic, it was postponed to March 2021 and was delivered virtually as ArLAR21 Jordan e-Congress [1]. This setup attracted the attention of many experts in the field. For the first time in ArLAR history, the French Society for Rheumatology participated greatly in the congress. Some lectures were delivered in French with a real-time English translation and a real-time French translation of the lectures in English. This increased the number of attendants from French-speaking countries in North Africa, creating a more language-friendly environment. ArLAR21 Jordan e-Congress was a big success despite an unusual epidemic, with around 1500 attendees worldwide.

The ArLAR23 congress was held in Kuwait in March 2023 in collaboration with the Kuwait Association of Rheumatologists (KAR). It was the first comeback to onsite congresses after the Amman virtual congress. ArLAR 23 witnessed great success with 530 attendees on site and 120 online attendees. It included 26 sessions, 11 workshops, and 170 speakers. There were 409 scientific papers submitted to the congress. There were remarkable onsite presentations from all the Arab countries. In addition, presidents of international rheumatology organizations, such as the European Alliance of Associations of Rheumatology (EULAR), the Asia Pacific League of Associations of Rheumatology (APLAR), and the African League of Associations of Rheumatology (AFLAR), met physically in a session called "The legendary meeting of rheumatologists across the globe." They shared their experiences and discussed the challenges they are facing in their organizations and geographic areas.

ArLAR 2025 was held in Algeria in April 2025. Sessions were held in English and French. The upcoming ArLAR27 is planned to be held in Iraq in 2027.

21.4.2 ArLAR College

ArLAR College was created in 2020 as the ArLAR Scientific Committee and ArLAR Board of Directors' initiative. The ArLAR Scientific Committee members run ArLAR College. The head of ArLAR College is the chairman of the ArLAR Scientific Committee. The ArLAR College is intended to execute the ArLAR objectives by gathering the efforts of all expert Arab rheumatologists in collaboration with the international rheumatology community via a series of meetings [1].

The objectives of ArLAR College are:

- To promote continuous medical education of ArLAR members in different rheumatology sectors through organizing regular webinars, workshops, and training.
- To mentor younger rheumatologists.
- To develop programs and projects aligned with the ArLAR College's objectives.

All members of the ArLAR Scientific Committee and ArLAR Board of Directors, presidents of the SIGs, and ArLAR past presidents (by default) can join the ArLAR College faculty. The ArLAR Scientific Committee and Board of Directors can recommend names of Arab rheumatologists to join the ArLAR College faculty, with the following criteria:

- Rheumatologists from the Arab countries, regardless of where they live or whether their Arab country of origin is a member of the ArLAR
- Rheumatologists who have established academic careers and are authors or co-authors of more than ten publications

Faculty members should express in writing their acceptance to be members of the ArLAR College faculty and accept the ArLAR College internal regulations and ArLAR bylaws. They should also express their fields of interest once they join ArLAR College.

The ArLAR College educational webinars are held regularly, usually one to two monthly webinars. The first webinar was held in July 2020. The average time of each webinar is around 70 min. Each webinar usually has two local Arab speakers and one international speaker to allow the mutual exchange of experience. The webinars are up-to-date with hot topics regarding rheumatic diseases, such as guidelines, management, research, and registries. Different SIGs also participate in ArLAR College with assigned webinars, including the ArLAR Francophone Group with real-time translation to English and the Pediatric Rheumatologist Arab Group (PRAG) with up-to-date pediatric rheumatology-related topics.

All webinars are recorded and uploaded on the ArLAR official website, making it accessible and convenient for rheumatologists who could not attend the webinars live. The average number of attendees is usually 200–250 from all over the world for each webinar.

ArLAR is committed to providing monthly educational webinars and planning new interactive and hands-on workshops such as speaker educational programs and SIGs programs with musculoskeletal radiology training courses, research, and registry formation workshops.

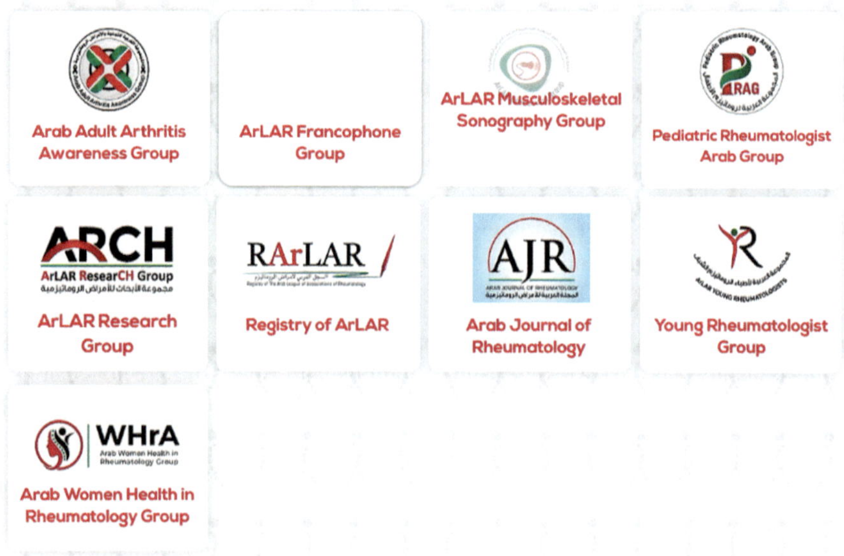

Fig. 21.1 Summary of ArLAR special interest groups with the official logo of each group

21.5 ArLAR Special Interest Groups (SIGs)

ArLAR has several nonprofit SIGs, which bring distinctive insight into different areas of rheumatology in the Arab world. SIGs represent a platform for developing ideas and collaboration among rheumatologists within their special interest areas. Generally, the groups play an important role in organizing various meetings and educational activities, conducting projects, publishing regional recommendations, and representing ArLAR in regional and international conferences (Fig. 21.1) [1, 2].

21.5.1 Arab Adult Arthritis Awareness (AAAA) Group

The Arab Adult Arthritis Awareness (AAAA) group was established in 2015 by independent rheumatologists interested in patient awareness and education about rheumatic diseases [1]. Founders have raised concerns that the Arab world is witnessing an increased prevalence and burden of arthritis. Every Arab country educates the public locally, which makes its impact on a narrow scale rather than an Arab-wide scale. Furthermore, many Arab patients have poor access to educational materials written in their native language. Because of the unmet needs, creating the AAAA committee was crucial. ArLAR approved AAAA as one of its official SIGs in 2019.

The group's mission is to be the collective voice of Arab rheumatologists to improve rheumatic disease awareness among the public.

The main goals of AAAA are:

- To create a rheumatologists' multi-country network and unify the efforts to obtain a higher impact of any awareness activity
- To promote public education about rheumatology as a specialty
- To raise awareness among the public and patients in the Arab region using a patient-centric and multi-country approach
- To train doctors who want to be involved in patient awareness, diagnosis, and referrals
- To raise awareness about methods of early diagnosis and treatment of arthritis. The activities are targeted toward patients, health educators, nurses, and doctors who are interested in patient education, diagnosis, and referrals
- To facilitate and encourage multidisciplinary arthritis care in Arab countries

The group aims to achieve this by:

- Conducting public awareness sessions about the rheumatology specialty.
- Organizing successful activities (patient support, research, conferences, awareness, etc...) in Arab countries
- Educating doctors interested in patient education, diagnosis, and referrals
- Educating nurses and health educators on the rheumatology topic
- Organizing educational days for patients according to the AAAA awareness days' calendar with the same unified theme across all the Arab countries

- Organizing awareness lectures on all comorbid diseases associated with arthritis
- Hosting events, including educational presentations, screening of informational materials, and walkathons
- Launching educational events through newspapers, TV shows, banners, contests for patients, and social media

The committee has established its responsibilities as follows:

- Writing a biannual consensus report with key recommendations on their working strategy
- Establishing vision, mission, and tactics with explicit goals
- Establishing policies and terms of reference
- Proposing guidelines on patient education
- Collecting a broad range of perspectives from and for each country
- Run surveys regarding patient education across Arab countries
- Obtaining an accurate, up-to-date snapshot status of the arthritis burden per country
- Writing a newsletter on a biannual basis and distributing it to physicians and patients to keep them up-to-date with the latest committee activities
- Disseminating the AAAA committee decisions, campaign material, and activity advertisements within their respective countries
- Leading awareness campaigns simultaneously and in collaboration with each participating country

21.5.2 ArLAR Francophone Group (ArFG)

The ArLAR Francophone Group (ArFG) is an autonomous group working under the umbrella of the ArLAR that was created on December 10, 2018. It was approved by the ArLAR Board of Directors in 2019 [1]. Partially or totally francophone Arab countries are represented at ArFG, including Algeria, Lebanon, Morocco, Syria, and Tunisia. The group is also open to francophone rheumatologists practicing in non-francophone Arab countries. ArFG aims to integrate Francophone Arab countries into the projects and activities of ArLAR.

The mission of the group is to:

- Represent the French-speaking Arab countries within ArLAR.
- Promote the activities of ArLAR in French so they are accessible to members of French-speaking countries.
- Organize scientific sessions in French during ArLAR congresses and seminars.
- Organize scientific activities (seminars, thematic workshops) in French-speaking countries.
- Provide French translations of ArLAR activities originally established in Arabic or English.
- Advance professional fellowship between Arab rheumatologists and the world.

- Promote research and training to improve the health of patients with rheumatic and musculoskeletal diseases, particularly in French-speaking countries.
- Collaborate with international French-speaking rheumatology organizations.

21.5.3 ArLAR Musculoskeletal Sonography (MSUS) Group

The group represents a platform for Arabic MSUS experts to engage and collaborate. Its main aim is to enhance the MSUS teaching and accreditation for the rheumatologists in the region to the international level within the Arabic region [1].

The objectives of the group are as follows:

- Spread the MSUS skills among the rheumatologists in the region.
- Facilitate the training of fellows and trainees within the Arabic region.
- Standardize the MSUS practice within the Arabic region according to international guidelines.
- Establish an accredited ArLAR-MSUS certification program and certify the rheumatologists in the region to practice MSUS.
- Conduct a regional MSUS-related research project.

The plan of the group is as follows:

- Organize regular accredited MSUS courses in the region, starting from basic to intermediate and targeting the advanced level.
- Collaborate with international bodies of MSUS, such as the EULAR and ACR, to implement their guidelines and accreditation standards.
- Publish articles related to MSUS practice and research.

The group has conducted its first “EULAR-endorsed MSUS basic course” during the ArLAR 2023 Congress. Fifty-five participants have participated in the course and been trained by regional and international instructors.

21.5.4 Pediatric Rheumatology Arab Group (PRAG)

The Pediatric Rheumatology Arab Group (PRAG) represents pediatric rheumatologists of the Arab countries at the ArLAR. The group’s main vision is to be the regional professional league for pediatric rheumatologists and present the members internationally [1].

The purpose of the group is to facilitate the above vision by:

- Promoting excellence in pediatric rheumatology care, education, and research
- Facilitating transmission and translation of research advances into daily care and adopting the best practices and guidelines

- Empowering patients and their families through addressing their specific needs to their governing bodies

21.5.5 Arab Research Group (ARCH)

Arab Research Group (ARCH) was formed in 2021. The ARCH group includes 16 voting members representing the 16 ArLAR countries, aiming to lead collaborative rheumatology research in the Arab countries by focusing on four main pillars:

(a) Research Projects: plan and conduct research projects on behalf of the ArLAR to serve the interests of the patients with rheumatic and musculoskeletal diseases, living in the Arab countries.
(b) Quality and infrastructure: support and promote high-quality collaborative research among the Arab countries and improve the research environment by ensuring compliance with international standards in both infrastructure and standard operating procedures.
(c) Motivation and support: motivate and assist young researchers in the Arab countries to conduct successful and high-standard research projects.
(d) Research Network: connect with the international rheumatology research teams, institutions, and companies to take part in their global clinical trials.

Since its establishment, the ARCH group has managed to publish several papers in peer-reviewed international journals and participate in important international projects that have helped enhance the recognition of ArLAR globally.

21.5.6 ArLAR Registry Group

The ArLAR Registry group was established in 2021, aiming to collect and generate electronic data across the Arab countries and, therefore, represent patients in the region [1].

It also aims at the following:

- Creating sub-registries for different Arab countries (local registries)
- Presenting data results in regional and international conferences
- Publishing in well-recognized journals
- Collaborating between the Arab countries to improve patient care via the registry

21.5.7 Arab Journal of Rheumatology

Arab Journal of Rheumatology (AJR) is the official scientific journal of ArLAR. The group was founded in 2021 and first published online in March 2023 as issue 1 [4].

It is a peer-reviewed journal that welcomes clinicians and researchers to submit original articles and experimental research in addition to interesting cases and smaller studies. It accepts and publishes high-quality medical articles related to rheumatology, immune disorders, osteoporosis, and rehabilitation medicine to disseminate scientific and clinical research that will advance knowledge and daily practice.

21.5.8 Young Rheumatologists Group

The first official group meeting was held on November 3, 2021.

A young rheumatologist is defined as having one of the following criteria:

- Residents or fellows in training programs
- Rheumatologists with less than 10 years of experience

The group's main aim is to organize educational activities and workshops for young rheumatologists and league members [1]. Furthermore, this group encourages young rheumatologists to contribute to national research and projects. The activities are held under the direct supervision of the scientific committee in collaboration with other SIGs.

The Young Rheumatologists Group had an impressive presence during the ArLAR 23 Kuwait Congress by organizing the musculoskeletal examination and joint injection workshop, which was well attended by fellows, internists, and other medical personnel from different specialties.

21.5.9 Arab Women's Health in Rheumatology Group (WHrA)

The Arab Women's Health in Rheumatology Group was established under the umbrella of the ArLAR in 2025. The group is dedicated to the interface between rheumatic and musculoskeletal diseases (RMD) and women's reproductive health across the Arab region. It was created to address the unique challenges that Arab women encounter in relation to fertility, pregnancy, postpartum care, and broader reproductive concerns when living with rheumatologic disease.

The group's mission is to raise awareness among both patients and healthcare professionals regarding the impact of RMDs on reproductive health while fostering a supportive and informed environment.

For patients, the group works to empower women to openly discuss issues related to fertility, preconception planning, pregnancy, and postpartum care. It also strives to promote understanding of family planning in the context of RMD and to ensure that accessible, culturally relevant, and linguistically appropriate educational resources are available.

For rheumatologists and other clinicians, the group aims to enhance knowledge, education, and support regarding reproductive health in the context of RMDs. It encourages the development of specialized clinics and services that integrate rheumatology with reproductive care. In addition, the group promotes the sharing of local data and clinical experiences, the adoption of best practices and international guidelines, and the establishment of collaborative networks across the Arab world. These efforts also serve to facilitate research and create opportunities for regionally relevant contributions to the global body of knowledge.

21.6 Role of Women in ArLAR

Over the years, women have proven their capabilities and equality to men in all aspects of life, including the workforce. The healthcare industry is no different, and the rheumatology field has shown a competitive share of women worldwide. As in other sectors, the number of women in rheumatology has risen over the years. Even though women face different challenges than men, female rheumatologists have shown a strong presence in the Arab world and in ArLAR since its establishment, closing the gender gap. There was no quota for their presence in different ArLAR committees, and over the years, their number has been increasing gradually and even recently surpassing the number of male rheumatologists [1, 3].

They formed most of the members. They have shown strong participation and engagement in all scientific activities and have been involved in different committees, SIGs, and leadership positions. Today, they hold executive management positions at the highest levels, representing 62.5% of chairperson positions of different SIGs of ArLAR [1]. The women's teams include a research team, the first Arab rheumatology journal, the electronic registry, and the first mass media campaign directed to millions in the Arab world [1]. Arab women had a significant role in leading the ArLAR. For example, one of the league's founders in the early 1990s was a female rheumatologist who later became the President of the 4th Pan Arab Society of Rheumatic Diseases congress [3]. In addition, the two immediate past presidents of ArLAR were women and led the league from 2021 to 2025.) [1, 3].

Despite the gender gaps in the Arab world and across different nations, ArLAR gave opportunities for female rheumatologists to reshape the specialty in the Arab world through their achievements. They were role models to other women in the healthcare industry.

21.7 Summary

The Arab League of Associations for Rheumatology (ArLAR) is a regional organization that meets the requirements and demands of adult and pediatric rheumatologists in the Arab world. It started in 1995 with only seven members. At the time of publishing this chapter, it consists of 16 members, with a target to include all 22 Arab countries.

Since its inception, ArLAR has accomplished many of the objectives that it set out to do. This includes extensive scientific activities such as the monthly ArLAR College webinars, the biannual regional congress, conducting international research published in well-recognized and peer-reviewed journals, arranging workshops, and creating the first rheumatology electronic registry gathering data from 16 countries in the Arab world.

ArLAR continues to achieve its vision to serve all rheumatologists and their patients in the Arab world and globally.

Acknowledgments Informed International for Events, ArLAR members, and Kuwait Association of Rheumatology (KAR) members.

Conflict of Interest The authors declare that they have no conflicts of interest.

References

1. Arab League of Associations of Rheumatology [Internet]. [Cited 2026 Jun 17]. Available from: https://www.arabrheumatology.org/.
2. Arab League of Associations of Rheumatology. Articles of Association. 2020.
3. Arab League of Associations of Rheumatology. ArLAR history video [Internet]. [Cited 2026 Jun 17]. https://www.instagram.com/info.arlar/.
4. Arab Journal of Rheumatology [Internet]. [Cited 2026 Jun 17]. Available from: https://journals.lww.com/ajrh/pages/default.aspx.

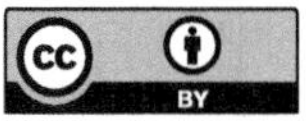

Chapter 22
Rheumatology Research in the Arab World

Hadeel Zaghloul, Hubaib Haider, and Thurayya Arayssi

Abstract The Arab League constitutes 22 countries located in Southwest Asia and North Africa, stretching from the Arabian Gulf in the east to the Atlantic Ocean in the west. Each country in the region has unique characteristics that affect public health priorities and disease burden. Rheumatology care and research vary significantly among Arab countries, but the overall rheumatology research output and impact remain limited. Some of the main barriers to conducting rheumatology research include a lack of vision, educational and training barriers, limited funding, limited collaborative efforts, and economic challenges. However, there is ample opportunity to improve rheumatology research in Arab countries to advance care within the region. In this chapter, we summarize the current global status of rheumatology research in the Arab region, highlight key barriers to high-quality rheumatology research, and propose a framework of recommendations to improve research output.

Keywords Rheumatology · Rheumatic Diseases · Arab countries · Bibliometrics · Biomedical Research · Research Support as Topic · International Cooperation · Clinical Trials as Topic · Health Policy · Research capacity building

H. Zaghloul · H. Haider · T. Arayssi (✉)
Weill Cornell Medicine-Qatar, Doha, Qatar
e-mail: hbz2002@qatar-med.cornell.edu; huh4001@qatar-med.cornell.edu; tha2002@qatar-med.cornell.edu

K. A. Alnaqbi, G. Aldabie (eds.), *Rheumatic Diseases in the Arab World*,
https://doi.org/10.1007/978-981-92-0967-5_22

22.1 Introduction

The Arab League is a voluntary association of 22 countries established to promote political unity among Arab nations and represent people's interests. These countries occupy a vast area in Southwest Asia and North Africa, stretching from the Arabian Gulf in the east to the Atlantic Ocean in the west. The 22 member countries are Algeria, Bahrain, Comoros, Djibouti, Egypt, Iraq, Jordan, Kuwait, Lebanon, Libya, Mauritania, Morocco, Oman, Palestine, Qatar, Saudi Arabia, Somalia, Sudan, Syria, Tunisia, the United Arab Emirates (UAE), and Yemen. The Arab countries have a population of over 400 million as of 2020 [1]. Although they share a common language (Arabic), each country has unique socio-cultural, historical, geopolitical, and economic characteristics that affect public health and the burden of disease and injury.

Medical research plays an essential role in economic growth, long-term sustainable development, standards of living, and quality of life. Governments of developed countries, such as the United States and European countries, have recognized this and increased research spending [2]. Arab countries, however, lag behind in the number of original research articles (particularly in high-impact journals) and citation frequency [3]. According to the 2025 Scimago Institutions Rankings, Arab nations' medical research output and overall impact remain limited [4]. Of the 1967 ranked universities and research institutions worldwide, only 59 are from Arab countries. The highest-ranking Arab institute (Jordan University Hospital) is ranked 95th [4]. In a comparative analysis, the total number of medical publications from all 22 Arab countries between 1996 and 2012 was 76,417 reports, approximately half of the output produced by Turkey alone and only 4% of publications produced by the United States [5].

The standard of rheumatology care and research across the 22 Arab countries varies considerably. Several factors contribute to this, including demographics, political stability, migration patterns, healthcare resource allocation, healthcare system implementation, and the number of qualified rheumatologists. Based on data from the Global Burden of Disease Study (GBD), there has been a clear shift in mortality patterns between 1990 and 2010, from deaths caused by communicable, maternal, neonatal, and nutritional causes to non-communicable diseases (NCDs) [6]. In recent decades, the prevalence of NCDs, including musculoskeletal diseases, has increased substantially in the Arab states, resulting in an epidemiological profile that closely resembles that of Western Europe and the United States [6]. This data collectively indicates an increasing need for medical research, particularly in NCDs, within Arab countries.

There is an excellent opportunity to improve rheumatology research in Arab countries and advance care within the region. In this chapter, we examine the current position of rheumatology research in the Arab world, identify barriers to conducting high-quality rheumatology research, and propose recommendations to improve research output. This chapter aims to help guide the future direction of rheumatology research in the Arab region.

Table 22.1 Biomedical and rheumatology research output from the Arab region

Author	Research investigated	Time period covered	Results
Biomedical research output			
Almuhaidib et al. [7]	Bibliometric analysis of medical research productivity, collaboration, and impact across 22 Arab countries	2017–2023	The Arab world contributed 2.72% to global medical research; publication output grew 87% from 2017 to 2022; 70% of research was from Saudi Arabia and Egypt; 66% of publications involved international collaboration
El Rassi et al. [8]	Medical research productivity for the 22 Arab countries	2007–2016	189 papers per million population were produced from the Arab countries (equivalent to about a quarter of the other world countries)
Tadmouri et al. [9]	MEDLINE-indexed biomedical publications from Arab countries	1988–2002	Arab countries produced less than 1% of biomedical citations
Rheumatology research output			
Jawad et al. [10]	Rheumatology research output from Arab institutions (PubMed/ MEDLINE)	2017–2021	Identified 10 leading countries; Qatar (P/P 6.48) and Tunisia (6.45) ranked highest per capita; Egypt had 282 publications (23 RCTs), and Saudi Arabia had 81 (no RCTs)
Bayoumy et al. [11]	Web of Science (WoS) Rheumatology publications from Arab countries	1976–2014	Arab countries published 944 rheumatology papers; the number of papers published increased by a factor of 2.77 every decade (95% CI: 2.75–2.78); citations increased by a factor of 2.36 every decade (0.96–5.82)
El Masri et al. [12]	Arab Behçet disease (BD) publications	2005–2019	Arab countries published 198 articles (0.1% of all studies published in this period)
El Masri et al. [13]	Arab Familial Mediterranean Fever (FMF) publications	2004–2019	Arab world's contribution is only 3.8% of all FMF publications

22.2 Bibliometric Data on Rheumatology Research in the Arab Countries

Bibliometric analysis is a method for assessing research in many widely used and accepted fields. It quantifies and evaluates research output and illustrates its growth and dissemination. Table 22.1 summarizes bibliometric studies conducted to describe the region's biomedical and rheumatology research output.

A study used bibliometric indicators to assess medical research productivity in the 22 Arab countries between 2007 and 2016 [8]. They found that the Arab world produced 189 papers per million population, equivalent to approximately one-quarter of that in other countries [8]. Qatar, Tunisia, Lebanon, and Kuwait were the four leading countries and produced more than 695 papers per million population, a value higher than the world average [8]. The average number of citations per paper was 9.2, which increased to 15 times for papers with international collaboration [8]. Another study investigating the number of MEDLINE-indexed publications from Arab countries between 1988 and 2002 found that Arab countries produced less than 1% of biomedical citations worldwide despite the availability of wealth and human resources [9]. Upon normalizing the results to population size, smaller countries such as Kuwait, the UAE, and Lebanon were found to be more productive than the larger publishing countries in the Arab world, such as Egypt and Saudi Arabia [9]. More recently, Almuhaidib et al. [7] extended this analysis to cover 2017–2023, revealing significant progress in the region's medical research landscape. The Arab world's contribution to global medical publications increased to 2.72%, with an 87% rise in annual research output during the study period. Qatar, Lebanon, and Saudi Arabia led per-capita output, while 70% of the region's total publications originated from Saudi Arabia and Egypt. The median citation impact (11.98) was nearly equivalent to the global average (12.02), and two-thirds (66%) of Arab publications involved international collaboration, underscoring growing regional integration and research visibility [7].

More specifically, for rheumatology research, several bibliometric studies have been conducted. In a study investigating rheumatology publications between 1976 and 2014, Web of Science (WoS) was searched, resulting in 944 rheumatology papers published during this period. Each decade, the number of papers published increased by a factor of 2.77 (95% CI: 2.75–2.78), and citations increased by a factor of 2.36 (95% CI: 0.96–5.82). In addition, this study found that although the total number of papers published in the top 10 rheumatology journals increased over time, their proportion decreased, indicating that the Arab region was not keeping pace with global research progress. Collaborative papers in the region increased over time [11].

Another study aimed to investigate the contribution of Arab countries to Behçet Disease (BD) publications [12]. BD was selected due to its high prevalence in the Arab world. PubMed was searched for publications between 2005 and 2019, and the number of publications was then normalized with respect to the average population size and gross domestic product (GDP). The results showed that 198 articles were published during this period, accounting for only 0.1% of all studies related to BD. Thus, it was concluded that despite the high prevalence of BD in Arab countries, research output is low, highlighting the need to increase BD research in the region [12].

In a third study estimating the contribution of Arab countries to research conducted on Familial Mediterranean Fever (FMF), PubMed was searched to identify all studies published between 2004 and 2019 [13]. Again, FMF was selected due to its high prevalence in Arabs. Similarly, the data were normalized with respect to the average population and GDP and compared to other non-Arab countries with high FMF prevalence [13]. The Arab countries' contribution was a mere 3.8% of all FMF-related publications compared with 24.9% produced solely by Turkey [13].

Tunisia had the highest productivity, followed by Lebanon when normalized to the average population and the GDP [13]. Similar to findings for BD, the study concluded that the prevalence of FMF in Arab countries did not match the research output on the topic.

More recently, Jawad et al. [10] provided an updated assessment of rheumatology research output in the Arab region between 2017 and 2021. Their analysis, based on PubMed/MEDLINE-indexed publications, revealed wide variability across Arab countries: Qatar and Tunisia recorded the highest publications per capita ratios (6.48 and 6.45, respectively), whereas Egypt led in total output with 282 papers (23 RCTs). Saudi Arabia produced 81 publications, primarily cross-sectional studies, but no randomized controlled trials. Notably, no rheumatology publications were found from Comoros, Djibouti, Libya, Mauritania, Palestine, or Somalia. The authors emphasized the urgent need for stronger investment, capacity building, and international collaboration to enhance the quality and impact of rheumatology research across the Arab world [10].

22.3 Status of Publications from the Arab Region

Although publications from some Arab countries have increased in quality and quantity over the past few decades, collectively, research from the Arab world still lags behind global research, as described previously. Despite its limitations, citation analysis can be used as an approximate measure of the scholarly impact of an article or scientist. The Science Citation Index (SCI) includes a relatively limited number of citations for studies from Arab countries compared to the rest of the world. This finding indicates that the scientific impact of published work may be limited [14]. Furthermore, the average number of citations per paper was 3.82 from the United States and 1.51 from South Korea. In contrast, the average number of citations per paper in the Arab region ranged from 0.01 to 0.99, remaining substantially lower than global averages. Similarly, many Arab scientific journals have limited standards and lack many fundamentals, such as objective peer review of the articles accepted for publication, and often resort to the publication of unedited proceedings of conferences and seminars [15]. In turn, most Arab scientists prefer to publish in peer-reviewed international journals. To identify the most impactful publications from Arab researchers in the last decade, we conducted a comprehensive search of the WoS database. This search aimed to identify publications on five common rheumatological diseases in Arab countries: rheumatoid arthritis, systemic lupus erythematosus, osteoarthritis, BD, and FMF. The search was then restricted to publications from the past 10 years and sorted by citation count. Table 22.2 summarizes the five most highly cited publications for each disease. The number of citations for the articles ranged from 9 to 250. Egypt accounted for the largest proportion of publications (44%), and only seven countries were represented among these studies. This finding indicates that research generated from the Arab world has a low global impact.

Table 22.2 Publications with the highest citations for rheumatoid arthritis, systemic lupus erythematosus, osteoarthritis, Behçet disease, and Familial Mediterranean fever from Arab countries

Author	Title	Year of publication	Journal	Country	Number of citations
Rheumatoid arthritis					
Khojah et al. [16]	Reactive oxygen and nitrogen species in patients with rheumatoid arthritis as potential biomarkers for disease activity and the role of antioxidants	2016	Free Radical Biology and Medicine	Saudi Arabia	79
Mosaad et al. [17]	Vitamin D receptor gene polymorphism as possible risk factor in rheumatoid arthritis and rheumatoid related osteoporosis	2014	Human Immunology	Egypt	55
Karray et al. [18]	Associations of vitamin D receptor gene polymorphisms FokI and BsmI with susceptibility to rheumatoid arthritis and Behçet's disease in Tunisians	2012	Joint Bone Spine	Tunisia	50
Hussein et al. [19]	Polymorphism in vitamin D receptor and osteoprotegerin genes in Egyptian rheumatoid arthritis patients with and without osteoporosis	2013	Molecular Biology Reports	Egypt	45
Ben Hamad et al. [20]	Association study of CARD8 (p.C10X) and NLRP3 (p. Q705K) variants with rheumatoid arthritis in French and Tunisian populations	2012	International Journal of Immunogenetics	Tunisia	36
Systemic lupus erythematosus					
Talaat et al. [21]	Th1/Th2/Th17/Treg cytokine imbalance in systemic lupus erythematosus (SLE) patients: Correlation with disease activity	2015	Cytokine	Egypt	250

(continued)

Table 22.2 (continued)

Author	Title	Year of publication	Journal	Country	Number of citations
Emerah et al. [22]	Role of vitamin D receptor gene polymorphisms and serum 25-hydroxyvitamin D level in Egyptian female patients with systemic lupus erythematosus	2013	Molecular Biology Reports	Egypt	34
Hammad et al. [23]	Interleukin-17A rs2275913, Interleukin-17F rs763780, and rs2397084 gene polymorphisms as possible risk factors in juvenile lupus and lupus related nephritis	2016	Autoimmunity	Egypt	28
Alamoudi et al. [24]	Pulmonary manifestations in systemic lupus erythematosus: Association with disease activity	2015	Respirology	Saudi Arabia	26
Abbas et al. [25]	Angiotensin-converting enzyme (ACE) serum levels and gene polymorphism in Egyptian patients with systemic lupus erythematosus	2012	Lupus	Egypt	22
Osteoarthritis					
El Hakeim et al. [26]	Fluoroscopic guided radiofrequency of genicular nerves for pain alleviation in chronic knee osteoarthritis: a single-blind randomized controlled trial	2018	Pain Physician	Egypt	41
Al-Daghri et al. [27]	Vitamin D status correction in Saudi Arabia: an experts' consensus under the auspices of the European Society for Clinical and Economic Aspects of Osteoporosis, Osteoarthritis, and Musculoskeletal Diseases (ESCEO)	2017	Archives of Osteoporosis	Saudi Arabia	41
Al Rashoud et al. [28]	Efficacy of low-level laser therapy applied at acupuncture points in knee osteoarthritis: a randomised double-blind comparative trial	2014	Physiotherapy	Saudi Arabia	39

(continued)

Table 22.2 (continued)

Author	Title	Year of publication	Journal	Country	Number of citations
Abd-Allah et al. [29]	Variation of matrix metalloproteinase 1 and 3 haplotypes and their serum levels in patients with rheumatoid arthritis and osteoarthritis	2012	Genetic Testing and Molecular Biomarkers	Egypt	31
Hussain et al. [30]	Efficacy and safety of co-administration of resveratrol with meloxicam in patients with knee osteoarthritis: a pilot interventional study	2018	Clinical Interventions in Aging	Iraq	27
Behçet disease					
Karray et al. [18]	Associations of vitamin D receptor gene polymorphisms FokI and BsmI with susceptibility to rheumatoid arthritis and Behçet's disease in Tunisians	2012	Joint Bone Spine	Tunisia	50
Safi et al. [31]	Neutrophils contribute to vasculitis by increased release of neutrophil extracellular traps in Behçet's disease	2018	Journal of Dermatological Science	Lebanon	38
Houman et al. [32]	Characteristics of neurological manifestations of Behçet's disease: a retrospective monocentric study in Tunisia	2013	Journal of Neurology and Neurosurgery	Tunisia	36
Talaat et al. [33]	Polymorphisms of interleukin 6 and interleukin 10 in Egyptian people with Behçet's disease	2014	Immunobiology	Egypt	35
Tizaoui et al. [34]	Vitamin D receptor TaqI and ApaI polymorphisms: a comparative study in patients with Behçet's disease and rheumatoid arthritis in Tunisian population	2014	Cellular Immunology	Tunisia	28

(continued)

Table 22.2 (continued)

Author	Title	Year of publication	Journal	Country	Number of citations
Familial Mediterranean fever					
Talaat et al. [35]	The expanded clinical profile and the efficacy of colchicine therapy in Egyptian children suffering from familial Mediterranean fever: a descriptive study	2012	Italian Journal of Pediatrics	Egypt	13
Moussa et al. [36]	Overlap of familial Mediterranean fever and hyper-IgD syndrome in an Arabic kindred	2015	Journal of Clinical Immunology	Qatar	12
Mansour et al. [37]	Molecular patterns of MEFV gene mutations in Egyptian patients with familial Mediterranean fever: a retrospective cohort study	2019	International Journal of Inflammation	Egypt	10
El Masri et al. [12]	Contribution of Arab countries to familial Mediterranean fever research: a PubMed-based bibliometric analysis	2022	Rheumatology International	Lebanon	9
Ait-Idir et al. [38]	The M694I/M694I genotype: a genetic risk factor of AA-amyloidosis in a group of Algerian patients with familial Mediterranean fever	2017	European Journal of Medical Genetics	Algeria	9

22.4 Barriers to Conducting Rheumatology Research in the Arab Countries

Arab researchers face many barriers to successfully conducting research in the region. Figure 22.1 summarizes the main barriers that scientists face when conducting research in the Arab world, and each is discussed below.

22.4.1 Lack of a Unified Research Vision

Progress in research productivity, knowledge distribution, and utilization of knowledge requires the establishment of national development strategies to realize a knowledge-based vision. However, a significant barrier to future research is the need for a unified vision at national and regional levels to guide future directions and set research agendas. Currently, medical research is not a national priority in many Arab states, and most research seeks to address research questions relevant to

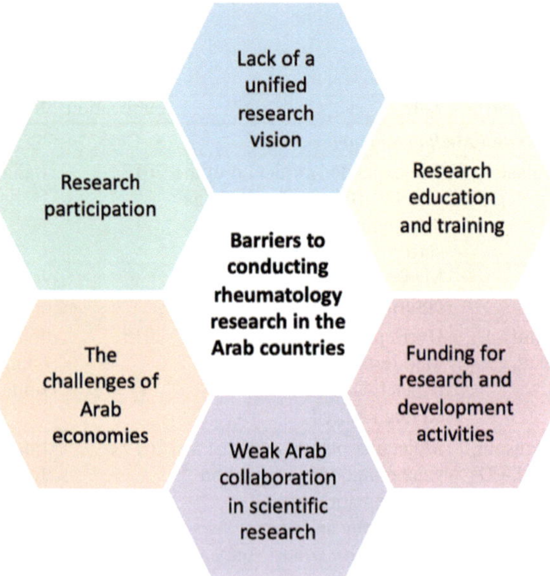

Fig. 22.1 The main barriers to conducting rheumatology research in the Arab world

developed countries. A recent study showed that a third of clinical trials sponsored by US-based companies were conducted in poor and low-income countries and did not target diseases prevalent in those countries [39]. Another study showed that only 10 of the 1556 new drugs produced between 1975 and 2004 targeted diseases of poor and low-income countries [40]. Therefore, healthcare systems, rather than pharmaceutical companies, should guide decisions on the high-priority areas for research within the region. Recently, developing countries have been calling for nationally prioritized research over industry-driven research. A unified regional vision would further strengthen these efforts.

22.4.2 Limited Research Education and Training

The lack of research education and adequate training is a significant barrier to conducting research in Arab countries. From a global perspective, universities are an essential determinant of the quality of a region's research infrastructure since most researchers receive research education and training from universities. However, Arab universities are often not supportive of research due to low-quality education that does not positively impact students' careers in research fields [41]. Education systems emphasize rote learning methods rather than encouraging critical thinking and provide education irrelevant to skills needed for thriving in research environments. Arab countries face a severe shortage of specialized research centers that provide research training and assistance [42]. Cross-sectional studies of medical students highlighted a scarcity of faculty willing to work with students on research projects and the inadequacy of high-quality research training [43, 44]. Gharaibeh and Mousa conducted a study at the Jordan University of Science and Technology in which 687 students filled out a survey that included questions about barriers faced by students conducting research [44]. "Lack of research supervision and guidance" was ranked the highest among the barriers [44]. Another qualitative study conducted on the challenges of carrying out research studies in Arab countries showed that more than 48% of physicians and clinical research coordinators and 60% of pharmacists identified inadequate training as a barrier to clinical research [45]. An adequate research infrastructure relies on the incoming generation of students developing a research-oriented mindset that ensures that the research cycle continues to bring innovative research ideas and proposals. However, Arab education systems have suffered from a "lack of scientific thinking training" since childhood, limiting research projects from having a multi-generational setup [46]. Research institutes in Arab countries are vulnerable to external pressures, as many have not inculcated a culture of "academic freedom and autonomy" [47]. This problem severely limits the ability of these research institutes to educate and train future researchers on pioneering scientific and social research projects. A critical shortcoming in research education is also highlighted by the fact that only 56% of family physicians currently involved in research projects reported having previously attended a research ethics course [48]. However, some encouraging examples have raised hope in the region in recent decades. For example, in Qatar, Weill Cornell Medicine's Continuing Professional Development (CPD) provides a research certificate program, while the Qatar National Research Fund (QNRF) provides various career development and funding opportunities. Still, overall research education and training in Arab countries suffer from their recipients' lack of awareness of key aspects of research, leading to compromised quality or, in some cases, a lack of published work.

22.4.3 Limited Funding for Research and Development Activities

Although developing countries bear the greatest burden in terms of disease in the world and would have the greatest benefit in reducing early mortality through research-based solutions, there is a lack of research and development activity to address this inequality. This is partly due to a lack of funding, which serves as a major barrier to conducting research in Arab countries. In an institutional mapping study, Mandil et al. found that a very small amount of national, regional, and international funding has been awarded to health research in the Middle East [49]. Moreover, Arab countries have the lowest gross expenditure on research and development compared to their GDP [50]. A cross-sectional study was conducted among students of three major Arab medical universities in Saudi Arabia, Bahrain, and Kuwait to assess barriers to participation in research. A self-administered questionnaire was distributed among students, and the response rate was 50% (213/423). Students perceived lack of funding and financial issues as major barriers to research participation [43]. This challenge shows how major universities in some of the wealthiest Arab countries reportedly suffer from a lack of funding for research. A 15-year bibliometric analysis of medical research in the Arab world in 2017 shows insufficient funding as a major reason for the gap in research output between Arab countries and the Western world. This research also points out the economic discrepancy between Arab countries, where low-income countries such as Yemen cannot prioritize research funding compared to oil-rich countries that can allocate more funds towards biomedical research [51]. Health Information Technology (HIT) is an essential part of the healthcare development of a region. HIT includes fields like electronic medical records (EMR) that serve as key resources in any region's medical research and development systems. Results of a systematic review conducted on the progress of HIT in Arab countries found that scarcity of funding was the main reason for the lack of HIT implementation by both government and private hospitals [52]. The lack of financial resources in Arab countries limits the region's ability to utilize such modern resources for research and healthcare infrastructure growth. Furthermore, a field study of Saudi Arabian hospitals to evaluate HIT and EMRs ranked lack of funding as the second most important barrier to medical infrastructure development in this field [53]. A bibliometric analysis of medical research productivity in Arab countries between 2007 and 2016 was conducted to assess trends in research productivity. The study concluded that medical research output in Arab countries lags behind global trends, despite improvement over the years, and highlighted inadequate funding as a major reason for Arab countries' low productivity in medical research. It highlighted the importance of international collaboration and the strengthening of national funding programs to reduce this gap in research productivity effectively [8]. Good quality higher education is essential to support high-quality research. Arab countries like Egypt, Jordan, and Tunisia suffer from a severe lack of funding in the higher education sector, which translates to poor research outcomes [54].

22.4.4 Weak Intra-Arab Scientific Collaboration

Sonnenwald has defined *scientific collaboration* as "an interaction taking place within a social context among two or more scientists that facilitates the sharing of meaning and completion of tasks with respect to a mutually shared, superordinate goal" [55]. Increased collaboration activity (number of authors, affiliations, and countries) is associated with an increased citation impact [56]. In a study assessing research productivity in the Arab states between 1980 and 2020, it was found that 49% of research from the Arab world resulted from international collaboration (mainly in Europe and North America), and these efforts were led by Saudi Arabia, Egypt, and Tunisia [57]. Intra-Arab research collaboration in research remains limited, with the exception of a few successful partnerships. Collaboration between Arab countries is vital for research on rheumatic diseases that are particularly prevalent in this region, such as FMF and BD. Collaboration between Arab researchers is necessary to generate a more significant impact and achieve generalizability of outcomes.

22.4.5 Economic Disparities and Competing National Priorities

The 22 Arab states occupy an area larger than that of Europe and the United States and are home to a population larger than that of the United States and marginally smaller than Western Europe. Although more than 60% of the world's oil reserves are present within the region, the region's overall economic status is less than desirable, and the degree of unemployment is high (ranging from 20% to 30%), particularly among the youth [58]. Individuals inhabiting the Arab states have unique characteristics specific to their genetics, geography, socio-cultural factors, economies, and ecosystems; therefore, it is not always possible to generalize findings from other regions of the world to the Arabic population. Most Arab countries have faced economic and political unrest in the past few decades, with some experiencing war and armed conflict, shifting research priorities toward humanitarian crises. The majority of countries in the Arab region are low- and middle-income [59] except for the members of the Arab Gulf Cooperative Council (GCC) countries (i.e., Bahrain, Kuwait, Oman, Qatar, Saudi Arabia, and the UAE). The healthcare systems are underdeveloped due to the adverse effects of political instability and military and social conflicts [60]. Due to economic constraints, research is a luxury in many low and middle-income countries. Scarce funds are mainly allocated to program implementation, leaving little to no room for funding research.

22.4.6 Limited Research Participation

The success of clinical studies depends on the recruitment of a sufficient number of participants. However, less than 10% of eligible individuals agree to participate in clinical trials [61]. A qualitative study conducted in Egypt found that although individuals valued the importance of medical research, most would only participate in research involving minimal risk [62]. Moreover, many associated the scientific designs of blinding and randomization with "experimentation" [62]. Recruitment into clinical trials can be challenging, particularly when a trial is conducted for the first time and requires a significant commitment from participants. A research study in Qatar suggested that most participants approached for research were willing to participate [63]. Despite this, the clinical trial density, defined as the number of clinical trial participants per million population, was less than 1 per million in the MENA region compared to 101 and 65 in North America and Western Europe, respectively [64]. Therefore, willingness to participate in a trial does not necessarily increase actual participation rates. The concept of clinical trials is relatively unfamiliar in the Arab world among both the general population and healthcare professionals. It is sometimes attached to the stigma that participants in a research study are disempowered and subjected to experimentation. Furthermore, because medical schools and hospitals in the region do not adequately train their graduates to conduct scientific research, clinicians may lack the motivation to encourage their patients to participate in clinical trials.

22.5 Recommendations for Improving Research Output in the Arab Countries

To improve rheumatology research output from the Arab region, we have developed a framework of recommendations to enhance research productivity. Figure 22.2 summarizes key recommendations to improve research productivity in the Arab world.

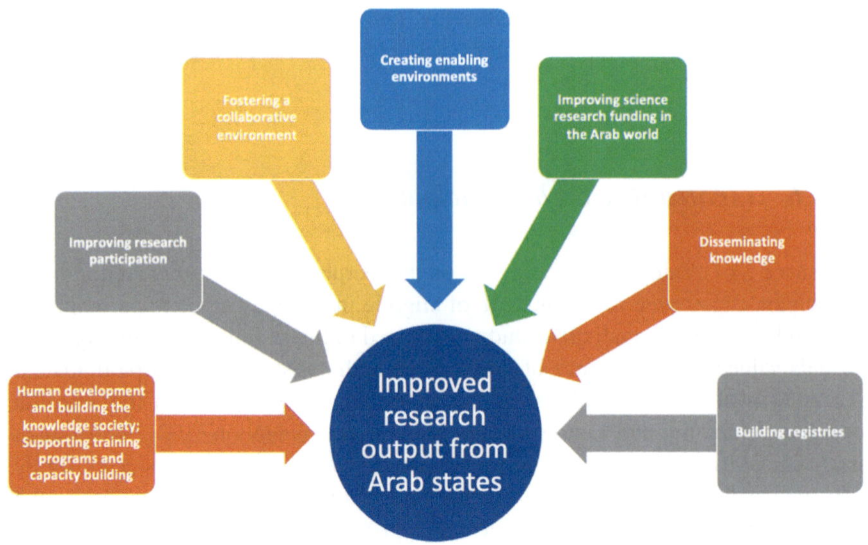

Fig. 22.2 Summary of recommendations to improve research output in the Arab states

22.5.1 Human Development and Building the Knowledge Society; Supporting Training Programs and Capacity Building

Capacity building in conducting medical research is vital to improve research output in the Arab states. Building scientific capacity entails much more than simply transferring science and technology from the developed to the developing world. The key to successful scientific capacity building relies heavily on human resources. Oliver et al. proposed conducting capacity building at the levels of individuals, research teams, organizations, and national systems [65]. Although some Arab states have witnessed waves of educational reform promoting research in the past few decades, these efforts have not been consistent across the entire region. Moreover, the effects of these changes have not been systematically studied or recorded. Teaching staff at Arab universities (who constitute the majority of researchers in the region) are burdened with large teaching loads (double that of teaching staff in Western universities). In fact, the research activity of Arab teaching staff rarely exceeds 5–10% of their total academic duties compared to 35–50% in European and American universities [15]. Therefore, more time and resources must be allocated to research training and activities in Arab academic institutions. Indeed, this is an encouraging finding that three-quarters of Arab physicians are interested in participating in research teams and networks [48]. Building research networks is widely recognized as essential to building research capacity [66]. Therefore, building networks and forums for communication between scientists interested in research is fundamental.

The lack of willingness of physicians to encourage their patients to participate in clinical studies may be due to a lack of time and incentives, as previously reported [67]. Barriers related to the system, including lack of rewards and recognition for physicians who are interested in research, must therefore be addressed. Additionally, the lack of protected time and space for research studies is another challenge for physicians in many busy clinical settings. Barriers to physician participation can be addressed through more formal education and training in research design and methodology for undergraduate and postgraduate trainees and reinforcement through continuing medical education. Additionally, financial incentives should be provided for conducting research activities. Hospitals and primary care centers must allocate protected space and time for clinical research.

22.5.2 Creation of Enabling Environments

Promoting biomedical research in the Arab region will require serious efforts, and all stakeholders, including scientists and decision-makers, must agree on several strategic goals. Governmental policies have a central role in effecting cultural shifts by reallocating resources to support national priorities. Therefore, governments must play a leading role in creating national and regional research strategies. The strategies should include upgrading research infrastructure (including regulatory and supervisory bodies and equipment), allocating sufficient funding, providing high-quality training, and promoting excellence. Additionally, Arab scientists employed abroad should be regarded as valuable assets and encouraged to return to their home countries. China has already set an example by recruiting qualified Chinese scientists from abroad (particularly from the USA) to increase research output by 330% [5]. Other institutional-level interventions include the provision of tenure, intramural funding programs, the establishment of doctoral and postdoctoral programs, and faculty compensation schemes that incentivize research.

22.5.3 Fostering a Collaborative Environment

Although most Arab research efforts are collaborative, they occur primarily with other regions, such as Europe and North America. There is no doubt that foreign investment and engagement should be encouraged and supported. However, it should be equally important for governments, academic institutions, and industry to promote collaboration among researchers from different Arab countries and generate knowledge with greater impact and broader implications. Collaboration between developed and developing countries is vital to fostering research development in less developed countries. Moreover, collaboration between the academic and industry sectors enhances innovation through knowledge transfer. Only Qatar and the UAE demonstrate significant university–industry cooperation, indicating limited levels of industrial development in the region [57]. Hence, greater efforts are needed to strengthen links between universities and industry. Establishing Arab research associations to create a forum for researchers to discuss common issues, establish collaborations across institutions and countries, promote rigorous research methods, and inform policy decisions would significantly enhance research productivity in the Arab world.

22.5.4 Improving Medical Research Funding in the Arab Region

Most research activities require ongoing funding, which may be perceived as a lower priority for many developing countries than other more pressing matters. Thus, to improve the Arab research output, national research funding programs need to be strengthened and expanded. Funding opportunities have increased over the past few decades, particularly in high-income countries (e.g., Qatar and the UAE) and middle-income countries (e.g., Egypt and Lebanon). These efforts should be sustained and expanded to additional countries in the region. Most international funding agencies encourage regional collaboration, which should be leveraged as an opportunity to secure funding. The pharmaceutical industry is also an important source that can provide research funding for Arab countries. While outsourcing and globalization of pharmaceutical clinical studies and trials are cost-effective and will remain essential, funding should also support investigator-initiated studies that benefit the local population.

22.5.5 Improving Research Participation

A research-oriented culture among the public needs to be established to enhance research participation. This step will require continued efforts to support the development of public awareness of research in medicine through interactive science and technology centers, exhibits, and events aiming at educating and engaging adults and children in areas of medicine that require further research. Ensuring the availability of well-trained Arabic-speaking researchers is needed to remove communication barriers with research participants. Incentivizing researchers to recruit participants can also enhance recruitment into research studies.

22.5.6 Dissemination of Knowledge

Translating research findings in the region into action on both societal and governmental levels is fundamental. To achieve this, research findings need to be communicated to governmental advisors and officials, including policymakers. Additionally, research findings should be communicated to the public. One way to disseminate knowledge could be through social media, which will raise public awareness and benefit both the author and the institution by making the publications more easily identifiable and accessible. This method may also increase citation impact [68]. One study examined the impact of specific altmetrics on citation rate. It showed that six of the eleven altmetrics assessed (tweets, Facebook wall posts, research highlights, blog mentions, mainstream media mentions, and forum posts) were associated with increased citations in medical and biological sciences [69].

22.5.7 Building Registries

The upcoming era of medical research is one of big data and data sharing. Digital health technologies such as EMRs will facilitate access to large datasets. To facilitate data sharing, creating and maintaining a pan-Arab research database for medical research (including rheumatology research) should thus be a priority. This step will require the input of all academic and non-academic institutions that conduct research in the region and the assistance and support of governmental and non-governmental organizations.

22.6 Conclusion

Rheumatological disorders are important causes of disability in the Arab region. Overall, rheumatology research output from the region is low, and efforts are needed to improve the quality and quantity of research. Patients with rheumatic disease residing in the Arab region have unique characteristics. Although the 22 Arab countries are geographically connected, there are considerable variations in research output due to many factors. All stakeholders must strive to improve rheumatology research in the region, which needs to be translated into improved rheumatology care. Although there are many barriers to conducting research, there are also great opportunities for improvement in the Arab region.

Conflict of Interest The authors have no conflicts of interest to declare.

References

1. Group WB. Population, total- Arab World. 2020.
2. Macilwain C. Science economics: what science is really worth. Nature. 2010;465(7299):682–4.
3. Benamer HT, Bakoush O. Arab nations lagging behind other Middle Eastern countries in biomedical research: a comparative study. BMC Med Res Methodol. 2009;9(1):1–6.
4. Scimago Institutions Rankings [Internet]. [cited 2025 Oct 22]. Available from: https://www.scimagoir.com/rankings.php?area=2700&ranking=(2025).
5. El-Azami-El-Idrissi M, Lakhdar-Idrissi M, Ouldim K, Bono W, Amarti-Riffi A, Hida M, et al. Improving medical research in the Arab world. Lancet. 2013;382(9910):2066–7.
6. Mokdad AH, Jaber S, Aziz MIA, AlBuhairan F, AlGhaithi A, AlHamad NM, et al. The state of health in the Arab world, 1990–2010: an analysis of the burden of diseases, injuries, and risk factors. Lancet. 2014;383(9914):309–20. https://doi.org/10.1016/S0140-6736(13)62189-3.
7. Almuhaidib S, Alqahtani R, Alotaibi HF, Saeed A, Alnasrallah S, Alshamsi F, et al. Mapping the landscape of medical research in the Arab world countries: a comprehensive bibliometric analysis. Saudi Med J. 2024;45(4):387–96. https://doi.org/10.15537/smj.2024.45.4.20230968.
8. El Rassi R, Meho LI, Nahlawi A, Salameh JS, Bazarbachi A, Akl EA. Medical research productivity in the Arab countries: 2007–2016 bibliometric analysis. J Glob Health. 2018;8(2):020411. https://doi.org/10.7189/jogh.08.020411.
9. Tadmouri GO, Bissar-Tadmouri N. Biomedical publications in an unstable region: the Arab world, 1988–2002. Lancet. 2003;362(9397):1766.
10. Jawad ASM, Hasbani GE, Uthman I. Rheumatology research in Arab countries. Saudi Med J. 2024;45(5):542. https://doi.org/10.15537/smj.2024.45.5.20240362.
11. Bayoumy K, MacDonald R, Dargham SR, Arayssi T. Bibliometric analysis of rheumatology research in the Arab countries. BMC Res Notes. 2016;9(1):393. https://doi.org/10.1186/s13104-016-2197-x.
12. El Masri J, El Hage S, Akoum A, Awaida I, Kourani F, Chanbour H, et al. Contribution of Arab countries to Behçet disease research: a PubMed-based bibliometric and altmetric analysis. Rheumatol Int. 2022;42(1):133–40. https://doi.org/10.1007/s00296-021-04990-5.
13. Masri DE, Alsaayed B, Masri JE, Zreika B, Chanbour H, Salameh P. Contribution of Arab Countries to Familial Mediterranean Fever Research: a PubMed-based bibliometric analysis. Rheumatol Int. 2022;42(1):95–100. https://doi.org/10.1007/s00296-021-04852-0.

14. ElObeidy A. Scientific system in the Arab region: from prestige towards development. Reg Sci Policy Pract. 2013;5(1):97–112.
15. UNDP. Arab knowledge report 2009: towards productive intercommunication for knowledge 2009.
16. Khojah HM, Ahmed S, Abdel-Rahman MS, Hamza A-B. Reactive oxygen and nitrogen species in patients with rheumatoid arthritis as potential biomarkers for disease activity and the role of antioxidants. Free Radic Biol Med. 2016;97:285–91. https://doi.org/10.1016/j.freeradbiomed.2016.06.020.
17. Mosaad YM, Hammad EM, Fawzy Z, Aal IAA, Youssef HM, ElSaid TO, et al. Vitamin D receptor gene polymorphism as possible risk factor in rheumatoid arthritis and rheumatoid related osteoporosis. Hum Immunol. 2014;75(5):452–61.
18. Karray EF, Ben Dhifallah I, Ben Abdelghani K, Ben Ghorbel I, Khanfir M, Houman H, et al. Associations of vitamin D receptor gene polymorphisms FokI and BsmI with susceptibility to rheumatoid arthritis and Behçet's disease in Tunisians. Joint Bone Spine. 2012;79(2):144–8. https://doi.org/10.1016/j.jbspin.2011.06.003.
19. Hussien YM, Shehata A, Karam RA, Alzahrani SS, Magdy H, El-Shafey AM. Polymorphism in vitamin D receptor and osteoprotegerin genes in Egyptian rheumatoid arthritis patients with and without osteoporosis. Mol Biol Rep. 2013;40(5):3675–80. https://doi.org/10.1007/s11033-012-2443-9.
20. Ben Hamad M, Cornélis F, Marzouk S, Chabchoub G, Bahloul Z, Rebai A, et al. Association study of CARD8 (p. C10X) and NLRP3 (p. Q705K) variants with rheumatoid arthritis in French and Tunisian populations. Int J Immunogenet. 2012;39(2):131–6.
21. Talaat RM, Mohamed SF, Bassyouni IH, Raouf AA. Th1/Th2/Th17/Treg cytokine imbalance in systemic lupus erythematosus (SLE) patients: correlation with disease activity. Cytokine. 2015;72(2):146–53.
22. Emerah AA, El-Shal AS. Role of vitamin D receptor gene polymorphisms and serum 25-hydroxyvitamin D level in Egyptian female patients with systemic lupus erythematosus. Mol Biol Rep. 2013;40(11):6151–62.
23. Hammad A, Mosaad YM, Hammad EM, Elhanbly S, El-Bassiony SR, Al-Harrass MF, et al. Interleukin-17A rs2275913, Interleukin-17F rs763780 and rs2397084 gene polymorphisms as possible risk factors in Juvenile lupus and lupus related nephritis. Autoimmunity. 2016;49(1):31–40.
24. Alamoudi OS, Attar SM. Pulmonary manifestations in systemic lupus erythematosus: association with disease activity. Respirology. 2015;20(3):474–80.
25. Abbas D, Ezzat Y, Hamdy E, Gamil M. Angiotensin-converting enzyme (ACE) serum levels and gene polymorphism in Egyptian patients with systemic lupus erythematosus. Lupus. 2012;21(1):103–10. https://doi.org/10.1177/0961203311418268.
26. Kamel EZ. Fluoroscopic guided radiofrequency of genicular nerves for pain alleviation in chronic knee osteoarthritis: a single-blind randomized controlled trial. Pain Physician. 2018;21:169–77.
27. Al-Daghri NM, Al-Saleh Y, Aljohani N, Sulimani R, Al-Othman AM, Alfawaz H, et al. Vitamin D status correction in Saudi Arabia: an experts' consensus under the auspices of the European Society for Clinical and Economic Aspects of Osteoporosis, Osteoarthritis, and Musculoskeletal Diseases (ESCEO). Arch Osteoporos. 2016;12(1):1. https://doi.org/10.1007/s11657-016-0295-y.
28. Al Rashoud AS, Abboud RJ, Wang W, Wigderowitz C. Efficacy of low-level laser therapy applied at acupuncture points in knee osteoarthritis: a randomised double-blind comparative trial. Physiotherapy. 2014;100(3):242–8. https://doi.org/10.1016/j.physio.2013.09.007.
29. Abd-Allah SH, Shalaby SM, Pasha HF, El-Shal AS, Abou El-Saoud AM. Variation of matrix metalloproteinase 1 and 3 haplotypes and their serum levels in patients with rheumatoid arthritis and osteoarthritis. Genet Test Mol Biomarkers. 2012;16(1):15–20.

30. Hussain SA, Marouf BH, Ali ZS, Ahmmad RS. Efficacy and safety of co-administration of resveratrol with meloxicam in patients with knee osteoarthritis: a pilot interventional study. Clin Interv Aging. 2018;13:1621.
31. Safi R, Kallas R, Bardawil T, Mehanna CJ, Abbas O, Hamam R, et al. Neutrophils contribute to vasculitis by increased release of neutrophil extracellular traps in Behçet's disease. J Dermatol Sci. 2018;92(2):143–50. https://doi.org/10.1016/j.jdermsci.2018.08.010.
32. Houman M-H, Bellakhal S, Salem TB, Hamzaoui A, Braham A, Lamloum M, et al. Characteristics of neurological manifestations of Behçet's disease: a retrospective monocentric study in Tunisia. Clin Neurol Neurosurg. 2013;115(10):2015–8. https://doi.org/10.1016/j.clineuro.2013.06.009.
33. Talaat RM, Ashour ME, Bassyouni IH, Raouf AA. Polymorphisms of interleukin 6 and interleukin 10 in Egyptian people with Behcet's disease. Immunobiology. 2014;219(8):573–82. https://doi.org/10.1016/j.imbio.2014.03.004.
34. Tizaoui K, Kaabachi W, Ouled Salah M, Ben Amor A, Hamzaoui A, Hamzaoui K. Vitamin D receptor TaqI and ApaI polymorphisms: a comparative study in patients with Behçet's disease and Rheumatoid arthritis in Tunisian population. Cell Immunol. 2014;290(1):66–71. https://doi.org/10.1016/j.cellimm.2014.05.002.
35. Talaat HSED, Mohamed MF, El Rifai NMM, Gomaa MA. The expanded clinical profile and the efficacy of colchicine therapy in Egyptian children suffering from familial mediterranean fever: a descriptive study. Ital J Pediatr. 2012;38(1):66. https://doi.org/10.1186/1824-7288-38-66.
36. Moussa T, Aladbe B, Taha RZ, Remmers EF, El-Shanti H, Fathalla BM. Overlap of familial Mediterranean fever and hyper-IgD syndrome in an Arabic kindred. J Clin Immunol. 2015;35(3):249–53. https://doi.org/10.1007/s10875-015-0140-x.
37. Mansour AR, El-Shayeb A, El Habachi N, Khodair MA, Elwazzan D, Abdeen N, et al. Molecular patterns of MEFV gene mutations in Egyptian patients with familial Mediterranean fever: a retrospective cohort study. Int J Inflamm. 2019;2019:2578760.
38. Ait-Idir D, Djerdjouri B, Bouldjennet F, Taha RZ, El-Shanti H, Sari-Hamidou R, et al. The M694I/M694I genotype: a genetic risk factor of AA-amyloidosis in a group of Algerian patients with familial Mediterranean fever. Eur J Med Genet. 2017;60(3):149–53. https://doi.org/10.1016/j.ejmg.2016.12.003.
39. Glickman SW, McHutchison JG, Peterson ED, Cairns CB, Harrington RA, Califf RM, et al. Ethical and scientific implications of the globalization of clinical research. N Engl J Med. 2009;360(8):816–23.
40. Chirac P, Torreele E. Global framework on essential health R&D. Lancet. 2006;367(9522):1560.
41. Anderson L. Fertile ground: the future of higher education in the Arab world. Soc Res Int Q. 2012;79(3):771–85.
42. Almansour S. The crisis of research and global recognition in Arab universities. Near Middle East J Res Educ. 2016;2016(1):1.
43. Amin TT, Kaliyadan F, Al Qattan EA, Al Majed MH, Al Khanjaf HS, Mirza M. Knowledge, attitudes and barriers related to participation of medical students in research in three Arab Universities. Educ Med J. 2012;4(1):47–55.
44. Gharaibeh A, Mousa YS. Should research thesis be a prerequisite for doctor of medicine degree? A cross-sectional study at Jordan university of science and technology. Int J Med Stud. 2014;2(1):8–12.
45. Sheblaq N, Al Najjar A. The challenges in conducting research studies in Arabic countries. Open Access J Clin Trials. 2019;11:57.
46. Aboshady OA, Gouda MA. Student research in Arab world: what is the current state? Saudi Med J. 2016;37(6):707.
47. Altbach PG. Peripheries and centers: research universities in developing countries. Asia Pac Educ Rev. 2009;10(1):15–27.

48. Romani MH, Hamadeh GN, Mahmassani DM, AlBeri AA, AlDabbagh AMY, Farahat TM, et al. Opportunities and barriers to enhance research capacity and outputs among academic family physicians in the Arab world. Prim Health Care Res Dev. 2016;17(1):98–104.
49. Mandil A, El Jardali F, El Feky S, Nour M, Al Abbar M, Bou Karroum L. Health research institutional mapping: an eastern Mediterranean regional perspective. EMHJ East Mediterr Health J. 2018;24(02):189–97.
50. Soete L, Schneegans S, Eröcal D, Angathevar B, Rasiah R. A world in search of an effective growth strategy. In: UNESCO science report: towards 2030; 2030. p. 20–55.
51. Fares MY, Fares J, Baydoun H, Fares Y. Sport and exercise medicine research activity in the Arab world: a 15-year bibliometric analysis. BMJ Open Sport Exerc Med. 2017;3(1):e000292.
52. Alsadan M, El Metwally A, Anna A, Jamal A, Khalifa M, Househ M. Health information technology (HIT) in Arab countries: a systematic review study on HIT progress. J Health Inform Dev Countries. 2015;9(2):32–49.
53. Khalifa M. Barriers to health information systems and electronic medical records implementation. A field study of Saudi Arabian hospitals. Procedia Comput Sci. 2013;21:335–42.
54. Galal A, Kanaan T. Financing higher education in Arab countries. Economic Research Forum (ERF) Policy research report 2010. p 29–47.
55. Sonnenwald DH. Scientific collaboration. Annu Rev Inf Sci Technol. 2007;41(1):643–81.
56. Bornmann L. Is collaboration among scientists related to the citation impact of papers because their quality increases with collaboration? An analysis based on data from F1000Prime and normalized citation scores. J Assoc Inf Sci Technol. 2017;68(4):1036–47.
57. Ahmad S, Ur Rehman S, Ashiq M. A bibliometric review of Arab world research from 1980–2020. Sci Technol Libr. 2021;40(2):133–53.
58. Dagher ZR, BouJaoude S. Science education in Arab states: bright future or status quo? Stud Sci Educ. 2011;47(1):73–101. https://doi.org/10.1080/03057267.2011.549622.
59. Qadir U, UN Development Programme (UNDP). Human development report 2015-work for human development. Pak Dev Rev. 2015;54(3):277–8.
60. Lancet T. GBD 2017: a fragile world. 2018.
61. Tanner A, Kim SH, Friedman DB, Foster C, Bergeron CD. Barriers to medical research participation as perceived by clinical trial investigators: communicating with rural and african american communities. J Health Commun. 2015;20(1):88–96. https://doi.org/10.1080/10810730.2014.908985.
62. Khalil SS, Silverman HJ, Raafat M, El-Kamary S, El-Setouhy M. Attitudes, understanding, and concerns regarding medical research amongst Egyptians: a qualitative pilot study. BMC Med Ethics. 2007;8(1):9. https://doi.org/10.1186/1472-6939-8-9.
63. Tohid H, Choudhury SM, Agouba S, Aden A, Ahmed LHM, Omar O, et al. Perceptions and attitudes to clinical research participation in Qatar. Contemp Clin Trials Commun. 2017;8:241–7. https://doi.org/10.1016/j.conctc.2017.10.010.
64. Nair SC, Ibrahim H, Celentano DD. Clinical trials in the Middle East and North Africa (MENA) region: grandstanding or grandeur? Contemp Clin Trials. 2013;36(2):704–10. https://doi.org/10.1016/j.cct.2013.05.009.
65. Oliver S, Bangpan M, Stansfield C, Stewart R. Capacity for conducting systematic reviews in low- and middle-income countries: a rapid appraisal. Health Res Policy Syst. 2015;13(1):23. https://doi.org/10.1186/s12961-015-0012-0.
66. van Weel C, Rosser WW. Improving health care globally: a critical review of the necessity of family medicine research and recommendations to build research capacity. Ann Fam Med. 2004;2(suppl 2):S5–S16.
67. Hummers-Pradier E, Scheidt-Nave C, Martin H, Heinemann S, Kochen MM, Himmel W. Simply no time? Barriers to GPs' participation in primary health care research. Fam Pract. 2008;25(2):105–12.
68. Xia J, Lynette Myers R, Kay Wilhoite S. Multiple open access availability and citation impact. J Inf Sci. 2011;37(1):19–28.
69. Thelwall M, Haustein S, Larivière V, Sugimoto CR. Do altmetrics work? Twitter and ten other social web services. PLoS One. 2013;8(5):e64841.

Chapter 23
Accreditation of Rheumatology Programs in the Arab World

Nafaja Alhasni, Hodan Hussein Jama, and Khalid A. Alnaqbi

Abstract Accreditation of rheumatology programs remains uncommon in the Arab world. It represents a formal process for recognizing excellence in the care of patients with rheumatic diseases and for promoting quality improvement in clinical practice. Several international accreditation models exist, including those offered by the European Alliance of Associations for Rheumatology (EULAR), the Asia Pacific League of Associations for Rheumatology (APLAR), and Joint Commission International (JCI). In this chapter, the authors review these accreditation models and describe their experience in achieving JCI Clinical Care Program Certification for four rheumatology programs (ankylosing spondylitis, systemic lupus erythematosus, rheumatoid arthritis, and juvenile idiopathic arthritis) at a hospital in the United Arab Emirates. This accreditation represents one of the early examples of rheumatology program certification outside the United States and may serve as a model for hospitals in Arab countries seeking similar accreditation. Finally, we outline essential steps for achieving successful accreditation.

Keywords Accreditation · Rheumatic and musculoskeletal diseases · Quality of care · Joint Commission International (JCI) · Clinical Care Program Certification · Health care quality improvement · Arab world

N. Alhasni · H. H. Jama
Sheikh Tahnoon bin Mohammed Medical City, SEHA/PureHealth, Al Ain, UAE
e-mail: hoabdi@seha.ae; nsalem@seha.ae

K. A. Alnaqbi (✉)
Rheumatology Division, Sheikh Tahnoon bin Mohammed Medical City, SEHA/PureHealth, Al Ain, UAE

Rheumatology Leader of Clinical Care Programs Certification (CCPC) for Rheumatology Programs at Al Ain Hospital (2018 to 2020), SEHA, Al Ain, UAE

Internal Medicine Department, College of Medicine and Health Sciences, UAE University, Al Ain, UAE
e-mail: kalnaqbi@seha.ae; kalnaqbi@gmail.com

K. A. Alnaqbi, G. Aldabie (eds.), *Rheumatic Diseases in the Arab World*,
https://doi.org/10.1007/978-981-92-0967-5_23

23.1 Introduction

Accreditation of rheumatology programs to establish a Center of Excellence (CoE) is an important strategy for promoting high-quality care, supporting continuous quality improvement, and maintaining international standards of practice within the field of rheumatology. Accreditation frameworks also contribute to strengthening patient safety systems and improving organizational processes in the management of rheumatic and musculoskeletal diseases (RMDs) [1]. In Arab countries, the landscape of healthcare accreditation is evolving, reflecting a growing emphasis on meeting global benchmarks and enhancing patient outcomes.

In this chapter, we examine the available international accreditation of rheumatology CoEs and research centers, with particular emphasis on experience from Arab countries. The authors also share their experience in achieving the accreditation for rheumatology programs at a hospital in the emirate of Abu Dhabi, United Arab Emirates (UAE).

23.2 The European Alliance of Associations for Rheumatology (EULAR) Center of Excellence in Rheumatology Research

The European Alliance of Associations for Rheumatology (EULAR) established the EULAR Center of Excellence in Rheumatology Research initiative to create a network of leading research centers and promote collaboration, training, and the exchange of scientific expertise across Europe [2]. To qualify for this designation, a rheumatology research unit consisting of a permanent team of investigators must demonstrate substantial scientific output. One of the key requirements is the accumulation of at least 400 impact factor points from original research publications in rheumatology or closely related fields over the preceding 5 years, with investigators from the center serving as first or senior/corresponding authors. Publications must be original research articles published in journals with an impact factor greater than four. Applicants must also provide evidence of research leadership, collaboration with other research groups, dissemination of research findings, and engagement of patients in research activities.

Notably, no rheumatology units from Arab countries are currently recognized as EULAR Centers of Excellence in Rheumatology Research.

23.3 The Asia Pacific League of Associations for Rheumatology (APLAR) Centers of Excellence

The Asia Pacific League of Associations for Rheumatology (APLAR) plays a significant role in advancing the standards of rheumatology care across the Asia-Pacific region. As of March 2026, several Arab countries are members of APLAR, including Syria, Iraq, Jordan, Kuwait, Saudi Arabia, Qatar, Oman, and the UAE. One of the APLAR key initiatives is the accreditation of Centers of Excellence, which are recognized for their exceptional contributions to clinical care, research, and education in rheumatology. APLAR has established a CoE certification program to recognize leading rheumatology institutions in the Asia-Pacific region that demonstrate high standards in clinical care, research, and education. Through this initiative, APLAR aims to develop a network of reference centers that promote best practices in the diagnosis, treatment, and management of RMDs and support the training of rheumatology professionals across the region [3].

Institutions applying for APLAR CoE certification are evaluated on multiple domains, including the quality of clinical services, research activities, and educational programs for healthcare professionals and patients. Certified centers are expected to contribute to regional capacity building by sharing best practices, supporting the implementation of APLAR guidelines, and participating in fellowship and exchange programs that facilitate training and collaboration among rheumatology centers. The CoE designation is valid for 3 years and may be renewed upon re-application and reassessment. Notably, no rheumatology centers from Arab countries currently hold APLAR Center of Excellence certification [3].

23.4 The Joint Commission International (JCI) Accreditation

The Joint Commission International (JCI) Accreditation is a United States-based non-profit organization that accredits healthcare organizations and programs. As of March 2026, numerous hospitals, both public and private, have received JCI accreditation in 11 Arab countries, with the largest number located in the UAE [4]. The JCI accreditation signifies that a healthcare institution meets the global standards of quality and patient safety, which are crucial for the effective delivery of clinical services.

The JCI accreditation offers Clinical Care Programs Certification (CCPC) for different clinical programs outside the United States, such as stroke, myocardial infarction, HIV, and psychiatric disorders [5]. Numerous healthcare facilities outside the United States have achieved such accreditation via JCI. Such accreditation implies a higher level of accrediting specific programs under a special status. The JCI accreditation for rheumatology programs represents a significant achievement in quality and patient safety standards for rheumatology care. None of the Arab countries, except the UAE, has achieved the JCI accreditation in rheumatology.

In the next section, we will discuss our journey to achieve the CCPC via the JCI at Al Ain Hospital, UAE.

23.4.1 Al Ain Hospital: Journey Towards Accreditation of Rheumatology Programs

The journey towards excellence in rheumatology care in Abu Dhabi has been marked by significant milestones. In early 2017, Al Ain Hospital took a pivotal step towards international recognition by initiating the process for CCPC accreditation for its rheumatology department. This decision aligns with the broader efforts to enhance rheumatology services in the emirate, as detailed in our comprehensive review of Abu Dhabi's rheumatology landscape [6]. The hospital's choice to pursue American CCPC accreditation was strategic, leveraging its existing JCI accreditation status. This decision reflects the growing emphasis on international standards and quality improvement in Abu Dhabi's healthcare sector, particularly in specialized fields like rheumatology.

23.4.1.1 Establishment of CCPC Team

A multidisciplinary CCPC team was formed, consisting of adult and pediatric rheumatologists, nurses, rehabilitation therapists, Information Technology (IT) specialists, and a clinical pharmacist. The purpose was to establish a collaborative framework for delivering comprehensive healthcare.

23.4.1.2 Strengths, Weaknesses, Opportunities, and Threats (SWOT) Analysis

Regular meetings were held to assess the current infrastructure of pediatric and adult rheumatology services using a Strengths, Weaknesses, Opportunities, and Threats (SWOT) analysis. At that time, rheumatology services included:

1. General pediatric rheumatology clinics
2. General adult rheumatology clinics
3. Specialized adult rheumatology clinics, including the Early Arthritis Clinic (established in 2013), the Connective Tissue Disease Clinic, and the Spondyloarthritis Clinic (both established in 2014)
4. Infusion Day Care, though lacking a formal manual for pharmacists and nurses
5. Inpatient consultations
6. A multidisciplinary team consisting of dietitians, physiotherapists, occupational therapists, and nurses who worked with rheumatologists but had limited experience and knowledge in rheumatology.

23.4.1.3 Main Chapters Required for Accreditation

We identified the patient population, met regularly with the team to assign tasks and provide updates, set a time frame, and allocated resources to define specific goals. The third edition of the JCI Survey Process Guide for CCPC was used for guidance [7], and the chapters included:

1. International Patient Safety Goals (IPSG): The program should establish processes to enhance patient safety by improving patient identification accuracy, verbal and telephone communication among caregivers, and reporting of critical diagnostic results. It should also implement procedures for handover communication and high-alert medication safety. Additional processes should ensure correct-site and correct-procedure practices, including a time-out before procedures. The program should adopt evidence-based hand-hygiene guidelines to reduce healthcare-associated infections and should implement a process to minimize the risk of patient harm from falls.
2. Program Leadership and Management (PLM): The program should define its mission, scope of services, and participation requirements in writing, ensuring they align with clinical practice guidelines (CPGs). The host organization should develop and implement a code of conduct. Reference materials are made easily accessible to clinical staff. The program identifies and assesses potential risks within the facility where it operates.
3. Delivering or Facilitating Clinical Care (DFC): The program should outline the patient assessment process, prioritize patient needs and risks based on age and development, and include a process for referrals and discharges according to ongoing patient needs.
4. Supporting Self-Management (SSM): Program materials should follow clinical practice guidelines and literature recommendations for effective interventions.
5. Clinical Information Management (CIM): The program should ensure standardization in the following areas:

   (a) Diagnosis and procedure codes are standardized and monitored.
   (b) Definitions, symbols, and abbreviations are standardized, with non-approved symbols and abbreviations identified and monitored.
   (c) Methods for adding comments, such as statements or addenda, into formal records are defined by the program.

6. Performance Measurement and Improvement (PMI): The program should identify and manage sentinel events, near-miss events, errors, or adverse events if they occur.

Furthermore, specific patient safety goals from the Abu Dhabi Department of Health, although not required for JCI accreditation, were also included [8]. These goals were:

1. Medication reconciliation.
2. Encourage patients' active involvement in their own care as a patient safety strategy.
3. Improving recognition and response to changes in a patient's condition.
4. Reduce the risk of hospital fires.

Four rheumatology programs were selected for CCPC accreditation: management of idiopathic juvenile arthritis, adult patients with ankylosing spondylitis, adult patients with systemic lupus erythematosus, and rheumatoid arthritis. Table 23.1 shows referral criteria, minimal testing requirements, key performance indicators (KPIs) before and after accreditation, and patient engagement. Developing such programs necessitated making significant steps, including:

1. Developing multidisciplinary clinical practice guidelines for each rheumatic disease with their respective reliable KPIs
2. Updating the scope of practice for pediatric and adult rheumatology services, rehabilitation, and nursing services
3. Developing a rheumatology nursing manual
4. Establishment of accredited rheumatology rounds held periodically
5. Educating and training nurses who were selected to work with rheumatologists
6. Conduct audits for quality assurance (to improve processes and outcomes, and sustain performance)
7. Developing satisfaction surveys for the CCPC team and patients.

23.4.1.4 Advancing Nursing Skills: Empowering CCPC Members

Given the absence of specialized rheumatology nurses in the country, we identified nurses interested in working in pediatric and adult rheumatology services. Nursing leadership provided essential support to these selected nurses, playing a pivotal role in the accreditation's success. To train and empower nurses who were part of the CCPC team, we implemented several key initiatives:

1. Enrollment in an online course to enrich their knowledge of rheumatic diseases and the administration of chemotherapeutic medications [9]
2. Provision of learning resources, including books such as *Core Curriculum for Rheumatology Nursing* and *Rheumatology Nursing Scope and Standards of Practice*, both published by the Rheumatology Nursing Society [10]
3. Training in the administration and scoring of patient-reported outcome measures related to various aspects of RMDs
4. Monitoring medication adherence and potential adverse events
5. Training patients and their caregivers in the administration of parenteral medications, such as biologics and methotrexate
6. Participation in public education activities and clinical research
7. Contribution to the development of educational pamphlets for patients
8. Participation in international awareness days related to RMDs

Table 23.1 Referral criteria, minimal testing requirements, key performance indicators before and after accreditation, and patient engagement measures for JCI-accredited rheumatology programs

	JIA	AS	RA	SLE
Minimum criteria for program referral	1. Joint pain 2. Joint swelling 3. Limping	1. Chronic back pain >3 months occurring at age < 45 years old, and improves with physical activity and NSAIDs, or does not improve with rest 2. Personal or family history of psoriasis, inflammatory bowel disease, or uveitis 3. Current or past history of peripheral arthritis (joint pain, swelling, or significant morning stiffness) and/or heel pain	1. Evidence of peripheral arthritis (joint pain, swelling, or morning stiffness >30 min) for more than 6 weeks 2. Positive rheumatoid factor and/or anti-CCP 3. High inflammatory markers (e.g., ESR or CRP)	1. Skin manifestations, e.g., rash (malar, butterfly, photosensitive), and/or ulcers (oral, genital, digital) 2. History of thrombosis (e.g., DVT or stroke or recurrent miscarriages) and/or Raynaud's phenomenon 3. Abnormal blood tests, e.g., anemia, thrombocytopenia, leukopenia, positive antinuclear test, positive dsDNA, low C3, low C4, or renal insufficiency
Minimum testing requirements	1. CBC 2. ESR or CRP	1. Routine blood tests: CBC, serum creatinine, AST, ALT, ESR, or CRP 2. ANA 3. ENA 4. C3 5. C4 6. dsDNA 7. Urinalysis with microscopy, protein/creatinine ratio, or 24-h urine for protein	1. Routine blood tests: CBC, serum creatinine, AST, ALT, ESR, or CRP 2. Rheumatoid factor 3. Anti-CCP antibodies 4. X-rays of involved joints, e.g., hands, knees, and feet	1. Routine blood tests: CBC, serum creatinine, AST, ALT, ESR, or CRP 2. HLA-B27 3. X-rays of lumbosacral spine and pelvis with hips, or sacroiliac joints, three views

(continued)

Table 23.1 (continued)

	JIA	AS	RA	SLE
KPI—Pre-accreditation	1. Referral to ophthalmology to screen for uveitis at diagnosis 2. Screen for varicella before starting Methotrexate 3. Methotrexate blood test monitoring (CBC, AST, ALT, and creatinine) every 2 months 4. Screen for TB before starting biologics	1. BASDAI every 4 months 2. CRP or ESR levels every 4 months 3. X-rays at baseline (including pelvis or hip or sacroiliac joint x-rays, and lumbosacral x-rays. Any missing test will result in a negative finding 4. Screening before starting biological treatment (hepatitis BsAg and hepatitis C antibody; QuantiFERON and chest x-rays). Any missing test will result in a negative finding	1. In active RA, measure ESR or CRP every 1–3 months. In inactive RA, measure ESR or CRP every 4–6 months 2. In active RA, measure DAS28 every 1–3 months. In inactive RA, DAS28 every 4–6 months 3. In active RA, blood tests to monitor DMARD toxicities are required every 1–3 months. In inactive RA, blood tests to monitor DMARD toxicities are required every 4–6 months (including CBC, ALT, AST, and creatinine). Any missing test will result in a negative finding 4. In active RA, screening before starting biological treatment (hepatitis BsAg and Hepatitis C antibody; QuantiFERON and chest X-rays) is required. Any missing test will result in a negative finding	1. SLEDAI score within 4 months 2. Lupus Serology (C3, C4, and dsDNA levels) within 4 months. Any missing test will result in a negative finding 3. Renal function (serum creatinine and urine tests) within 4 months. Any missing test will result in a negative finding 4. Drug adherence within 4 months

KPI—post accreditation	1. Referral to ophthalmology to screen for uveitis at diagnosis 2. Screen for varicella before starting Methotrexate 3. Blood tests monitoring while the patient is on Methotrexate (CBC, AST, ALT, and creatinine) every 2 months 4. Screening before starting biological treatment (QuantiFERON and chest x-rays) 5. Functional self-assessment on initial visit and within 3 months of entry to the program 6. Referrals to physical therapy at initial visit 7. Pneumococcal vaccination within 3 months of entry to the program	1. BASDAI within 3 months of entry to the program (once diagnosis is confirmed) 2. CRP or ESR levels within three months of entry to the program (once diagnosis is confirmed) 3. X-rays at baseline (including pelvis or hip or sacroiliac joint x-rays, and lumbosacral x-rays). Any missing test will result in a negative finding 4. Tuberculosis screening before starting biological treatment (QuantiFERON and chest x-rays). Any missing test will result in a negative finding 5. Functional self-assessment (such as BASFI) at initial visit (when the diagnosis is confirmed) and within 3 months of entry to the program (once diagnosis is confirmed) 6. Referrals to physical therapy at initial visit (once diagnosis is confirmed) 7. Pneumococcal vaccination within 3 months of entry to the program (once diagnosis is confirmed) 8. Cardiovascular risk screening assessment within 3 months of entry to the program (once diagnosis is confirmed)	1. Measure DAS28 within 3 months of entry to the program (once diagnosis is confirmed) 2. Blood tests (CBC, AST, ALT, and creatinine) to monitor DMARDs toxicities every 3–4 months. Any missing tests will result in a negative finding 3. Screening before starting biological treatment (QuantiFERON and chest x-rays). Any missing test will result in a negative finding 4. Functional self-assessment (such as HAQ) at initial visit (when the diagnosis is confirmed) and within 3 months of entry to the program (once diagnosis is confirmed) 5. Referrals to physical therapy at initial visit (once diagnosis is confirmed) 6. Pneumococcal vaccination within 3 months of entry to the program (once diagnosis is confirmed) 7. Cardiovascular risk screening assessment within 3 months of entry to the program (once diagnosis is confirmed)	1. SLEDAI score every 3–4 months 2. Functional self-assessment (e.g., HAQ) at initial visit (once diagnosis is confirmed) and within 3 months of entry to the program 3. Referrals to physical therapy at initial visit (once diagnosis is confirmed) if the patient complains of joints symptoms 4. Pneumococcal vaccination within 3 months of entry to the program (once diagnosis is confirmed) 5. Cardiovascular risk screening assessment within 3 months of entry to the program (once diagnosis is confirmed) 6. Screening before starting biological treatment (QuantiFERON and chest x-rays). Any missing test will result in a negative finding

(continued)

Table 23.1 (continued)

	JIA	AS	RA	SLE
Measures to engage patients in their care	1. Provision of educational pamphlets on disease and medications 2. Patient satisfaction 3. Issuing Certificate of Adherence for patients who are adherent to their medications and appointments 4. Issuing Certificate of Achievement for patients, parents of a child with rheumatic disease, or caregivers who pass the training course for self-injection at home			

Abbreviations: *AS* Ankylosing Spondylitis, *BASDAI* Bath Ankylosing Spondylitis Disease Activity Index, *BASFI* Bath Ankylosing Spondylitis Functional Index, *CBC* Complete Blood Count, *CRP* C-reactive Protein, *DAS28* Disease Activity in 28 Joints Score, *DMARDs* Disease-Modifying Antirheumatic Drugs, *DVT* Deep Venous Thrombosis, *ENA* Extractable Nuclear Antigen, *ESR* Erythrocyte Sedimentation Rate, *HAQ* Health Assessment Questionnaire, *JIA* Juvenile Idiopathic Arthritis, *KPIs* Key Performance Indicators, *RA* Rheumatoid Arthritis, *SLE* Systemic Lupus Erythematosus, *SLEDAI* Systemic Lupus Erythematosus Disease Activity Index, and *TB* Tuberculosis

9. Ensuring up-to-date vaccination, including influenza, pneumococcus, and hepatitis B vaccines
10. Coordination of care with other healthcare providers, including the management of referrals to and from rheumatology clinics
11. Opportunities to present at rheumatology departmental meetings, intra-city educational meetings, the monthly and annual meetings of the Emirates Society for Rheumatology, and the APLAR annual meeting in Dubai (October 2017). These experiences helped build their knowledge, communication skills, and confidence in co-managing RMDs alongside rheumatologists
12. Issuance of business cards to enhance professional identity
13. Participation in a preceptorship at St. Thomas' Hospital in Dublin, Ireland, in 2018, sponsored by the Emirates Society for Rheumatology, where they shared their experiences in caring for patients with RMDs [6]
14. Establishment of a hotline to facilitate communication with patients and improve accessibility

23.4.1.5 Development of Rheumatology Nursing Manual

One of our major objectives of the accreditation was to develop a Rheumatology Nursing Manual for rheumatology clinics and infusion day care. Despite extensive searches across various databases and personal communications with prominent rheumatologists worldwide, particularly in Arab countries, we were unable to find any existing rheumatology nursing manuals. As a result, the CCPC team decided to create a comprehensive manual addressing key aspects of rheumatology nursing.

The final manual covered essential topics related to infusion day care, including checklists for infusion protocols of all intravenous (IV) medications used in rheumatology services, such as biologic drugs, anti-osteoporosis drugs, pulse glucocorticoids, cyclophosphamide, and iron. It also provided guidelines for pre- and post-infusion care. Additionally, the manual provided checklists to ensure patient adherence to medications and to support the safe home administration of injections by patients or their caregivers at home. These checklists also ensured standardized nursing documentation in the electronic medical record (EMR).

23.4.1.6 Enhancement of Electronic Medical Record (EMR)

Enhancing the EMR is essential for improving the care of patients with RMDs [11]. Several key steps were taken to ensure this improvement, including:

1. Development of a specialized rheumatology workflow within the EMR, including calculators for measuring patient-reported outcomes and various disease--related aspects.
2. Creation of a Pre-Requisite Biologic Form in collaboration with the insurance company (Daman, the largest health insurance company in the UAE).
3. Implementation of order sets for infusion drugs (e.g., immunosuppressive drugs, IV immunoglobulin (IVIG), and IV anti-osteoporosis drugs).

23.4.1.7 Additional Measures to Improve Quality of Care

Additional steps were taken to improve the quality of patient care, including:

1. Development of clinic forms, such as a survey for new patients, a visit summary checklist, travel letters for patients carrying subcutaneous medications to facilitate airport procedures, and consent forms for email communication between healthcare professionals and patients
2. Monitoring rheumatologists' productivity, measured by relative value units (RVUs), and assessing the financial aspects of patient care, such as revenues and claim denials
3. Auditing nurses' documentation by rheumatologists in both the ambulatory clinics and infusion day care
4. Auditing rheumatologists' documentation by nurses in both the ambulatory clinics and infusion day care
5. Publication of an electronic Newsletter with contributions from the CCPC team
6. Creation of patient pamphlets on diseases and medications, available in both Arabic and English
7. Implementation of patient awareness initiatives in locations, such as the municipality and the outpatient department
8. Organization of accredited continuous medical education (CME) activities to raise awareness about rheumatology programs among healthcare professionals, such as internists, orthopedic surgeons, neurosurgeons, nephrologists, and family physicians
9. Issuance of a Certificate of Adherence to patients who consistently adhere to their medications and appointments
10. Issuance of a Certificate of Achievement to patients, parents of children with RMDs, or caregivers who complete the self-injection training course
11. Development of patient satisfaction questionnaires for both pediatric and adult patients, with regular monitoring of the results and the creation of action plans when needed
12. Organization of JCI awareness fairs for healthcare professionals at Al Ain Hospital to familiarize them with the CCPC accreditation process

23.4.1.8 The Day of the Accreditation Survey

The accreditation survey for Al Ain Hospital's rheumatology programs was conducted by two experienced surveyors from the USA. This face-to-face evaluation aimed to verify the implementation of CPGs over the preceding 12 months and ensure patient safety in the clinics. The survey process included several key components, including:

1. Assessment of CCPC team qualifications
2. Review of closed medical records
3. Patient tracers: Surveyors requested specific scenarios related to the CPGs, such as patients with spondylitis and uveitis, or lupus with anti-phospholipid antibody syndrome
4. Evaluation of the patient journey, including referral, program clinic registration, pediatric or adult rheumatology encounters, interactions with allied healthcare professionals (nurses, dietitians, rehabilitation services), pharmacy visits, and infusion day care experiences. This comprehensive assessment involved visiting various clinic locations and service areas
5. Face-to-face interviews with patients enrolled in the rheumatology programs

The surveyors provided constructive feedback upon completion of the survey. Following their evaluation, all four rheumatology programs at Al Ain Hospital were awarded an initial 3-year JCI accreditation in April 2019. This achievement marked a significant milestone, representing one of the first rheumatology programs outside the USA to receive JCI accreditation. This milestone underscored the hospital's commitment to maintaining high standards of care and patient safety in its rheumatology services.

23.4.1.9 Post-accreditation Activities

Following the accreditation, several key initiatives were implemented to further enhance rheumatology care, including:

1. Clarification of selected points within the four CPGs
2. Fine-tuning of existing KPIs and development of new ones
3. Utilization of the EMR system to ensure documentation of selected KPIs
4. Establishment of a dedicated rheumatology nursing education clinic, among the first of its kind in the region, providing structured education and support for adult patients with RMDs
5. Participation of nurses in regional conferences, such as the 3rd Abu Dhabi Geriatric Senior Citizens Conference in April 2019
6. Organization of the first Rheumatology Nursing Preceptorship Course in the Gulf region at Al Ain Hospital in December 2019. Nursing attendees participated in hands-on workshops led by rheumatology nurses and rheumatologists. Sessions covered topics including:

    - Calculation of various scores used in rheumatology
    - Improving patient adherence
    - Managing challenging patient interactions
    - Co-management of RMDs during pregnancy
    - Vaccination protocols for rheumatology patients

7. Contribution of a rheumatology nurse to the APLAR Pulse newsletter, with an article in February 2020 titled "*New Horizon in the UAE: Rheumatology Nurse*." [12]

23.4.1.10 Intra-Cycle Review of Rheumatology Programs

After receiving accreditation, regular audits were conducted and sent to JCI headquarters in the USA. On 31 October 2019, JCI approved the intra-cycle review reports submitted by the Quality Department of Al Ain Hospital. In April 2020, at the onset of the COVID-19 pandemic, the hospital was converted into a COVID-19 center. By September 2020, the rheumatology service had merged with a nearby tertiary hospital, Tawam Hospital. Due to the restructuring of the rheumatology programs, the accreditation could no longer be sustained.

23.4.2 Essential Steps for Successful Rheumatology Program Accreditation

Our experience in accrediting rheumatology programs provided valuable insights into the accreditation process. Figure 23.1 illustrates the phases of the JCI accreditation process for rheumatology programs, highlighting the systematic approach required.

The process of achieving successful accreditation begins with a clear vision aimed at obtaining international or regional recognition for the rheumatology department or program. This vision should be clearly communicated to and supported by the entire multidisciplinary team. Key steps include:

1. Ensuring the team is equipped with the necessary knowledge and skills to understand and implement the accreditation plan
2. Delegating specific responsibilities to team members to promote accountability and engagement in the accreditation process
3. Orchestrating collaborative efforts among different disciplines to ensure a coordinated and effective approach to meeting accreditation standards

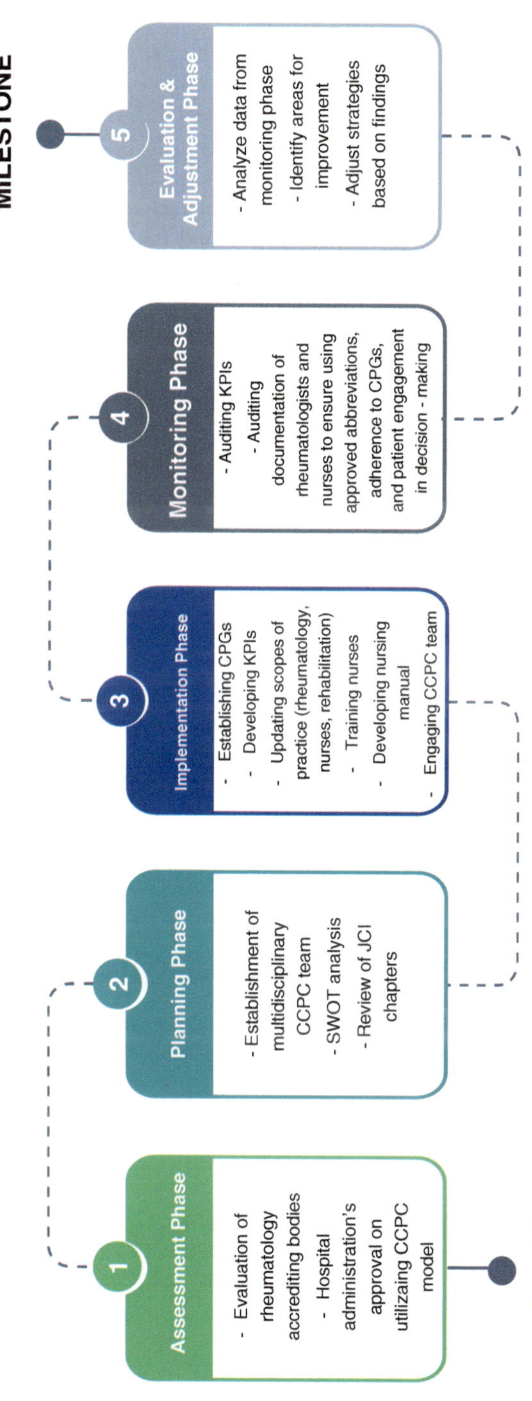

Fig. 23.1 Phases of the JCI accreditation process for rheumatology programs. CCPC Clinical Care Program Certification, CPGs Clinical Practice Guidelines, JCI Joint Commission International, KPIs Key Performance Indicators, and SWOT Strengths, Weaknesses, Opportunities, and Threats

23.5 Conclusion

The landscape of rheumatology accreditation in the Arab world is evolving. International standards set by organizations such as EULAR, APLAR, and JCI can be used as models.

The JCI accreditation model aims to improve rheumatology practice standards, focusing on patient safety, program management, clinical care delivery, self-management support, information management, and performance improvement. The successful JCI accreditation of Al Ain Hospital's rheumatology programs in April 2019, making it one of the first rheumatology centers outside the United States to achieve this recognition, demonstrates the potential of Arab institutions to meet international standards.

However, challenges remain. The absence of a specialized Arab accrediting body for rheumatology highlights the need for regional initiatives. Establishing such a body, tailored to the unique healthcare landscape of Arab countries while maintaining international standards, should be a priority for advancing rheumatology care in the region.

Furthermore, the lack of specialized rheumatology nurses in the Arab world presents both a challenge and an opportunity. Developing specialized nursing programs in rheumatology could significantly enhance patient care and support the accreditation process.

As the field of rheumatology in the Arab world continues to grow, focusing on accreditation and specialized training will be essential. These efforts will not only improve the quality of care for patients with rheumatic diseases but also position Arab countries as leaders in rheumatology care and research on the global stage.

Acknowledgments We extend our sincere gratitude to the Senior Management of Al Ain Hospital (2017–2020) and the many professionals who contributed to our rheumatology accreditation journey.

Senior Management
- Mr. Humaid bin Amhi Almansoori, Chief Executive Officer
- Dr. Ghazala Balhaj, Chief Medical Officer

Rheumatology Team
- Dr. Jamal Teir, Consultant Adult Rheumatologist
- Dr. Elsadegh Sherif, Consultant Pediatric Rheumatologist

Nursing Team
- Marlize Seaman
- Susan Oakley
- Rahma Abdulla Alsawafi
- Paula Ryan
- Ebtissam Abdalmniem
- Ekhlas Taha Mohammed
- Fatimah Salmeen Almenhali
- Chandreshkumar Gupta

Pharmacy Team
- Dr. Mohammed Tashtoush
- Dr. Zohdi Abu Shabaan

Quality Department
- Huriya El Qasass
- Letha Joseph Louis
- Mini Susan Sunil
- Aji Jose

Information Technology Department
- Fatima Alneyadi
- Khalifa Saeed Alshamsi
- Dr. Marri Subhash Reddy

Their collective dedication and efforts were instrumental in achieving this important milestone in rheumatology care at Al Ain Hospital.

Conflict of Interest None.

Disclaimer The views and opinions expressed in this chapter are those of the authors and do not necessarily reflect the official policy or position of their affiliated institutions or organizations. In addition, ChatGPT (version 5.2, OpenAI) was used solely for language editing and structural refinement. All scientific content, interpretations, and conclusions are the author's own.

References

1. Alhawajreh MJ, Paterson AS, Jackson WJ. Impact of hospital accreditation on quality improvement in healthcare: a systematic review. PLoS One. 2023;18(12):e0294180. https://doi.org/10.1371/journal.pone.0294180.
2. EULAR Centres of Excellence in Rheumatology Research. [cited 2026 May 16]. Available from: https://www.eular.org/eular-centres-of-excellence.
3. Application for APLAR Center of Excellence. [cited 2026 May 16]. Available from: https://aplar.org/collaboration/center-of-excellence/new-application/.
4. Joint Commission International: Who We Are – JCI-Accredited Organizations. 2026. [cited 2026 May 16]. Available from: https://www.jointcommission.org/en/about-us/recognizing-excellence/find-accredited-international-organizations.
5. Joint Commission International: Certification – Clinical Care Program Certification. 2026. [cited 2026 May 16]. Available from: https://www.jointcommission.org/en/certification/clinical-care-program.
6. Alnaqbi KA, Fazal F, Namas R. From sand to excellence: a deep dive into Abu Dhabi's rheumatology landscape. Mediterr J Rheumatol. 2024;35(1):73–82. https://doi.org/10.31138/mjr.011123.fst.
7. Joint Commission International Survey Process Guide for Clinical Care Program Certification. 3rd ed. Oakbrook Terrace (IL); 2014.
8. Policy for Quality and Patient Safety- Version 1: Health Authority Abu Dhabi. 2017.
9. Canterbury District Health Board. Antineoplastic drug administration for the non-cancer setting. [cited 2026 May 16]. Available from: https://edu.cdhb.health.nz/Hospitals-Services/Health-Professionals/Cytotoxic-Biotherapy/Pages/Antineoplastic%20Drug-Administration-for-Non-Cancer-Areas.aspx.

10. The Rheumatology Nurses Society (RNS). [cited 2026 May 16]. Available from: https://rnsnurse.org.
11. Schmajuk G, Yazdany J. Leveraging the electronic health record to improve quality and safety in rheumatology. Rheumatol Int. 2017;37(10):1603–10. https://doi.org/10.1007/s00296-017-3804-4.
12. Asia Pacific League of Associations for Rheumatology (APLAR). Voice of APLAR. [cited 2026 May 16]. Available from: https://aplar.org/publication/voice-of-aplar/.

Chapter 24
Pediatric Rheumatology in the Arab World

Soad Hashad, Djohra Hadef, and Buthaina Al Adba

Abstract Pediatric rheumatology is a relatively new specialty in the Arab world. It is still a growing field in which the number of centers and specialists is gradually increasing in these countries. Unfortunately, few published data are describing pediatric rheumatology in the Arab world. Therefore, we sought to provide an overview of pediatric rheumatology services in these countries, as well as to assess the published papers from Arab countries in this field. We gathered the information by conducting an online questionnaire on "SurveyMonkey." We distributed the survey's link via email and WhatsApp to the pediatric Arab rheumatology group. The responses provide an idea of the pediatric rheumatology practice.

Data on academic pediatric rheumatology activities in the Arab world are scarce. In this chapter, we will highlight some of the remarkable publications that described the incidence and prevalence of juvenile idiopathic arthritis, which is one of the most common diseases in pediatric rheumatology in the Arab world, autoinflammatory conditions and some of the basic science publications. We will also focus on some challenges that pediatric rheumatology services face, such as a shortage of pediatric rheumatologists, limited access to diagnostic laboratory and medications, and the referral system. New emerging topics such as the COVID pandemic and telemedicine health in pediatric rheumatology will be discussed as well.

S. Hashad
Peditratic Rheumatology, University of Tripoli, Tripoli, Libya
e-mail: Soadhashad@hotmail.com

D. Hadef
Pediatric Rheumatology, Batna 2 University, Batna, Algeria
e-mail: d.hadef@univ-batna2.dz

B. Al Adba (✉)
Pediatric Rheumatology, Sidra Medicine, Doha, Qatar
e-mail: Baladba@sidra.org; Buthainaalathba@gmail.com

K. A. Alnaqbi, G. Aldabie (eds.), *Rheumatic Diseases in the Arab World*,
https://doi.org/10.1007/978-981-92-0967-5_24

Keywords Pediatric rheumatology · Rheumatic diseases · Juvenile idiopathic arthritis · Child · Adolescent · Autoinflammatory diseases · Familial Mediterranean fever · Health services accessibility · Telemedicine · Transition to adult care

24.1 Introduction

From the first cases of chronic arthritis in children described in 1897 by George Still to the era of modern biotherapy, pediatric rheumatology (PR) has seen unprecedented progress and a broad evolution. PR is a subspecialty that has its own priorities and distinct practices. Indeed, some adult rheumatologists may regard pediatric rheumatic diseases as identical to the adult rheumatic diseases; nevertheless, they are often quite different [1]. Furthermore, adult rheumatologists have limited skills in dealing with multiple pediatric issues, such as pain, use of anti-rheumatic drugs in children, the art of dealing with parents, and handling school problems [1].

It was only until 1990 that the PR was officially recognized as a subspecialty in several countries, such as the USA and the UK [2], which was a necessary first and crucial step towards managing pediatric rheumatic diseases more efficiently, bearing in mind the ongoing increase in the number of children suffering from this disease. There are roughly 6–7 million children suffering from rheumatic illness globally, with the world's population being 6809.7 million, and children making up 30% of the population. The prevalence of rheumatic disease ranges from 2500 to 3000 cases per million children. Most of these kids (78% of them) reside in Asia and Africa [3].

After the foundation of the PR, the next challenging mission was to introduce it around the world. This mission was carried out with great ardor by different international workforce and associations such as the Pediatric Rheumatology International Trial Organization (PRINTO), the Pediatric Rheumatology European Society (PReS), the International League of Associations of Rheumatology (ILAR), the European Alliance of Associations of Rheumatology (EULAR), and the American College of Rheumatology (ACR).

The ultimate goal of the PR workforce is to reduce morbidity by giving children access to care and better clinical outcomes. Despite its low profile and low mortality rate, rheumatic disease, according to the World Health Organization (WHO), has a significant impact on morbidity and is "the major cause of morbidity throughout the world, having a substantial influence on health and quality of life, and imposing an enormous burden on health systems" [4]. To achieve thismission, promoting pediatric rheumatology as a subspecialty in the whole world becomes a crucial necessity.

The Arab League consists of 22 nations, with a total population of approximately 473 million people as of 2023, and a significant portion of this population is young, with adolescents and youth (aged 10–24) accounting for about 27% of the total [5].

Table 24.1 The Prevalence and incidence of different pediatric rheumatology diseases from some Arabic countries

References	Region	Disease	Prevalence	Incidence
Abdwani, 2015 [6]	Oman	JIA	20/100,000	2/100,000
Al Mayouf, 2021 [7]	Africa and the Middle East	JIA	3.8–400/100,000	
AlKhars, 2022 [8]	Gulf region	JIA	20/100,000	
Jaber, 2002 [9]	Arab community in Palestine	Behçet's disease	12/10,000	
Al Dhanhani, 2016 [10]	UAE	SLE	103/100,000	8.6/100,000

Abbreviations: *JIA* juvenile idiopathic arthritis, *SLE* systemic lupus erythematosus

There are more than 30 inflammatory pediatric rheumatic diseases, such as Juvenile Idiopathic Arthritis (JIA), systemic lupus erythematosus (SLE), scleroderma, vasculitis, juvenile dermatomyositis, periodic fever syndromes, sarcoidosis, Sjogren syndrome, and rare diseases. In Arab countries, the estimated prevalence of pediatric rheumatology disease is not fully understood, as there are few published epidemiological studies in the region. More studies and the establishment of Internet-based registries are needed to address the prevalence and the true burden of this disease in Arab countries. Examples of the available data are shown in Table 24.1, which summarizes the epidemiological data from the region on JIA, Behcet disease, and SLE.

It is important to note that the nations of Africa and the Middle East represent a broad range of races, socioeconomic situations, and climatic conditions [7]. Despite the proximity of 15 nations, there are significant differences in the quality of rheumatology research and care among them. This variability is influenced by a number of variables, including the amount of government funding for healthcare services, national demography, the healthcare system, the availability of skilled rheumatologists, and political stability [11].

As data on PR are scarce in the Arab world, we conducted an online questionnaire via SurveyMonkey (Table 24.2) to get more information regarding the pediatric rheumatology service in the region. We distributed the questionnaire's link via email and WhatsApp to the pediatric Arab rheumatology group. Among the 22 Arab countries, we got responses from 26 centers from 16 countries. The reasons behind the lack of response include:

- Absence of pediatric rheumatologists in some countries, such as Somalia, Mauritania, Iraq, Lebanon, and Yemen (though we were able to get data regarding their service from some of the adult rheumatologists in these respective countries, as they are covering pediatric service).
- We did not have any information or contact details in Djibouti and Islands of Comoros.

Though we used the survey in describing the pediatric rheumatology service in these countries, these responses may not reflect the true pediatric rheumatology service in

Table 24.2 Content of questions sent through SurveyMonkey

Content of questions
Number of pediatric rheumatologists in your center
Number of pediatric rheumatologists in other centers in your city /country (Governmental and private hospitals, if available). Kindly name the centers
Number of pediatric rheumatology clinics per week in your center
Availability of any sub-specialized clinic in pediatric rheumatology at your center. If yes, what are they?
Number of cases per year seen in rheumatology pediatric clinics in your center. Mention any available statistics
Available data on the prevalence of pediatric rheumatic disease in your country/city like juvenile idiopathic arthritis (JIA), SLE, etc.
International clinical trial (in the past or present) in which your center is/was a recruiting center. If yes, how many? If published (please attach publications) or mention trials in progress
Fellowship program at your center. If yes, how many rheumatology fellows are graduating from your program per year?
Any publication by your center describing your service? Please attach
Does your center have a pediatric rheumatology association? Kindly name the association?
Any difficulty in accessing rheumatic drugs at your center? e.g., NSAIDs, DMARDs, biologic drugs
Any certain system for referrals to the pediatric rheumatology service at your center?
Do you face any difficulty in the availability of laboratory tests at your center? e.g., antibodies (ANA, rheumatoid factor, anti-CCP, etc.), genetic testing (for periodic fever syndrome and other autoinflammatory), and genetic markers (HLA-B27, HLA-B51, etc.)
Any difficulty in accessing images for diagnosis and monitoring at your center? e.g., CT, CT angiography, MRI, MRA, and Positron Emission Tomography (PET)
Are musculoskeletal radiologists available at your center?
Are the patients paying for care and treatment at your center?

Abbreviations: *NSAIDs* nonsteroidal anti-inflammatory drugs, *DMARD* disease-modifying anti-rheumatic drugs, *ANA* antinuclear antibody, *anti-CCP* anti-cyclic citrullinated peptide antibody, *CT* computed tomography, *MRI* magnetic resonance imaging, *MRA* magnetic resonance angiography

the Arab world due to the small number of participants. However, it helps us understand more about PR services, which might be similar to neighboring countries.

24.2 Challenges in Pediatric Rheumatology Care in the Arab World

- *Awareness of Pediatric Rheumatic Diseases in Arab countries*

Pediatric musculoskeletal medicine (pMSK) is very important and should be integral to core pediatric clinical teaching. As with all other core skills, it should be delivered by general pediatricians and primary care physicians. To deliver the best pMSK clinical teaching, there is a need to 'teach the teachers' within pediatrics and primary care medicine. This will require input from specialists within pediatric rheumatology [12]. Multiple studies have demonstrated that recent residency graduates and general pediatricians report a lack of confidence in their clinical skills when

Table 24.3 Evidence of inadequacies of undergraduate RMD education in different regions

Region	Inadequacies of undergraduate RMD education
Egypt	>80% of surveyed pediatric practitioners ($n = 297$) reported low confidence in performing MSK physical examinations; therefore, 75% achieved an unsatisfactory score in the assessment [14].
Saudi Arabia	Overall knowledge of osteoarthritis among surveyed health practitioners was found to be inadequate (only 50% of responses were correct) [15].
USA	MSK clinical instruction continues to be underrepresented in undergraduate curricula. MSK clerkships were found to only present in 15% of medical schools (mean of 2 ± 1 weeks), and clinical MSK medicine selectives were only offered in 34% of medical schools [16].
UK	The evaluation of the MSK system was found to be consistently overlooked or performed in an unsatisfactory manner during the admission of children to four separate hospitals. Low self-reported MSK assessment confidence was seen among specialist registrars, and none could recollect learning pediatric MSK examination techniques during their undergraduate training [12].

Abbreviations: *RMD* rheumatic and musculoskeletal disease, *MSK* musculoskeletal

evaluating and treating children with musculoskeletal complaints [13]. Raising awareness of pMSK in the medical community and among the public is crucial to improving referral behavior and avoiding diagnostic delays and improper management. Meaningful progress in improving pediatric rheumatology teaching has since been made by virtue of global initiatives, such as the WHO, which endorsed a global campaign, Bone and Joint Decade (BJD) (2000–2010). A key priority for the BJD was to increase the education of all healthcare practitioners working in MSK medicine [14]. Table 24.3 demonstrates the evidence of inadequacies of undergraduate Rheumatic and Musculoskeletal Disease (RMD) education in different regions, including the Arabic region.

- *Number of Pediatric Rheumatologists in Arab Countries*

  Overall, there is a shortage of pediatric rheumatologists both in developed and developing countries. There are no published statistics with regard to the number of pediatric rheumatologists in Arab countries. From our survey, there is no accurate number of pediatric rheumatologists; there are roughly more than 170 pediatric rheumatologists and more than 50 pediatric rheumatology centers in the Arabic region. These numbers, though, are not accurate, demonstrating a shortage of pediatric rheumatologists in our region, affecting the rheumatology care in children and adolescents. In contrast, there are currently only an estimated 280–300 pediatric rheumatologists in the US, and eight states that do not have any [13].

- *Access to Pediatric Rheumatology Care in Arab Countries*

  The rationale for early referral is based on a window of opportunity early in the disease course that may alter the natural history of the disease process. Evidence supporting earlier and more aggressive medical intervention is growing [17]. Access issues for children and adolescents with rheumatology are significant and indicate worse disease outcomes. All children with JIA must be evaluated by a pediatric rheumatology team within 10 weeks of the onset of symptoms and within 4 weeks of referral, according to standards of care [18]. There is limited access to pediatric rheumatology care worldwide, including the Arab region. There are no data regarding access to medical care and medical coverage for children with rheumatic disease in Arab countries. A recently published paper looked at access to care for JIA patients through a pediatric rheumatology clinic in the UAE [19]. They divided their patients into two groups: Emirati-Emirates, who are native Emirati children and hold Emirati nationality and therefore have full access to free medical care; and non-Emirati-Emirates, who represent other nationalities that can get medical care either through insurance or a governmental pathway with justifications. Sixty-six patients with JIA were identified: 33 Emirates and 33 non-Emirates (3% represented other Arabs, 50% South Asians, and 8% other expatriates, including Westerners and East Asians). They concluded that both groups got access to the rheumatology service; however, delay in presentation to pediatric rheumatology was identified in their population. Such delay could have been attributed to access to care, lack of awareness, clinical skills, professional networks, and, in addition to geographical factors.

A referral system may aid the pediatrician in identifying patients who require early referral to a rheumatology service. In our survey, 11 out of 26 centers used an online referral system. Long wait times and travel distances are obstacles to pediatric rheumatology referrals; therefore, physicians opt for alternatives like self-care or sending patients to other specialists who may or may not be well-trained to treat rheumatic disorders.

The type of health care insurance coverage may play a major role in delivering medical care. In the Arab region, there are well-built insurance systems, but mainly used in the private sector. In the Emirati study [19], the type of healthcare insurance coverage did not affect the number of patients who received biological therapy once patients were seen in the pediatric rheumatology service. However, the total number of patients in that study was small. In our survey, 14 out of 26 centers in 16 different Arabic countries have pediatric rheumatology services free for citizens. The others stated that the payment for non-citizens was either by insurance or self-pay, especially in Gulf countries. Few Arab countries have free medical access to all governmental hospitals.

- *Access to Diagnostic Tools in Pediatric Rheumatology Care in Arab Countries*

The main challenge in pediatric rheumatic diseases is establishing early diagnosis in order to start management. Access to laboratory tests, particularly genetic testing (e.g., HLA-B27, HLA-B51, Mediterranean fever gene (MEFV), and other genetic mutations) and advanced imaging modalities (e.g., CT, CT angiography, MRI), is challenging in some Arabic countries. In our survey, 50% of the centers stated they have difficulties either in accessing some imaging tests or genetic testing/markers, while none of the Gulf countries identified such difficulty. Fifty percent of these centers have at least one musculoskeletal radiologist.

- *Availability of Anti-Rheumatic Drugs in Arab Countries*

  Government expenditure on healthcare services influences the practice of rheumatology in the Middle East [11]. In less prosperous countries, there is limited access to anti-rheumatic medications. On the other hand, in some countries with fast-growing economies, the government predominantly funds rheumatology services or has fully implemented a health insurance system that provides coverage. This grants easy access to rheumatologists and treatment for citizens and non-citizens [11]. A recent publication identified a severe shortage of pediatric rheumatology drug supply in different centers [20]. Fifty percent of centers that answered our survey identified some difficulty in accessing biologic treatment, while none of the Gulf countries had such difficulty.

24.3 Risk Factors for Rheumatic Diseases Arab Children

The main goals of researching the genetics of rheumatic diseases are to understand the etiopathogenesis of the diseases, develop a diagnostic tool, and to discover genetic predictors of diseases [21]. Several autoinflammatory diseases are single-gene disorders like Familial Mediterranean Fever (FMF). Many genetic studies on MEFV mutation were established in Arab countries [22]: Algeria [23–26], Morocco [27], Tunisia [28], Egypt [29–34], Palestine [35], Jordan [36–38], Lebanon [39, 40], and Syria [41].

In JIA, substantial contribution to disease risk is likely attributed to gene-environment interactions and environmental factors. The role of environmental factors in JIA, such as breastfeeding, infection and smoking, is less clear [41]. Identifying environmental factors associated with JIA could help develop new therapeutic modalities and assist in patient counseling and risk stratification. The availability of high-quality data in JIA is limited, and there are no studies from Arab countries.

24.3.1 Telemedicine Health: Expand the Reach of Pediatric Rheumatologists

Delivery of healthcare facilities to remote areas has been made a reality with the advancement of the health business and technology. Telemedicine is not only being used for diagnosing and treating illnesses, but it has also led to the elaboration of plentiful health-related educational resources [42]. Telehealth services were launched with the emergence of the Coronavirus Disease 19 (COVID-19) pandemic in 2020; however, it is still underutilized. Even though this high demand may decline once the pandemic has ended, the need for telehealth services will most likely persist in the future [42]. In 2014, only seven pediatric rheumatology clinics in the US had telemedicine capability, with only three clinics ever reporting using it [43]. The Arab League of Associations for Rheumatology (ArLAR) developed in 2021 the Best Practice Guidelines (BPG) for the use of Telehealth in Rheumatology in the Arab region, which provide rheumatologists with an approach to the most consistent, productive, and rational methodologies that utilize telehealth [44]. Although Arab countries share a common culture and language, there are some discrepancies in the quality of life, education, and availability of healthcare facilities. This mainly depends on the status of Gross Domestic Product (GDP) and political stability. Furthermore, the difference in the quality of life between different Arab nations creates a gap of inaccessibility to the healthcare system for all. Telemedicine in this region can be a key factor in achieving sustainable developmental goals and promoting well-being for all, at all ages [42].

24.4 Research and Education in Pediatric Rheumatology in the Arab World

- *Training and Fellowship Programs*

  While pediatric rheumatology fellowship programs have been well established in Western countries, it is still developing in Arab countries. There are no published data investigating the pediatric rheumatology fellowship programs in Arab countries, though these programs exist in a few Arab countries. In the USA, pediatric rheumatology training programs have existed since the 1970s, and in the early 1990s, the training was formalized into a three-year training program by the American College of Graduate Medical Education (ACGME) [45]. As far as we know, none of the programs in Arab countries is accredited by ACGME. However, some programs (e.g., in the UAE) have adopted structured training based on the ACGME curriculum and are currently in the process of getting accreditation.

  According to our survey response, nine out of 25 (36%) centers in the Arab countries have fellowship programs with 1–2 graduated fellows every 1–2 years. The program's duration ranged from 2 to 3 years. Their programs include inpatient and outpatient services (2–4 clinics /week) in addition to research activities. In our survey, the subspeciality pediatric rheumatology clinic is well-established in seven centers out of 25, for example, Lupus Clinic, Auto-inflammatory Clinic, and Juvenile Dermatomyositis Clinic. There is a wide variation in clinical practice among pediatric rheumatologists across Arab countries; therefore, pediatric rheumatology programs differ based on the local practice. The fellows are exposed to common pediatric diseases such as SLE, JIA, dermatomyositis, and more unique autoinflammatory conditions in our area, such as FMF. At the time of writing this chapter, there are no official subspecialty programs available in pediatric rheumatology in Arab countries. After completing the fellowship program, some of the fellows will have the opportunity to work in the same country or work outside the country. The establishment of a local, comprehensive, hands-on pediatric rheumatology fellowship training program may be a better strategy to decrease the patient-to-doctor ratio, eventually leading to an improvement in overall childhood-onset rheumatic disease outcomes.

- *Research Activities*

Pediatric rheumatology research is a crucial step in advancing knowledge of the pathophysiological basis of various rheumatic diseases and treatment options, in addition to improving clinical practice. Thus, international networks and study groups were formed to facilitate research, such as the Childhood Arthritis and Rheumatology Research Alliance (CARRA) and the PRINTO. A Pediatric Rheumatology of Arab Group (PARG) was established and officially recognized in 2016 as a special interest group of the ArLAR.

There are still limited data regarding research activities in pediatric rheumatology in the Arab world. We are not aware of any published clinical trials in pediatric rheumatology in the Arab region. The following section will briefly discuss some descriptive papers.

Migowa and colleagues described the pediatric rheumatology services in Africa that exist in ten of 54 countries (five out of ten are Arabic countries) [46]. In one center in Egypt, they see 600 inpatients and 8000 outpatients per year. In two centers in Libya, up to 70 inpatients are being seen in addition to 1100 outpatients per year. In three centers in Tunisia, 150 inpatients and 600 outpatients per year are being evaluated. In Algeria, 30 inpatients and 100 outpatients are being seen in one center per year. In Sudan, one center is seeing 100 inpatients and 400 outpatients per year.

Looking at specific disease epidemiology, a recent study summarized the available data on the prevalence of JIA and its subtypes in Africa and the Middle East [47]. The prevalence of JIA in Africa and the Middle East was in the lower range of the global estimate (3.8–400 per 100,000). The lowest prevalence was in Africa, with a prevalence rate of less than 3.43 per 100,000 and less than 22 per 100,000 in the Gulf area. The findings of this review support that the most prevalent subtype in Africa and the Middle East is the oligoarticular JIA subtype, followed by polyarticular rheumatoid factor-negative and systemic subtype. Most of the Saudi Arabia studies reported systemic JIA subtype to be the most frequent subtype.

A higher incidence of systemic JIA was associated with large familial clusters in Saudi Arabia, especially in the southe. Familial JIA suggests an autosomal recessive mode of inheritance with specific mutations in genetic markers like LACC1 [48].

A recently published paper from a tertiary center in the UAE recruited 138 JIA patients and found the JIA prevalence to be 32/100,000 in that cohort. The frequencies of subtypes were as follows: oligoarticular (55%), polyarticular JIA (25%), enthesitis-related arthritis (ERA) (7%), psoriatic arthritis (6%), systemic JIA (5%), and undifferentiated JIA (2%). A diagnostic delay was found in ERA and undifferentiated JIA, with a mean of 11.4 and 7.5 months, respectively. About 73% of patients were on methotrexate and 49% received biologic treatment [49].

An interesting paper published by the Pediatric Rheumatology Arab Group (PRAG) looked at the cumulative articular and extra-articular damage in 14 pediatric rheumatology centers from seven Arab countries in children with JIA [50]. In this cohort, the cumulative damage was common, particularly in JIA patients with their siblings emphasizing the role of consanguinity in the pathogenesis.

A multicenter study by the same PARG group looked at the pattern and the diagnostic evaluation of systemic autoinflammatory diseases (SAID) other than FMF among 144 Arab children followed at ten tertiary Arab pediatric rheumatology clinics in different Arabic countries. It was found that the most frequent monogenic SAID were *LACC1*-mediated monogenic disorders, and the most frequent multifactorial SAID was chronic recurrent multifocal osteomyelitis (CRMO). In addition, growth failure was the most frequent accrual damage, followed by cognitive impairment in that cohort [51].

The Juvenile Arthritis Multidimensional Assessment Report (JAMAR) is a new parent/patient-reported outcome measure that enables a thorough assessment of the disease status in children with JIA. JAMAR was cross-culturally adapted to Arabic patients and their parents and was validated as part of the multi-center project conducted by the PRINTO [52]. The Arabic version of JAMAR discriminated well between healthy subjects and JIA patients and is a valid instrument for the assessment of children with JIA in clinical practice and research.

A cross-sectional study included 109 pediatric patients with a diagnosis of FMF followed at a single center in Cairo, where 95 of those patients had a positive MEFV mutation (87.16%). The most frequent mutations in Egyptian patients were E148Q (24 patients, 25.3%), V726A (19 patients, 20%), M680I (19 patients, 20%), M694V (17/95 patients, 17.9%), and M694I (7 patients, 7.4%).

They reported that patients with the E148Q mutation had a higher response to colchicine therapy. On the other hand, people with M694V mutations were reported to have more severe illnesses [53].

Basic science research is still growing in the Arab world; however, few interesting basic science papers have been published in the Arab pediatric rheumatology region. One of these papers looked at serum IL-18 levels in 59 Iraqi patients with JIA and 58 matched controls [54]. The results revealed a significantly increased IL-18 in JIA patients compared to controls. A similar increased level was observed in subgroups of patients characterized according to gender, laboratory (rheumatoid factor, C-reactive protein), and clinical profile (i.e., juvenile arthritis disease activity score 27 or JADAS27, type of medication, and JIA subtypes). There was a significant positive correlation between JADAS27 and IL-18 level. The study suggested that IL-18 is a significant biomarker that supports the diagnosis of JIA.

Another basic research paper assessed the level of serum Interleukin-35, Interleukin-36, and the Interleukin-35/Interleukin-36 ratio in 51 patients with JIA and 46 healthy controls [55]. In comparison to the control group, JIA children exhibited notably higher serum IL-36 levels ($p = 0.002$), while they had significantly lower serum IL-35 levels and IL-35/IL-36 ratio ($p = 0.002$, $p < 0.001$, respectively). Moreover, the positive correlation between the IL-35/IL-36 serum ratio and JADAS-27 indicated a good measure of disease outcome. Additionally, the IL-35/

IL-36 serum ratio demonstrated higher sensitivity and specificity in comparison to absolute cytokine levels.

24.5 Pediatric Rheumatology Associations in the Arab World

The majority of Arab rheumatologists are members of pediatric and adult local rheumatology associations. The ArLAR is a non-profit organization that was founded in March 1995 originally as the Pan-Arab Society of Rheumatic Diseases. This name was changed later in November 2018 to ArLAR. There have been 13 biennial congresses held in different Arab countries since it was founded. Pediatric Rheumatology of Arab Group (PARG) was established and was officially recognized in 2016 as a special interest group. The main objective of this group is to promote excellence in pediatric rheumatology clinical care and research within the region through collaborative work among PRAG members, in addition to fostering scientific partnership and collaboration with international pediatric rheumatology associations and networks [56].

Many Arab pediatric rheumatologists are members of international associations such as PRINTO, the Pediatric Rheumatology European Society (PReS), ILAR, EULAR, ACR, and the Pediatric Society of the African League Against Rheumatism (PAFLAR). All of these associations focus mainly on the education of pediatric rheumatologists and pediatric rheumatology patients and promote research through their conferences.

24.6 Transition to Adult Care

Transition to adult care has a high impact on adolescents and young adults with rheumatic diseases. Many of our adult colleagues are uncomfortable caring for young adults, especially those with pediatric-onset disease. In the Western world, there are several published recommendations that guide rheumatologists in how to successfully transition and transfer young adult patients with childhood-onset rheumatic disease [57–60]. According to a recent European survey, the majority (99%) of pediatric rheumatologists reported that a formalized process of transitional care is essential, whereas (25%) of the participants reported that their centers did not provide transitional care [61]. Almost all published studies on transitional care in rheumatology patients were performed in developed countries; therefore, relevant data from developing countries are limited. In the Arab region, such data still need to be developed. The current transition practice in the Arab world is individualized as per the institute.

One of the published research conducted by Abdwani and colleagues examined the transition-ready abilities of adolescents and young adults with childhood-onset rheumatic illnesses in Oman using a cross-cultural adaptation of the UNC TRxANSITION scale [62]. This 32-question scale measures health care transition in ten domains, including knowledge about diagnosis or treatment, diet, reproductive health, school/work, insurance, ability to self-manage, and identification of new health providers.

Eighty-one Omani adolescents and young adults with chronic childhood-onset rheumatic diseases were recruited. They emphasized that the transition readiness in Oman is low when compared to Western countries, indicating the necessity to introduce a healthcare transition preparation initiative for children and adolescents with chronic rheumatologic diseases.

Many challenges contribute to the poor transition of care. For example, in many pediatric rheumatology fellowship programs, there is no formal training in transition of care. Furthermore, there is a cultural difference between pediatric and adult health care. For instance, pediatric providers are skillful in dealing with the child and parent, whereas the adult physician is more likely to hold the young adult patient responsible for self-management. In addition, this age group often is not interested in health advice, and treatment adherence which is a serious concern. In the Arabic culture, these young adults are not fully oriented to their disease, which may affect their care, especially since their parents may no longer be involved. Therefore, cooperation between pediatric and adult rheumatologists will help overcome these challenges. We strongly believe that regional guidelines and policies must be established to address the transfer and transition of care in line with international recommendations. It is very important while developing these recommendations to consider our culture, population, and the most common rheumatic diseases in our region.

24.6.1 Vaccination in Pediatric Rheumatology in the Arab World

No studies were published about the safety, immunogenicity, and coverage rate of vaccines from Arab countries.

24.7 COVID-19 Pandemic

The COVID pandemic in 2020 has severely affected the world. It was evident that children infected with SARS-CoV-2 remain mostly asymptomatic or mildly symptomatic. Nevertheless, a post-infectious disease (multi-system inflammatory syndrome in children, MIS-C) was described for the first time in 2020 in Europe. MIS-C is a critical and potentially life-threatening complication of COVID-19 in pediatric patients.

On March 2, 2020, Saudi Arabia reported the discovery of the first verified case of pediatric COVID-19 [63]. Since that time, a wide range of Arab reports have contributed to painting a clear picture of the various ways in which children with COVID-19 might present and develop [64–72]. One paper from Saudi Arabia looked at 390 pediatric cases with COVID and found that the majority were asymptomatic or had mild symptoms, and only around one-third of them required hospital admissions. Compared with international reports, the percentage of their asymptomatic and those with mild symptoms (75.4%) was slightly lower than in two previous major meta-analyses (98% and 96%) [63]. The information about MISC has been expanded by several additional Arabic research studies, which have also validated the clinical profiles and laboratory traits outlined in the literature [73–76].

A recent multicenter cohort from the UAE looked at the genetic and clinical characteristics of 45 patients with multisystem inflammatory syndrome in children (MIS-C) of Middle East origin [77]. They recruited 45 MIS-C patients in all, and 25 controls. In 36 patients, mucocutaneous and gastrointestinal manifestations were identified; cardiac findings were reported in 22 patients; and neurologic signs were reported in 14 patients. Nineteen patients were found to have rare, likely harmful heterozygous variations in immune-related genes, including TLR3, TLR6, IL22RA2, IFNB1, and IFNA6. Of these, seven patients had multiple variants. Compared to controls, patients had a higher enrichment of genetic variations (29 versus 3, P 0.001). Patients with these variants tended to experience treatment resistance (eight patients with genetic findings vs three patients without genetic findings received two doses of intravenous immunoglobulin), and earlier disease onset (seven patients with genetic findings vs two patients. The findings of this cohort analysis imply that MIS-C illness may be caused by uncommon, probably harmful genetic variations [77].

Many studies from the Arabic world were published on COVID and MIS-C, including papers from the UAE [64, 73, 77], Saudi Arabia [65–71, 74, 75], Syria [78], Qatar [79, 80], and Egypt [67, 81, 82].

24.8 Conclusion

Although several publications on pediatric rheumatology in the Arab world are available, further regional collaboration is needed to establish registries and develop working groups that can guide improvements in the management of pediatric rheumatic diseases. The shared cultural and historical background among Arab populations also provides an important opportunity for collaborative research on a range of rheumatic diseases, particularly autoinflammatory diseases.

Acknowledgments We would like to acknowledge the following centers for their participation in our survey:

Tanta University Hospital (Tanta, Egypt), Bagdad Teaching Hospital Medical City (Bagdad, Iraq), Queen Rania Children's Hospital (Aman, Jordan), King Saud Medical City (Medina, KSA), Children Specialized Hospital - King Fahad Medical City (Medina, KSA), King Faisal Specialist Center (Riyadh, KSA), King Abdulaziz Hospital (Jeddah, KSA), King Abdullah Specialized Children Hospital (Riyadh, KSA), Sabah Hospital (Kuwait), Al Adan Hospital (Ahmadi Health Governate, Kuwait), Hotel Dieu de France (Beirut, Lebanon), Benghazi Children's Hospital (Benghazi, Libya), Tripoli Children's Hospital (Tripoli, Libya), Child University Hospital A. Harouchi (Ibn Rochd, Casablanca, Morocco), Royal hospital (Muscat, Oman), Makasses Hospital (Jerusalem, Palestine), Sidra Medicine (Doha, Qatar), Children's University Hospital (Damascus, Syria), Kassab institute (Tunis, Tunesia), Tawam hospital (Al Ain, UAE), Jalila Hospital (Dubai, UAE), Sheikh Khalifa Medical City (Abu Dhabi, UAE), Sheikh Shakhbout Medical City (Abu Dhabi, UAE), Ahmed Gassim Children's Hospital (Khartoum, Sudan), and University Hospital Center of Batna (Algeria).

Conflict of Interest The authors have no conflicts of interest to declare.

References

1. Spencer CH. Why should pediatric rheumatology be recognized as a separate subspecialty: an open letter to medical councils and government agencies. Pediatr Rheumatol Online J. 2007;5:21.
2. Antón J, Lovillo MC, Cuadros EN. Paediatric rheumatology: where we are coming from and where we are going. An Pediatr (Barc). 2020;92(3):121–3.
3. Henrickson M. Policy challenges for the pediatric rheumatology workforce: Part III. The international situation. Pediatr Rheumatol. 2011;9:26.
4. WHO Scientific Group on the Burden of Musculoskeletal Conditions at the Start of the New Millennium. World Health Organization: The burden of musculoskeletal conditions at the start of the new millennium: report of a WHO scientific group. Geneva: World Health Organization; 2003.
5. Youth in the Arab world [Internet]. Wikipedia; [Last updated 2025 Oct 8, cited 2026 Jun 17]. Available from: https://en.wikipedia.org/wiki/Youth_in_the_Arab_world.
6. Abdwani R, Abdalla E, Al-Abrawi S, Al-Zakwani I. Epidemiology of juvenile idiopathic arthritis in Oman. Pediatr Rheumatol Online J. 2015;13:33. https://doi.org/10.1186/s12969-015-0030-z.
7. Al-Mayouf SM, Al Mutairi M, Bouayed K, Habjoka S, Hadef D, Lotfy HM, et al. Epidemiology and demographics of juvenile idiopathic arthritis in Africa and Middle East. Pediatr Rheumatol. 2021;19(1):166.
8. Alkhars F, Almutairi N, Al-Malouf SM. Demographic similarity and variability between patients with juvenile idiopathic arthritis in the Gulf Cooperation Council Countries. Ann Rheumatol Autoimmun. 2022;2(1):1–5.
9. Jaber L, Milo G, Halpern GJ, Krause I, Weinberger A. Prevalence of Behçet's disease in an Arab community in Israel. Ann Rheum Dis. 2002;61(4):365–6.
10. Al Dhanhani AM, Agarwal M, Othman YS, Bakoush O. Incidence and prevalence of systemic lupus erythematosus among the native Arab population in UAE. Lupus. 2017;26(6):664–9.
11. Watad A, Al-Saleh J, Lidar M, Amital H, Shoenfeld Y. Rheumatology in the Middle East in 2017: clinical challenges and research. Arthritis Res Ther. 2017;19(1):149.
12. Jandial S, Rapley T, Foster H. Current teaching of paediatric musculoskeletal medicine within UK medical schools - a need for change. Rheumatology. 2009;48(5):587–90.

13. Guglielmo-Roxby T, Louissaint V, Ettinger A, Llanos A, Cahill E, Chefitz D, et al. Assessment of resident knowledge in pediatric rheumatology. Glob Pediatr Health. 2021;8:2333794X211062020.
14. Al Maini M, Al Weshahi Y, Foster HE, Chehade MJ, Gabriel SE, Al Saleh J, et al. A global perspective on the challenges and opportunities in learning about rheumatic and musculoskeletal diseases in undergraduate medical education: White paper by the World Forum on Rheumatic and Musculoskeletal Diseases (WFRMD). Clin Rheumatol. 2020;39(3):627–42.
15. Homoud AH. Knowledge, attitude, and practice of primary health care physicians in the management of osteoarthritis in Al-Jouf province, Saudi Arabia. Niger Med J. 2012;53(4):213.
16. DiGiovanni BF, Sundem LT, Southgate RD, Lambert DR. Musculoskeletal medicine is underrepresented in the American medical school clinical curriculum. Clin Orthop Relat Res. 2016;474(4):901–7.
17. Demoruelle MK, Deane KD. Treatment strategies in early rheumatoid arthritis and prevention of rheumatoid arthritis. Curr Rheumatol Rep. 2012;14(5):472–80.
18. McErlane F, Foster HE, Carrasco R, Baildam EM, Alice Chieng SE, Davidson JE, et al. Trends in paediatric rheumatology referral times and disease activity indices over a ten-year period among children and young people with juvenile idiopathic arthritis: results from the childhood arthritis prospective study. Rheumatology. 2016;55(7):1225–34.
19. Khawaja K, Al-Maini M. Access to pediatric rheumatology care for juvenile idiopathic arthritis in The United Arab Emirates. Pediatr Rheumatol Online J. 2017;15(1):41.
20. Migowa AN, Hadef D, Hamdi W, Mwizerwa O, Ngandeu M, Taha Y, et al. Pediatric rheumatology in Africa: thriving amidst challenges. Pediatr Rheumatol. 2021;19(1):1–6.
21. Brown MA, Li Z. Polygenic risk scores and rheumatic diseases. Chin Med J. 2021;134(21):2521–4.
22. El-Shanti H, Majeed HA, El-Khateeb M. Familial Mediterranean fever in Arabs. Lancet. 2006;367:101624.
23. Ait-Idir D, Djerdjouri B. Differential mutational profiles of familial Mediterranean fever in North Africa. Ann Hum Genet. 2020;84(6):423–30.
24. Ait-Idir D, Khilan A, Djerdjouri B, El-Shanti H. Spectrum of mutations and carrier frequency of familial Mediterranean fever gene in the Algerian population. Rheumatology (Oxford). 2011;50(12):2306–10.
25. Ait-Idir D, Djerdjouri B, Bouldjennet F, Taha RZ, El-Shanti H, Sari-Hamidou R, et al. The M694I/M694I genotype: a genetic risk factor of AA-amyloidosis in a group of Algerian patients with familial Mediterranean fever. Eur J Med Genet. 2017;60(3):149–53.
26. Ait-Idir D, Bouldjennet F, Taha R, El-Shanti H, Djerdjouri B. Prevalence of Mediterranean fever gene mutations in clinically suspected FMF patients in Algeria. Pediatr Rheumatol Online J. 2015;13(S1):P94.
27. Belmahi L, Sefiani A, Fouveau C, et al. Prevalence and distribution of MEFV mutations among Arabs from the Maghreb patients suffering from familial Mediterranean fever. C R Biol. 2006;329:714.
28. Chaabouni HB, Ksantini M, M'Rad R, et al. MEFV mutations in Tunisian patients suffering from familial Mediterranean fever. Semin Arthritis Rheum. 2007;36:397401.
29. El-Garf A, Salah S, Iskander I, Salah H, Amin SN. MEFV mutations in Egyptian patients suffering from familial Mediterranean fever: analysis of 12 gene mutations. Rheumatol Int. 2010;30(10):1293–8. https://doi.org/10.1007/s00296-009-1140-z.
30. El Gezery DA, Abou-Zeid AA, Hashad DI, El-Sayegh HK. MEFV gene mutations in Egyptian patients with familial Mediterranean fever. Genet Test Mol Biomarkers. 2010;14(2):263–8.
31. Brahim GH, Khalil FA, Mostafa F, Fawzy MS, Said M, Omar AE, et al. Analysis of common MEFV mutations in Egyptian patients with familial Mediterranean fever: molecular characterisation of the disease. Br J Biomed Sci. 2010;67(4):202–7.
32. Al-Haggar MS, Yahia S, Abdel-Hady D, Al-Saied A, Al-Kenawy R, Abo-El-Kasem R. Phenotype-genotype updates from familial Mediterranean fever database registry of Mansoura University Children' Hospital, Mansoura, Egypt. Indian J Hum Genet. 2014;20(1):43–50.

33. Ali FT, Elhady MM, Abbas HH, Mandouh AY. The spectrum of MEFV gene mutations and genotype-phenotype correlation in Egyptian patients with familial Mediterranean fever. Int J Res Med Sci. 2017;5(4):1388.
34. Mansour AR, El-Shayeb A, El Habachi N, Khodair MA, Elwazzan D, Abdeen N, et al. Molecular patterns of MEFV gene mutations in Egyptian patients with familial Mediterranean fever: a retrospective cohort study. Int J Inflam. 2019;2019:2578760.
35. Ayesh SK, Nassar SM, Al-Sharef WA, et al. Genetic screening of familial Mediterranean fever mutations in the Palestinian population. Saudi Med J. 2005;26:7327.
36. Medlej-Hashim M, Rawashdeh M, Chouery E, et al. Genetic screening of fourteen mutations in Jordanian familial Mediterranean fever patients. Hum Mutat. 2000;15:384.
37. Medlej-Hashim M, Serre J-L, Corbani S, Saab O, Jalkh N, Delague V, et al. Familial Mediterranean fever (FMF) in Lebanon and Jordan: a population genetics study and report of three novel mutations. Eur J Med Genet. 2005;48(4):412–20.
38. Majeed HA, El-Khateeb M, El-Shanti H, Rabaiha ZA, Tayeh M, Najib D. The spectrum of familial Mediterranean fever gene mutations in Arabs: report of a large series. Semin Arthritis Rheum. 2005;34(6):813–8.
39. Sabbagh AS, Ghasham M, Abdel Khalek R, Greije L, Shammaa DMR, Zaatari GS, et al. MEFV gene mutations spectrum among Lebanese patients referred for familial Mediterranean fever work-up: experience of a major tertiary care center. Mol Biol Rep. 2008;35(3):447–51. https://doi.org/10.1007/s11033-007-9105-3.
40. El Roz A, Ghssein G, Khalaf B, Fardoun T, Ibrahim J-N. Spectrum of MEFV variants and genotypes among clinically diagnosed FMF patients from southern Lebanon. Med Sci. 2020;8(3):35.
41. Jarjour RA, Jamra RA. Mutations of familial Mediterranean fever in Syrian patients and controls: evidence for high carrier rate. Gene Rep. 2017;6:87–92.
42. Waqas A, Mehmood S, Jawwad AM, Pittam B, Kundu S, Correia JC, et al. Telemedicine in Arab countries: innovation, research trends, and way forward. Front Digit Health. 2021;2:610837.
43. Riebschleger MP, Tootoo J, Mroczek A, Clark S. A163: alternative mechanisms of care delivery in pediatric rheumatology: to what extent do they expand the reach of pediatric rheumatologists? Arthritis Rheumatol. 2014;66(S11):S211.
44. Ziade N, Hmamouchi I, el Kibbi L, Daou M, Abdulateef N, Abutiban F, et al. Telehealth in rheumatology: the 2021 Arab league of rheumatology best practice guidelines. Rheumatol Int. 2022;42(3):379–90.
45. Patwardhan A, Henrickson M, Laskosz L, Duyenhong S, Spencer CH. Current pediatric rheumatology fellowship training in the United States: what fellows actually do. Pediatr Rheumatol Online J. 2014;12:8.
46. Migowa AN, Hadef D, Hamdi W, Mwizerwa O, Ngandeu M, Taha Y, Ayodele F, Webb K, Scott C. Pediatric rheumatology in Africa: thriving amidst challenges. Pediatr Rheumatol Online J. 2021;19(1):69.
47. Al-Mayouf SM, Al Mutairi M, Bouayed K, Habjoka S, Hadef D, Lotfy HM, Scott C, Sharif EM, Tahoun N. Epidemiology and demographics of juvenile idiopathic arthritis in Africa and Middle East. Pediatr Rheumatol Online J. 2021;19(1):166.
48. Al Marri M, Qari A, Al-Mayouf SM. Juvenile idiopathic arthritis in multiplex families: longitudinal follow-up. Int J Rheum Dis. 2017;20(7):898–902.
49. Khawaja K, Kalas R, Almasri N. Subtype frequency, demographic features, treatment and outcome of Juvenile Arthritis in one Centre in Abu Dhabi in The United Arab Emirates. Pediatr Rheumatol Online J. 2023;21(1):14.
50. Al-Mayouf SM, Hashad S, Khawaja K, Alrasheedi A, Abdwani R, Abushhaiwia A, AlSuwaiti M, Alzyoud R, Al Abrawi S, Asiri A, Alshaikh M, Sharif E, Muzaffer M, Alsewairi W, Zlenti M, Kawaja E, Almutairi M, Majeed M, Lotfy H, AlMarri M, Almutairi N, Pediatric Arab Rheumatology Group. Cumulative damage in juvenile idiopathic arthritis: a multicenter study from the pediatric rheumatology Arab group. Arthritis Care Res (Hoboken). 2021;73(4):586–92.

51. Al-Mayouf SM, Almutairi A, Albrawi S, Fathalla BM, Alzyoud R, AlEnazi A, et al. for Pediatric Arab Rheumatology Group (PRAG). Pattern and diagnostic evaluation of systemic autoinflammatory diseases other than familial Mediterranean fever among Arab children: a multicenter study from the Pediatric Rheumatology Arab Group (PRAG). Rheumatol Int. 2020;40(1):49–56.
52. Al-Mayouf SM, AlE'ed A, Muzaffer M, Consolaro A, Bovis F, Ruperto N, Paediatric Rheumatology International Trials Organization (PRINTO). The Arabic version of the Juvenile Arthritis Multidimensional Assessment Report (JAMAR). Rheumatol Int. 2018;38(Suppl 1):43–9.
53. Talaat HS, Sheba MF, Mohammed RH, Gomaa MA, Rifaei NE, Ibrahim MFM. Genotype mutations in Egyptian children with familial Mediterranean fever: clinical profile, and response to colchicine. Mediterr J Rheumatol. 2020;31(2):206–13.
54. Al-bassam WW, Ad'hiah AH, Mayouf KZ. Biomarker significance of Interleukin-18 in juvenile idiopathic arthritis. Iraqi J Sci. 2020;61(12):3200–7.
55. Jamal QW, Alubaidi G, Humadi YA. Level of Interleukin-35, Interleukin-36, and the Interleukin-35/Interleukin-36 ratio in juvenile idiopathic arthritis. Open Access Maced J Med Sci. 2021;9(A):741–7.
56. Arab League of Associations for Rheumatology (ArLAR) - Pediatric Rheumatologist Arab Group [Internet]. [Cited 2026 Jun 17]. Available from: https://www.arabrheumatology.org/pediatric-rheumatologist-arab-group.
57. Foster HE, Minden K, Clemente D, Leon L, McDonagh JE, Kamphuis S, Berggren K, van Pelt P, Wouters C, Waite-Jones J, Tattersall R, Wyllie R, Stones SR, Martini A, Constantin T, Schalm S, Fidanci B, Erer B, Demirkaya E, Ozen S, Carmona L. EULAR/PReS standards and recommendations for the transitional care of young people with juvenile-onset rheumatic diseases. Ann Rheum Dis. 2017;76(4):639–46.
58. McManus M, White P, Barbour A, Downing B, Hawkins K, Quion N, Tuchman L, Cooley WC, McAllister JW. Pediatric to adult transition: a quality improvement model for primary care. J Adolesc Health. 2015;56(1):73–8.
59. Walter M, Kamphuis S, van Pelt P, de Vroed A, Hazes JMW. Successful implementation of a clinical transition pathway for adolescents with juvenile-onset rheumatic and musculoskeletal diseases. Pediatr Rheumatol Online J. 2018;16(1):50.
60. Walter M, Hazes JM, Dolhain RJ, van Pelt P, van Dijk A, Kamphuis S. Development of a clinical transition pathway for adolescents in The Netherlands. Nurs Child Young People. 2017;29(9):37–43.
61. Clemente D, Leon L, Foster H, Carmona L, Minden K. Transitional care for rheumatic conditions in Europe: current clinical practice and available resources. Pediatr Rheumatol Online J. 2017;15:49.
62. Abdwani R, Al Sabri R, Al Hasni Z, Rizvi S, Al Wahshi H, Al Lawati B, Al Abrawi S, Wali Y, Al Sadoon M. Transition readiness in adolescents and young adults with chronic rheumatic disease in Oman: today's needs and future challenges. Pediatr Rheumatol Online J. 2022;20(1):27.
63. Al-Tawfiq JA, Memish ZA. COVID- 19 in the eastern Mediterranean region and Saudi Arabia: prevention and therapeutic strategies. Int J Antimicrob Agents. 2020;55:105968.
64. Ennab F. Clinical characteristics of children with COVID-19: a multicenter study in The United Arab Emirates. J Pediatr Infect Dis Soc. 2021;7:S17–8.
65. Albuali WH, AlGhamdi AA, Aldossary SJ, AlHarbi SA, Al Majed SI, Alenizi A, et al. Clinical profile, risk factors and outcomes of ric COVID-19: a retrospective cohort multicentre study in Saudi Arabia. BMJ Open. 2022;12(3):e053722.
66. Mosalli RM, Kobeisy SAN, Al-Dajani NM, Ateeg MA, Ahmed MA, Meer WM, et al. Coronavirus disease in children: a single-center study from western Saudi Arabia. Int J Pediatr. 2021;2021:9918056.
67. Shaiba LA, Altirkawi K, Hadid A, Alsubaie S, Alharbi O, Alkhalaf H, et al. COVID-19 disease in infants less than 90 days: case series. Front Pediatr. 2021;9:674899.

68. Kari JA, Shalaby MA, Albanna AS, Alahmadi TS, Sukkar SA, MohamedNur HAH, et al. Coronavirus disease in children: a multicentre study from the Kingdom of Saudi Arabia. J Infect Public Health. 2021;14(4):543–9.
69. AlMayouf A, AlShahrani D, AlGhain S, AlFaraj S, Bashawri Y, AlFawaz T, et al. Clinical characteristics, laboratory findings, management, and outcome of severe Coronavirus disease 2019 in children at a tertiary care center in Riyadh, Saudi Arabia: a retrospective study. Front Pediatr. 2022;10:865441.
70. AlGhamdi A, Al Talhi Y, Al Najjar A, Sobhi A, Al Juaid A, Ibrahim A, et al. Epidemiology, clinical characteristics and risk factors of COVID-19 among children in Saudi Arabia: a multicenter chart review study. BMC Pediatr. 2022;22(1):86.
71. Duabie B, Alfattani A, Althawadi S, Taha A, Javaid HA, Mobarak O, et al. Epidemiological characteristics, clinical course, and laboratory investigation of pediatric COVID-19 patients in a tertiary Care Center in Saudi Arabia. Int J Pediatr Adolesc Med. 2022;9:153.
72. Saleh NY, Aboelghar HM, Salem SS, Ibrahem RA, Khalil FO, Abdelgawad AS, et al. The severity and atypical presentations of COVID-19 infection in pediatrics. BMC Pediatr. 2021;21(1):144.
73. Rajebhosale P, Mohamed M, Swilem M, Abdelmogheth A, Nabawi M, Farahat AA, et al. Clinical profile and immediate outcome of the multisystem inflammatory syndrome in children: retrospective observational single center study from The United Arab Emirates. J Pediatr Crit Care. 2022;9(4):116.
74. Harbi A, Kobeisy S, Elsayed SAN, Mehdawi HMM, Abdulrahman RS, Akef WKA, et al. Pediatric COVID-19 and MIS-C patients in Jeddah, Saudi Arabia: clinical, laboratory and radiological aspects. J Biomed Sci. 2021;9:1–4.
75. Al-Harbi S, Yasser M, Uddin M. Clinical characteristics and outcomes of Multisystem Inflammatory Syndrome in Children (MIS-C): a national multicenter cohort in Saudi Arabia. Curr Pediatr Res. 2021;25(9):904–13.
76. Ibrahim HM, Mohammad SA, Fouda E, Abouelfotouh K, Habeeb NM, Rezk AR, et al. Clinical characteristics and pulmonary computerized imaging findings of critically ill Egyptian patients with multisystem inflammatory syndrome in children. Glob Pediatr Health. 2022;9:2333794X221085386.
77. Abuhammour W, Yavuz L, Jain R, Abu Hammour K, Al-Hammouri GF, El Naofal M, Halabi N, Yaslam S, Ramaswamy S, Taylor A, Wafadari D, Alsarhan A, Khansaheb H, Deesi ZO, Varghese RM, Uddin M, Al Suwaidi H, Al-Hammadi S, Alkhaja A, AlDabal LM, Loney T, Nowotny N, Al Khayat A, Alsheikh-Ali A, Abou Tayoun A. Genetic and clinical characteristics of patients in the Middle East with multisystem inflammatory syndrome in children. JAMA Netw Open. 2022;5(5):e2214985.
78. Zaino J, Bakri A, Al Sayed Ahmad A, Hadba G. An Arab adolescent with multisystem inflammatory syndrome associated with COVID-19: a report from Syria. Avicenna J Med. 2021;11(4):221–4.
79. Magboul S, Khalil A, Hassan M, Habra B, Alshami A, Khan S, et al. Multisystem inflammatory syndrome in children (MIS-C) related to COVID-19 infection in the State of Qatar: association with Kawasaki-like illness. Acta Biomed. 2022;92(6):e2021543.
80. Hasan MR, Al Zubaidi K, Diab K, Hejazi Y, Bout-Tabaku S, Al-Adba B, Al Maslamani E, Janahi M, Roscoe D, Lopez AP, Tang P. COVID-19 related multisystem inflammatory syndrome in children (MIS-C): a case series from a tertiary care pediatric hospital in Qatar. BMC Pediatr. 2021;21(1):267. https://doi.org/10.1186/s12887-021-02743-8.
81. Hussein S, Khamis Y, Magdy R, Masoud M. COVID-19 in children: clinical presentations and outcomes in Fayoum Governorate, Egypt. Arch Pediatr Infect Dis. 2021;10(2):e112798.
82. Morsy HK, Tohamy NS, Abd El Ghaffar HM, Sayed R, Sabri NA. COVID-19 in children: an approach for multisystem inflammatory syndrome. Egypt Pediatr Assoc Gaz. 2021;69(1):33. https://doi.org/10.1186/s43054-021-00082-y.

Chapter 25
Pharmacoeconomics of Rheumatic Diseases in the Arab World

Nicole Gebran, Lamia AlHajri, Abdulrazaq S. Al-Jazairi, and Solaiman Alhawas

Abstract Pharmacologic therapy constitutes an integral part of managing rheumatologic diseases, with a diversity of available options from simple molecules to complex biologics and a trending rise in the cost of therapy accompanying novel innovations. The application of pharmacoeconomic principles is thus of particular significance regarding drug therapy selection in rheumatology. Additionally, there is current global interest in adopting new health technology assessment models and value-based approaches to care delivery. The Arab world is no different, with potential country-specific roadmaps in draft or the initial phases of implementation involving key stakeholders from regulators, payers, manufacturers, health economists, and healthcare providers. This chapter will define basic concepts in health economics, shed light on rheumatologic disease burden and budget impact, and explore approaches to cost-effective therapies. We conclude with recommendations to support the adoption of biosimilars as cost-effective treatment alternatives, highlight barriers to their adoption, and suggest means to strengthen pharmacovigilance as the way forward.

Keywords Cost-effectiveness · Health technology assessment · Biosimilars · Health economics · Pharmacoeconomics · Value-based care · Rheumatology · Cost-utility · Cost-benefit · Cost-minimization

N. Gebran (✉)
Pharmacy Department, Dubai Health, Mohammed Bin Rashid University of Medicine and Health Sciences, Dubai, UAE
e-mail: nigebran@dubaihealth.ae

L. AlHajri
Higher Colleges of Technology, Dubai, UAE
e-mail: lalhajri@hct.ac.ae

A. S. Al-Jazairi
King Faisal Specialist Hospital and Research Center, Riyadh, Saudi Arabia
e-mail: ajazairi@kfshrc.edu.sa

S. Alhawas
Saudi Food and Drug Authority, Riyadh, Saudi Arabia
e-mail: Smhawas@sfda.gov.sa

K. A. Alnaqbi, G. Aldabie (eds.), *Rheumatic Diseases in the Arab World*,
https://doi.org/10.1007/978-981-92-0967-5_25

25.1 Basic Principles in Health Economics

Health economics covers an increasingly important aspect of the assessment of disease burden. It has become an essential discipline to explore how therapeutic innovations can be made available to physicians and patients in our constrained economic environment by estimating the benefits and costs of healthcare interventions.

Pharmacoeconomics is defined as the description and analysis of costs of pharmaceuticals and pharmaceutical services and their impact on individuals, health care systems, and society. It is a division of outcomes research. However, not all outcomes research is pharmacoeconomic. The difference is that outcomes research not only takes into account the clinical and cost impact of healthcare but also the outcomes from a patient's perspective [1].

Ideally, the evaluation of drug therapy and associated services should include an assessment of clinical, economic, and humanistic outcomes. Clinical outcomes are medical events resulting from a disease state or medical treatment. Economic outcomes are defined as direct, indirect, and intangible costs compared with the consequences of treatment alternatives. Humanistic outcomes are the consequences of a disease or treatment on a patient's functional status or quality of life measured along several dimensions (e.g., physical function, social functioning, general health perceptions, and well-being). Pharmacoeconomic evaluation strives to assess the value of pharmaceutical products and services to the healthcare system by simultaneously incorporating and balancing all these outcomes [1].

25.1.1 Economic Outcomes Assessment

25.1.1.1 Costs

Traditional cost containment measures are not always synonymous with improved patient care. Hence, there has been a recent diversion in attention toward demonstrating the value of healthcare, considering various cost categories: direct, indirect, and intangible costs defined below. This provides a more accurate estimate of the total economic impact of a treatment option on a specific population, organization, or patient.

Direct costs can be medical or non-medical costs. Medical costs include medical products and services used for the prevention, detection, and treatment of a disease (e.g., hospitalization, medications, diagnostics, and supplies). Non-medical costs include services resulting from the illness but do not involve purchasing medical services (e.g., special food, transportation, and family care). Direct costs can be further divided into fixed (overhead) and variable costs. While fixed costs (e.g., rent, electricity) are typically excluded from pharmacoeconomic evaluations, variable costs are included as a function of volume. There is controversy around whether personnel costs should be considered fixed or variable. However, at this time of "rightsizing," administrators often view personnel as variable costs [2].

Indirect costs are the costs of morbidity and mortality resulting from the illness (e.g., lost productivity and premature death), which can be evaluated through either the human capital method or the less favored willingness-to-pay method. The human capital approach estimates morbidity and mortality losses based on an individual's earning capacity and the value of life tied to income. The willingness-to-pay approach relies on what the patients explicitly declare, how much they are willing to spend for an illness.

Intangible costs relate to non-financial outcomes of disease, including but not limited to the cost of pain, suffering, and grief. These are the most difficult costs to measure and are typically identified in economic analysis but not quantified. These costs can be either presented as a caveat or translated into a common unit of outcome measure, such as quality-adjusted life-year (QALY) [2].

By definition, incremental costs are the extra costs required to purchase another unit of effect, while opportunity costs are the value of the alternative foregone [2].

25.1.2 Consequences

Pharmacoeconomic studies compare therapeutic alternatives in terms of units of output (outcomes) per unit of input (costs). The manner by which positive and negative consequences are measured and assessed determines the difference among the various pharmacoeconomic methodologies. The benefits of drug therapy are defined in terms of beneficial effects on the patient [2].

Positive consequences may be defined as life years gained, disability days avoided, functional status, and well-being. Negative consequences can include disease exacerbations, medication side effects, treatment failure, and death [2].

The essence of pharmacoeconomic evaluation is balancing costs and consequences, the objective of which is to provide the relative value of treatment alternatives. Such analysis can be performed from different perspectives, including those of the patient, provider, payer, or society [2].

25.1.3 Methods of Economic Assessment

Pharmacoeconomic evaluations may be full or partial. Full evaluations generally include cost-minimization analysis (CMA), cost-benefit analysis (CBA), cost-effectiveness analysis (CEA), and cost-utility analysis (CUA). Partial evaluations compare either costs or outcomes. However, they do not compare both in one analysis. An example includes cost-outcome analysis (COA), which compares only the costs of alternatives [3].

25.1.3.1 Cost of Illness

The cost of illness (COI) identifies and estimates the overall cost of a disease in a defined population. This analysis measures the direct and indirect costs associated with specific diseases or illnesses, often referred to as disease burden. The cost burden of various chronic diseases, including rheumatologic conditions, is estimated across the globe and in various countries. The relative value of a treatment or prevention strategy can be measured by identifying an illness's direct and indirect costs. COI is not used to compare alternative treatments but to identify the financial burden of the disease; hence, the value of the prevention or treatment therapies can be measured against the disease costs [3].

25.1.3.2 Cost-Minimization Analysis

Cost-minimization analysis (CMA) compares treatment alternatives that are equal in efficacy but differ in cost. The underlying assumption is that treatment alternatives are therapeutically equivalent, outcomes are not compared, and the main focus is to determine the least costly alternative in monetary value. CMA only demonstrates the cost savings of one treatment over another; a typical example of where CMA is used would be when brand name products are compared with generic equivalents or when comparing drugs within the same therapeutic class with equivalent safety and efficacy. However, the cost comparison is extended beyond direct acquisition cost to include the relevant cost of preparing, administering, and monitoring the drugs [3].

25.1.3.3 Cost-Benefit Analysis

Cost-benefit analysis (CBA) is a method used to evaluate both costs and benefits, with both valued in monetary units. Thus, when comparing the two treatment alternatives, the alternative with the highest cost-benefit ratio or net benefit, which is more commonly used, would be considered the most efficient use of resources. To appropriately use the CBA methodology, it should be possible to compare the outcomes of treatment alternatives in monetary terms. It is particularly useful when allocating scarce funds to completing programs or therapies [3].

25.1.3.4 Cost-Effectiveness Analysis

Cost-effectiveness analysis (CEA) is used when comparing treatment alternatives that are not therapeutically equivalent or when it is not desirable or possible to express outcomes in monetary value. CEA provides a more comprehensive evaluation methodology where cost is measured in monetary units while outcomes are expressed in terms of reaching a specific therapeutic objective. A product or service may be considered cost-effective compared to a competing alternative if one of the following three conditions are satisfied: a cost-effective alternative is less expensive and at least as effective as the alternative or more costly but provides additional benefit that is worth the extra cost or less expensive and less effective in instances where the extra benefit is not worth the additional cost. Cost-effectiveness is synonymous with cost optimization and may not necessarily imply cost reduction. It provides the means to promote and embrace the most efficient drug therapy. Making formulary addition decisions between two or more drugs can best illustrate this concept [3].

25.1.3.5 Cost-Utility Analysis

Cost-utility analysis (CUA) is used whenever assessing patient preference or quality of life is desirable to measure outcomes of competing treatment alternatives. In CUA, costs are measured in monetary units, while outcomes are typically measured in quality-adjusted life years (QALYs). This method helps compare life-extending treatments, such as cancer, but is still associated with high rates of side effects. Additionally, CUA is used to compare treatments associated with high morbidity rather than mortality, such as the treatment of arthritis. CUA is usually expressed as cost per QALYs gained. QALYs represent the number of full years of full health valued as equivalent to the years experienced. For example, a full year in a disease-free patient is 1 QALY, whereas one in a patient on dialysis could be 0.5 QALY with a significantly lower value. However, these measures are often too complex; hence, CUA may be limited in application, especially from an institutional perspective [3].

25.1.4 Pharmacoeconomic Application in Formulary Management

A drug formulary is the list of medications that a healthcare institution or system chooses to maintain in stock within its facilities and that are usually covered by various health plans. It is often viewed as a cost containment tool. However, the purpose of formularies today is to optimize therapeutic outcomes while controlling costs. Accordingly, formulary management decisions should consider humanistic outcomes, extending beyond safety, efficacy, and cost evaluations of drug acquisition in order to assess the value of a healthcare service or product.

Formulary management decisions may result in formulary inclusion of the new drug, its exclusion, its inclusion with restrictions, deletion of formulary alternatives, curtailing non-formulary use, and directing physician prescribing through institutional guidelines. Economic data can provide critical support for these various formulary decision options.

25.1.4.1 Clinical Practice Guidelines and Drug Use Policy

In our current cost-conscious healthcare environment, it may not be sufficient to determine the treatment alternatives that are the best value or the most cost-effective. It is also important to determine the best way to use these treatment alternatives in hospitals and healthcare settings. Developing medication use guidelines, policies, and protocols can assist in influencing prescribing and promoting the most cost-effective and desirable use of medications. In the US, the Agency for Health Care Policy and Research (AHCPR) has sought to standardize the parameters of medical care nationally by decreasing procedural variance, improving therapeutic outcomes, and increasing the appropriateness of the medical services paid for by third-party insurance payers. At governmental, institutional, and organizational levels, policies regarding the appropriate use of health care products or services are made. These may be implemented to promote the use of the most cost-effective product or service, namely, pharmaceuticals. Successful policies may have a significant impact on influencing prescribing patterns and provide high-quality patient care for the available resources. Efforts are ongoing in the Arab world to introduce value-based health policies and agreements. These are mostly being carried out at the governmental level, such as the Ministry of Health in Saudi Arabia or the Departments of Health in Abu Dhabi and the Dubai Health Authority in the United Arab Emirates (UAE). A successful medication policy should result from pharmacoeconomic evaluations for its development, strategic oversight in its implementation, and multimodal education for its sustainability. A successful policy relies on the chosen pharmacoeconomic data, implementation, and education strategies [4].

25.1.5 Health Technology Assessment

Health Technology Assessment (HTA) uses modeling and systematic review methods to explore whether interventions are cost-effective, thus emphasizing the role of health economists. HTAs use modeling involving multidisciplinary expert panels to draw conclusions and make recommendations to stakeholders. The model inputs should preferably result from a systematic review. Based on these models, cost-effectiveness analysis is used to compare the costs and outcomes of alternative policy options and is considered a tool for assessing value for money. Alongside affordability, cost-effectiveness ratios and thresholds, budget impact, feasibility, and other important contextual criteria could be used. It is important to note that using thresholds as isolated decision rules can lead to wrong decisions. Depending on the decision-making context, HTAs often consider societal, ethical, or legal contexts. However, HTAs differ from guideline development. While HTAs often lead to coverage decisions focusing on the results of economic evaluations, guidelines make recommendations focusing on health benefits and harms, relying on formalized consensus judgments and contextual factors. HTAs and guideline development can involve a broad group of stakeholders but often differ in who initiates them (e.g., industry for HTAs and professional societies for guidelines) [4, 5].

25.1.5.1 Capacity Building

HTA is still in the early stages of development in the Arab world. The International Society of Health Economics and Outcomes Research (ISPOR) conducted its first Middle East and North Africa (MENA) regional conference in Dubai in September 2018. Several satellite meetings were arranged during the ISPOR Dubai 2018 conference, including the 2nd MENA Health Policy Forum. Outcomes of an electronically distributed survey before and during the conference indicated potential roadmaps that countries in the region could implement over the following 10 years. Preliminary survey results were presented during the conference in a policy panel with senior HTA experts from Egypt, Jordan, Kuwait, Lebanon, and Tunisia. It was noted that HTA capacity building in the region has to be strengthened by more graduate and postgraduate programs. Increased institutionalization and public budget are necessary success factors for HTA implementation. Additionally, efforts should strengthen local evidence and data in Arab countries, which translates to the extended use of regional patient registries and payers' databases. Duplication of efforts may be reduced when national HTA implementation is integrated into the healthcare system through international collaboration. HTA roadmaps are not transferable without accounting for country size, economic status, public health priorities, and the adopted healthcare financing systems [5].

25.1.6 Driving Access to Innovative Therapies

Accelerated access to innovative therapies at affordable prices has been a growing global challenge. While the World Health Organization (WHO) strives to provide equal access to essential medicines, innovative medicines remain in the hands of manufacturers and patent holders, with high medicine prices reportedly the main barrier to overcome in healthcare systems. Furthermore, healthcare expenditure is directly related to the gross domestic product (GDP); hence, developed countries are more likely to have a higher health budget and, therefore, better access to innovative medicines than developing countries [6].

Over the years, models for solutions have been adopted by regulatory authorities, albeit with limited data. The pathway of medication approval is lengthy and consists of the development, evaluation, authorization, access, reimbursement, and adequate benefit-safety monitoring through registries. Regulatory bodies, on one end, are making efforts to get the processes to work. Manufacturers, on the other end, are required to show excellence in reporting and fulfilling payer-specific needs by demonstrating their new medicines' real-world value. The challenge is to optimally integrate this with HTA processes, organization, and outcomes. To that end, certain countries are recently deciding to use a more multi-criteria decision analysis (MCDA)-attributed HTA, which is better suited to evaluate the value of healthcare interventions, particularly for high-cost oncology and orphan drugs.

Furthermore, managed entry agreements (MEAs) pose an excellent solution for access to innovative medicines. MEAs were introduced as a tool to mitigate the uncertainty attributed to economic evaluations and budget impact analysis, accounting for real-world evidence. Manufacturers are keen on value-based MEA to better position their products on the market. More research is needed worldwide, particularly in the Arab region, to better position safety, prioritize value elements, and establish a standard MCDA structure. Additionally, more effort should be directed toward sharing data among countries to prevent duplicate work and fasten submission processes. Increasing attention to safety in MCDAs and MEAs will increase the trust of health authorities and improve access for the manufacturers and availability of safe and effective drugs for patients [6].

25.2 Economic Burden of Rheumatic Diseases

The significant socioeconomic impact of rheumatic diseases remains a public concern and a worldwide challenge despite being intensively discussed in the literature [7–10]. Accordingly, many studies were published to assess the economic burden of rheumatic diseases [7–10]. However, literature unraveled that the cost-of-illness studies in rheumatology are usually restricted to a specific condition, for example, rheumatoid arthritis (RA), osteoarthritis, ankylosing spondylitis, and more [11] and are country/region-specific [12]. It is well recognized that despite the similarities in pharmacological treatments, there is a significant variation between the conditions falling under rheumatic diseases, as further discussed in the text. It was also observed that more studies focused on RA compared to other rheumatic conditions. Furthermore, different countries and regions have variations in the organization of care, treatment patterns, health insurance systems, GDP, inflation rate, and other economic values. The instability of the economy also added another layer of complexity. Thus, the economic analyses of published studies are less generalizable due to the aforementioned observations. In other words, what appears to be cost-effective in a certain region or a specific year might not be cost-effective in another region or a different year.

The following section will shed light on the economic evaluations and analyses carried out concerning various rheumatic diseases available in the literature. Specifically, this section will discuss the analyses carried out on direct (medical and non-medical) and indirect costs. Given that studies from the Middle East or the Arab World are scarce, this chapter, unlike published literature, is not intended to draw a comparison between different treatment modalities or methods to assess the cost-effectiveness. However, it aims to tabulate the common findings and observations from published studies and literature to serve as a reference point for future cost-effectiveness studies conducted in the Middle East and Arab world.

25.2.1 Direct Cost

Direct costs in rheumatic diseases included multiple components and items such as drugs or pharmacological interventions; non-pharmacological interventions (surgeries and devices); costs of diagnosis (imaging and laboratory tests); emergency visits; inpatient and outpatient care (including costs of traveling/transportation); visits to healthcare professionals other than physicians (physical therapists, occupational therapists, social workers, and psychologists); admission to extended-care facilities (nursing home or rehabilitation unit); and other healthcare-related costs (home remodeling and home care) [8]. However, drugs and outpatient visits are two major contributors to direct costs. A systematic review of 36 studies conducted in North America, Europe, and East Asia found that the annual direct costs of patients with RA were between $401 and $67,306, with medications being consistently the main component of direct cost [8]. In Saudi Arabia, the average annual direct cost in 2020 was approximately 38,596 ± 3055 Saudi Arabian Riyal (SAR) per patient, which was mainly due to medications [13]. Unfortunately, we did not find statistics on the direct cost of rheumatic diseases in Arab countries. In another region, two studies from the United States (US) showed that for patients with generalized osteoarthritis, the annual costs in Euros were between 7300 and 9399, with medications and primary care visits being the major contributors [14, 15]. In ankylosing spondylitis patients, $24,978 was the mean annual total healthcare cost during 2018 in the US, and this was largely driven by medication costs and outpatient visits [16]. Therefore, it is worth discussing the two main items that consistently contribute to the direct cost, as seen in the successive section.

25.2.1.1 The Biological Disease-Modifying Antirheumatic Drugs (bDMARD)

Over the past two decades, there has been a major improvement in the pharmacological agents used in the treatment of rheumatic diseases, as listed in Table 25.1. This is mainly due to the availability of disease-modifying antirheumatic drugs (DMARDs), specifically the biological ones (bDMARDs) [17, 18]. These agents 'biologics,' are also costly; in fact, five times more expensive than the conventional DMARDs [17, 18]. Hence, these agents are causing an increase in the direct costs [19, 20]; for example, the Australian government expenditure during 2014 increased to A$383 million due to the use of bDMARDs [21]. A similar observation was seen in the US, emphasizing the huge burden these agents are imposing on the system [22, 23]. However, the price of biologics is not only higher than that of other treatment options, but has also continued to rise [22, 24]. For instance, since 2013, the price of etanercept increased by 80%, adalimumab by 70%, and tofacitinib by 44.3% [25]. But biologics whose patents have expired by now lowered their price.

Although bDMARDs have drastically increased the expenditure, studies also confirmed that using these agents has significantly improved patient outcomes and,

Table 25.1 Pharmacological treatment of common rheumatologic diseases [26–36]

Drug	RA	PsA	AxSpA	JIA	SLE
csDMARD					
Methotrexate	x	x	x	x	x
Hydroxychloroquine	x			x	x
Leflunomide	x	x		x	
Sulfasalazine	x	x	x	x	
Cyclosporine		x		x	x
Mycophenolate					x
Cyclophosphamide				x	x
bDMARD					
Anakinra				x	
Canakinumab				x	
Etanercept	x	x	x	x	
Adalimumab	x	x	x	x	
Infliximab	x	x	x	x	
Certolizumab pegol	x	x	x	x	
Golimumab	x	x	x	x	
Tocilizumab	x			x	
Sarilumab	x				
Abatacept	x	x		x	
Rituximab	x			x	x
Secukinumab		x	x		
Ixekizumab		x	x		
Ustekinumab		x			
Guselkumab		x			
Risankizumab		x			
Belimumab					x
Anifrolumab					x
tsDMARD					
Tofacitinib	x	x	x		
Baricitinib	x				
Upadacitinib	x	x	x		
Filgotinib	x				
Apremilast		x			

csDMARD conventional synthetic disease-modifying antirheumatic, *bDMARD* biologic disease-modifying antirheumatic, *tsDMARD* targeted synthetic disease-modifying antirheumatic, *RA* Rheumatoid arthritis, *PsA* Psoriatic Arthritis, *AxSpA* Axial Spodyloarthritis, *JIA* Juvenile idiopathic Arthritis, *SLE* Systemic Lupus Erythematosus

accordingly, the associated economic burden of rheumatic diseases [20]. Whereas lowering the disease activity and achieving remission were found to be associated with a lower overall cost [26]. It is worth mentioning that disease activity is measured using various tools, which might show different outcomes. For example, assessing different aspects of RA includes Clinical Disease Activity Index (CDAI),

Disease Activity Score in 28 joints (DAS28), Health Assessment Score (HAQ)-II, Patient Activity Scale (PAS) II, 10-Item Patient-Reported Measure of Physical Function (PROMIS PF10a), Routine Assessment of Patient Index Data 3 (RAPID 3), and Simplified Disease Activity Index (SDAI) [27]. In the US, the medical costs for RA patients in remission were $8594 compared to non-remission patients ($10,002) based on data obtained between 2007 and 2019 [28]. In addition, using biological DMARDs was associated with a significant reduction in hospitalization costs over time [8]. Hence, these medications are now a cornerstone of the treatment of rheumatic diseases.

25.2.1.2 Mitigating the Costs Associated with Using bDMARDs

One of the methods by which bDMARD-related costs can be reduced is to shift patients to subcutaneous dosage forms instead of infusions. Subcutaneous injections are associated with a 50% lower administration cost than infusions, as patients mostly administer the injections themselves [37]. Accordingly, there is less cost due to the price of the subcutaneous drug itself in comparison to the infusion and a reduction in outpatient-associated costs (including costs of traveling/transportation). Another method assessed for its cost-effectiveness is switching treatments (cyclers) [38]. For example, a Swedish study on patients with inflammatory arthritis who were on subcutaneous TNF inhibitors showed that after 12 months, cyclers had a significant increase in their non-treatment costs ($1.135) compared to patients on persistent therapy who managed to lower their non-treatment costs [38].

Technology also provides an ample opportunity to reduce the cost. For example, when relapsed ankylosing spondylitis patients were compared to new achievers of inactive disease or low disease activity, the new achievers underwent more online patient assessments through the Smartphone Management System [39]. Furthermore, the smartphone system helped solve 29% of problems that required outpatient visits [39]. In fact, using effective medications to lower disease activity not only helps lower the overall cost but also heightens the utilization of technology (telemedicine and mobile health) [39]. Although some studies showed more preference for face-to-face consultations with rheumatologists, being in a low disease activity state increases the chances of using telemedicine, which helps reduce the costs of outpatient visits [40]. Furthermore, the acceptability of telemedicine, especially during the pandemic (COVID-19), increased among users due to the cumulative experience as most rheumatologists used telemedicine for the first time during the pandemic [41]. This facilitated changing the perceptions and preferences toward virtual consultations and, accordingly, not just reduced the cost but also heightened accessibility of patients to healthcare and rheumatologists [41–43]. Yet, the disparity between countries in telehealth laws, legislation, and guidelines remains a stumbling block in the Arab region [44].

The availability of biosimilar drugs is also a critical step in the right direction. This will be discussed in more detail in the biosimilars section below.

25.2.1.3 Pharmacoeconomic Studies Should Be Evaluated Critically

Studies evaluating the cost-effectiveness of DMARDs are heterogeneous, using different willingness-to-pay thresholds (quality-adjusted life years; QALY), perspectives (payer or societal), GDP, costs of studied medications, different disease activity, especially at baseline, outcomes, intensities of treatment, and responses to treatments. Hence, results of studies should not be taken at face value but rather should incorporate all these factors when attempting to draw conclusions [45–50]. To illustrate, when the willingness-to-pay threshold is €35,000 per QALY, biologics do not seem cost-effective among conventional DMARD-naïve patients or patients with an insufficient response to conventional DMARDs. However, when the threshold is €50,000 to 100,000 per QALY, biologics might be cost-effective among patients with an inadequate response to the conventional DMARDs [48]. In another example, tofacitinib, as initial third-line therapy, was an effective cost-saving strategy (€337,489 per QALY foregone) in patients with moderate to severe RA and inadequate responses to TNF inhibitors [51].

Additionally, a recent study conducted in China showed that when the willingness-to-pay threshold is 3 times the average GDP per capita, using a combination of etanercept with methotrexate is less cost-effective compared to triple DMARDs [52]. The GDP used in this study was around ¥165,960.0 for the years 2016 and 2017. Hence, findings of studies should be examined critically and holistically to assess their suitability for adaptation.

25.2.2 *Indirect Costs*

25.2.2.1 Loss of Productivity

Indirect costs refer to productivity losses due to morbidity and mortality, incurred by the individual, family, society, or employer [8]. Direct cost is similar to the indirect cost, which contributes massively to the cost structure in patients with rheumatic diseases. A study found that disability and absenteeism (sick leave) make up the majority of the cost structure (direct and indirect) of patients with rheumatic diseases <65 years old [9]. Furthermore, in a systematic review, nine studies measured the annual indirect cost in RA patients and found that the cost ranged between $595 and $22,444 [8]. These studies also confirmed that absenteeism and work disability were the two major components of indirect costs [8].

Furthermore, an analysis of indirect costs among patients with RA in Romania showed that, at the cohort level, the annual cost of temporary work loss due to sick leave was €4653.6, while the cost of permanent work incapacity due to early retirement was €214530. Therefore, the economic burden is not limited to temporary productivity loss due to sick leave, but also includes early retirement before the legal retirement age, which is a major concern and a substantial economic burden on individuals, countries, and governments [53]. In another example, the incremental non-healthcare costs of osteoarthritis in Hong Kong in 2011 ranged from €432 [54] to €11,956 [55] per year. A major observation was that the overall indirect cost was much lower when the cost of productivity losses due to work absences was excluded [56]. Hence, this confirms the major contribution of loss in productivity toward the indirect costs' structure. On the other hand, presenteeism, defined as presenting to work without being productive, is another crucial concept that must be explored [57]. Although rarely estimated in studies, presenteeism accounted for 8.8% and 92.9% of indirect costs in the Danish and Japanese studies, respectively [58, 59].

25.2.2.2 Lack of Standardization

Further to the observations mentioned in the section on direct cost, which are also valid for the indirect cost, it was noted that studies in the literature have variations in terms of the components contributing to the indirect cost, which makes it challenging to draw comparisons or consensus. The heterogeneity was also seen in the definitions of the components contributing to the indirect cost (e.g., loss of productivity, absenteeism, presenteeism, and more). Additionally, studies assessed the direct and indirect costs separately. However, the indirect costs cannot be disentangled from the (used or implemented) treatment modalities and the direct costs. Whereas it was found that over 2 years, the sick leave costs were €717 in rheumatoid arthritis, psoriatic arthritis, and ankylosing spondylitis patients on persistent treatment compared to €1241 in the non-persistent cohort [60]. Hence, when assessing cost-effectiveness, all types of costs should be assessed in relation to each other.

25.2.3 *The Way Forward for Research*

There is a limited number of cost-effectiveness studies and economic analyses conducted in the Arab world. Hence, this chapter aims to shed light on the common findings related to studies conducted elsewhere, serving as a reference point for future studies conducted in the Arab world. Research should examine all types of costs holistically, as these cannot be disentangled and are highly interrelated. Lowering disease activity by using an optimal treatment is of prime importance to achieve optimal outcomes for patients' health, maintenance of productivity, and avoidance of early retirement. Therefore, cost-effectiveness studies should focus on how to continue utilizing costly DMARDs and reduce the associated costs using various methods that suit the socio-ecological context of the Arab world. Furthermore, there is a need for standardization of definitions and tools, as elaborated earlier, to enable conducting studies and systematically assessing the findings.

25.3 Adoption and Experience with Biosimilar Drugs in Arab Countries

A biosimilar is a biological medicine highly similar to a previously approved reference medicine, with no clinically meaningful differences in structure, biological activity, safety, quality, and efficacy [61]. A reference product is "the single biological product, already approved by the Food and Drug Administration (FDA), against which a proposed biosimilar product is compared" [62].

An interchangeable biosimilar is a biosimilar that meets FDA standards for interchangeability through the submission of additional data on the impact of switching or alternating with the originator product. Therefore, it is expected to pose a similar clinical effect to the originator with no increase in the risk [63]. The purple book has been the primary source to locate all registered and interchangeable biosimilars in the US [64].

25.3.1 Guideline Recommendations, Extrapolation, and Interchangeability

The introduction of biosimilars in recent years has been a game-changer in reducing total healthcare expenditure, particularly in rheumatology. The adoption of biosimilars is associated with price reductions ranging from 10% to 50%, with most studies reporting price reductions of 12–25% [65], resulting in considerable direct cost savings.

The US FDA has approved interchangeable biosimilars that may be substituted with the reference product by pharmacists (subject to state law); however, unless approved as such, a prescribed biosimilar may not be interchanged or substituted without authorization from the prescribing physician [66]. In August 2022, ranibizumab-eqrn was the first biosimilar deemed interchangeable with the originator product without requesting additional systematic switching studies. The decision was based on robust data (analytical, clinical, and manufacturing) evaluation that concluded the inability of switching studies to show the risk for the particular medication [67]. This highlights that interchangeability is evaluated case by case. In most Arab countries, biosimilars are prescribed by physicians following a discussion with the patient and are not interchangeable unless auto-substitution by a pharmacist is authorized through institutional policies or pharmacy and therapeutics committees. The extrapolation of approved indications from originators to biosimilar products is considered acceptable by many authorities, including the European Medicines Agency (EMA), where consideration of EMA-specific criteria is required [68, 69]. In past months, the EMA and Heads of Medicine Agency (HMA) published a joint statement to confirm the interchangeability of biosimilars approved in the European Union with originators or equivalent biosimilars from a scientific perspective. Therefore, it is not required to conduct additional systematic switch studies to support interchangeability at the prescribers' level. Guidelines also vary in recommendations. In patients with RA, ACR guidelines consider biosimilars equivalent to FDA-approved originators [30], yet recommend the continuation of originator TNFi over mandating switching to biosimilars in adults with stable AS [33].

25.3.2 Biosimilars in Rheumatology in the Arab World

In Arab countries, studies on perception, knowledge, and attitude toward biosimilars in rheumatology are scarce and indicate a knowledge gap. In the UAE, the adoption of biosimilars in rheumatology has been relatively slower than in other disciplines, with a general lack of confidence from the prescribers' end to switch stable patients on originator products to biosimilars and a reluctance to start treatment-naïve patients on the biosimilar product. In Saudi Arabia, a cross-sectional survey assessed rheumatologists' perception of biosimilars and non-medical switching (NMS). One-hundred forty-three rheumatologists completed the survey [70]. Sixty-nine (48.3%) participants believed their knowledge about biosimilars was adequate. In addition, the availability of an adequate level of evidence to approve biosimilars for the studied and extrapolated indications of the originator products was reported by 88 (61.5%) and 69 (48.3%) participants, respectively [67]. Moreover, 88 (61.5%) respondents believed there are cost savings resulting from NMS, while 81 (56.6%) respondents reported willingness to perform NMS. Perceived knowledge about biosimilars and published evidence among 43 (30.07%) participants who tried biosimilars was inadequate in 8 (18.6%) and 9 (20.9%), respectively. In addition, knowledge of extrapolation and the totality of evidence concept was inadequate in 18 (41.9%) and 20 (46.5%), respectively. NMS was thought to be associated with harm and not supposed to result in cost savings among 29 (67.4%) and 23 (53.5%) participants. Most participants used biosimilars as part of automatic switching as authorized by their Pharmacy and Therapeutics Committee [70, 71]. Gulf consensus-based recommendations on the use of biosimilars in inflammatory arthritis have been developed and will be submitted soon in a peer-reviewed journal.

25.3.3 Biosimilar Experience Outside Rheumatology

Few studies from Tunisia, Jordan, and Iraq about biosimilar experience were identified [69, 72–74]. In Tunisia, the perception of biosimilars was assessed among 107 out of 150 invited hematologists and oncologists. Approximately 23% of physicians were completely against the substitution and interchangeability of biosimilars with originator products. In addition, 11% were totally against biosimilar prescribing. On the other hand, about 89% of physicians preferred prescribing biosimilars. The preference among 69% of these physicians was dependent on patient cases. Most physicians supported policies encouraging biosimilar use and believed that biosimilars provided better access and resulted in lower costs. However, 16% thought these drugs carry a higher risk of side effects or are less effective [72]. In another study, 65% of surveyed health care providers felt that they were not well informed about biosimilars [73]. In Jordan, a survey among pharmacists highlighted the presence of adequate knowledge about the concept of biosimilars [73]. In Iraq, a major problem for biosimilar introduction was the lack of guidelines on the uptake. However, the implementation of "Basis and Guidelines for the Registration of Proposed Biosimilars in Iraq" in 2019 improved biosimilar uptake. Barriers included a lack of healthcare provider awareness of biosimilars [74]. In the hematology and oncology setting in the UAE, the conversion rate of some biologics to biosimilars in certain facilities reached almost 80% in 2022 (personal communication).

25.3.4 Barriers to Biosimilar Adoption

Published literature on barriers to the adoption of biosimilars among rheumatologists is scarce. A study in Saudi Arabia showed that the most common barriers were lack of availability of long-term data (79%), absence of national treatment guidelines recommending biosimilars (54.5%), inadequate safety or efficacy profile (45.5%), uncertainties related to similarity to the original molecule (38.5%), and absence of local data (38.5%). Other barriers included doubts in the product manufacturers, limited cost savings, and the absence of a need for biosimilars [70].

Outside rheumatology, a few publications highlighted barriers in Arab countries. Studies from Tunisia and Iraq stressed the importance of healthcare providers' awareness [72–74]. In addition to educational activities, an effort is highly needed to resolve uncertainties about safety and/or efficacy [72]. In addition, a regulation for biosimilars was a previous barrier in Iraq and a current barrier in Tunisia [72, 74]. Additional efforts targeting healthcare providers are needed to enhance knowledge and awareness about biosimilars [75].

Other barriers highlighted in international studies included switching stable patients, extrapolation of efficacy and safety without clinical trial data, doubts about quality and manufacturing processes, immunogenicity, and patient perception [76–79]. In addition, decentralization of decisions, lack of incentives, and limited involvement of healthcare professionals are considerable barriers [78].

25.3.5 Suggested Recommendations to Adopt Biosimilars

Based on literature evaluation and the author's experience, we recommend the following actions to enhance adoption and switch to biosimilars [76–79]:

(A) *At a National Level*

1. Establish national guidelines for the registration of biosimilars.
2. Establish national disease management guidelines and policies to promote the use of biosimilars in rheumatic diseases.
3. Promote collaboration among manufacturers, decision-makers, insurance companies, hospital leaders, and healthcare provider champions to support the use of biosimilars (i.e., regulations, incentives, and sharing of other countries' experiences).
4. Establish disease registries to capture real-world data on biosimilar experience within Arab countries.
5. Implement the utilization of health technology assessment (HTA) to answer ambiguity related to the extrapolation of biosimilar indications.

(B) *At the Level of Decision-Makers*

1. Involve all key stakeholders in the decision-making process (e.g., administration, physicians, pharmacists, supply chain, health economists, nurses, etc.).
2. Understand the concerns of healthcare providers to implement targeted improvement strategies.
3. Establish robust policies, protocols, or guidelines for handling biosimilars and automatic substitution under a Pharmacy and Therapeutics Committee or equivalent.
4. Thoroughly discuss decisions for extrapolation of indications and switching (e.g., in rheumatology, consider initiating biosimilars on treatment-naïve patients as a start) and restrict prescribing and dispensing accordingly by pharmacy and therapeutics or equivalent committees.
5. Avoid the introduction of multiple biosimilars for the same originator product within the same institution. This may negatively impact pharmacovigilance tracking.
6. Ensure consistency of supply through the manufacturer and supply chain to avoid multiple switches within the same year.
7. Establish a structured team led by physicians and pharmacists to provide periodic educational activities to all healthcare providers on biosimilars, including published real-world evidence.
8. Prepare educational material for patients to enhance communication.
9. Establish a strategy to incentivize adherent healthcare providers.
10. Update the electronic prescribing system (e.g., order sentences, label information, and barcode). When the originator and the biosimilar are available, adding the brand name to order sentences is suggested.

(C) *Ongoing Monitoring of Biosimilars*

1. Obtain inquiries and feedback from end-users within the first few months to optimize targeted educational activities for healthcare providers and patients.

2. Request a prospective medication utilization evaluation (MUE), especially for first-time biosimilars, and discuss results to capture low utilization, cost savings, and any safety concerns if needed.
3. Enrich local data through collaboration between health economists and healthcare providers in generating real-world evidence.
4. Promote reporting of encountered adverse drug events and product manufacturing quality issues to regulatory authorities.
5. Conduct periodic webinars through regulatory authorities and pharmacovigilance centers at hospitals to share results and receive inquiries.

25.3.6 Traceability and Pharmacovigilance

Biosimilars are handled as biological products and carry immunogenicity risks, which may lead to therapy failure or the development of adverse drug reactions [80, 81]. Special consideration should be given to ensure appropriate tracking for these products. In addition, safety concerns may arise due to incomplete nomenclature, and therefore, using the brand name is highly recommended. In many Arab countries, policies governing post-commercialization pharmacovigilance measures exist. However, supply and usage monitoring are not adequately regulated [82]. Studies on the pharmacovigilance of biosimilars are very scarce. A published abstract from Saudi Arabia assessed the traceability of insulin glargine and its biosimilar products. Authors found that 47.3% of spontaneously reported adverse reactions lack the batch number and 2.7% of reports lack the brand name [83].

25.3.7 Economic Evaluation and Real-World Evidence

Collaboration between health economists and healthcare providers to generate local real-world evidence within Arab countries is growing. In patients with rheumatic diseases, a single budget impact analysis of switching originator rituximab to a biosimilar product was identified. The total projected cost saving from switching patients with RA for the 13 included Arab countries was more than seven million (−1,040,000–180,000 per country) [84]. However, more studies provided real-world data for biosimilars used in oncology and diabetes (e.g., rituximab, filgrastim, and insulin) [85–87].

25.4 Conclusion

Efforts to establish a coherent healthcare ecosystem that nurtures value-based and evidence-based therapies for rheumatic diseases are maturing in Arab countries. Future collaborations at national and regional levels are the way forward to support building health economic data and real-world evidence that drives informed, cost-effective clinical decision-making forward.

Conflicts of Interest The authors have no conflicts of interest to declare.

Disclaimer The views expressed in this chapter are those of the authors.

References

1. Kozma CM, Reeder CE, Schulz RM. Economic, clinical, and humanistic outcomes: a planning model for pharmacoeconomic research. Clin Ther. 1993;15:1121–32. discussion 1120
2. Wong JB. Chapter 3: Principles of health economics and application to rheumatic disorders. In: Hochberg MC, Silman AJ, Smolen JS, et al., editors. Rheumatology. 6th ed. Philadelphia: Mosby. p. 20–6.
3. Meltzer MI. Introduction to health economics for physicians. Lancet. 2001;358:993–8.
4. Schünemann HJ, Reinap M, Piggott T, et al. The ecosystem of health decision making: from fragmentation to synergy. Lancet Public Health. 2022;7:e378–90.
5. Fasseeh A, Karam R, Jameleddine M, et al. Implementation of health technology assessment in the Middle East and North Africa: comparison between the current and preferred status. Front Pharmacol. 2020;11:15.
6. Fens T, van Puijenbroek EP, Postma MJ. Efficacy, Safety, and economics of innovative medicines: the role of multi-criteria decision analysis and managed entry agreements in practice and policy. Front Med Technol. 2021;3:629750. https://doi.org/10.3389/fmedt.2021.629750.
7. Fautrel B, Guillemin F. Cost of illness studies in rheumatic diseases. Curr Opin Rheumatol. 2002;14:121–6.
8. Hsieh P-H, Wu O, Geue C, et al. Economic burden of rheumatoid arthritis: a systematic review of literature in biologic era. Ann Rheum Dis. 2020;79:771–7.
9. Huscher D, Merkesdal S, Thiele K, et al. Cost of illness in rheumatoid arthritis, ankylosing spondylitis, psoriatic arthritis and systemic lupus erythematosus in Germany. Ann Rheum Dis. 2006;65:1175–83.
10. Yelin E. Chapter 32: Economic burden of rheumatic diseases. In: Firestein GS, Budd RC, Gabriel SE, et al., editors. Kelley and Firestein's textbook of rheumatology. 6th ed. Elsevier; 2017. p. 486–95.
11. van den Akker-van Marle ME, Chorus AMJ, Vliet Vlieland TPM, et al. Cost of rheumatic disorders in The Netherlands. Best Pract Res Clin Rheumatol. 2012;26:721–31.
12. Kobelt G. Thoughts on health economics in rheumatoid arthritis. Ann Rheum Dis. 2007;66:iii35–9.
13. Alghamdi A, Alsaif K, Alsahli M, et al. PMS14 economic burden of rheumatoid arthritis in Saudi Arabia: a single-center cost of illness study. Value Health. 2020;23:S594.
14. Berger A, Bozic K, Stacey B, et al. Patterns of pharmacotherapy and health care utilization and costs prior to total hip or total knee replacement in patients with osteoarthritis. Arthritis Rheum. 2011;63:2268–75.

15. White AG, Birnbaum HG, Janagap C, et al. Direct and indirect costs of pain therapy for osteoarthritis in an insured population in the United States. J Occup Environ Med. 2008;50:998–1005.
16. Walsh JA, Song X, Kim G, et al. Healthcare utilization and direct costs in patients with ankylosing spondylitis using a large US administrative claims database. Rheumatol Ther. 2018;5:463–74.
17. Gleason PP, Alexander GC, Starner CI, et al. Health plan utilization and costs of specialty drugs within 4 chronic conditions. J Manag Care Pharm JMCP. 2013;19:542–8.
18. Nurmohamed MT, Dijkmans BAC. Efficacy, tolerability and cost effectiveness of disease-modifying antirheumatic drugs and biologic agents in rheumatoid arthritis. Drugs. 2005;65:661–94.
19. Hresko A, Lin J, Solomon DH. Medical care costs associated with rheumatoid arthritis in the US: a systematic literature review and meta-analysis. Arthritis Care Res. 2018;70:1431–8.
20. Wailoo A, Hock ES, Stevenson M, et al. The clinical effectiveness and cost-effectiveness of treat-to-target strategies in rheumatoid arthritis: a systematic review and cost-effectiveness analysis. Health Technol Assess Winch Engl. 2017;21:1–258.
21. Hopkins AM, Proudman SM, Vitry AI, et al. Ten years of publicly funded biological disease-modifying antirheumatic drugs in Australia. Med J Aust. 2016;204:64–8.
22. Yazdany J, Dudley RA, Chen R, et al. Coverage for high-cost specialty drugs for rheumatoid arthritis in medicare Part D. Arthritis Rheumatol (Hoboken NJ). 2015;67 https://doi.org/10.1002/art.39079.
23. Westhovens R, Annemans L. Costs of drugs for treatment of rheumatic diseases. RMD Open. 2016;2:e000259.
24. Kobelt G, Woronoff A-S, Richard B, et al. Disease status, costs and quality of life of patients with rheumatoid arthritis in France: the ECO-PR study. Joint Bone Spine. 2008;75:408–15.
25. Rheumatoid arthritis drug costs nearly doubled in 5 years [Internet]. GoodRx; 2019. [cited 2026 Jun 17]. Available from: https://www.goodrx.com/conditions/rheumatoid-arthritis/rheumatoid-arthritis-drug-prices-nearly-doubled-in-5-years.
26. Curtis JR, Fox KM, Xie F, et al. The economic benefit of remission for patients with rheumatoid arthritis. Rheumatol Ther. 2022;9(5):1329–45. https://doi.org/10.1007/s40744-022-00473-6. Epub 2022 Jul 14
27. England BR, Tiong BK, Bergman MJ, et al. 2019 Update of the American College of Rheumatology Recommended Rheumatoid Arthritis Disease Activity Measures. Arthritis Care Res. 2019;71:1540–55.
28. Bergman M, Zhou L, Patel P, et al. Healthcare costs of not achieving remission in patients with rheumatoid arthritis in the United States: a retrospective cohort study. Adv Ther. 2021;38:2558–70.
29. DiPiro J, Yee G, Posey LM, et al. Pharmacotherapy: a pathophysiologic approach, eleventh edition. 11th ed. New York: McGraw Hill/Medical; 2020.
30. Fraenkel L, Bathon JM, England BR, et al. 2021 American College of Rheumatology Guideline for the treatment of rheumatoid arthritis. Arthritis Rheumatol. 2021;73:1108–23.
31. Smolen JS, Landewé RBM, Bijlsma JWJ, et al. EULAR recommendations for the management of rheumatoid arthritis with synthetic and biological disease-modifying antirheumatic drugs: 2019 update. Ann Rheum Dis. 2020;79:685–99.
32. Regel A, Sepriano A, Baraliakos X, et al. Efficacy and safety of non-pharmacological and non-biological pharmacological treatment: a systematic literature review informing the 2016 update of the ASAS/EULAR recommendations for the management of axial spondyloarthritis. RMD Open. 2017;3:e000397.
33. Ward MM, Deodhar A, Gensler LS, et al. 2019 Update of the American College of Rheumatology/Spondylitis Association of America/Spondyloarthritis Research and Treatment Network Recommendations for the Treatment of Ankylosing Spondylitis and Nonradiographic Axial Spondyloarthritis. Arthritis Rheumatol Hoboken NJ. 2019;71:1599–613.

34. Gossec L, Baraliakos X, Kerschbaumer A, et al. EULAR recommendations for the management of psoriatic arthritis with pharmacological therapies: 2019 update. Ann Rheum Dis. 2020;79:700–12.
35. Singh JA, Guyatt G, Ogdie A, et al. 2018 American College of Rheumatology/National Psoriasis Foundation Guideline for the Treatment of Psoriatic Arthritis. Arthritis Rheumatol. 2019;71:5–32.
36. Onel KB, Horton DB, Lovell DJ, et al. 2021 American College of Rheumatology Guideline for the treatment of juvenile idiopathic arthritis: recommendations for nonpharmacologic therapies, medication monitoring, immunizations, and imaging. Arthritis Care Res. 2022;74:505–20.
37. Heald A, Bramham-Jones S, Davies M. Comparing cost of intravenous infusion and subcutaneous biologics in COVID-19 pandemic care pathways for rheumatoid arthritis and inflammatory bowel disease: a brief UK stakeholder survey. Int J Clin Pract. 2021;75:e14341.
38. Dalén J, Luttropp K, Svedbom A, et al. Healthcare-related costs associated with switching subcutaneous tumor necrosis factor-α inhibitor in the treatment of inflammatory arthritis: a retrospective study. Adv Ther. 2020;37:3746–60.
39. Ji X, Wang Y, Ma Y, et al. Improvement of disease management and cost effectiveness in Chinese patients with ankylosing spondylitis using a smart-phone management system: a prospective cohort study. Biomed Res Int. 2019;2019:2171475.
40. Sloan M, Lever E, Harwood R, et al. Telemedicine in rheumatology: a mixed methods study exploring acceptability, preferences and experiences among patients and clinicians. Rheumatology. 2022;61:2262–74.
41. Chock EY, Putman M, Conway R, et al. Experience with telemedicine among rheumatology clinicians during the COVID-19 pandemic: an international survey. Rheumatol Adv Pract. 2022;6:rkac039.
42. Cuomo G, Masini F, Gjeloshi K, et al. Ab0905-Hpr telemedicine in rheumatology at time of Covid pandemic. Ann Rheum Dis. 2021;80:1475.
43. Tang W, Inzerillo S, Weiner J, et al. The impact of telemedicine on rheumatology care. Front Med (Lausanne). 2022;9:876835. https://doi.org/10.3389/fmed.2022.876835.
44. Ziade N, Hmamouchi I, el Kibbi L, et al. Telehealth in rheumatology: the 2021 Arab league of rheumatology best practice guidelines. Rheumatol Int. 2022;42:379–90.
45. Curtis JR, Schabert VF, Harrison DJ, et al. Estimating effectiveness and cost of biologics for rheumatoid arthritis: application of a validated algorithm to commercial insurance claims. Clin Ther. 2014;36:996–1004.
46. Curtis JR, Chastek B, Becker L, et al. Cost and effectiveness of biologics for rheumatoid arthritis in a commercially insured population. J Manag Care Spec Pharm. 2015;21:318–29.
47. Eriksson JK, Karlsson JA, Bratt J, et al. Cost-effectiveness of infliximab versus conventional combination treatment in methotrexate-refractory early rheumatoid arthritis: 2-year results of the register-enriched randomised controlled SWEFOT trial. Ann Rheum Dis. 2015;74:1094–101.
48. Joensuu JT, Huoponen S, Aaltonen KJ, et al. The cost-effectiveness of biologics for the treatment of rheumatoid arthritis: a systematic review. PLoS One. 2015;10:e0119683.
49. Kvamme MK, Lie E, Uhlig T, et al. Cost-effectiveness of TNF inhibitors vs synthetic disease-modifying antirheumatic drugs in patients with rheumatoid arthritis: a Markov model study based on two longitudinal observational studies. Rheumatology (Oxford). 2015;54:1226–35.
50. van der Velde G, Pham B, Machado M, et al. Cost-effectiveness of biologic response modifiers compared to disease-modifying antirheumatic drugs for rheumatoid arthritis: a systematic review. Arthritis Care Res. 2011;63:65–78.
51. Navarro F, Martinez-Sesmero JM, Balsa A, et al. Cost-effectiveness analysis of treatment sequences containing tofacitinib for the treatment of rheumatoid arthritis in Spain. Clin Rheumatol. 2020;39:2919–30.

52. Shi Z-C, Fei H-P, Wang Z-L. Cost-effectiveness analysis of etanercept plus methotrexate vs triple therapy in treating Chinese rheumatoid arthritis patients. Medicine (Baltimore). 2020;99:e16635.
53. Codreanu C, Mogoşan C, Popescu C, et al. Analysis of the indirect costs of rheumatoid arthritis in Romania. Biomed Res Int. 2019;2019:9343812.
54. Woo J, Lau E, Lau CS, et al. Socioeconomic impact of osteoarthritis in Hong Kong: utilization of health and social services, and direct and indirect costs. Arthritis Rheum. 2003;49:526–34.
55. Gupta S, Hawker GA, Laporte A, et al. The economic burden of disabling hip and knee osteoarthritis (OA) from the perspective of individuals living with this condition. Rheumatology. 2005;44:1531–7.
56. Puig-Junoy J, Ruiz ZA. Socio-economic costs of osteoarthritis: a systematic review of cost-of-illness studies. Semin Arthritis Rheum. 2015;44:531–41.
57. Goetzel RZ, Long SR, Ozminkowski RJ, et al. Health, absence, disability, and Presenteeism cost estimates of certain physical and mental health conditions affecting U.S. employers. J Occup Environ Med. 2004;46:398–412.
58. Søgaard R, Sørensen J, Linde L, et al. The significance of presenteeism for the value of lost production: the case of rheumatoid arthritis. Clin Outcomes Res CEOR. 2010;2:105–12.
59. Sruamsiri R, Mahlich J, Tanaka E, et al. Productivity loss of Japanese patients with rheumatoid arthritis - a cross-sectional survey. Mod Rheumatol. 2018;28:482–9.
60. Ziegelbauer K, Kostev K, Hübinger M, et al. The impact of non-persistence on the direct and indirect costs in patients treated with subcutaneous tumour necrosis factor-alpha inhibitors in Germany. Rheumatol Oxf Engl. 2018;57:1276–81.
61. European Medicines Agency. Biosimilar medicines: overview [Internet]. [cited 2026 Jun 17]. Available from: https://www.ema.europa.eu/en/human-regulatory-overview/biosimilar-medicines-overview.
62. US Food and Drug Administration. Biological product definitions [Internet]. [cited 2026 Jun 17]. Available from: https://www.fda.gov/files/drugs/published/Biological-Product-Definitions.pdf.
63. US Food and Drug Administration. Biosimilars info sheet level 1: foundational concepts [Internet]. Silver Spring: US Food and Drug Administration; 2022. [cited 2026 Jun 17]. Available from: https://www.fda.gov/media/154911/download.
64. US Food and Drug Administration. Center for Drug Evaluation and Research. Purple book: lists of licensed biological products with reference product exclusivity and biosimilarity or interchangeability evaluations [Internet]. Silver Spring: US Food and Drug Administration; 2020. [cited 2026 Jun 17]. Available from: https://www.fda.gov/drugs/therapeutic-biologics-applications-bla/purple-book-lists-licensed-biological-products-reference-product-exclusivity-and-biosimilarity-or.
65. Mulcahy AW, Predmore Z, Mattke S. The cost savings potential of biosimilar drugs in the United States [Internet]. Santa Monica: RAND Corporation; 2014. [cited 2026 Jun 17]. Available from: https://www.rand.org/pubs/perspectives/PE127.html.
66. U.S. Food and Drug Administration. Biosimilar and interchangeable biologics: more treatment choices [Internet]. 2023. [cited 2026 Jun 17]. Available from: https://www.fda.gov/consumers/consumer-updates/biosimilar-and-interchangeable-biologics-more-treatment-choices.
67. US Food and Drug Administration. Biologic product definitions [Internet]. [cited 2026 Jun 17]. Available from: https://www.accessdata.fda.gov/drugsatfda_docs/nda/2022/761165Orig1s000MultidisciplineR.pdf.
68. European Medicines Agency. Biosimilar medicines can be interchanged [Internet]. 2022. [cited 2026 Jun 17]. Available from: https://www.ema.europa.eu/en/news/biosimilar-medicines-can-be-interchanged.

69. European Medicines Agency. Biosimilars in the EU: Information guide for healthcare professionals [Internet]. 2019. [cited 2026 Jun 17]. Available from: https://www.ema.europa.eu/en/documents/leaflet/biosimilars-eu-information-guide-healthcare-professionals_en.pdf.
70. Omair MA, Almadany R, Omair MA, et al. Perception of biosimilar biologics and non-medical prescription switching among rheumatologists: a Saudi Society for Rheumatology Initiative. Saudi Pharm J. 2022;30:39–44.
71. Mysler E, Azevedo VF, Danese S, et al. Biosimilar-to-biosimilar switching: what is the rationale and current experience? Drugs. 2021;81:1859–79.
72. Hadoussa S, Bouhlel M, Soussi MA, et al. Perception of hematologists and oncologists about the biosimilars: a prospective Tunisian study based on a survey. J Oncol Pharm Pract. 2020;26:124–32.
73. Mhiri A, Khemakhem M, Kalboussi N, et al. Knowledge and perceptions of biosimilar medicines by health professionals in Tunisia. Ann Pharm Fr. 2022;80:327–39.
74. Al-Kinani KK, Ibrahim MJ, Al-Zubaidi RF, et al. Iraqi regulatory authority current system and experience with biosimilars. Regul Toxicol Pharmacol. 2020;117:104768.
75. Sarnola K, Merikoski M, Jyrkkä J, et al. Physicians' perceptions of the uptake of biosimilars: a systematic review. BMJ Open. 2020;10:e034183.
76. Demirkan FG, Sönmez HE, Lamot L, et al. Embracing change: an international survey study on the beliefs and attitudes of pediatric rheumatologists towards Biosimilars. BioDrugs Clin Immunother Biopharm Gene Ther. 2022;36:421–30.
77. Aragon Cuevas O, Hedrich CM. Biosimilars in pediatric rheumatology and their introduction into routine care. Clin Immunol Orlando Fla. 2020;216:108447.
78. Edgar BS, Cheifetz AS, Helfgott SM, et al. Overcoming barriers to biosimilar adoption: real-world perspectives from a national payer and provider initiative. J Manag Care Spec Pharm. 2021;27:1129–35.
79. Lobo F, Río-Álvarez I. Barriers to biosimilar prescribing incentives in the context of clinical governance in Spain. Pharm Basel Switz. 2021;14:283.
80. Francescon S, Fornasier G, Baldo P. Biosimilar oncology drugs in Europe: regulatory and pharmacovigilance considerations. Oncol Ther. 2016;4:173–82. https://doi.org/10.1007/s40487-016-0028-9.
81. European Commission. What you need to know about biosimilar medicinal products: a consensus information document. Brussels: European Commission; 2013. [cited 2026 Jun 17]. Available from: https://ec.europa.eu/docsroom/documents/8242.
82. Alnaqbi KA, Barquin P, Bellanger A, Brill A, Castañeda Hernández G, Clopés Estela A, Delgado Sánchez O, García Alfonso P, Gyger P, Heinrich D, Hezard G, Kakehasi A, Koehn C, Mariotte O, Pérez Tapia SM, Pistollato M, Mennini F, Ross-Stewart K, Saada R, Sasaki T, Simoens S, Tambassis G, Thill M, Werutsky G, Wilsdon T. Biosimilars: A global roadmap for policy sustainability. 2022. [cited 2026 Jun 17]. Available from: https://biosimilarsroadmap.com.
83. Alrubaish F, Alhawas S, Alnuaim A, Alfadel N. Traceability of insulin glargine innovator and its biosimilar products' adverse drug event reports in Saudi Arabia (abstract). International Society for Pharmacoepidemiology (ISPE) Annual Meeting; 2022 Aug 24–28; Copenhagen, Denmark.
84. Almaaytah A. Budget impact analysis of switching to rituximab's biosimilar in rheumatology and cancer in 13 countries within the Middle East and North Africa. Clinicoecon Outcomes Res. 2020;12:527–34. https://doi.org/10.2147/CEOR.S265041.

85. Alwan AF, Abdulsahib MA, Abbas DD, Abdulsattar SA, Ensaif RT. Efficacy and safety of biosimilar rituximab (ZytuxTM) in newly diagnosed patients with non-Hodgkin lymphoma and chronic lymphocytic leukemia. Hematol Rep. 2020;12(3):8296. https://doi.org/10.4081/hr.2020.8296.
86. Al-Rabayah AA, Al Mashni O, Hanoun E, et al. Effectiveness and safety of Filgrastim (Neupogen™) versus Filgrastim-aafi (Nivestim™) in primary prophylaxis of chemotherapy-induced febrile neutropenia: an observational cohort study. Drugs Real World Outcomes. 2022;9(4):589–95. https://doi.org/10.1007/s40801-022-00312-8.
87. AlRuthia Y, Bahari OH, Alghnam S, et al. Real-world impact of switching from insulin glargine (Lantus®) to Basaglar® and potential cost saving in a large public healthcare system in Saudi Arabia. Front Public Health. 2022;10:852721. https://doi.org/10.3389/fpubh.2022.852721.

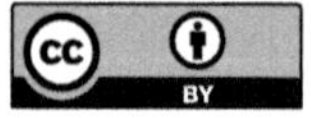

Chapter 26
Perspectives of Arab Patients on Rheumatic Diseases

Shaimaa Alasfour, Nida Abul, and Khalid A. Alnaqbi

Abstract Rheumatic diseases (RDs) present a substantial health challenge in the Arab world, affecting millions of individuals and families across the region. RDs impact patients physically, psychologically, socially, and financially, similar to their counterparts worldwide, despite cultural differences that may influence disease activity and prognosis.

Addressing the unique unmet needs of RD patients in the Arab world is crucial. Some patient-initiated advocacy groups aim to raise public awareness and promote patient education. Enhanced public awareness efforts are needed to support Arab patients living with RDs, while rheumatologists should strive to better understand and evaluate the impact of RDs on patients' overall quality of life. This chapter explores the perspective of Arab patients living with RDs toward their illness.

Keywords Arab patients · Rheumatic diseases · Rheumatic and musculoskeletal diseases · Patient perspectives · Quality of life · Patient-reported outcomes · Medication adherence · Health literacy · Cultural beliefs · Patient advocacy

26.1 Introduction

Rheumatic diseases (RDs) represent a major public health challenge across the Arab world, with prevalence rates varying between countries and influenced by economic, cultural, and socioeconomic factors. This chapter aims to explore the perspectives of patients living with RDs in the Arab region through a review of the

S. Alasfour (✉) · N. Abul
Kuwait Lupus Group, Kuwait City, Kuwait
e-mail: drshaimaa00@gmail.com; nida1045@gmail.com

K. A. Alnaqbi (✉)
Rheumatology Division, Sheikh Tahnoon bin Mohammed Medical City, SEHA/ PureHealth, Al Ain, UAE

College of Medicine and Health Sciences, UAE University, Al Ain, UAE
e-mail: kalnaqbi@seha.ae

K. A. Alnaqbi, G. Aldabie (eds.), *Rheumatic Diseases in the Arab World*,
https://doi.org/10.1007/978-981-92-0967-5_26

existing literature. Given the limited availability of epidemiological data on rheumatic diseases in Arab countries, this exploration is both timely and relevant.

Beyond addressing prevalence, the chapter examines the impact of RDs on patients' quality of life (QOL), their knowledge and beliefs about disease management, and their unmet needs within healthcare systems. It also highlights the growing role of patient advocacy groups across the region that provide education, psychosocial support, and community engagement. By presenting these insights, the chapter seeks to enhance rheumatologists' understanding of their patients' experiences and expectations, thereby facilitating more effective communication, shared decision-making, and patient-centered care in the Arab region.

26.2 Impact of Rheumatic Diseases on Arab Patients

RDs, like any chronic illness, impact patients' QOL, which encompasses diverse aspects of an individual's life, ranging from physical well-being and financial stability to their ability to manage life challenges and engage in social activities or networks [1, 2]. These aspects can be broadly categorized as physical, psychological, social, and financial.

Chronic systemic autoimmune disorders, such as rheumatoid arthritis (RA) or systemic lupus erythematosus (SLE), are characterized by articular and extra-articular manifestations, affecting various organs and increasing mortality and morbidity rates among patients [3, 4].

26.2.1 Pain and Limitations of Physical Function

High disease activity, often manifested as pain in most rheumatic diseases, can significantly impair physical function. For example, recent studies have highlighted limitations in physical activity among RA patients due to pain or disability. In a Moroccan study involving married women, RA was associated with a divorce rate of 10%. Additionally, 67% of patients reported sexual problems, and many Moroccan women with RA encountered challenges in carrying out household tasks. These women also experienced limitations in participating in social activities, such as attending weddings and funerals [5]. Furthermore, an observational study conducted in Lebanon on RA patients demonstrated that RA was linked to decreased physical and mental abilities, as well as lower overall QOL [6].

Studies have shown that patients with RA in different countries report varying levels of pain, fatigue, and disability, which are not always aligned with clinical measures of disease severity. Recognizing these cultural differences is key to understanding how RA affects patients' daily lives and their interactions with healthcare providers in the Arab world [7, 8].

Moreover, multiple factors contribute to a decline in the QOL of patients with RA. These factors include advanced age, unemployment, limited educational attainment, increased joint pain, prolonged osteoarthritis, and other health issues, as observed in a study from Palestine [9].

In gout, the severity of pain resulting from attacks can impede patients' ability to concentrate and perform tasks efficiently. The frequency with which a patient's diet triggers gout attacks can also impact their capacity to work and engage in physical activities. Furthermore, the nature of a patient's occupation can influence their productivity, particularly if it involves physical exertion that may be hindered by gout. Additionally, age is a determining factor as it can affect a patient's overall vitality and their ability to recuperate from gout attacks [10].

In SLE, a study by Robinson and colleagues showed that recurrent lupus flares, measured by frequent hospitalizations and visits to the emergency department, were associated with reduced productivity and impaired activity [3].

In psoriatic arthritis (PsA), Egyptian patients experiencing enthesitis in both upper and lower regions report worsened QOL and increased work impairment. Enthesitis can cause discomfort, pain, and limited mobility, affecting daily activities and overall well-being. This adverse impact on QOL may be due to enthesitis' persistent nature and its association with other PsA symptoms like joint pain, fatigue, and skin manifestations [11].

26.2.2 *Fatigue in Rheumatic Diseases*

Fatigue is a commonly reported complaint in patients with RDs. Patients often describe fatigue as feeling worn out, tired, exhausted, slow-moving, less energetic, struggling to concentrate, and feeling sleepy. Patients feel a profound fatigue in their bodies, making all tasks appear challenging to accomplish. They experience an overwhelming sensation of physical exhaustion that may even necessitate assistance with minor movements [12].

Severe fatigue, disrupted sleep, and depression are frequently observed in RA patients. This was recently found in an Egyptian study, implying that fatigue may not only be attributed to RA activity but could also arise from a combination of factors, including depression and sleep disturbances [13].

The prevalence of persistent fatigue is high among individuals with RD. Approximately 66% of Moroccan patients with ankylosing spondylitis (AS) reported severe fatigue [14]. Similarly, up to 44% of Saudi patients with primary Sjögren's syndrome had a positive fatigue score based on the Fatigue Severity Scale [15].

Fatigue has a significant impact on women, both mentally and physically. However, the description of fatigue can vary depending on cultural influences, including the patient's religion, country of residence, and cultural background. A study conducted among Egyptian patients revealed that they predominantly reported experiencing physical fatigue rather than mental fatigue, with a higher prevalence among women compared to men. Fatigue can have a significant impact on women's intimate lives and sexual function, prompting some to explore coping strategies such as suggesting their husbands remarry (a practice specific to Arabic and Islamic cultures) [12]. These findings highlight the multifaceted nature of fatigue and its impact on women in different cultural contexts. Strikingly, physical fatigue was more prevalent among patients from highly developed countries than those from less developed countries with lower incomes [16].

26.2.3 Mental Health Disorders in Rheumatic Diseases

RDs frequently impose a significant burden on mental well-being, with depression and anxiety commonly emerging as prevailing manifestations. Depression can manifest as low mood, low self-esteem, fatigue, insomnia, psychomotor dysfunction, recurrent negative thoughts, and difficulty concentrating. Patients with chronic autoimmune diseases, such as RA, are nearly twice as likely to suffer from depression compared to the general population [17]. In some cases, depression may even appear early in the disease course.

In Egyptian patients with early RA, depression and anxiety scores were significantly higher than in healthy controls, with approximately one-quarter (26.9%) meeting criteria for anxiety [18]. A cross-sectional study from the Kingdom of Saudi Arabia (KSA) reported depression in 16% of RA patients and anxiety in 23% [19]. Likewise, a large meta-analysis including 139,875 participants demonstrated a significantly elevated risk of anxiety among individuals with RA compared to those without the disease [20].

Mental health involvement is also substantial in SLE: around 25% of patients experience depression and 37% experience anxiety [21]. Depression in SLE correlates with disease duration, activity, and the extent of organ damage, contributing to considerable impairment in overall quality of life [22].

Beyond RA and SLE, studies from the Arab region reveal that patients with other RDs, such as psoriasis and RA, frequently exhibit comorbidities including metabolic syndrome, cardiovascular disease, and obesity, all of which are associated with a greater psychological burden, particularly depression and anxiety [23–25]. This highlights the complex bidirectional interaction between physical health and emotional well-being.

Mental disorders can interfere with treatment adherence [26] and impair coping with stress and pain, resulting in reduced function, social withdrawal, and greater emotional distress [27]. In Moroccan patients with AS, disease activity was the strongest predictor of fatigue, with psychological factors such as depression, anxiety, and sleep disturbance also contributing significantly [14]. Additionally, a cross-sectional study from Syria found that nearly half of AS patients exhibited clinically significant depressive symptoms, and over one-third had clinically significant anxiety [28].

The emotional challenges experienced by patients with PsA are equally profound. Many Arab patients report feelings of sadness, worry, isolation, and, in some cases, thoughts of self-harm due to the persistent impact of the disease. They often feel misunderstood or not taken seriously, even by healthcare professionals. Visible skin involvement may lead to embarrassment, self-consciousness, and social withdrawal, further worsening psychological distress. Many PsA patients also experience diminished self-esteem and perceive themselves as inferior to others, intensifying the emotional burden of the disease [29].

In summary, mental health disorders are prevalent in RD patients and can significantly impact their overall well-being and QOL. Understanding and addressing these challenges are essential for providing comprehensive care to individuals living with rheumatic diseases.

26.2.4 Financial Burden of Rheumatic Diseases

The economic and financial burden of RDs can be divided into direct costs (healthcare services) and indirect costs (productivity), which are influenced by the economic status of the country, total population, and personal income. In countries with high economic growth, such as the Gulf countries (e.g., Kuwait), citizens often benefit from free healthcare services and access to advanced treatments, including biological therapies [7]. In contrast, limited social welfare support, low socioeconomic status, and inadequate health insurance coverage further add to the financial burden of patients with RA, as reported in a Moroccan study [5].

Similarly, a recent survey of patients with psoriasis and PsA in Gulf countries found that those with plaque psoriasis and PsA incurred substantially higher out-of-pocket expenses across most cost categories—particularly for healthcare visits (USD 448 vs 173), nonprescription medications (USD 323 vs 154), makeup, and special clothing (USD 137 vs 52), and psychological counseling (USD 174 vs 60). Collectively, these findings emphasize the substantial economic burden that rheumatic and related diseases impose on patients across different socioeconomic settings [30].

26.2.5 Stigma

The stigma associated with RDs impacts patients' lives. RDs can affect patients' general appearance through different manifestations, such as joint deformities in RA and skin manifestations in scleroderma and PsA, making patients more susceptible to health-related stigma [31–34]. In a cross-sectional survey of patients with chronic RDs, higher levels of anticipatory stigma, particularly work-related stigma, were associated with poorer medication adherence, emphasizing how stigma can directly influence treatment behavior and outcomes [31]. Another study found that higher internalized stigma was significantly associated with lower self-esteem and suggested that stigma may impede treatment adherence and help-seeking behavior [32].

Stigma can be conceptualized in two forms: *public stigma* (behaviors and attitudes toward people with a stigmatized condition) [35] and *self-stigma* (the internalization of negative stereotypes leading to reduced self-esteem and self-efficacy) [36]. For example, a Saudi study of psoriatic patients found that the majority reported significant stigmatization; those with lower QOL reported higher levels of perceived stigma and poorer life satisfaction [37]. A global survey by the World Lupus Federation revealed that limited public awareness and widespread misconceptions contribute substantially to stigma and prejudice towards people living with SLE [38].

In a Gulf-region survey of patients with psoriasis and PsA, 73% reported experiencing stigma or discrimination. The most common experiences included being asked if they were contagious (40%), being stared at in public (22%), feeling that others did not understand the impact of the disease (29%), withdrawing from social activities (22%), self-isolation (19%), and fearing that others might refuse to shake their hand (17%) [30].

26.3 Impact of the COVID-19 Pandemic on Patients with Rheumatic Diseases

In response to the COVID-19 pandemic, the World Health Organization (WHO) declared a global public health emergency in March 2020 [39]. Individuals with RDs are particularly vulnerable to infections due to being immunocompromised, placing them at a higher risk compared to the general population [40]. A study conducted by the Arab Adult Arthritis Awareness (AAAA) group examined the impact of COVID-19 on Arab RD patients and highlighted the adverse effects on the continuity of their healthcare. Challenges accessing hospitals and clinics during lockdowns and the loss of income resulting from job losses were identified as significant obstacles [41]. Additionally, patients with RDs experienced a decline in their QOL compared to healthy individuals and an increased risk of mental health disorders. There was also a shortage of medications, especially hydroxychloroquine, as it was initially promoted as a potential treatment and prevention for COVID-19 [41, 42]. These findings emphasize the unique physical, psychological, and financial challenges faced by RD patients during the pandemic [43].

26.4 Knowledge and Awareness of Arab Patients About Rheumatic Diseases

Arab patients' attitudes and beliefs toward RDs are influenced by several factors, including age, educational level, socioeconomic status, and psychosocial factors. A persistent misconception is that all RDs fall under the umbrella term "rheumatism." Many patients mistakenly believe that these conditions should be managed by orthopedic specialists and view rheumatology and orthopedics as the same field of practice.

In KSA, a recent study from Jeddah demonstrated poor public knowledge about gout [44]. Similarly, a systematic review and meta-analysis of ten cross-sectional studies involving 6703 participants reported that 83.5% of the public had heard of osteoarthritis, 54.5% knew about RA, and 80.4% were familiar with gout. However, knowledge about disease causes, risk factors, and treatment options remained limited. The authors concluded that while general awareness of common arthritic conditions appears acceptable, significant gaps persist in detailed understanding, emphasizing the need for targeted educational initiatives [45].

In the Gulf countries, a recent survey of patients with psoriasis and PsA found that 63% were familiar with the term "psoriatic disease," with awareness highest among those affected by both conditions. Patients with both manifestations were also more aware of associated comorbidities than those with psoriasis alone, highlighting the value of patient education and disease-specific awareness programs [30].

In Iraq, a survey from the Kurdistan region revealed that 87.6% of respondents had limited knowledge about RDs. Greater awareness was significantly associated with a higher educational level, regular physical activity, and a family history of RDs. Notably, 53.3% were uncertain about the ineffectiveness of herbal remedies as stand-alone treatments, and 47.1% believed that orthopedic physicians were the main providers for RDs [46].

In Lebanon, a nationwide cross-sectional study found that most respondents lacked adequate information about RA and AS, with many incorrectly assuming that orthopedic surgeons were responsible for treating these conditions. These findings underscore the importance of national public awareness campaigns about RDs [47].

In Egypt, a large multicenter survey across four governorates reported limited public knowledge about common RDs—including RA, SLE, crystal-induced arthritis, and osteoarthritis. Higher awareness was positively correlated with female sex, higher educational attainment, marital status, urban residence, unemployment, and a family history of RDs [48].

26.5 Beliefs of Arab Patients About Rheumatic Diseases

Culture, education level, and awareness strongly influence patients' beliefs about the causes and treatment of RDs. Many patients associate RDs with a familial predisposition and believe that these conditions may remain hidden for some time [49]. Consequently, when contemplating marriage or starting a family, such inherited concerns can provoke significant anxiety and hesitation.

To explore these perceptions more systematically, the first and largest online survey specifically developed for Arab patients with RDs was conducted to assess their perspectives and experiences with these conditions [50]. It was constructed using a combination of validated methodologies, including clinimetric sensibility assessment, the Open-Source Metric for Measuring Arabic Narratives (OSMAN) to evaluate readability, and the Checklist for Reporting Internet E-Surveys (CHERRIES) to ensure methodological rigor. A total of 456 participants were included in the analysis, the majority of whom were female (81.4%) and aged 25–44 years (63.4%). The most commonly reported RDs were SLE, RA, and AS. Figure 26.1 summarizes the perceived causes of RDs, and patients' main concerns. The most frequently used sources of patient education were rheumatologists (83.6%), internet search engines (71.3%), and social media accounts of rheumatologists (63.6%). Other resources included patient support groups (41.7%), awareness events (22.4%), and research associations (22.4%), while 2.9% relied on other sources. About one-third (33.3%) reported believing in and using alternative medicine.

Beyond this regional survey, global and regional evidence further illustrates how patients' beliefs and fears shape their experience of rheumatic diseases. A recent systematic review on fears among RA patients found that beliefs strongly influenced psychological well-being, adherence to therapy, and coping patterns. The predominant fears centered on pharmacologic treatment and the prospect of disability [51].

Interestingly, these concerns are not limited to Arab populations. Many patients across cultures share magico-religious interpretations of their illnesses, viewing them as divine punishment for their sins or inappropriate behavior, or outcomes of witchcraft or the evil eye. Among Arab patients newly diagnosed with RDs, such beliefs often lead them to pursue nonmedical therapies, including consulting traditional healers, using herbal remedies, reading holy texts, or engaging in prayer [52].

Misconceptions about specific diseases are also common. For example, an Egyptian study found that 85.3% of participants believed that gout frequently causes heel pain, a misconception not consistent with clinical reality [53].

Medication-related beliefs also play a pivotal role in treatment adherence. Negative perceptions—such as doubts about medication efficacy or concerns about side effects—can lead to nonadherence, while positive beliefs, including trust in physicians and confidence in therapy, are associated with improved outcomes [54]. Cultural and social contexts further shape these beliefs, underscoring the importance of clear communication and patient education. Interventions aimed at

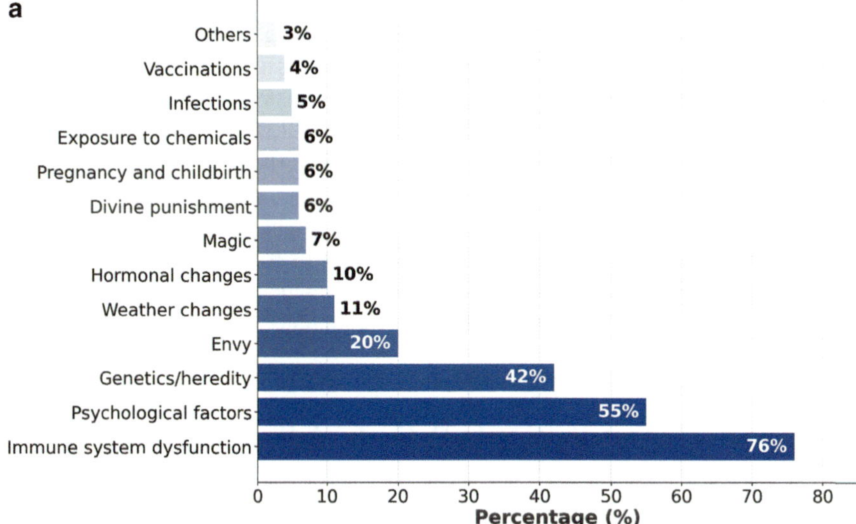

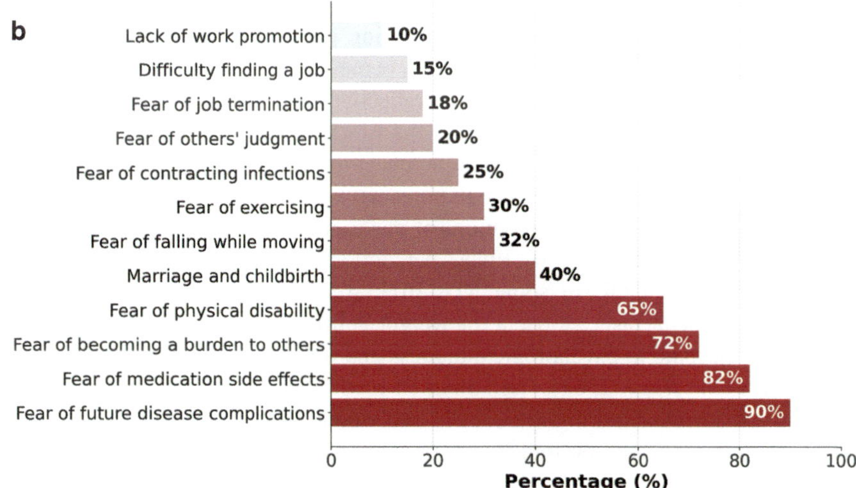

Fig. 26.1 (**a**) Perceived causes of rheumatic and musculoskeletal diseases from respondents' perspectives, and (**b**) Main concerns of patients with rheumatic diseases. (Adapted and reproduced from Alnaqbi et al. [50]. © Springer Nature 2025. Reproduced with permission)

addressing misconceptions and enhancing communication are likely to improve adherence and health outcomes.

Evidence from different populations with RDs presents a mixed picture of medication-related beliefs. Many patients with RDs expressed confidence in their prescribed medications' ability to maintain remission and improve QOL, although concerns about long-term adverse effects persisted [54]. Conversely, a Moroccan study reported that over one-third of patients with chronic inflammatory RDs believed that medication was not essential for maintaining health, with 51.3% citing long-term side effects as their main concern. Factors associated with these beliefs included lower educational level, methotrexate use, catastrophizing (the tendency to focus on worst-case outcomes), and trust in physicians [55].

In summary, misconceptions and fears regarding rheumatic diseases remain common, even among patients receiving care from a rheumatologist. A recent study among individuals with RA and spondyloarthritis highlighted the persistence of misconceptions and fears regarding the disease and its treatment, emphasizing the need for open, empathetic communication between patients and healthcare professionals to address misinformation and enhance adherence and outcomes [56].

26.6 Factors Contributing to Patients' Adherence and Satisfaction

Adherence, defined by the World Health Organization as the degree to which a person's behavior corresponds with the agreed treatment recommendations from a healthcare provider [57], is crucial for ensuring patient satisfaction. Conversely, treatment satisfaction describes how patients perceive their therapy as meeting their functional and QOL needs, based on their reflective assessment of treatment effects and care experience [58].

Several factors influence patients' adherence, including age, with older patients generally exhibiting better adherence than younger ones, as well as their beliefs and awareness about the disease, perceptions of treatment necessity, and concerns about potential adverse effects [59, 60]. Illness perceptions have also been shown to influence health-related QOL in some RDs [61]. Additionally, outward appearance changes (e.g., facial rash, alopecia, or weight gain) in patients with RDs such as SLE may contribute to psychological distress and treatment discontinuation due to body-image concerns [62, 63]. High doses of corticosteroids can lead to changes in body image, such as Cushingoid features and weight gain, which may cause emotional disturbances and prompt some patients to discontinue their medication [62, 63].

Poor adherence to treatment also carries a significant economic burden in terms of global healthcare costs and patients' QOL [64]. For example, in the United States, an estimated one-third to two-thirds of hospital admissions and hospitalizations are due to poor adherence to medications [65]. Additionally, the route of medication administration and the number of medications required influence patient adherence, with fewer medications prescribed correlating with better adherence. Biologics and new anti-rheumatic medications have shown higher rates of adherence, likely due to factors such as route of administration, scheduled dosing, and significant improvements in disease activity perceived by patients [66, 67]. On the other hand, despite the current advancements in the treatment of many RDs, the Arab region continues

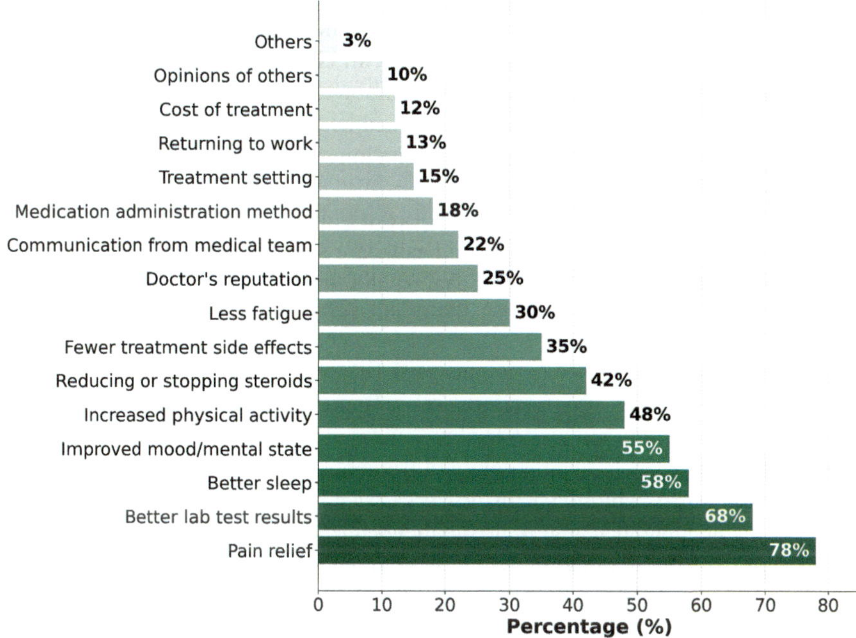

Fig. 26.2 Factors influencing satisfaction with treatment provided by rheumatologists (Adapted and reproduced from et al. [50]. © Springer Nature 2025. Reproduced with permission)

to have limited data regarding its prevalence and severity. This lack of understanding prevents patients from seeking timely and appropriate assistance. Many patients prefer oral over injectable medication options, and the emergence of novel oral targeted therapy holds the potential to alleviate these challenges for patients and care providers [68].

Furthermore, disease-related factors, such as disease duration and activity, functional disability, health-related QOL, and comorbidities like depression, obesity, and fibromyalgia, are associated with decreased patient satisfaction [69]. In addition, a large cross-sectional survey among Arab patients with RDs revealed the main factors that influence satisfaction with treatment (Fig. 26.2) [50]. A cross-sectional study conducted in Tunisia among RA patients identified predictive factors influencing treatment satisfaction. These factors included satisfaction with the attending physician, participation in treatment decisions, and the impact of RA [70]. Similarly, a study from Palestine on RA patients found a correlation between health-related QOL and treatment satisfaction [71].

26.7 Definition of Disease Flares by Arab Patients

Patients experience and describe flares differently depending on the type of RD, the nature of symptoms, and the flare's duration. Flares may last from a few days to several weeks, months, or even years [72].

In SLE, flares can present with nonspecific symptoms, such as hair loss or fever, that may mimic alternative diagnoses and therefore require careful evaluation [73]. In contrast, RA flares typically present with morning stiffness, increased joint pain, joint swelling, and limitations in daily functioning [72].

Medication-related behaviors are important contributors to disease exacerbations. In SLE, self-discontinuation or poor adherence to treatment has been associated with more severe flares, greater risk of organ damage, and increased hospitalization rates [74, 75]. Similarly, other studies have shown that dose reduction or stopping therapy remains a leading trigger of SLE flares [76].

Across different RDs, several common triggers have been identified, including psychological stress, emotional disturbances, sleep disruption, infections, inadequate treatment adherence, and limited patient education [74–79].

Findings from our regional survey of Arab patients further highlight how patients conceptualize flares. The most frequently cited descriptors of flare or relapse were joint pain (95.4%), limited mobility (87.9%), mood swings or irritability (80.9%), and joint swelling (73.5%). Additional features included fever (42.1%), absence from work (41.0%), skin rash (30.9%), and infections (29.8%). Patients also reported fatigue, morning stiffness, eye pain, difficulty concentrating, sleep disturbance, and headaches as part of their flare experience [50].

26.8 Healthcare Needs of Arab Patients with Rheumatic Diseases

Arab patients with RDs share many needs with patients globally, including early diagnosis, prevention of organ or joint damage, and improved QOL. However, these needs are influenced by various factors, both medical and related to the disease itself and nonmedical such as socioeconomic status and availability of a supportive healthcare system [80].

One significant challenge faced by Arab patients is delayed diagnosis, which can result from nonspecific initial symptoms. For example, a study conducted in KSA revealed delays of up to two years in diagnosing patients with RA [81]. In contrast, the diagnosis timeline in Morocco was approximately 20 weeks [82]. The level of public awareness is an essential factor impacting the needs of Arab patients. Insufficient knowledge about RDs among patients highlights the need for increased awareness campaigns [47]. This awareness can encourage patients to seek treatment from rheumatologists rather than other specialists and ensure better adherence to treatment plans. In addition, patients with an established diagnosis of RDs need to be aware of the chronic nature of their diseases. For example, some patients with RA discontinue their treatment when symptoms improve [80].

Furthermore, patients' emotional needs are often overlooked in Arab countries due to cultural stigma and limited clinic time. Many patients may feel ashamed to share their feelings, and healthcare providers may not have the opportunity to assess emotional well-being adequately [8, 83].

Additionally, female Arab patients may face unique challenges in choosing a rheumatologist, influenced by factors such as family pressure, cultural norms, and religious beliefs. This decision-making process is multifaceted and influenced by various factors, including professionalism, availability, waiting time, the physician's location, popularity, the physician's presence on social media and advertising practices, and the patient's economic status [84].

The healthcare system in Arab countries can directly and indirectly influence patients' needs in several ways, including accessibility (services, medications, tests), affordability, insurance coverage, quality of care, and health policy and governance.

For instance, there is a shortage of rheumatologists in Arab countries, with an estimated 0.84 rheumatologists per 100,000 inhabitants [85]. This scarcity contributes to delays in diagnosis and treatment, with waiting times for initial visits sometimes exceeding three months. Additionally, in Egypt, heavy reliance on the private healthcare sector increases the financial burden on patients, leading to challenges in affording medications and follow-up care [86].

In many Arab countries, limited rheumatology expertise among nonspecialist providers and restricted access to specialist care, particularly outside major urban centers, contribute to substantial unmet needs in the management of RDs [80, 82]. In addition, the economic and political stability of the country plays a significant role in meeting patients' needs. In countries affected by war and conflict, government priorities often focus on these crises rather than addressing the needs of patients with RDs or even those with illnesses affecting a large portion of the population, such as diabetes mellitus. Conversely, wealthier countries typically have excellent healthcare systems, providing medications and services, along with offering options like early medical retirement with full salary or reduced working hours for patients.

In conclusion, addressing the healthcare needs of Arab patients with RDs requires a multifaceted approach that considers cultural, socioeconomic, and healthcare system factors. By improving awareness, prioritizing RDs similar to other noncommunicable diseases in healthcare policies, increasing access to rheumatologists, and addressing emotional needs, healthcare systems can better meet the diverse needs of patients in the Arab region.

26.9 Patient Advocacy Groups in the Arab World

A patient support group includes individuals sharing similar life experiences and concerns about specific conditions. Support groups serve a variety of purposes, including educating patients and their family members, allowing sharing of illness experiences, providing support and strength to members, raising public awareness, fundraising [87], supporting and stimulating clinical and scientific research, providing peer-to-peer support, and using social media platforms as a way to advertise their events.

Patient advocacy is not a new concept in Arab countries. However, it tends to focus on common health conditions, such as breast cancer, by supporting patients and raising awareness.

26.9.1 The Arab Adult Arthritis Awareness (AAAA) Group

The Arab League of Associations for Rheumatology (ArLAR) is the leading organization of rheumatologists in the Arab world. The primary objectives are to enhance medical care for individuals with rheumatic diseases, promote research in this field, and promote the education and training of healthcare professionals. Additionally, it strives to enhance the QOL for patients while promoting professional and scientific collaboration at both regional and global levels [88].

One of ArLAR's important initiatives is the establishment of the Arab Adult Arthritis Awareness (AAAA) Group. This initiative aims to address the unique needs of Arabic-speaking patients by providing reliable information in Arabic. This group empowers rheumatology patients through awareness, comprehensive education, patient engagement, and ongoing support by providing trusted resources to engage and empower patients from different Arab regions. Additionally, it focuses on patient-centered care and responds to patients' needs and desires to improve their QOL. Moreover, this group raises awareness through virtual events [89].

26.9.2 Friends of Arthritis

Friends of Arthritis was a nonprofit organization established in 2021 under the Health Education Department of the Supreme Council for Family Affairs in Sharjah, United Arab Emirates. Its activities focused on disease education, screening, and prevention of various rheumatic diseases, aiming to raise public awareness, facilitate early detection of joint disorders, and promote overall physical and mental well-being. The organization also worked to educate patients about arthritis, provide psychological support to patients and their families, and offer financial assistance to those in need. In addition, Friends of Arthritis organized several community walkathons and public awareness events to encourage engagement and healthy lifestyles [90, 91]. The organization remained active until its formal dissolution in July 2025.

26.9.3 Middle East Arthritis Foundation

Founded in 2006, this nonprofit foundation is dedicated to assisting patients unable to afford their treatment. It aims to raise awareness and educate about arthritis in the UAE, organizing events such as World Arthritis Day and the Walkathon for Arthritis [92].

26.9.4 Kuwait Patient Support Groups

The Kuwait Lupus Group was established following a suggestion from a physician who herself battles lupus on a recurring basis. This group serves as a platform where lupus patients from diverse backgrounds, united by their shared experience, can come together to share their stories, offer mutual support, and uplift one another during challenging times. Despite facing lupus, this group encourages patients to take control of their diseases instead of letting the disease control their lives. The mission of the group is to provide support to lupus patients and their families, raise awareness about the condition, and stay informed about relevant topics related to lupus. Its vision is to enhance understanding of lupus by offering a reliable platform with up-to-date, unbiased information.

The group aims to create a space where both new and seasoned lupus warriors, along with their families, can openly discuss and share their experiences, ensuring proper representation both locally and internationally. Since its inception in 2015, the group has achieved significant milestones, including organizing annual celebrations of International Lupus Day through public awareness initiatives and participating in national and regional rheumatology conferences and symposiums. The group remains active on social media such as Instagram [93].

In Kuwait, patients have established additional support groups aimed at providing emotional support, raising awareness, and identifying individuals affected by specific rheumatological conditions. These groups include the Scleroderma and Rheumatoid Support Groups, which were initiated and organized by patients themselves. Through workshops and social gatherings, these groups have effectively heightened awareness about their respective conditions.

26.9.5 *Oman Lupus Group*

The Oman Lupus group was initiated by a single patient who initially maintained anonymity on social media due to societal stigma. After receiving consent to create a WhatsApp support group, efforts were made to expand membership. The group quickly grew, gaining recognition across Gulf countries. In 2022, it participated in the second rheumatology conference of the Gulf Cooperation Council (GCC) in Oman.

Lupus Oman aims to expand its reach across various regions of Oman, offering education about the disease and support to patients and caregivers. Its main goal is to ensure lupus patients, regardless of gender or age, feel supported and informed [94].

26.10 Conclusion

Rheumatic diseases (RDs) impose significant physical, social, mental, and financial burdens on patients in the Arab world. Addressing different aspects of managing RD patients is essential to mitigate these burdens and enhance patient satisfaction and adherence to treatment plans. Unique beliefs among Arab patients regarding their chronic autoimmune diseases and the definition of disease flares warrant discussion and consideration in patient care. Further research in the Arab world is necessary to explore these issues and enhance the understanding of healthcare professionals involved in RD management.

While some patient advocacy groups exist in the Arab world, the establishment of more organizations is needed to provide comprehensive educational and psychological support to patients.

Authors' Conflict of Interest Declaration The authors declare that they have no conflicts of interest.

References

1. Katz P, Nelson W, Daly R, Topf L, Connolly-Strong E, Reed M. Patient-reported lupus flare symptoms are associated with worsened patient outcomes and increased economic burden. J Manag Care Spec Pharm. 2020;26(3):275–83. https://doi.org/10.18553/jmcp.2020.26.3.275.
2. Chaigne B, Chizzolini C, Perneger T, Trendelenburg M, Huynh-Do U, Dayer E, et al. Impact of disease activity on health-related quality of life in systemic lupus erythematosus: a cross-sectional analysis of the Swiss Systemic Lupus Erythematosus Cohort Study (SSCS). BMC Immunol. 2017;18(1):17. https://doi.org/10.1186/s12865-017-0200-5.
3. Robinson D, Aguilar D, Schoenwetter M, Dubois R, Russak S, Ramsey-Goldman R, et al. Impact of systemic lupus erythematosus on health, family, and work: the patient perspective. Arthritis Care Res (Hoboken). 2010;62(2):266–73. https://doi.org/10.1002/acr.20077.

4. Murimi-Worstell IB, Lin DH, Nab H, Kan HJ, Onasanya O, Tierce JC, et al. Association between organ damage and mortality in systemic lupus erythematosus: a systematic review and meta-analysis. BMJ Open. 2020;10(5):e031850. https://doi.org/10.1136/bmjopen-2019-031850.
5. Rkain H, Allali F, Jroundi I, Hajjaj-Hassouni N. Socioeconomic impact of rheumatoid arthritis in Morocco. Joint Bone Spine. 2006;73(3):278–83. https://doi.org/10.1016/j.jbspin.2005.03.021.
6. Awada S, Ajrouche R, Shoker M, Al-Hajje A, Rachidi S, Zein S, Bawab W. Rheumatoid arthritis in the Lebanese adults: impact on health-related quality of life. J Epidemiol Glob Health. 2019;9(4):281–7. https://doi.org/10.2991/jegh.k.190820.001.
7. Al-Herz A, Saleh K, Al-Awadhi A, Al-Kandari W, Hasan E, Ghanem A, et al. Accessibility to biologics and its impact on disease activity and quality of life in patients with rheumatoid arthritis in Kuwait. Clin Rheumatol. 2021;40(5):1759–65. https://doi.org/10.1007/s10067-020-05444-2.
8. Omair MA, Erdogan A, Tietz N, Alten R. Physical and emotional burden of rheumatoid arthritis in Saudi Arabia: an exploratory cross-sectional study. Open Access Rheumatol. 2020;12:337–45. https://doi.org/10.2147/OARRR.S284734.
9. Al-Jabi SW, Seleit DI, Badran A, Koni A, Zyoud SH. Impact of sociodemographic and clinical characteristics on functional disability and health-related quality of life in patients with rheumatoid arthritis: a cross-sectional study from Palestine. Health Qual Life Outcomes. 2021;19:241. https://doi.org/10.1186/s12955-021-01874-x.
10. Ali MM, Mosbah SK, Abo El-Fadl NM. Factors affecting quality of life and work productivity among patients with gout. Am J Nurs Res. 2019;7(2):128–35. https://doi.org/10.12691/ajnr-7-2-4.
11. Fahmi DS, Makarm WK, Zaghlol R. Burden of enthesitis on the quality of life and work productivity in psoriatic arthritis patients. Egypt Rheumatol Rehabil. 2022;49:58. https://doi.org/10.1186/s43166-022-00157-7.
12. Mortada M, Abdul-Sattar A, Gossec L. Fatigue in Egyptian patients with rheumatic diseases: a qualitative study. Health Qual Life Outcomes. 2015;13:134. https://doi.org/10.1186/s12955-015-0304-7.
13. Hammam N, Hammam N, Gamal RM, Rashed AM, El-Fetoh NA, Mosad E, et al. Fatigue in rheumatoid arthritis patients: association with sleep quality, mood status, and disease activity. Reumatol Clin (Engl Ed). 2020;16(5 Pt 1):339–44. https://doi.org/10.1016/j.reuma.2018.07.010.
14. Aissaoui N, Rostom S, Hakkou J, Berrada Ghziouel K, Bahiri R, Abouqal R, et al. Fatigue in patients with ankylosing spondylitis: prevalence and relationships with disease-specific variables, psychological status, and sleep disturbance. Rheumatol Int. 2012;32(7):2117–24. https://doi.org/10.1007/s00296-011-1928-5.
15. AlEnzi F, Alqahtani B, Alhamad EH, Daghestani M, Tashkandy Y, Othman N, Alshahrani K, Paramasivam MP, Halwani R, Omair MA. Fatigue in Saudi patients with primary Sjögren's syndrome and its correlation with disease characteristics and outcome measures: a cross-sectional study. Open Access Rheumatol. 2020;12:303–8. https://doi.org/10.2147/OARRR.S284985.
16. Hifinger M, Putrik P, Ramiro S, Keszei A, Hmamouchi I, Dougados M, et al. In rheumatoid arthritis, country of residence has an important influence on fatigue: results from the multinational COMORA study. Rheumatology (Oxford). 2016;55(4):735–44. https://doi.org/10.1093/rheumatology/kev395.
17. Lwin M, Serhal L, Holroyd C, Edwards CJ. Rheumatoid arthritis: the impact of mental health on disease: a narrative review. Rheumatol Ther. 2020;7(3):457–71. https://doi.org/10.1007/s40744-020-00217-4.
18. Abu Al-Fadl EMA, Ismail MA, Thabit M, El-Serogy Y. Assessment of health-related quality of life, anxiety and depression in patients with early rheumatoid arthritis. Egyptian Rheumatologist. 2014;36(2):51–6. https://doi.org/10.1016/j.ejr.2013.12.004.
19. Baghdadi LR, Alhassan MK, Alotaibi FH, Alsuwaida AA, Shehadah AE, Alzahrani MT. Effect of type of disease-modifying antirheumatic drugs on depression and anxiety of patients with

rheumatoid arthritis in Saudi Arabia: a cross-sectional study. Front Psych. 2023;14:1184720. https://doi.org/10.3389/fpsyt.2023.1184720.
20. Qiu X-J, Zhang X-L, Cai L-S, et al. Rheumatoid arthritis and risk of anxiety: a meta-analysis of cohort studies. Clin Rheumatol. 2019;38:2053–61. https://doi.org/10.1007/s10067-019-04502-8.
21. Zhang L, Fu T, Yin R, Zhang Q, Shen B. Prevalence of depression and anxiety in systemic lupus erythematosus: a systematic review and meta-analysis. BMC Psychiatry. 2017;17(1):70. https://doi.org/10.1186/s12888-017-1234-1.
22. Figueiredo-Braga M, Cornaby C, Cortez A, Bernardes M, Terroso G, Figueiredo M, et al. Depression and anxiety in systemic lupus erythematosus. Medicine (Baltimore). 2018;97(28):e11376. https://doi.org/10.1097/MD.0000000000011376.
23. Alenazy AE, Alenazy AES, Alanazi MS, Alshammari MN. Prevalence, comorbidities and management of psoriasis in Saudi Arabia: a review. J Pharm Res Int. 2021;33(44B):321–7. https://doi.org/10.9734/JPRI/2021/v33i44B32682.
24. Fragoulis GE, Evangelatos G, Tentolouris N, Fragkiadaki K, Panopoulos S, Konstantonis G, et al. Higher depression rates and similar cardiovascular comorbidity in psoriatic arthritis compared with rheumatoid arthritis and diabetes mellitus. Ther Adv Musculoskelet Dis. 2020;12:1759720X20976975. https://doi.org/10.1177/1759720X20976975.
25. Shand G, Fuller DT, Lufkin L, Lovelett C, Pal N, Mondal S, et al. A stronger association of depression with rheumatoid arthritis in presence of obesity and hypertriglyceridemia. Front Epidemiol. 2023;3:1216497. https://doi.org/10.3389/fepid.2023.1216497.
26. DiMatteo M, Lepper HS, Croghan TW. Depression is a risk factor for noncompliance with medical treatment: meta-analysis of the effects of anxiety and depression on patient adherence. Arch Intern Med. 2000;160(14):2101–7. https://doi.org/10.1001/archinte.160.14.2101.
27. Katz PP, Yelin EH. Activity loss and the onset of depressive symptoms: do some activities matter more than others? Arthritis Rheum. 2001;44(5):1194–202. https://doi.org/10.1002/1529-0131(200105)44:5<1194::AID-ANR203>3.0.CO;2-6.
28. Safiah MH, Kalalib Al Ashabi K, Haj-Abow T, Alchallah MO, Khalayli N, et al. Exploring associations with depressive and anxiety symptoms among Syrian patients with ankylosing spondylitis undergoing biological treatment: A cross-sectional study. Medicine (Baltimore). 2024;103(14):e37708. https://doi.org/10.1097/MD.0000000000037708.
29. El-Moselhy EA, Hagrass SAA, Mohammed AES, Abd-Alrhman TM, Alnabawy AA, Mosalam A. Psychosocial impact and quality of life among adult Egyptian patients with psoriatic arthritis. Egypt J Hosp Med. 2017;66:237–47. https://doi.org/10.12816/0034659.
30. Albreiki F, Alfalasi A, Al-Otaibi M, Ameen A, Bazali A, Steinhoff M, Al Hashmi S, Al-Lafi A. Patient awareness and perspectives on psoriatic disease: results of the psoriasis and beyond survey from the Gulf region. J Dermatolog Treat. 2025;36(1):2485254. https://doi.org/10.1080/09546634.2025.2485254.
31. Myung G, Harada N, Fong S, Aquino-Beaton C, Fong C, Fang M. Stigma and medication adherence in patients with rheumatic disease. J Psychosom Res. 2019;125:109791. https://doi.org/10.1016/j.jpsychores.2019.109791.
32. Corker E, Henderson R, Lempp H, Brown J. Internalised stigma in people with rheumatoid arthritis: a cross-sectional study to establish the psychometric properties of the ISMI-RA. BMC Musculoskelet Disord. 2016;17:244. https://doi.org/10.1186/s12891-016-1089-5.
33. Jewett LR, Hudson M, Malcarne VL, Baron M, Thombs BD, Canadian Scleroderma Research Group. Sociodemographic and disease correlates of body image distress among patients with systemic sclerosis. PLoS One. 2012;7(3):e33281. https://doi.org/10.1371/journal.pone.0033281.
34. Dimitrov D, Matusiak Ł, Szepietowski JC. Stigmatization in Arabic psoriatic patients in The United Arab Emirates - a cross sectional study. Postepy Dermatol Alergol. 2019;36(4):425–30. https://doi.org/10.5114/ada.2018.80271.

35. Antoniou J. Shunned: Discrimination against people with mental illness. By Graham Thornicroft. Oxford University Press. 2006. 328pp. £24.95 (pb). ISBN 0198570988. Br J Psychiatry. 2008;192(3):237. https://doi.org/10.1192/bjp.bp.106.031377.
36. Corrigan P, Watson A, Barr L. The self-stigma of mental illness: implications for self-esteem and self-efficacy. J Soc Clin Psychol. 2006;25(8):875–84. https://doi.org/10.1521/jscp.2006.25.8.875.
37. Soliman MM. Feeling of stigmatization and satisfaction with life among Arabic psoriatic patients. Saudi Pharm J. 2020;28(12):1868–73. https://doi.org/10.1016/j.jsps.2020.11.013.
38. World Lupus Federation. Lupus knows no boundaries e-report: global e-report highlights the physical, economic and social impacts of Lupus [Internet]. Washington, DC: World Lupus Federation; 2017 [updated 2018 May 22; cited 2026 Jun 17]. Available from: https://worldlupusfederation.org/global-e-report/.
39. Wang C, Horby P, Hayden F, Gao G. A novel coronavirus outbreak of global health concern. Lancet. 2020;395(10223):470–3. https://doi.org/10.1016/S0140-6736(20)30250-6.
40. Kiltz U, Celik A, Tsiami S, Buehring B, Baraliakos X, Andreica I, Kiefer D, Braun J. Are patients with rheumatic diseases on immunosuppressive therapies protected against preventable infections? A cross-sectional cohort study. RMD Open. 2021;7(1):e001499. https://doi.org/10.1136/rmdopen-2020-001499.
41. Ziadé N, el Kibbi L, Hmamouchi I, Abdulateef N, Halabi H, Hamdi W, et al. Impact of the COVID-19 pandemic on patients with chronic rheumatic diseases: a study in 15 Arab countries. Int J Rheum Dis. 2020;23(11):1550–7. https://doi.org/10.1111/1756-185X.13960.
42. Tharwat S, Zohdy Mohamed S, Kamal Nassar M. Challenges of Egyptian patients with systemic lupus erythematosus during the COVID-19 pandemic. Reumatologia. 2021;59(4):237–43. https://doi.org/10.5114/reum.2021.108620.
43. Hassan M, Mostafa D, Abdelhady E, Sarhan S, Abdelghani M, Seleem D. Psychosocial and clinical impact of COVID-19 pandemic and its relationship to the quality of life in patients with rheumatoid arthritis: a cross-sectional study. Egypt Middle East Current Psychiatry. 2022;29(1) https://doi.org/10.1186/s43045-022-00184-2.
44. Alzain MA, Bazuhair MA, Alharthi MS, Alamoudi WA, Saleh BH, Hebaishi S, et al. Public knowledge and awareness of gout among adults in Jeddah, Saudi Arabia: a cross-sectional study. Medicine (Baltimore). 2025;104(16):e42192. https://doi.org/10.1097/MD.0000000000042192.
45. Ghaddaf AA, Alomari MS, AlHarbi FA, Alquhaibi MS, Alsharef JF, Alsharef NK, et al. Public awareness about arthritic diseases in Saudi Arabia: a systematic review and meta-analysis. Int Orthop. 2023;47(12):3013–29. https://doi.org/10.1007/s00264-023-05725-w.
46. Hawezy G, Mahmood KA, Media SK, Ahmed SK. The level of awareness and predictors about rheumatic diseases in Kurdistan region-Iraq: an online community-based survey. Discov Public Health. 2025;22:425. https://doi.org/10.1186/s12982-025-00823-z.
47. Menassa J, Bou Nassar D, El Naboulsi F, El Naggar E, Sunna N, Ghoubar M. Public awareness of rheumatoid arthritis and ankylosing spondylitis in Lebanon. Open Rheumatol J. 2022;16(1):221130. https://doi.org/10.2174/18743129-v16-e221130-2022-7.
48. Elsabae OEM, Habib HM, Abady WA, Radwan AR, Shaat RM, Gharbia OM, et al. Evaluation of general public awareness, knowledge and attitude about common rheumatic diseases in Egypt: a multicenter study. Egypt Rheumatol Rehabil. 2023;50:48. https://doi.org/10.1186/s43166-023-00216-7.
49. Stack RJ, Stoffer M, Englbrecht M, Mosor E, Falahee M, Simons G, et al. Perceptions of risk and predictive testing held by the first-degree relatives of patients with rheumatoid arthritis in England, Austria and Germany: a qualitative study. BMJ Open. 2016;6(6):e010555. https://doi.org/10.1136/bmjopen-2015-010555.
50. Alnaqbi KA, Alaswad M, Alasfour S. Patient perspectives on rheumatic and musculoskeletal diseases: insights from a large-scale survey. Clin Rheumatol. 2025;44(4):1457–66. https://doi.org/10.1007/s10067-025-07388-x.

51. Palominos PE, Gasparin AA, de Andrade NPB, Xavier RM, da Silva Chakr RM, Igansi F, et al. Fears and beliefs of people living with rheumatoid arthritis: a systematic literature review. Adv Rheumatol. 2018;58(1):1. https://doi.org/10.1186/s42358-018-0001-4.
52. Taïeb O, Bricou O, Baubet T, Gaboulaud V, Gal B, Mouthon L, et al. Patients' beliefs about the causes of systemic lupus erythematosus. Rheumatology (Oxford). 2010;49(3):592–9. https://doi.org/10.1093/rheumatology/kep430.
53. Daifallah O, Moshrif A, Khalifa H, Ali R. Awareness and attitude of Egyptian population towards gout. Egypt J Orthop Res. 2021;2(2):87–94.
54. Neame R, Hammond A. Beliefs about medications: a questionnaire survey of people with rheumatoid arthritis. Rheumatology (Oxford). 2005;44(6):762–7. https://doi.org/10.1093/rheumatology/keh587.
55. Taik FZ, Mansouri NE, Bensaid R, Adnine A, Amar A, Fourtassi M, et al. Beliefs of Moroccan patients with chronic inflammatory rheumatic diseases regarding medication: related factors and correlation with therapeutic adherence. BMC Rheumatol. 2024;8(1):45. https://doi.org/10.1186/s41927-024-00419-1.
56. Berenbaum F, Chauvin P, Hudry C, Mathoret-Philibert F, Poussiere M, De Chalus T, et al. Fears and beliefs in rheumatoid arthritis and spondyloarthritis: a qualitative study. PLoS One. 2014;9(12):e114350. https://doi.org/10.1371/journal.pone.0114350. Erratum in: PLoS One. 2015 Mar 05;10(3):e0119056. doi:10.1371/journal.pone.0119056.
57. World Health Organization. Adherence to long-term therapies: evidence for action [Internet]. Geneva: World Health Organization; 2003 [cited 2026 Jun 17]. Available from: https://www.paho.org/sites/default/files/WHO-Adherence-Long-Term-Therapies-Eng-2003.pdf.
58. Ermeidis C, Dimitroulas T, Pourzitaki C, Voulgari PV, Kouvelas D. Perceived treatment satisfaction in patients with systemic rheumatic diseases treated with biologic therapies: results of a self-reported survey. Rheumatol Int. 2023;43(6):1151–9. https://doi.org/10.1007/s00296-023-05280-y.
59. Smolen J, Gladman D, McNeil H, Mease P, Sieper J, Hojnik M, et al. Predicting adherence to therapy in rheumatoid arthritis, psoriatic arthritis or ankylosing spondylitis: a large cross-sectional study. RMD Open. 2019;5(1):e000585. https://doi.org/10.1136/rmdopen-2017-000585.
60. McCulley C, Katz P, Trupin L, Yelin EH, Barton JL. Association of Medication Beliefs, self-efficacy, and adherence in a diverse cohort of adults with rheumatoid arthritis. J Rheumatol. 2018;45(12):1636–42. https://doi.org/10.3899/jrheum.171339.
61. Berner C, Erlacher L, Fenzl K, Dorner T. A cross-sectional study on self-reported physical and mental health-related quality of life in rheumatoid arthritis and the role of illness perception. Health Qual Life Outcomes. 2018;16(1):238. https://doi.org/10.1186/s12955-018-1064-y.
62. Hale ED, Radvanski DC, Hassett AL. The man-in-the-moon face: a qualitative study of body image, self-image and medication use in systemic lupus erythematosus. Rheumatology (Oxford). 2015;54(7):1220–5. https://doi.org/10.1093/rheumatology/keu448.
63. Hale E, Treharne G, Norton Y, Lyons A, Douglas K, Erb N, et al. 'Concealing the evidence': the importance of appearance concerns for patients with systemic lupus erythematosus. Lupus. 2006;15(8):532–40. https://doi.org/10.1191/0961203306lu2310xx.
64. Burkhart P, Sabaté E. Adherence to long-term therapies: evidence for action. J Nurs Scholarsh. 2003;35(3):207. https://doi.org/10.1016/S1474-5151(03)00091-4.
65. Brown M, Bussell J, Dutta S, Davis K, Strong S, Mathew S. Medication adherence: truth and consequences. Am J Med Sci. 2016;351(4):387–99. https://doi.org/10.1016/j.amjms.2016.01.010.
66. Tolu S, Rezvani A, Karacan I, Bugdayci D, Küçük H, Bucak Ö, et al. Self-reported medication adherence in patients with ankylosing spondylitis: the role of illness perception and medication beliefs. Arch Rheumatol. 2020;35(4):495–505. https://doi.org/10.46497/ArchRheumatol.2020.7732.

67. Goh H, Kwan Y, Seah Y, Low L, Fong W, Thumboo J. A systematic review of the barriers affecting medication adherence in patients with rheumatic diseases. Rheumatol Int. 2017;37(10):1619–28. https://doi.org/10.1007/s00296-017-3763-9.
68. Al Emadi S, Hammoudeh M, Mounir M, Mueller RB, Wells AF, Sarakbi HA. An assessment of the current treatment landscape for rheumatology patients in Qatar: Recognising unmet needs and moving towards solutions. J Int Med Res. 2017;45(2):733–43. https://doi.org/10.1177/0300060516686872.
69. Schäfer M, Albrecht K, Kekow J, Rockwitz K, Liebhaber A, Zink A, et al. Factors associated with treatment satisfaction in patients with rheumatoid arthritis: data from the biological register RABBIT. RMD Open. 2020;6(3):e001290. https://doi.org/10.1136/rmdopen-2020-001290.
70. Miladi S, Belhadj W, Boussaa H, Yasmine M, Leith Z, Abdelghani KB, et al. Patient satisfaction with medication in rheumatoid arthritis: an unmet need. Reumatologia. 2023;61(1):38–44. https://doi.org/10.5114/reum/161575.
71. Abu Hamdeh H, Al-Jabi SW, Koni A, et al. Health-related quality of life and treatment satisfaction in Palestinians with rheumatoid arthritis: a cross-sectional study. BMC Rheumatol. 2022;6(1):19. https://doi.org/10.1186/s41927-022-00251-5.
72. Bykerk V, Shadick N, Frits M, Bingham C, Jeffery I, Iannaccone C, et al. Flares in rheumatoid arthritis: frequency and management. J Rheumatol. 2013;41(2):227–34. https://doi.org/10.3899/jrheum.121521.
73. Adamichou C, Bertsias G. Flares in systemic lupus erythematosus: diagnosis, risk factors and preventive strategies. Mediterr J Rheumatol. 2017;28(1):4–12. https://doi.org/10.31138/mjr.28.1.4.
74. Zeng X, Zheng L, Rui H, Kang R, Chen J, Chen H, et al. Risk factors for the flare of systemic lupus erythematosus and its influence on prognosis: a single-center retrospective analysis. Adv Rheumatol. 2021;61(1) https://doi.org/10.1186/s42358-021-00202-7.
75. Tharwat S, Shaker EA. Adherence patterns to medications and their association with subsequent hospitalization in adult Egyptian patients with systemic lupus erythematosus. Lupus. 2023;32(11):1335–44. https://doi.org/10.1177/09612033231198826.
76. Zhang L, Luan W, Geng S, Ye S, Wang X, Qian L, et al. Lack of patient education is risk factor of disease flare in patients with systemic lupus erythematosus in China. BMC Health Serv Res. 2019;19(1) https://doi.org/10.1186/s12913-019-4206-y.
77. Yılmaz V, Umay E, Gündoğdu İ, Karaahmet ZÖ, Öztürk AE. Rheumatoid arthritis: are psychological factors effective in disease flare? Eur J Rheumatol. 2017;4(2):127–32. https://doi.org/10.5152/eurjrheum.2017.16100.
78. Al Juffali LA, Almalag H, Alalem S, Alamairah S, Omair MA. Patients' perceptions of rheumatoid arthritis and their behaviour towards medications in Saudi Arabia: a qualitative study. BMJ Open. 2025;15(3):e084057. https://doi.org/10.1136/bmjopen-2024-084057.
79. Potestio L, Lauletta G, Tommasino N, Portarapillo A, Salsano A, Battista T, et al. Risk factors for psoriasis flares: a narrative review. Psoriasis (Auckl). 2024;14:39–50. https://doi.org/10.2147/PTT.S323281.
80. Almoallim H, Al Saleh J, Badsha H, Ahmed H, Habjoka S, Menassa J, et al. A review of the prevalence and unmet needs in the management of rheumatoid arthritis in Africa and the Middle East. Rheumatol Ther. 2020;8(1):1–16. https://doi.org/10.1007/s40744-020-00252-1.
81. Hussain W, Noorwali A, Janoudi N, Baamer M, Kebbi L, Mansafi H, et al. From symptoms to diagnosis: an observational study of the journey of rheumatoid arthritis patients in Saudi Arabia. Oman Med J. 2016;31(1):29–34.
82. El Zorkany B, AlWahshi H, Hammoudeh M, Al Emadi S, Benitha R, Al Awadhi A, et al. Suboptimal management of rheumatoid arthritis in the Middle East and Africa: could the EULAR recommendations be the start of a solution? Clin Rheumatol. 2012;32(2):151–9. https://doi.org/10.1007/s10067-012-2153-7.
83. Khatib HE, Alyafei A, Shaikh M. Understanding experiences of mental health help-seeking in Arab populations around the world: a systematic review and narrative synthesis. BMC Psychiatry. 2023;23:324. https://doi.org/10.1186/s12888-023-04827-4.

84. Bornstein B, Marcus D, Cassidy W. Choosing a doctor: an exploratory study of factors influencing patients' choice of a primary care doctor. J Eval Clin Pract. 2001;6(3):255–62. https://doi.org/10.1046/j.1365-2753.2000.00256.x.
85. Ziade N, Hmamouchi I, Haouichat C, Baron F, Al Mayouf S, Abdulateef N, et al. The rheumatology workforce in the Arab countries: current status, challenges, opportunities, and future needs from an ArLAR cross-sectional survey. Rheumatol Int. 2023;43(12):2281–92. https://doi.org/10.1007/s00296-023-05427-x.
86. Fasseeh A, ElEzbawy B, Adly W, ElShahawy R, George M, Abaza S, ElShalakani A, Kaló Z. Healthcare financing in Egypt: a systematic literature review. J Egypt Public Health Assoc. 2022;97(1):1. https://doi.org/10.1186/s42506-021-00089-8.
87. Hu A. Reflections: the value of patient support groups. Otolaryngol Head Neck Surg. 2017;156(4):587–8. https://doi.org/10.1177/0194599817697030.
88. Arab League of Associations for Rheumatology (ArLAR). About ArLAR. [Internet]. [cited 2026 Jun 17]. Available from: https://www.arabrheumatology.org/about-arlar/.
89. El Kibbi L, Halabi H, Masri B, Hmamouchi I, Metawee M, Alnaqbi K, et al. Shaping awareness about rheumatic and musculoskeletal diseases in the Arab region: the Arab Adult Arthritis Awareness Group initiative. Arab J Rheumatol. 2024;2(1):1–6. https://doi.org/10.4103/ajr.ajr_3_24.
90. Sharjah Events. Friends-of-Arthritis-Patients (9th Charitable Marathon) – Event Archive. [Internet]. Sharjah (UAE): SharjahEvents.ae; 2022 Mar 16 [cited 2026 Jun 17]. Available from: https://cms.sharjahevents.ae/en/organizer/friends-of-arthritis-patients/.
91. Emirates News Agency (WAM). Friends of Arthritis Patients to launch 11th marathon on February 25 [Internet]. Abu Dhabi (UAE): WAM; 2024 Feb 23 [cited 2026 Jun 17]. Available from: https://www.wam.ae/en/article/b1pkkp7-friends-arthritis-patients-launch-11th-marathon.
92. Middle East Arthritis Foundation. [Internet]. [cited 2026 Jun]. Available from: https://arthritis.ae/.
93. Kuwait Lupus Group (@lupusgroup) [Internet]. Kuwait City: Instagram; [cited 2026 Jun 17]. Available from: https://www.instagram.com/lupusgroup/.
94. Yousuf K. Lupus Oman kick-starts awareness. Oman Observer [Internet]. 2022 May 24 [cited 2026 Jun 17]. Available from: https://www.omanobserver.om/article/1119712/oman/lupus-oman-kick-starts-awareness.

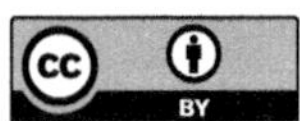

Chapter 27
Complementary and Alternative Medicine Use in Rheumatic Diseases in the Arab World

Noria Ghulam Nabi, Hazem Taifour, Khalid A. Alnaqbi, and Yossra Suliman

Abstract The chronic nature of rheumatic diseases and their direct influence on patients' quality of life (i.e., fatigue and pain) have urged patients to utilize different complementary and alternative medicine (CAM) modalities as a natural way of dealing with their chronic conditions. Examples of CAM include acupuncture, cupping, homeopathy, Chinese or Oriental medicine, and herbal/dietary supplements. In this chapter, we will discuss commonly used complementary alternative medicine modalities and their use and safety in rheumatic diseases, with a particular remark on studies conducted in the Arab region.

Keywords Complementary medicine · Alternative medicine · Hijamah · Cupping · Herbal medicine · Acupuncture · Homeopathy · Rheumatic diseases · Arab world · Safety

---

N. G. Nabi
Department of Internal Medicine, Sheikh Tahnoon bin Mohammed Medical City, SEHA/PureHealth, Al Ain, UAE
e-mail: nooriya.afghan@gmail.com

H. Taifour
Department of Medicine, Rochester Regional Health/Unity Hospital, Rochester, NY, USA
e-mail: h.taifour@outlook.com

K. A. Alnaqbi (✉)
Rheumatology Division, Sheikh Tahnoon bin Mohammed Medical City, SEHA/ PureHealth, Al Ain, UAE

Internal Medicine Department, College of Medicine and Health Sciences, UAE University, Al Ain, UAE

College of Medicine, RAK Medical and Health Sciences University, Ras Al Khaimah, UAE
e-mail: kalnaqbi@gmail.com

Y. Suliman (✉)
Rheumatology Department, Mediclinic—Al Ain Hospital, Al Ain, UAE

Faculty of Medicine, Assiut University, Assiut, Egypt
e-mail: dr.yossra@gmail.com

K. A. Alnaqbi, G. Aldabie (eds.), *Rheumatic Diseases in the Arab World*,
https://doi.org/10.1007/978-981-92-0967-5_27

27.1 Introduction

Complementary and alternative medicine (CAM) has expanded dramatically lately in developed and developing countries. Examples of CAM include acupuncture, cupping, Ayurveda, homeopathy, Chinese or Oriental medicine, and herbal/dietary supplements. In the Arab region, there is limited research on this topic, and physicians have little knowledge about it, often approaching CAM therapies with prejudice [1]. Not long ago, what was recognized as CAM was referred to as "quackery." As it blends evidence-based therapies worldwide into regular practice, many people now refer to this treatment as integrative medicine [2].

Rheumatic disorders are chronic diseases with a wide range of clinical features, but common symptoms such as joint pain and fatigue significantly influence the patient's quality of life (QOL) and necessitate significant effort to manage. Furthermore, due to the chronic nature of the disease, patients dealing with these conditions may need to take medication for extended durations, possibly indefinitely. As a result, many individuals turn to CAM approaches for relief [3].

CAM modalities vary per country, based on local traditions and popular CAM. In Saudi Arabia, CAM practices are largely associated with cultural and religious beliefs. Rituals such as the use of honey, camel milk, Zamzam water, olive oil, cupping, and skin cauterization are commonly observed in Saudi Arabia and are rooted in Quranic traditions and Sunnah teachings. As a result, a ministerial decree established a center for complementary and alternative medicine to serve as a reference center for all conditions connected to CAM, regulate CAM practices within healthcare services, and deploy evidence-based CAM alongside traditional therapy [4].

In this chapter, we will discuss commonly used CAM modalities and their use in rheumatic disease, with a particular remark on studies done in the Arab region.

27.2 Epidemiology

Rheumatic and musculoskeletal conditions are often linked to reduced productivity and a lower QOL. Conventional treatments for these conditions typically involve medications that can suppress the immune system, although some individuals may not respond well to these medications.

Patients with autoimmune diseases often turn to alternative treatment options like CAM. A study in Saudi Arabia aimed to assess the prevalence and types of CAM use among individuals with rheumatoid arthritis (RA) and the factors influencing their choice. The study found that 67% of the 438 patients had used CAM for their RA, with females constituting 92% of CAM users. Common CAM products included supplements, honey, ginger, turmeric, and black seeds. Additionally, 45% of participants believed CAM to be safe, and 90% recognized the potential additional benefits of CAM [4].

These findings highlight the significant prevalence of CAM utilization among RA patients, indicating a widespread belief in the supplementary advantages of these approaches for managing their condition.

In 2013, a study conducted in the UAE revealed that one-third of patients utilized CAM for diverse reasons, with 72% of them not seeking advice from a physician beforehand. Therefore, integrating discussions or inquiries about CAM usage into the clinical history could be crucial for gaining a deeper understanding of the patient's health status and assessing the safety of the CAM approach [5].

27.3 Types of Complementary and Alternative Medicine (CAM)

27.3.1 Acupuncture

Acupuncture is a concept based on the application of small needles in the form of pressure specifically to certain areas of the body. Originating from Chinese traditional medicine, acupuncture is grounded in philosophical concepts such as vital energy. It aims to unblock channels or regulate the flow of excess energy, thereby promoting overall wellness [6]. Acupuncture has been utilized in the management of various clinical disorders, including RA [7]. The American College of Physicians recognizes it as a treatment option for alleviating low back pain [8].

Furthermore, among students at the University of Sharjah (UAE), acupuncture, along with cupping, was identified as a preferred CAM method for pain relief [9].

27.3.2 Bee Venom

Bee venom therapy has been suggested to have therapeutic benefits dating back to ancient times. It encompasses various treatment methods such as live bee stings, bee venom injections, and bee venom acupuncture (BVA, or apipuncture). The last method involves the injection of diluted, pure bee venom into specific acupoints [10]. It is believed that BVA exerts multiple pharmacological effects, including analgesic, anti-inflammatory, antiarthritic, and anti-cancer properties, through different pathways such as stimulating the central inhibitory and excitatory systems and modulating the immune system. Animal studies and clinical observations have indicated the analgesic properties of BVA. Research suggests that bee venom may possess antiarthritic, anti-inflammatory, and analgesic effects by inhibiting the production of cyclo-oxygenase-2 and phospholipase A2, as well as reducing the levels of tumor necrosis factor (TNF), interleukins (IL-1 and IL-6), nitric oxide, and reactive oxygen species [11].

27.3.3 Cupping (Hijama)

Cupping therapy, Hijama in Arabic, was first used in Egypt 3500 years BC, as documented in hieroglyphic writing. In addition to ancient Egyptians, Chinese culture, Arabic medicine, Greek medicine, Prophetic medicine, and recent European and American medicine have all practiced different types of cupping [12].

Traditionally aimed at pain relief, cupping therapy has been applied to a wide range of medical conditions. However, it is important to note that not all medical conditions can be treated with cupping. While various forms of cupping therapy are available, including dry cupping, wet cupping (with bloodletting), moving cupping, and fire cupping, the wet and dry types are the most commonly utilized. Cupping serves four primary purposes: alleviating pain, reducing inflammation, modulating the immune system, and adjusting hematologic parameters. Cupping promotes an anti-inflammatory effect mainly through nitric oxide-mediated vasodilation [13]. A previous report suggested that wet cupping effectively reduces levels of total cholesterol, low-density lipoprotein (LDL) cholesterol, triglycerides, uric acid, inflammatory markers, and immunoglobulin antibodies (such as the rheumatoid factor) [14].

Cupping was a widely favored method for treating gout and arthritis in Italy [15]. Furthermore, a recent systematic review provides evidence that bloodletting therapy, including wet cupping, may improve symptoms and reduce inflammation in patients with gouty arthritis [16].

Furthermore, a systematic literature review (SLR) and meta-analysis indicate that herbal medicines for external use may offer a safe and effective alternative for managing pain and symptoms associated with acute gouty arthritis. Nonetheless, due to variations in interventions, outcomes, and potential regional biases, additional high-quality clinical trials are necessary to confirm these findings [17].

In the case of ankylosing spondylitis, a recent SLR and meta-analysis found only weak evidence supporting the benefits of cupping therapy, indicating the need for further research in this area [18].

27.3.4 Cauterization (Al-Kaiy)

Al-Kaiy, the Arabic term for cauterization, refers to the practice of applying a heated metal rod to specific skin areas to treat various medical conditions, such as osteoarthritis (OA) and sciatica. Historically, it has also been used to rapidly stop bleeding. The perception and utilization of cauterization vary across different cultures; some view it as a method for treating resistant diseases, while others believe it treats ailments caused by demonic possession, necessitating the use of cauterization for a cure. This practice dates back to ancient civilizations, including the Egyptians, as mentioned in the Ebers Papyrus around 1550 BC Cauterization was a common treatment approach in Greek, Indian, and Ancient Chinese medicinal traditions as well

[19]. Notably, traditional Arabic cauterization was practiced even before the advent of Islam [20].

A study published in 1989 highlighted its widespread use in Saudi Arabia, reporting a prevalence rate of 22% among children visiting a pediatric orthopedic clinic [21]. Patients with polio and those with neurological diseases such as cerebral palsy, congenital hypotonia, and congenital hydrocephalus are the most commonly cauterized [20].

A survey in Libya was administered to 50 participants who had undergone cauterization for various diseases, revealing that most (60%) participants were not educated. About 90% followed the advice of their parents or relatives. The main reasons were their desire for a rapid improvement of their symptoms and that medical treatment takes too long a time before noticing beneficial effects, with a possibility of failure or a need to undergo many tests. Additionally, about 64% of patients did not see any benefit of cauterization and experienced side effects such as disfigurement or keloids [22].

27.3.5 Herbal Medicine

According to a review study published in 2019, around 80% of the Arab population has used herbal remedies for the treatment of various medical conditions, including arthritis. This is primarily due to the inflammatory nature of arthritis and the hypothesized anti-inflammatory effect of these herbs [23].

Some herbal remedies commonly used for managing arthritis include borage seed oil, capsaicin, curcumin, flaxseed oil, Asphodelus aestivus, Citrullus colocynthis, Thapsia garganica, Marrubium alysson, Peganum harmala, Solanum nigrum, and Thymus capitatus. Borage seed oil, derived from the borage plant and historically utilized in the Mediterranean region for both culinary and medicinal purposes, is notably rich in gamma-linolenic acid (GLA), which has been associated with various health benefits [24].

Capsaicin, extracted from chili peppers, possesses burning and pungent properties. Its high absorption rate of around 94%, whether taken orally or applied topically, contributes to its effectiveness in providing pain relief when consumed in appropriate doses and at appropriate times [25].

Curcumin, found in turmeric, serves as an active pigment with diverse therapeutic properties, including anti-inflammatory, antioxidant, anti-cancer, and immunomodulatory effects. It functions through various cellular pathways, inhibiting pro-inflammatory proteins and interfering with the actions of tumor necrosis factor (TNF) alpha and its receptors, thus reducing inflammation [26]. A recent systematic literature review on curcumin showed scientific evidence suggesting that turmeric extract (approximately 1000 mg/day of curcumin) may be effective in managing arthritis. Nevertheless, the limited number of randomized controlled trials (RCTs), small overall sample size, and variable methodological quality of the included studies prevent drawing firm or definitive conclusions [27].

Flaxseed, an ancient plant with a long history of commercial use, has gained recent attention for its potential health benefits. Flaxseed is increasingly recognized for its potential health advantages due to its rich content of omega-3 fatty acids, fiber, and antioxidants [28].

A cross-sectional national survey conducted among 448 participants across the UAE found that approximately 99% used herbal medicines, with the majority being aged between 18 and 24 years and predominantly female (70%). Respondents with chronic diseases were significantly less likely to use herbal medicine, at just 11%. Most users of herbal medicine believed these products to be harmless, attributing their safety to their natural origins.

Despite the promising properties of these herbal remedies commonly used in the Arab world [29], research on their effectiveness in managing arthritis in Arabic patients remains limited [1].

27.3.6 Gold

Archaeological records and historical accounts suggest that gold was used medicinally in ancient civilizations. In the 8th century CE, Jābir ibn Hayyān, known as Geber in European historical records, produced soluble gold compounds by dissolving gold in aqua regia. Later alchemical traditions regarded potable gold, or aurum potabile, as an elixir with broad remedial and life-prolonging properties. In the fifteenth century, Paracelsus advocated for its use alongside mercury as an elixir of life [30]. Gold thiolate compounds used in medicine include myocrisin, myochrisin/mychrisis, solganol, sanocrysin, sanochrisin/crisalbine/aurothion, allocrysine/allochrysin krysolgan, and auranofin. These compounds have been historically employed to treat various diseases, including leprosy, epilepsy, systemic lupus erythematosus (SLE), skin diseases such as pemphigus and discoid lupus, inflammatory bowel diseases, and certain cancers affecting organs such as the tongue and lung [31].

Gold clusters created from biomolecules, particularly peptides, have attracted considerable interest as novel gold nanomaterials due to their excellent biocompatibility and beneficial biological properties. Historically administered parenterally, gold is systemically distributed following chronic use, with its concentration varying considerably. Tissues like bone marrow, liver, and spleen exhibit notably higher gold levels compared to synovium and cartilage, suggesting that therapeutic effects may be achieved with relatively small amounts of gold at these sites [32]. Despite its empirical use in RA treatment in the past, the precise mechanism of action in these patients remains incompletely understood [31].

Interestingly, a case report showed a 49-year-old woman with poly-articular psoriatic arthritis affecting all proximal interphalangeal (PIP) joints of both hands except the left PIP joint of the finger with the ring. On physical examination, there was no evidence of arthritis in the left ring finger PIP joint. No joint damage was observed in the PIP joint of the left ring finger by musculoskeletal ultrasound and

MRI of the small joints of the hand. All other PIP joints in both hands had a high degree of joint damage secondary to chronic psoriasis. Therefore, it is postulated that wearing a gold ring may have a protective effect against inflammatory arthritis [33].

Unfortunately, no studies were found on gold use for the treatment of rheumatic diseases in the Arab countries.

27.3.7 Homeopathy

Homeopathy was founded by Dr. Samuel Hahnemann in the eighteenth century with the principle of "likes being able to treat likes". It activates the immune system, combating illnesses which could be extracted from herbs, metals, or poisons, considered safe when given in very dilute amounts. The mechanism of action of homeopathic remedies is not fully understood [34]. Studies conducted on homeopathy as a treatment for rheumatic diseases in the Arab world are limited.

27.3.8 Glucosamine and Chondroitin Sulfate

Glucosamine, chondroitin, and collagen are utilized in promoting joint well-being, aimed at preventing injuries commonly associated with sports activities, such as OA, among athletes. Researchers evaluated the effect of glucosamine on urine markers of collagen type II synthesis (assessed by urine CP II) and breakdown (assessed by urine CTX-II) in young athletes (rugby and soccer players) and non-athlete controls paired for age. After of treatment with glucosamine 1.5 or 3 g/day, the biomarkers' levels of collagen breakdown in the athletes had returned to the levels of the control subjects, and three months after discontinuation of treatment, these levels had again increased. Conclusive outcomes need to be tested in larger studies [35]. Another study randomized the athletes to receive either 2 g/day of glucosamine or a placebo supplement. After three months of treatment, the urine CTX-II levels had significantly decreased in the glucosamine group but not in the placebo group [36]. These studies suggested that high doses of glucosamine (2–3 g per day) positively affect cartilage metabolism in vivo, therefore confirming the effect observed in vitro, where glucosamine inhibited matrix metalloproteinase production and chondrocyte apoptosis [37].

In a recent meta-analysis of randomized trials on glucosamine and chondroitin sulfate, 26 articles were included. Chondroitin versus placebo was compared, and chondroitin was shown to alleviate joint pain symptoms and improve function. Glucosamine showed a dramatic effect on stiffness improvement compared to placebo. However, the combination therapy did not show enough evidence to be superior to placebo. Additionally, there was no significant difference in the incidence of adverse events compared with placebo [38]. Nevertheless, the American College of

Rheumatology (ACR) recommendations for the management of OA published in 2019 reported that both glucosamine and chondroitin sulfate are strongly recommended against for patients with knee and hip OA but conditionally recommended for patients with hand OA [39], suggesting that more evidence is needed to support their use in OA patients.

27.4 CAM in Some Rheumatic Diseases

27.4.1 Rheumatoid Arthritis (RA)

RA is an inflammatory autoimmune arthritis and is associated with a more significant burden for individuals and healthcare systems [4]. A cross-sectional study in Saudi Arabia among 438 patients was conducted and reported that 67% of RA patients had used CAM to treat their RA. Females were the majority of CAM users (92.1%). Among the CAM therapies used, vitamin D (47%) was the most used, followed by calcium (37%), honey (15%), ginger (13%), turmeric (11%), black seeds (8%), and fenugreek (7%) [4]. Another Saudi study by Al-Zahim et al. reported that honey, black seeds, anise, green tea, and myrrh were the most utilized complementary and alternative medicines for other diseases in Saudi Arabia [40].

In the following section, we will discuss available studies of CAM use in RA.

27.4.1.1 Acupuncture

A recent review of 43 studies investigating the efficacy of acupuncture for RA concluded that acupuncture, whether used alone or alongside other treatments, benefits RA patients. It enhances their QOL and overall function without any reported side effects. The therapeutic effects of acupuncture were attributed to its anti-inflammatory, antioxidative, and immune system regulatory properties. Despite its widespread use, the exact mechanism of action of acupuncture remains a topic of ongoing discussion [7].

While an anti-inflammatory effect is commonly proposed, the precise mechanisms, including potential impacts on inflammatory responses, blood flow enhancement, and muscle relaxation, are still largely speculative [41].

27.4.1.2 Bee Venom Acupuncture (BVA)

An SLR was published to evaluate studies about bee venom on RA. A total of 304 potentially relevant studies were reported; based on only one RCT that met the inclusion criteria, BVA significantly improved joint pain, swollen joint counts, tender joint counts, C-reactive protein, and erythrocyte sedimentation rate (ESR) but was not shown to improve morning stiffness compared to placebo. However, the quality of evidence is low, as it is based on only one trial. Therefore, further studies are necessary to provide stronger evidence [10].

27.4.1.3 Cupping (Hijama)

Published research on the effect of cupping on RA patients showed some immunomodulatory effects and reported that cupping significantly reduced the pain and laboratory markers of RA activity. Additionally, it tends to modulate the activity of the innate immune response, especially the natural killer cells. However, more studies are still needed to validate such results [42].

A study conducted in Egypt on 50 RA patients found that wet cupping decreases pain and the laboratory indicators of RA activity. Additionally, this treatment appears to regulate the innate immune system activity, particularly natural killer cells, and the adaptive cellular immune response through the soluble interleukin 2 receptor (SIL-2R), which could be utilized in assessing disease progression and prognosis. Furthermore, when combined with conventional therapy, cupping has the potential to reduce rheumatoid factor levels in RA beyond what conventional therapy alone can achieve [43].

Cupping has been demonstrated to reduce serum ferritin levels, an inflammatory marker that is elevated in many autoimmune diseases, including RA [44].

27.4.1.4 Herbal Medicine

A 2003 SLR on the use of herbal medicines in treating RA revealed moderate evidence supporting the efficacy of GLA, present in certain herbal remedies, in improving pain, tender joint counts, and stiffness. However, for most herbal medicines, only one RCT was available, providing limited evidence. Additional research is necessary to further assess their effectiveness, safety, and possible interactions with other medications [45].

Borage Seed Oil

Two randomized controlled trials (RCTs) examined the efficacy of borage seed oil for RA. The first RCT compared 1.4 g/day of GLA, administered as borage seed oil, with placebo capsules containing cottonseed oil. At the end of the 6-month treatment period, patients who received borage seed oil showed significant improvement ($p < 0.05$) compared to those in the placebo group in terms of joint tenderness counts and scores, joint swelling scores, global physician assessment, and pain. Although the sample size is too small to draw a definitive conclusion (n = 37), these findings suggest a possible supportive role in disease activity control in RA patients [46].

In the second RCT, 56 RA patients received either 2.8 g/day of GLA from borage seed oil or a placebo. At the end of 6 months, patients treated with borage seed oil showed significant improvement compared to placebo patients in the tender joint count, swollen joint count, tender joint score, and pain score [47]. Larger studies are needed to confirm these findings. Additionally, no studies investigated borage seed oil use in RA patients in the Arab world.

Capsaicin

In a study involving 31 RA patients and 70 OA patients experiencing moderate to severe joint pain, participants were randomly assigned to apply either topical capsaicin (0.025%) or a vehicle cream (placebo) four times daily for 4 weeks. At the end of the 4 weeks, there was a notable disparity in the reduction of patient pain scores between the treatment and control groups, with a 57% reduction from baseline among RA patients and a 33% among OA patients. A burning sensation at the site of the capsaicin application was reported by 44% of those in the treatment group [48].

Curcumin (Diferuloyl Methane)

An SLR of the literature evaluating the effectiveness of curcumin in RA included 10 RCTs. Curcumin showed promise in the management of RA, offering potential benefits in reducing inflammation levels and alleviating clinical symptoms. The proposed inflammatory mechanisms of curcumin in RA patients are the inhibition of the mitogen-activated protein kinase family, activator protein-1, extracellular signal-regulated protein kinase, and nuclear factor kappa B. However, the authors addressed the need for more robust, well-controlled studies with larger patient cohorts to substantiate these findings [49].

Although it is widely used in the Arab countries, curcumin has not been investigated in the treatment of rheumatic diseases in the Arab world.

Flaxseed Oil

In a study involving 22 RA patients who received 30 g/day of either flaxseed or placebo oil for 3 months, no significant changes were found between the two groups. All patients continued taking non-steroidal anti-inflammatory drugs (NSAIDs) [50]. Although flaxseed oil is widely used in the Arab world, there is a lack of research on its efficacy in rheumatic diseases.

Evening Primrose Oil

A study focusing on the impact of primrose oil involved 49 patients with mild RA who were randomly assigned to receive primrose oil, a combination of primrose oil and fish oil, or a placebo (liquid paraffin) [51]. An intent-to-treat analysis after 12 months revealed no significant change in clinical measurements for any group. However, a considerably higher percentage of patients in the treatment groups reported subjective improvement than those in the placebo group (94% vs. 30%). Additionally, a significant proportion of primrose oil patients (73%) and primrose oil/fish oil patients (80%) reduced or stopped their NSAIDs compared to placebo patients ($p < 0.05$).

In a 6-month double-blind placebo-controlled study involving 40 RA patients, GLA at 540 mg/day was supplemented, with 19 patients receiving evening primrose oil and 21 receiving olive oil. No patients ceased NSAID therapy, but some reduced their dosage. Results showed that GLA may provide modest RA improvements [52].

Lastly, a trial involving 18 RA patients investigated the effects of primrose oil (20 mL/day) compared to olive oil (20 mL/day) over 3 months. No significant changes in the clinical variables were observed [53].

The conflicting results of different studies call for conducting larger studies to demonstrate the effect of primrose oil in the management of RA. To date, no studies on evening primrose oil have been conducted in the Arab world.

27.4.1.5 Homeopathy

In a 6-month RCT involving 112 RA patients who continued their background medications (disease-modifying anti-rheumatic drugs and NSAIDs), the outcomes related to articular index, erythrocyte sedimentation rate (ESR), and morning stiffness were comparable between those receiving active homeopathy and those given a placebo. The study did not provide evidence supporting the idea that active homeopathy has a beneficial effect on RA symptoms [54].

27.4.1.6 Gold

Chrysotherapy refers to the use of gold-based drugs, which are available in different complexes with mostly injectable formulations for the treatment of RA and other autoimmune conditions. Case histories based on 2166 RA patients who received gold compounds for periods ranging from 1 to 13 years revealed variable side effects, affecting 45% of patients and necessitating discontinuation of treatment. These side effects included hematologic abnormalities (e.g., thrombocytopenia, leukopenia, and aplastic anemia); proteinuria due to nephropathy; high accumulations of gold; chrysiasis (blue-gray skin discoloration); dermatitis; enterocolitis; and psychiatric and neurological complications, as well as organ damage affecting the kidneys, lungs, liver, and parotid glands. The proposed mechanism is that it has anti-inflammatory and immunomodulatory activity. Despite 70 years of empirical use in RA treatment in the past, the precise mechanism of action in these patients remains incompletely understood [31].

In a study, a gold cluster incorporating glutathione ($Au_{29}SG_{27}$), referred to as GA, was synthesized. This cluster demonstrated the ability to effectively inhibit both inflammation and bone damage in collagen-induced arthritis in rats, offering promising prospects for RA treatment. The results suggested that GA restores bone health by decreasing bone degradation and suppressing inflammation, displaying a therapeutic effect that varied based on dosage [55].

In another study conducted by Mulherin et al., gold was observed to delay erosion in individuals who wore gold rings with 25 non-wearers, utilizing standard hand radiographs to quantify joint erosion in both the metacarpophalangeal (MCP) and PIP joints. The results suggest less joint erosion observed in the left ring of the ring bearer with RA and possibly adjacent MCP joints. These data support the hypothesis that gold can move "downstream" from the gold ring through the skin and local lymphatic vessels to nearby MCP joints, delaying joint erosion. These results supported the hypothesis that gold rings can affect local joint erosion [56]. However, further controlled studies are warranted to assess these results.

In conclusion, the scarcity of RCTs in CAM use in RA treatment with relatively small sample sizes poses a major limitation in assessing the evidence for their use in RA treatment. Larger studies with appropriate sample sizes investigating various types of CAM in RA treatment will help draw definitive conclusions [57]. Furthermore, the 2022 ACR recommendations for diet and integrative interventions in RA suggest prioritizing adherence to established dietary guidelines without relying on dietary supplements. The authors favor the Mediterranean-style diet over supplement use and also endorse weight loss, mind-body techniques, acupuncture, and massage as beneficial approaches [58].

27.4.2 Systemic Lupus Erythematosus (SLE)

SLE is an autoimmune multi-systemic inflammatory disease associated with various manifestations affecting systems such as the skin, blood, liver, lungs, kidneys, and heart. It is often characterized by the presence of autoantibodies and antibody-immune complexes that can lead to tissue damage. Disease flares in SLE patients occur irregularly and unpredictably [59]. Most individuals with SLE experience significant fatigue and discomfort, which can impact their work productivity and ability to carry out daily activities [60, 61].

Based on the authors' experiences, we will briefly discuss the types of CAM that are commonly used in the Arab region.

27.4.2.1 Herbal Medicine

Various natural molecules and their derivatives have been reported to have beneficial effects. These include curcumin, baicalin, antroquinonol, mangiferin, emodin, salvianolic acid A, the total glycosides of paeony, triptolide, and artemisinin. They interact with immune mediators, cytokines, and transcription factors [62].

Furthermore, omega-6 and omega-3 polyunsaturated fatty acids have been shown to decrease levels of anti-dsDNA antibodies, TNF-alpha, interleukins, and CRP. However, the limited number of clinical trials makes it challenging to conduct a meta-analysis of reported herbal medicines [62].

Nevertheless, caution is advised regarding the ingredients of herbal medicines, as they may worsen lupus symptoms. A case report involved a 29-year-old woman with SLE who developed biopsy-proven lupus nephritis after taking an unregistered herbal supplement. The renal biopsy was consistent with the International Society of Nephrology/Renal Pathology Society (ISN/RPS) 2003 classification, specifically Class IV-S (A/C) and V, along with secondary membranoproliferative glomerulonephritis. Her renal condition did not improve after stopping the herbal supplement, necessitating immunosuppressive treatment. Following one cycle of IV cyclophosphamide, remission was achieved, allowing for a gradual reduction in steroid dosage [63].

Additionally, there is a lack of available data from the Arab region regarding the use of these treatment modalities in lupus patients.

27.4.2.2 Acupuncture

Due to the chronic nature of SLE, patients tend to seek alternative therapies alongside conventional immunosuppressive medications [62]. A recent SLR and meta-analysis showed that combining acupuncture with conventional medications is an effective and safe treatment for SLE, though the findings are limited by the small, variable quality of the studies included, introducing heterogeneity and bias [64]. Furthermore, another study evaluated the effectiveness of acupuncture combined with the antiemetic medication ondansetron in managing nausea and vomiting induced by cyclophosphamide infusions in 39 patients with rheumatic diseases (including 11 with SLE). The acupuncture group reported significantly reduced severity of nausea 24 and 48 hours post-infusion and significantly reduced the number of vomiting episodes following infusion. However, the small sample size and lack of a placebo group make the study difficult to generalize the results [65]. We could not identify a study on the efficacy of acupuncture among lupus patients in the Arab region.

27.4.2.3 Minerals and Vitamins

Certain minerals, such as calcium, iron, selenium, and zinc, along with vitamins A, B, C, D, and E, have demonstrated the potential to offer positive effects for individuals with lupus [62].

Vitamin D deficiency occurs commonly in SLE patients with risk factors including sun avoidance, use of sunblock creams, ethnicities (e.g., of African origin), lupus nephritis, and medications such as antimalarials and oral glucocorticosteroids [66, 67].

Two studies from Saudi Arabia and one study from the UAE revealed a high prevalence of vitamin D deficiency among patients with SLE [66–68], with rates of 90% in active disease compared to 85% in inactive disease [67]. Patients with SLE are at an increased risk of experiencing 25(OH) vitamin D deficiency when they have low serum C3 and C4 levels and elevated anti-dsDNA levels. While no correlation was found between 25(OH) vitamin D levels and active disease as assessed by the Systemic Lupus Erythematosus Disease Activity Index 2000 (SLEDAI-2 K) score, significant associations were observed between 25(OH) vitamin D levels, anti-dsDNA, and C4 levels [67].

Furthermore, studies examining the effect of vitamin D supplementation on various aspects of SLE, such as fatigue and serology (C3, C4, and dsDNA), have yielded conflicting results, as summarized in Table 27.1 [68–78]. These discrepancies may arise from several factors. Firstly, the small sample sizes in some studies may lead to underpowered results. Secondly, many studies lacked a placebo control group, which is crucial for assessing the actual effect of the supplement. Thirdly, despite adherence to supplementation protocols, many patients did not achieve the target vitamin D levels, possibly due to the risk factors previously mentioned. Fourthly, non-adherence to vitamin D intake and the influence of geographical location on vitamin D synthesis and status were also notable complicating factors. Fifthly, most studies did not account for interferon-alpha plasma levels and gene expression, both of which are known to be elevated in SLE patients with vitamin D deficiency, as highlighted by researchers [70, 73, 78]. This complex interplay of factors underscores the need for more rigorous and comprehensive studies to clarify the role of vitamin D in managing SLE.

Petri et al. found that higher levels of vitamin D were modestly but significantly associated with an improved urine protein-to-creatinine ratio, suggesting a role in reducing renal morbidity [70]. In contrast, this association was not observed in the study by Pakchotanon et al. [77].

Replenishing vitamin D in deficient patients is supported by various studies as a treatment option. A range of doses has shown some degree of success, including daily doses from 2,000 to 8,000 IU) IU, weekly doses of 50,000 U accompanied by twice-daily calcium-vitamin D (200 U), and 1200 IU/day over a period of 3 months. Following this period, it is recommended to reassess serum vitamin D levels to evaluate the adequacy of supplementation [70, 76, 78].

Recent SLR and meta-analysis have demonstrated that vitamin D supplementation can significantly reduce the SLEDAI score and increase C3 levels. However, changes in anti-dsDNA and C4 levels were not significant. Additionally, the impact of vitamin D supplementation on fatigue among SLE patients remains unclear [79].

Table 27.1 Summary of lupus outcome measures following vitamin D supplementation

Study Authors	Study type, year of publication	Country	Total number of participants	Time of assessment (weeks)	Fatigue	Outcome measure(s)	C3 and C4	dsDNA
Ruiz- Irastorza et al. [69]	Observational, 2010	Spain	80	104.4	Improved**	No correlation with SLEDAI-2 K and SDI	–	–
Petri et al. [70]	Prospective, 2013	USA	1006	128	–	↓PGA** and ↓SELENA-SLEDAI (only for 25 OH vitamin D level < 40 ng/mL)**	↑C3** and ↑C4** intra-patients comparison	No correlation
Andreoli et al. [71]	Prospective unblinded randomized, cross-over, 2015	Italy	34	104.4	–	No correlation with SLEDAI-2 K	No correlation	No correlation
Lima et al. [72]	RCT, 2016	Brazil	60	24	Improved**	↓ SLEDAI** ↓ ECLAM**	–	↓**
Karimzadeh et al. [73]	RCT (active and placebo arms), 2017	Iran	90	24	–	No correlation with SLEDAI-2 K	No correlation	–
Wahono et al. [74]	RCT (active and placebo arms), 2017	Indonesia	39	12	–	No correlation with SLEDAI	No correlation	No correlation
Al-Kushi et al. [75]	Prospective interventional, 2018	KSA	81	24	–	No correlation with SLEDAI-2 K	No correlation	No correlation
Rifa'i et al. [76]	Open-label RCT, 2018	Indonesia	39	12	Improved **	↓ SLEDAI**	–	–
Pakchotanon et al. [77]	RCT, 2020	Thailand	104	24	–	No correlation with SLEDAI-2 K, flare, HAQ, UPCR	No correlation	No correlation
Magro et al. [78]	Prospective open-label study, 2021	Malta	31	52	Improved *	↓ SLEDAI-2 K**	–	↓**

(continued)

Table 27.1 (continued)

Study Authors	Study type, year of publication	Country	Total number of participants	Time of assessment (weeks)	Fatigue	Outcome measure(s)	C3 and C4	dsDNA
Ali and Alalawi [68]	Retrospective, 2023	UAE	150	208.6	–	↓ SLEDAI-2 K**	–	–

Data synthesized from references [68–78]

Abbreviations: *ECLAM* European Consensus Lupus Activity Measurement, *HAQ* health assessment questionnaire, *KSA* Kingdom of Saudi Arabia, PGA: patient global assessment, *SDI* Systemic Lupus International Collaborating Clinics/American College of Rheumatology Damage Index, *SELENA-SLEDAI* Safety of Estrogens in Lupus Erythematosus National Assessment version of the Systemic Lupus Erythematosus Disease Activity Index, *SLEDAI-2K* Systemic Lupus Erythematosus Disease Activity Index 2000, *SLR* systematic literature review, *UAE* United Arab Emirates, *UPCR* urine protein/creatinine ratio, *USA* United States of America

* Non-significant, ** Significant

27.4.2.4 Omega 3 Fatty Acids

DHA and EPA are the omega-3 polyunsaturated fatty acids with the highest biological activity. Multiple studies evaluated fish oil/omega-3 for SLE. The effect of omega-3 on endothelial dysfunction was evaluated in an RCT in 60 patients with SLE. Patients in the omega-3 group took four capsules per day compared to placebo (olive oil) capsules. Endothelial dysfunction measured by the brachial artery's flow-mediated dilation (FMD) was the primary outcome measure. FMD improved from baseline to 12 weeks and 24 weeks in the omega-3 fatty acid group ($p = 0.002$ and $p < 0.001$, respectively), and there were no significant improvements in FMD in the placebo group. Secondary outcomes, including disease activity measures such as the British Isles Lupus Assessment Group (BILAG) and Systemic Lupus Activity Measure-Revised (SLAM-R) scores, showed significant improvement from baseline to 12 weeks [80].

On the other hand, a meta-analysis revealed that omega-3 appears to have a significant but small effect on reducing lupus activity, particularly noticeable in patients with active disease at baseline. Additionally, it suggests that omega-3 fatty acids may offer therapeutic advantages when combined with immunosuppressive regimens [81].

27.4.3 Fibromyalgia (FM)

Fibromyalgia (FM) is a chronic pain condition characterized by widespread pain and discomfort, often referred to as a 'central sensitization syndrome' resulting from biochemical abnormalities in the central nervous system. It frequently coexists with other disorders such as irritable bowel syndrome and depression. Recent recommendations from both EULAR and Egyptian guidelines advocate for the utility of CAM in managing FM, with acupuncture, meditative movement, exercise, and multi-component therapy being highlighted as effective approaches. Other modalities like massage, homeopathy, and cognitive behavioral therapy also show promise, albeit with varying levels of evidence [82, 83].

The efficacy of CAM in treating FM is further supported by the findings of a recent network meta-analysis, which included 41 studies involving 2877 participants. This analysis demonstrated the significant effectiveness of CAM with a high safety profile. Notably, combinations of acupuncture and massage therapy were found to improve pain. Additionally, umbilical acupuncture decreased the number of tender points, while electroacupuncture effectively alleviated insomnia symptoms. Furthermore, abdominal acupuncture therapy demonstrated superiority in improving depression symptoms and mental status [84].

Incorporating CAM alongside conventional treatments offers a holistic approach to FM management, potentially enhancing symptom relief. Evidence from an online survey reveals that combining CAM with prescription or over-the-counter medications leads to improved QOL and reduced pain levels compared to pharmacologic treatment alone. Moreover, those exclusively using CAM reported significantly lower pain levels compared to those solely using pharmacologic treatment [85].

A meta-analysis revealed that combining acupuncture and cupping therapy surpasses conventional medications in both reducing pain and improving depression scores among FM patients [86]. In addition, an SLR found that acupoint stimulation therapy, encompassing both acupuncture and cupping, is effective in treating FM when compared to medications. However, larger trials with more rigorous designs than those previously conducted are required to draw definitive conclusions [87].

Furthermore, studies exploring the use of medical cannabis in FM treatment have shown promising results. A prospective observational study reported a high treatment response rate (81%) and significant pain reduction after 6 months of medical cannabis use, albeit with mild side effects like dizziness, dry mouth, and gastrointestinal symptoms [88]. Similarly, a retrospective study found substantial improvements in FM symptoms with medical cannabis, with 50% of patients discontinuing other therapies altogether. The mean duration of cannabis treatment was 10.4 months. Adverse effects were mild and were reported by 30% of patients. Despite the small sample size, these findings suggest a potential role for medical cannabis, calling for further well-designed studies to validate its efficacy [89].

27.4.4 Osteoarthritis (OA)

OA is a highly prevalent degenerative disease of cartilage and joints. It frequently presents as pain and stiffness in the affected joint, limiting the patient's ability to perform daily activities. The use of CAM in the treatment of OA has been evaluated.

A meta-analysis encompassed 30 trials investigating the effects of marine oil, containing docosahexaenoic acid (DHA) and eicosapentaenoic acid (EPA), on pain (primary outcome), function, and inflammation (secondary outcomes). Among these trials, five specifically assessed the impact of marine oil on patients with OA. However, the analysis concluded that there was insufficient evidence to assess the effect of marine oil in patients with OA [90].

A large prospective study comprising 4470 individuals with or at risk of knee OA found that higher fiber intake, particularly meeting the recommended daily average intake of 25 grams, was associated with lower odds of being in high-pain groups [91]. Another large prospective study, which involved 2092 patients diagnosed with radiographic knee OA, revealed that higher consumption of monounsaturated and polyunsaturated fatty acids was associated with a delay in the progression of joint space narrowing compared to higher fat intake [92].

There are limited RCTs on the effect of CAM in OA patients in the Arab region. A prospective study conducted in Egypt divided knee OA patients into 3 groups: 25 in the acupuncture group, 25 in the homeopathy group (receiving Arnica Montana, Ruta graveolans, and Rhus toxicodendron), and 25 in the control group (continuing only on their previous medications). By the end of week 6, both acupuncture and homeopathy proved efficacious in decreasing pain and improving knee function. However, acupuncture demonstrated notably superior effectiveness compared to homeopathy. Limitations of the study included a small sample size and a short follow-up period [93].

27.4.4.1 Glucosamine/Chondroitin Sulfate

Data on the efficacy of glucosamine/chondroitin sulfate in treating OA present a complex picture, with findings that are often conflicting. Initially, several RCTs demonstrated a symptomatic improvement with glucosamine/chondroitin sulfate in knee OA that was superior to placebo and comparable to NSAIDs [94, 95]. However, the Osteoarthritis Research Society International (OARSI) has classified the efficacy of glucosamine as 'uncertain.' This assessment stems from the variability in effect sizes, which range from low (0.17 [0.05–0.28]) to moderate (0.47 [0.23–0.72]), influenced by the study's quality and the type of glucosamine used (hydrochloride vs. sulfate) [96].

Subsequent comprehensive reviews, including multiple meta-analyses and SLRs, have indicated that glucosamine and chondroitin sulfate yield only small effect sizes on outcomes such as pain relief and functional improvement in OA patients [97]. Notwithstanding, more recent meta-analyses have specifically underscored the symptomatic efficacy of glucosamine sulfate, noting its moderate effect size, which aligns closely with those reported for other symptomatic OA treatments, particularly NSAIDs [98].

An interesting contribution from an Egyptian study comparing the clinical efficacy of topical versus oral forms of glucosamine/chondroitin sulfate found both to be safe and equally effective in alleviating knee pain and stiffness [99].

In conclusion, while glucosamine/chondroitin sulfate may not offer significant benefits for OA broadly, it does provide some relief for knee OA. Notably, improvements in pain and analgesic effects manifest after several weeks of treatment and can last for weeks after discontinuing the treatment. This pattern differs from a placebo effect and aligns with the characteristics of symptomatic slow-acting drugs for osteoarthritis (SYSADOAs) [98].

27.4.4.2 Acupuncture

For patients with knee OA who have an inadequate response to standard medical therapy and are not surgical candidates, other pain management strategies, such as acupuncture, may be considered. A rigorous systematic review and meta-analysis concluded that acupuncture provides statistically significant improvements in pain and physical function compared to sham acupuncture and no-acupuncture control groups, supporting its role as an effective complementary therapy for managing knee OA [100].

27.4.4.3 Cupping (Hijama)

An SLR analyzing 7 RCTs concluded that there is only weak evidence supporting the effectiveness of cupping therapy in enhancing treatment efficacy and physical function for patients with knee OA [101]. Similarly, another SLR, which examined 5 studies, found weak evidence that cupping therapy contributes to pain reduction and improvement in physical function in knee OA patients [102].

On a broader scale, a recent meta-analysis incorporating 19 eligible studies on the combined approach of acupuncture and collaterals cupping therapy for knee OA concluded that this traditional Chinese medicine technique is both effective and safe for treating knee OA [103].

27.4.4.4 Homeopathy

A study conducted in Egypt evaluated the efficacy of homeopathy in 30 patients with knee OA. Participants were administered a 6-week course of oral homeopathic remedies, including Arnica Montana, Ledum Palustre, Rhus Tox, and Ruta Graveolens, with ascending potency levels. There was significant improvement in pain, tenderness, knee flexion, QOL, serum levels of enkephalin, interleukin-4, and ESR. Limitations of the study included a small sample size, a short follow-up period, and the absence of a control group [104].

27.4.4.5 Curcuma

Almost all products containing Curcuma consistently showed statistically significant enhancements in endpoints related to OA compared to a placebo. In comparison with active controls, Curcuma-containing products exhibited similar effectiveness to NSAIDs and potentially to glucosamine. However, the small sample size of the reviewed studies, poor overall study design, and differences in baseline characteristics make the generalizability of these studies a challenge [105].

27.5 Safety and Adverse Events of CAM

Despite the impression regarding CAM that it can be beneficial without adverse effects, many complications have been documented in the literature because of CAM.

Acupuncture needles may cause injury to vulnerable internal tissues such as the viscera, pleura, and blood vessels. Despite their rarity, acupuncture-related pneumothorax and pericardial effusion have been reported in the literature. Improper sterilization or failure to properly dispose of the acupuncture needles can result in the transmission of infections like HIV or hepatitis. However, local skin infections are the most common side effect. Many herbals have been reported to cause allergic reactions. However, only 0.2% of cases required hospital admission [106].

Furthermore, some herbal medications cause drug-induced liver injury (DILI), and some have been found to trigger lupus nephritis [63, 107].

27.6 Conclusion

Throughout history, ancient civilizations have harnessed various therapies now recognized as complementary and alternative medicine (CAM). Even today, modern medicine incorporates age-old practices such as herbal medicine, acupuncture, cupping, and cauterization into therapeutic regimes. This is particularly relevant in the realm of rheumatic diseases, where patients often endure chronic conditions, and some may find limited relief from conventional medications.

Surveys across various Arab countries have indicated that CAM is commonly used, underscoring the urgent need for clinical trials to evaluate these practices scientifically. Although existing research on CAM has indicated potential benefits for rheumatic disease sufferers, there is a critical need for further studies—particularly in the Arab world. These studies should aim for larger sample sizes and rigorous methodologies to comprehensively assess the benefits and risks of CAM alongside conventional treatments.

The establishment of dedicated research centers for CAM within the Arab world represents a crucial step toward a deeper understanding of these therapies. Such efforts can potentially transform patient care in rheumatology, offering more holistic and effective treatment paradigms that blend the best of traditional and modern approaches.

Conflict of Interest Declaration The authors declare they have no conflicts of interest.

References

1. Aboushanab TS, AlSanad S. Cupping therapy: an overview from a modern medicine perspective. J Acupunct Meridian Stud. 2018;11(3):83–7.
2. Rajbhandary R, Bhangle S, Patel S, Sen D, Perlman A, Panush RS. Perspectives about complementary and alternative medicine in rheumatology. Rheum Dis Clin. 2011;37(1):1–8.
3. Gözcü E, Çakmak İ, Öz B, Karataş A, Akar ZA, Koca SS. Complementary alternative medicine in rheumatic diseases: causes, choices, and outcomes according to patients. Eur J Rheumatol. 2021;9(1):36–41.
4. Almuhareb AM, Alhawassi TM, Alghamdi AA, Omair MA, Alarfaj H, Alarfaj A, et al. Prevalence of complementary and alternative medicine use among rheumatoid arthritis patients in Saudi Arabia. Saudi Pharm J. 2019;27(7):939–44.
5. Muttappallymyalil J, Sreedharan J, John L, John J, Mehboob M, Mathew A, et al. Self-reported use of complementary and alternative medicine among the health care consumers at a tertiary care center in Ajman, United Arab Emirates. Ann Med Health Sci Res. 2013;3(2):215.

6. Van Hal M, Dydyk AM, Green MS. Acupuncture [updated 2023 Jul 24; Internet]. Treasure Island: StatPearls Publishing; 2024 Jan– [cited 2025 Oct 29]. Available from: https://www.ncbi.nlm.nih.gov/books/NBK532287/.
7. Chou PC, Chu HY. Clinical efficacy of acupuncture on rheumatoid arthritis and associated mechanisms: a systemic review. Evid Based Complement Alternat Med. 2018:8596918. https://doi.org/10.1155/2018/8596918.
8. Qaseem A, Wilt TJ, McLean RM, Forciea MA; Clinical Guidelines Committee of the American College of Physicians; Denberg TD, et al. Noninvasive treatments for acute, subacute, and chronic low back pain: a clinical practice guideline from the American College of Physicians. Ann Intern Med. 2017;166(7):514–30. https://doi.org/10.7326/M16-2367.
9. Ibrahim O, Rashrash M, Soliman S. Perception and utilization of complementary and alternative medicine (CAM) among University of Sharjah (UOS) students. Bull Fac Pharm Cairo Univ. 2019;57(1):82–7.
10. Lee JA, Son MJ, Choi J, Jun JH, Kim JI, Lee MS. Bee venom acupuncture for rheumatoid arthritis: a systematic review of randomized clinical trials. BMJ Open. 2014;4(11):e006140.
11. Avalo Z, Barrera MC, Agudelo-Delgado M, Tobón GJ, Cañas CA. Biological effects of animal venoms on the human immune system. Toxins. 2022;14(5):344. https://doi.org/10.3390/toxins14050344.
12. Qureshi NA, Ali GI, Abushanab TS, El-Olemy AT, Alqaed MS, El-Subai IS, et al. History of cupping (Hijama): a narrative review of literature. J Integr Med. 2017;15(3):172–81. https://doi.org/10.1016/S2095-4964(17)60339-X.
13. Al-Bedah AMN, Elsubai IS, Qureshi NA, Aboushanab TS, Ali GIM, El-Olemy AT, et al. The medical perspective of cupping therapy: effects and mechanisms of action. J Tradit Complement Med. 2019;9(2):90–7. https://doi.org/10.1016/j.jtcme.2018.03.003.
14. El Sayed SM, Baghdadi H, Abou-Taleb A, Mahmoud HS, Maria RA, Ahmed NS, Helmy Nabo MM. Al-hijamah and oral honey for treating thalassemia, conditions of iron overload, and hyperferremia: toward improving the therapeutic outcomes. J Blood Med. 2014;(5):219–37. https://doi.org/10.2147/JBM.S65042.
15. Turk JL, Allen E. Bleeding and cupping. Ann R Coll Surg Engl. 1983;65(2):128–31.
16. Li SH, Hu WS, Wu QF, Sun JG. The efficacy of bloodletting therapy in patients with acute gouty arthritis: a systematic review and meta-analysis. Complement Ther Clin Pract. 2022;46:101503. https://doi.org/10.1016/j.ctcp.2021.101503.
17. Choi SH, Song HS, Hwang J. Herbal medicine for external use in acute gouty arthritis: a PRISMA-compliant systematic review and meta-analysis. Medicine (Baltimore). 2023;102(37):e34936. https://doi.org/10.1097/MD.0000000000034936.
18. Ma SY, Wang Y, Xu JQ, Zheng L. Cupping therapy for treating ankylosing spondylitis: the evidence from systematic review and meta-analysis. Complement Ther Clin Pract. 2018;32:187–94. https://doi.org/10.1016/j.ctcp.2018.07.001.
19. Nayab M. History of Amal-i-Kaiyy (cauterization) and its indications according to the shapes of instruments: a review. Int J Med Health Res. 2017;3(3):60–1.
20. Aboushanab T, AlSanad S. An Ethnomedical perspective of Arabic traditional cauterization. Al-Kaiy Adv J Soc Sci. 2019;4(1):18–23. https://doi.org/10.21467/ajss.4.1.18-23.
21. Watt HG. Cutaneous cautery (Al Kowi): a study in pediatric orthopedic clinic in central Saudi Arabia. Ann Saudi Med. 1989;9:475–8.
22. Farid MK, El-Mansoury A. Kaiy (traditional cautery) in Benghazi, Libya: complications versus effectiveness. Pan Afr Med J. 2015;22:98. https://doi.org/10.11604/pamj.2015.22.98.6399.
23. Nwabichie CC, Al Washali AY, Abuaisha AA, Albishty MM, Ismail S, Manaf RA. The use of herbal medicine in Arab countries: a review. Int J Public Health Clin Sci. 2017;4(5):1–13.
24. Casas-Cardoso L, Mantell C, Obregón S, Cejudo-Bastante C, Alonso-Moraga Á, de la Ossa EJM, de Haro-Bailón A. Health-promoting properties of borage seed oil fractionated by supercritical carbon dioxide extraction. Foods. 2021;10(10):2471. https://doi.org/10.3390/foods10102471.

25. Fattori V, Hohmann MS, Rossaneis AC, Pinho-Ribeiro FA, Verri WA. Capsaicin: current understanding of its mechanisms and therapy of pain and other pre-clinical and clinical uses. Molecules. 2016;21(7):844. https://doi.org/10.3390/molecules21070844.
26. Coelho MR, Romi MD, Ferreira DMTP, Zaltman C, Soares-Mota M. The use of curcumin as a complementary therapy in ulcerative colitis: a systematic review of randomized controlled clinical trials. Nutrients. 2020;12(8):2296. https://doi.org/10.3390/nu12082296.
27. Daily JW, Yang M, Park S. Efficacy of turmeric extracts and curcumin for alleviating the symptoms of joint arthritis: a systematic review and meta-analysis of randomized clinical trials. J Med Food. 2016;19(8):717–29. https://doi.org/10.1089/jmf.2016.3705.
28. Goyal A, Sharma V, Upadhyay N, Gill S, Sihag M. Flax and flaxseed oil: an ancient medicine & modern functional food. J Food Sci Technol. 2014;51(9):1633–53. https://doi.org/10.1007/s13197-013-1247-9.
29. Al Mazrouei N, Al Meslamani AZ, Alajeel R, Alghadban G, Ansari N, Al Kaabi M, Sadeq A, Ibrahim R, Ibrahim OM. The patterns of herbal medicine use in The United Arab Emirates; a national study. Pharm Pract. 2022;20(3):2698. https://doi.org/10.18549/PharmPract.2022.3.2698.
30. Norton S. A brief history of potable gold. Mol Interv. 2008;8(3):120–3. https://doi.org/10.1124/mi.8.3.1. PMID: 18693188.
31. Eisler R. Chrysotherapy: a synoptic review. Inflamm Res. 2003;52(12):487–501.
32. Balfourier A, Kolosnjaj-Tabi J, Luciani N, Carn F, Gazeau F. Gold-based therapy: from past to present. Proc Natl Acad Sci USA. 2020;117(37):22639–48. https://doi.org/10.1073/pnas.2007285117.
33. Hlaing T, Ramteke S, Binymin K. Gold finger: metal jewellery as a disease modifying anti-rheumatic therapy! Case Rep Med. 2009;2009:1–2.
34. Kaplan B. Homoeopathy: 1—what is it? Prof Care Mother Child. 1994;4(5):151–2.
35. Nagaoka I, Tsuruta A, Yoshimura M. Chondroprotective action of glucosamine, a chitosan monomer, on the joint health of athletes. Int J Biol Macromol. 2019;132:795–800.
36. Tsuruta A, Horiike T, Yoshimura M, Nagaoka I. Evaluation of the effect of the administration of a glucosamine-containing supplement on biomarkers for cartilage metabolism in soccer players: a randomized double-blind placebo controlled study. Mol Med Rep. 2018;18(4):3941–8.
37. Henrotin Y, Mobasheri A, Marty M. Is there any scientific evidence for the use of glucosamine in the management of human osteoarthritis? Arthritis Res Ther. 2012;14(1):201.
38. Zhu X, Sang L, Wu D, Rong J, Jiang L. Effectiveness and safety of glucosamine and chondroitin for the treatment of osteoarthritis: a meta-analysis of randomized controlled trials. J Orthop Surg Res. 2018;13(1):170.
39. Kolasinski SL, Neogi T, Hochberg MC, Oatis C, Guyatt G, Block J, et al. 2019 American College of Rheumatology/Arthritis Foundation guideline for the management of osteoarthritis of the hand, hip, and knee. Arthritis Rheumatol. 2020;72(2):220–33. https://doi.org/10.1002/art.41142. Erratum in: Arthritis Rheumatol. 2021;73(5):799.
40. Al-Zahim AA, Al-Malki NY, Al-Abdulkarim FM, Al-Sofayan SA, Abunab HA, Abdo AA. Use of alternative medicine by Saudi liver disease patients attending a tertiary care center: prevalence and attitudes. Saudi J Gastroenterol. 2013;19:75–80.
41. Meng YH, Yang WB, Don BQ. Clinical observation of modified DuhuoJisheng decoction combined with acupuncture and moxibustion in the treatment of rheumatoid arthritis. Inf Trad Chin Med. 2018;35(01):58–62.
42. Hasbani GE, Jawad A, Uthman I. Cupping (Hijama) in rheumatic diseases: the evidence. Mediterr J Rheumatol. 2021;32(4):316–23.
43. Ahmed SM, Madbouly NH, Maklad SS, Abu-Shady EA. Immunomodulatory effects of blood letting cupping therapy in patients with rheumatoid arthritis. Egypt J Immunol. 2005;12(2):39–51.

44. Baghdadi H, Abdel-Aziz N, Ahmed NS, Mahmoud HS, Barghash A, Nasrat A, Nabo MM, El Sayed SM. Ameliorating role exerted by Al-Hijamah in autoimmune diseases: effect on serum autoantibodies and inflammatory mediators. Int J Health Sci (Qassim). 2015;9(2):207–32.
45. Soeken KL. Herbal medicines for the treatment of rheumatoid arthritis: a systematic review. Rheumatology (Oxford). 2003;42(5):652–9.
46. Leventhal LJ, Boyce EG, Zurier RB. Treatment of rheumatoid arthritis with gammalinolenic acid. Ann Intern Med. 1993;119:867–73.
47. Zurier RB, Rossetti RG, Jacobson EW, DeMarco DM, Liu NY, Temming JE, et al. gamma-Linolenic acid treatment of rheumatoid arthritis. A randomized, placebo-controlled trial. Arthritis Rheum. 1996;39(11):1808–17. https://doi.org/10.1002/art.1780391106.
48. Deal CL, Schnitzer TJ, Lipstein E, Seibold JR, Stevens RM, Levy MD, et al. Treatment of arthritis with topical capsaicin: a double-blind trial. Clin Ther. 1991;13(3):383–95.
49. Kou H, Huang L, Jin M, He Q, Zhang R, Ma J. Effect of curcumin on rheumatoid arthritis: a systematic review and meta-analysis. Front Immunol. 2023;14:1121655. https://doi.org/10.3389/fimmu.2023.1121655.
50. Nordström DCE, Honkanen VEA, Nasy Y, Antila E, Friman C, Konttinen YT. Alpha-linolenic acid in the treatment of rheumatoid arthritis. A double-blind, placebo-controlled and randomized study: flaxseed vs safflower seed. Rheumatol Int. 1995;14:231–4.
51. Brzeski M, Madhok R, Capell HA. Evening primrose oil in patients with rheumatoid arthritis and side-effects of non-steroidal anti-inflammatory drugs. Br J Rheumatol. 1991;30:370–2.
52. Belch JJF, Ansell D, Madhok R, O'Dowd A, Sturrock RD. Effects of altering dietary essential fatty acids on requirements for non-steroidal anti-inflammatory drugs in patients with rheumatoid arthritis: a double-blind placebo controlled study. Ann Rheum Dis. 1988;47:96–104.
53. Jäntti J, Seppälä E, Vapaataol H, Isomäki H. Evening primrose oil and olive oil in treatment of rheumatoid arthritis. Clin Rheumatol. 1989;8:238–44.
54. Fisher P, Scott DL. A randomized controlled trial of homeopathy in rheumatoid arthritis. Rheumatology (Oxford). 2001;40(9):1052–5.
55. Yuan Q, Zhao Y, Cai P, He Z, Gao F, Zhang J, Gao X. Dose-dependent efficacy of gold clusters on rheumatoid arthritis therapy. ACS Omega. 2019;4(9):14092–9.
56. Mulherin DM, Struthers GR, Situnayake RD. Do gold rings protect against articular erosion in rheumatoid arthritis? Ann Rheum Dis. 1997;56(8):497–9.
57. Macfarlane GJ, El-Metwally A, De Silva V, Ernst E, Dowds GL, Moots RJ. Evidence for the efficacy of complementary and alternative medicines in the management of rheumatoid arthritis: a systematic review. Rheumatology (Oxford). 2011;50(9):1672–83.
58. England BR, Smith BJ, Baker NA, Barton JL, Oatis CA, Guyatt G, et al. 2022 American College of Rheumatology Guideline for exercise, rehabilitation, diet, and additional integrative interventions for rheumatoid arthritis. Arthritis Care Res (Hoboken). 2023;75(8):1603–15. https://doi.org/10.1002/acr.25117.
59. Ameer MA, Chaudhry H, Mushtaq J, Khan OS, Babar M, Hashim T, Zeb S, Tariq MA, Patlolla SR, Ali J, Hashim SN, Hashim S. An overview of systemic lupus erythematosus (SLE) pathogenesis, classification, and management. Cureus. 2022;14(10):e30330. https://doi.org/10.7759/cureus.30330.
60. Yuen HK, Cunningham MA. Optimal management of fatigue in patients with systemic lupus erythematosus: a systematic review. Ther Clin Risk Manag. 2014;10:775–86.
61. Al Dhanhani AM, Gignac MA, Su J, Fortin PR. Work disability in systemic lupus erythematosus. Arthritis Rheum. 2009;61(3):378–85. https://doi.org/10.1002/art.24347.
62. Pasdaran A, Hassani B, Tavakoli A, Kozuharova E, Hamedi A. A review of the potential benefits of herbal medicines, small molecules of natural sources, and supplements for health promotion in lupus conditions. Life (Basel). 2023;13(7):1589. https://doi.org/10.3390/life13071589.
63. Abdul Rashid AM, Abd Ghani F, Inche Mat LN, et al. Herbal medication triggering lupus nephritis - a case report. BMC Complement Med Ther. 2020;20:163. https://doi.org/10.1186/s12906-020-02971-y.

64. Wang H, Wang B, Huang J, Yang Z, Song Z, Zhu Q, Xie Z, Sun Q, Zhao T. Efficacy and safety of acupuncture therapy combined with conventional pharmacotherapy in the treatment of systemic lupus erythematosus: a systematic review and meta-analysis. Medicine (Baltimore). 2023;102(40):e35418. https://doi.org/10.1097/MD.0000000000035418.
65. Josefson A, Kreuter M. Acupuncture to reduce nausea during chemotherapy treatment of rheumatic diseases. Rheumatology (Oxford). 2003;42(10):1149–54.
66. Damanhouri LH. Vitamin D deficiency in Saudi patients with systemic lupus erythematosus. Saudi Med J. 2009;30(10):1291–5.
67. Attar SM, Siddiqui AM. Vitamin D deficiency in patients with systemic lupus erythematosus. Oman Med J. 2013;28(1):42–7. https://doi.org/10.5001/omj.2013.10.
68. Ali N, Alalawi F. Vitamin D status and SLE disease activity among Dubai Hospital lupus patients. Eur J Clin Med. 2023;4(2):18–24. https://doi.org/10.24018/clinicmed.2023.4.2.251.
69. Ruiz-Irastorza G, Gordo S, Olivares N, Egurbide MV, Aguirre C. Changes in vitamin D levels in patients with systemic lupus erythematosus: effects on fatigue, disease activity, and damage. Arthritis Care Res (Hoboken). 2010;62(8):1160–5. https://doi.org/10.1002/acr.20186.
70. Petri M, Bello KJ, Fang H, Magder LS. Vitamin D in systemic lupus erythematosus: modest association with disease activity and the urine protein-to-creatinine ratio. Arthritis Rheum. 2013;65(7):1865–71. https://doi.org/10.1002/art.37953.
71. Andreoli L, Dall'Ara F, Piantoni S, Zanola A, Piva N, Cutolo M, Tincani A. A 24-month prospective study on the efficacy and safety of two different monthly regimens of vitamin D supplementation in pre-menopausal women with systemic lupus erythematosus. Lupus. 2015;24(4–5):499–506. https://doi.org/10.1177/0961203314559089.
72. Lima GL, Paupitz J, Aikawa NE, Takayama L, Bonfa E, Pereira RM. Vitamin D supplementation in adolescents and young adults with juvenile systemic lupus erythematosus for improvement in disease activity and fatigue scores: a randomized, double-blind, Placebo-Controlled Trial Arthritis Care Res (Hoboken). 2016;68(1):91–8. https://doi.org/10.1002/acr.22621.
73. Karimzadeh H, Shirzadi M, Karimifar M. The effect of Vitamin D supplementation in disease activity of systemic lupus erythematosus patients with Vitamin D deficiency: a randomized clinical trial. J Res Med Sci. 2017;22(1):4.
74. Wahono CS, Diah Setyorini C, Kalim H, Nurdiana N, Handono K. Effect of *Curcuma xanthorrhiza* supplementation on systemic lupus erythematosus patients with hypovitamin D which were given vitamin D_3 towards disease activity (SLEDAI), IL-6, and TGF-β1 serum. Int J Rheumatol. 2017;2017:7687053. https://doi.org/10.1155/2017/7687053.
75. Al-Kushi AG, Azzeh FS, Header EA, ElSawy NA, Hijazi HH, Jazar AS, Ghaith MM, Alarjah MA. Effect of vitamin D and calcium supplementation in patients with systemic lupus erythematosus. Saudi J Med Med Sci. 2018;6(3):137–42. https://doi.org/10.4103/sjmms.sjmms_134_17.
76. Rifa'i A, Kalim H, Kusworini K, Wahono CS. Effect of vitamin D supplementation on disease activity (SLEDAI) and fatigue in systemic lupus erythematosus patients with hypovitaminosis D: An open clinical trial. Indones J Rheumatol. 2018;8(2).
77. Pakchotanon R, Lomarat W, Narongroeknawin P, Chaiamnuay S, Asavatanabodee P. Randomized double-blind controlled trial to evaluate efficacy of vitamin D supplementation among patients with systemic lupus erythematosus. J Southeast Asian Med Res. 2020;4(1):24–32. https://doi.org/10.55374/jseamed.v4i1.57.
78. Magro R, Saliba C, Camilleri L, Scerri C, Borg AA. Vitamin D supplementation in systemic lupus erythematosus: relationship to disease activity, fatigue and the interferon signature gene expression. BMC Rheumatol. 2021;5(1):53. https://doi.org/10.1186/s41927-021-00223-1.
79. Irfan SA, Ali AA, Shabbir N, Altaf H, Ahmed A, Thamara Kunnath J, Divya Boorle NVL, Miguel AK, Loh CC, Gandrakota N, Ali Baig MM. Effects of vitamin D on systemic lupus erythematosus disease activity and autoimmunity: a systematic review and meta-analysis. Cureus. 2022;14(6):e25896. https://doi.org/10.7759/cureus.25896. PMID: 35844337; PMCID: PMC9278795.

80. Wright SA, O'Prey FM, McHenry MT, Leahey WJ, Devine AB, Duffy EM, et al. A randomised interventional trial of omega-3-polyunsaturated fatty acids on endothelial function and disease activity in systemic lupus erythematosus. Ann Rheum Dis 2008;67(6):841–848. doi:https://doi.org/10.1136/ard.2007.077156.
81. Duarte-García A, Myasoedova E, Karmacharya P, Hocaoğlu M, Murad MH, Warrington KJ, Crowson CS. Effect of omega-3 fatty acids on systemic lupus erythematosus disease activity: a systematic review and meta-analysis. Autoimmun Rev. 2020;19(12):102688. https://doi.org/10.1016/j.autrev.2020.102688.
82. Macfarlane GJ, Kronisch C, Dean LE, Atzeni F, Häuser W, Fluß E, et al. EULAR revised recommendations for the management of fibromyalgia. Ann Rheum Dis. 2017;76(2):318–28. https://doi.org/10.1136/annrheumdis-2016-209724.
83. El Miedany Y, Gadallah N, Mohasseb D, Gaballah NM, El Zohiery AK, Hassan M, et al. Consensus evidence-based clinical practice recommendations for the management of fibromyalgia. Egypt Rheumatol Rehabil. 2022;49:30. https://doi.org/10.1186/s43166-022-00129-x. Erratum in: Egypt Rheumatol Rehabil. 2022;49:38. doi:10.1186/s43166-022-00137-x.
84. Ye G, Miao R, Chen J, Huang J, Jiang M. Effectiveness of complementary and alternative medicine in fibromyalgia syndrome: a network meta-analysis. J Pain Res. 2024;17:305–19. https://doi.org/10.2147/JPR.S439906.
85. Pfalzgraf AR, Lobo CP, Giannetti V, Jones KD. Use of complementary and alternative medicine in fibromyalgia: results of an online survey. Pain Manag Nurs. 2020;21(6):516–22.
86. Cao H, Liu J, Lewith GT. Traditional Chinese Medicine for treatment of fibromyalgia: a systematic review of randomized controlled trials. J Altern Complement Med. 2010;16(4):397–409. https://doi.org/10.1089/acm.2009.0599.
87. Cao H, Li X, Han M, Liu J. Acupoint stimulation for fibromyalgia: a systematic review of randomized controlled trials. Evid Based Complement Alternat Med. 2013;2013:362831. https://doi.org/10.1155/2013/362831.
88. Sagy I, Bar-Lev Schleider L, Abu-Shakra M, Novack V. Safety and efficacy of medical cannabis in fibromyalgia. J Clin Med. 2019;8(6):807. https://doi.org/10.3390/jcm8060807.
89. Habib G, Artul S. Medical cannabis for the treatment of fibromyalgia. J Clin Rheumatol. 2018;24:255–8.
90. Senftleber NK, Nielsen SM, Andersen JR, Bliddal H, Tarp S, Lauritzen L, et al. Marine oil supplements for arthritis pain: a systematic review and meta-analysis of randomized trials. Nutrients. 2017;9(1):42. https://doi.org/10.3390/nu9010042.
91. Dai Z, Lu N, Niu J, et al. Dietary fiber intake in relation to knee pain trajectory. Arthritis Care Res (Hoboken). 2017;69(9):1331–9. https://doi.org/10.1002/acr.23158.
92. Lu B, Driban JB, Xu C, et al. Dietary fat intake and radiographic progression of knee osteoarthritis: data from the osteoarthritis initiative. Arthritis Care Res (Hoboken). 2017;69(3):368–75. https://doi.org/10.1002/acr.22952.
93. Mobasher S, Badr Eldin A, El-Zohiery A, Ibrahim S, Mohamed M, Abdalla A. Acupuncture versus homeopathy as a complementary therapy in patients with knee osteoarthritis. Egypt J Rheumatol Clin Immunol. 2014;2(1):45–51.
94. Noack W, Fischer M, Förster KK, Rovati LC, Setnikar I. Glucosamine sulfate in osteoarthritis of the knee. Osteoarthr Cartil. 1994;2(1):51–9. https://doi.org/10.1016/s1063-4584(05)80006-8.
95. Pavelká K, Gatterová J, Olejarová M, Machacek S, Giacovelli G, Rovati LC. Glucosamine sulfate use and delay of progression of knee osteoarthritis: a 3-year, randomized, placebo-controlled, double-blind study. Arch Intern Med. 2002;162(18):2113–23. https://doi.org/10.1001/archinte.162.18.2113.
96. Bannuru RR, Osani MC, Vaysbrot EE, Arden NK, Bennell K, Bierma-Zeinstra SMA, et al. OARSI guidelines for the non-surgical management of knee, hip, and polyarticular osteoarthritis. Osteoarthr Cartil. 2019;27(11):1578–89. https://doi.org/10.1016/j.joca.2019.06.011.

97. Gwinnutt JM, Wieczorek M, Rodríguez-Carrio J, Balanescu A, Bischoff-Ferrari HA, Boonen A, et al. Effects of diet on the outcomes of rheumatic and musculoskeletal diseases (RMDs): systematic review and meta-analyses informing the 2021 EULAR recommendations for lifestyle improvements in people with RMDs. RMD Open. 2022;8(2):e002167. https://doi.org/10.1136/rmdopen-2021-002167.
98. Conrozier T, Lohse T. Glucosamine as a treatment for osteoarthritis: what if it's true? Front Pharmacol. 2022;13.
99. Hammad YH, Magid HR, Sobhy MM. Clinical and biochemical study of the comparative efficacy of topical versus oral glucosamine/chondroitin sulfate on osteoarthritis of the knee. Egypt Rheumatol. 2015;37(2):85–91.
100. Manyanga T, Froese M, Zarychanski R, Abou-Setta A, Friesen C, Tennenhouse M, et al. Pain management with acupuncture in osteoarthritis: a systematic review and meta-analysis. BMC Complement Altern Med. 2014;14:312. https://doi.org/10.1186/1472-6882-14-312.
101. Li J-Q, Guo W, Sun Z-G, Huang QS, Lee EY, Wang Y, et al. Cupping therapy for treating knee osteoarthritis: the evidence from systematic review and meta-analysis. Complement Ther Clin Pract. 2017;28:152–60.
102. Wang Y-L, An C-M, Song S, Lei F-L, Wang Y. Cupping therapy for knee osteoarthritis: a synthesis of evidence. Complement Med Res. 2018;25(4):249–5.
103. Zhang Li-Hui ZY-C, Zhang Li-Hui ZY-C. Systematic evaluation and meta-analysis of acupuncture and collaterals cupping therapy for Knee Osteoarthritis. TMR Mod Herb Med. 2019;2(1):36–47.
104. El Gendy A, Monir R, Zikri EN, Ali MA, Abdel-Wahhab KG, Fouad S, et al. Therapeutic effectiveness of oral homeopathic remedy in management of knee osteoarthritis via attenuation of oxidative and inflammatory pathway. Egyptian Pharm J. 2024.
105. Perkins K, Sahy W, Beckett RD. Efficacy of curcuma for treatment of osteoarthritis. J Evid Based Complement Altern Med. 2016;22(1):156–65.
106. Niggemann B, Grüber C. Side-effects of complementary and alternative medicine. Allergy. 2003;58(8):707–16.
107. Ballotin VR, Bigarella LG, Brandão ABM, Balbinot RA, Balbinot SS, Soldera J. Herb-induced liver injury: systematic review and meta-analysis. World J Clin Cases. 2021;9(20):5490–513. https://doi.org/10.12998/wjcc.v9.i20.5490.

Chapter 28
War, Conflict, and Rheumatic Diseases in the Arab World

Sami Salman, Sima Abu Al-Saoud, Arwa Aljohi, Ziryab Imad Taha Mahmoud, Khalid A. Alnaqbi, and Mira Merashli

Abstract War and violence have become part of daily life in many areas of the Middle East and North Africa (MENA), including some Arab countries, with profound consequences for both mental and physical health.

Civil wars, prolonged political instability, large-scale refugee crises, the COVID-19 pandemic, and escalating economic challenges in several low- and

S. Salman
College of Medicine, University of Baghdad, Baghdad, Iraq
e-mail: ssshihab2@gmail.com

S. A. Al-Saoud
Department of Pediatrics, Division of Pediatric Rheumatology, Al-Quds University, Faculty of Medicine, Makassed Hospital, Jerusalem, Palestine
e-mail: ssaud@staff.alquds.edu

A. Aljohi
Rheumatology and Rehabilitation, Alsheikh Othman polyclinic, Aden, Yemen
e-mail: aljohiarwa@gmail.com

Z. I. T. Mahmoud
Department of Internal Medicine, University of Bahri, Khartoum, Sudan

Merowe Medical City, Merowe, Sudan
e-mail: Ziryab2008@yahoo.com

K. A. Alnaqbi
Division of Rheumatology, Sheikh Tahnoon bin Mohammed Medical City, SEHA / PureHealth, Al Ain, UAE

Internal Medicine Department, College of Medicine & Health Sciences, UAE University, Al Ain, UAE

College of Medicine, RAK Medical and Health Sciences University, Ras Al Khaimah, UAE
e-mail: kalnaqbi@gmail.com

M. Merashli (✉)
Department of Internal Medicine, Division of Rheumatology, American University of Beirut, Beirut, Lebanon
e-mail: mm116@aub.edu.lb

K. A. Alnaqbi, G. Aldabie (eds.), *Rheumatic Diseases in the Arab World*,
https://doi.org/10.1007/978-981-92-0967-5_28

middle-income countries across the region have had catastrophic effects on population health. Physicians working in conflict settings have been forced to fundamentally alter their practice, often rationing limited resources, working in primitive conditions, and adapting treatment approaches under extreme constraints. Data specifically addressing rheumatic diseases in the Arab world during periods of war and conflict remains scarce. Nevertheless, rates of non-communicable diseases and their associated risk factors, including musculoskeletal disorders, have steadily increased across the MENA region over recent decades.

Rheumatologists in conflict-affected Arab countries frequently report increases in post-infectious reactive arthritis, complex regional pain syndrome, post-traumatic musculoskeletal injuries, and stress-related fibromyalgia. However, these trends remain insufficiently documented in the literature. Treatment interruptions, disruption of vaccination programs, destruction of sanitation infrastructure, increased disease burden, reduced access to healthcare facilities, and shortages of healthcare professionals due to migration have collectively had devastating effects on already fragile health systems.

Public health policies and responses by international health organizations have often been slow and insufficiently aligned with the complex social, economic, and political realities faced by countries in the MENA region.

To mitigate the health consequences of war, each country requires a tailored and adaptable healthcare strategy, supported by continuous monitoring and evaluation. At the same time, sustained diplomatic efforts remain essential to prevent conflict and to protect populations from the profound and lasting health consequences of war.

Keywords Armed conflict · Rheumatic and musculoskeletal diseases · Health systems · Arab countries · Noncommunicable diseases · Health services accessibility · Refugees · Conflict-affected settings · COVID-19

28.1 Introduction

The Arab world comprises 22 countries that together form the League of Arab States. These countries can be classified according to their economic characteristics as well as their geographic location [1]. From a geographic perspective, Arab states are commonly grouped into four regions. The Gulf Cooperation Council (GCC) includes Bahrain, Kuwait, Oman, Qatar, Saudi Arabia, and the United Arab Emirates. The Eastern Arab region (Mashriq) includes Jordan, Iraq, Syria, Lebanon, Palestine, and Egypt. North Africa (the Maghreb) comprises Algeria, Libya, Mauritania, Morocco, and Tunisia. The southern group includes Yemen, Djibouti, Somalia, Comoros, and Sudan.

The population of the Arab nations in 2024 is estimated at over 492.6 million people, representing approximately 6% of the world's population [2, 3]. Collectively,

Arab countries contribute around 5% of global gross domestic product (GDP), reflecting substantial demographic weight but a relatively modest share of global economic output [4].

Despite the common historical, cultural, linguistic, and religious backgrounds of the Arab region, deep patterns of division and polarization exist across many Arab countries, largely driven by political, geographical, and sociological differences. Notably, suffering in the Arab world has arisen from both internal and external pressures [1].

In this context, liberation from colonization following the Second World War came at a high cost for many Arab countries. The long-term consequences have affected multiple sectors, including education, healthcare, and economic development. Prolonged conflicts, often linked to disputes over land and identity, have contributed to persistent instability. As a result, humanitarian consequences have included large-scale displacement, economic hardship, and increased mortality and morbidity [5].

Consequently, the burden of non-communicable diseases (NCDs) has risen across the Arab world, contributing to a growing global health impact. This includes an increased prevalence of rheumatic and musculoskeletal diseases (RMDs), mental health disorders, and post-traumatic health injuries [6].

The consequences of war on health are diverse. Violence leads not only to death and physical and psychosocial disabilities but also to indirect effects such as displacement, loss of livelihood, and deterioration of living conditions. These factors, in turn, have a profound impact on access to healthcare.

This chapter explores how war and protracted conflict affect the organization and delivery of care for patients with RMDs in selected Arab countries. Based on the authors' experience and the best available evidence, we focus on Palestine, Lebanon, Syria, Iraq, Yemen, Sudan, and Somalia, where conflict-related disruption has significantly strained healthcare systems and access to specialty care.

28.2 Challenges Facing Rheumatic Care in Conflict-Affected Regions

The Arab Spring, which began in late 2010, along with subsequent conflicts, has affected nearly all countries in the MENA region [7]. While much of the attention has focused on security and political developments, these events have had profound consequences for population health. Immediate impacts include deaths and injuries, large-scale population displacement, and damage to essential infrastructure, leading to restricted access to healthcare facilities. In addition, conflicts have resulted in increased psychological stress and mental health disorders, shortages of medical supplies, and major disruptions to medical training and education at all levels. Addressing these challenges requires targeted efforts to strengthen health systems and develop sustainable solutions to improve healthcare delivery in conflict-affected Arab countries [8].

28.2.1 Palestine

Rheumatology practice in Palestine, similar to other developing countries in the region, faces numerous challenges related to the healthcare system, medical workforce, availability of medications, political instability, access to healthcare services, and limited research funding. Additionally, the interruption of electricity with frequent power cuts and shortage of fuel affected the functionality of the health services [9–11].

28.2.1.1 Healthcare System

The Palestinian healthcare system operates under persistent structural constraints that limit its capacity to deliver comprehensive and equitable care [10, 12]. Health infrastructure remains fragile, characterized by a limited number of hospital beds, chronic shortages of essential medications, insufficient medical equipment, and constrained diagnostic and therapeutic services [10, 12]. These challenges affect healthcare accessibility across the West Bank, Gaza Strip, and East Jerusalem, with disparities particularly pronounced in conflict-affected and underserved areas [10, 12, 13]. These system constraints may contribute to delayed diagnosis and treatment initiation, potentially increasing disease burden among patients with RMDs.

Healthcare services in the Palestinian territory are delivered through four main providers: the Palestinian Ministry of Health (MoH), the United Nations Relief and Works Agency for Palestine Refugees in the Near East (UNRWA), Palestinian non-governmental organizations (NGOs), and the private sector [14]. The Palestinian MoH, established in 1994 following the Oslo Accords, serves as the primary provider of public healthcare services, particularly primary care, and plays a central role in health system governance and planning. UNRWA, established in 1949, continues to provide essential health services to registered Palestinian refugees, particularly through its primary healthcare network. Following the October 2023 war in Gaza, however, severe operational disruptions have significantly affected UNRWA's service capacity, resulting in marked disruption of services and reduced access to many health centers, particularly in Gaza [15]. Palestinian NGOs and the private sector complement these services, with NGOs playing a particularly important role in service delivery, especially in the Gaza Strip [14]. Variability in coverage and service delivery across providers may hinder the implementation of standardized treatment protocols, particularly for patients with chronic diseases requiring continuous pharmacologic management. Furthermore, the large refugee population places additional strain on an already weakened healthcare system, disproportionately affecting patients with RMDs who require long-term monitoring and sustained access to specialized therapies.

Ongoing political instability, movement restrictions, and recurrent episodes of armed conflict have further strained the healthcare system, resulting in damage to health facilities, disruption of supply chains, and limitations on the availability of specialized services. Recent assessments by international health agencies have highlighted worsening shortages of medical supplies, constrained referral pathways, and increasing pressure on already limited healthcare resources. These systemic challenges collectively undermine the continuity and quality of care for patients with chronic diseases, including RMDs.

28.2.1.2 Health Workforce

The health workforce in Palestine is limited, particularly in rheumatology. Overall physician density is estimated at 2.8 per 1000 population [16], with only 18 practicing rheumatology specialists serving a population of over five million; most rheumatologists are based in the West Bank and East Jerusalem. Pediatric rheumatology care was introduced relatively recently, in 2017, and is currently provided by only two pediatric rheumatologists nationwide.

Palestine also faces a persistent shortage of nurses, driven by long-standing resource constraints and challenging working conditions. Studies report widespread understaffing, heavy workloads, and limited infrastructure across healthcare settings. The density of nurses and midwives is estimated at 25.7 per 10,000 population, which remains below the national Sustainable Development Goal target of 39, with the Ministry of Health serving as the primary employer of the nursing workforce [17]. There are currently no rheumatology nurse practitioners or rheumatology assistants.

Rheumatology education and training capacity remain insufficient to meet population needs. A formal rheumatology training program was established in 2017, but it has the capacity to train only one physician per year. Combined with limited resources and restricted access to essential medications, including several biologic therapies, these workforce constraints continue to affect the optimal management of patients with RMDs.

28.2.1.3 Accessibility to Healthcare

Access to rheumatology care in Palestine remains constrained. Most rheumatologists are concentrated in major urban centers, which limits access to specialized care for patients living in rural areas. In addition, a substantial proportion of advanced and tertiary healthcare services, including subspecialty care, are centralized in East Jerusalem. For patients from the West Bank and Gaza Strip, reaching these facilities often requires going through complex permit systems, checkpoints, and physical barriers, resulting in long travel times, financial burden, and missed appointments [13].

Movement restrictions have a particularly severe impact on patients from the Gaza Strip. According to World Health Organization (WHO) monitoring, a large proportion of patient referrals from Gaza are directed to East Jerusalem hospitals, yet access is frequently delayed or denied through the permit system. In recent years, permit approval rates for Gaza patients have declined to approximately 60%, while only 34% of companion permit applications have been approved, resulting in many patients missing scheduled appointments due to delayed responses, security interviews, or permit denials [13]. These barriers significantly affect continuity of care, follow-up, and disease monitoring for patients with chronic RMDs. Following the October 2023 war in Gaza, however, referral pathways to East Jerusalem and other tertiary centers in the West Bank were halted, further limiting access to specialized care and advanced therapeutic services for patients with chronic RMDs.

In addition to geographic and political barriers, the financial burden of rheumatology care places further strain on patients and their families. Similar to other chronic diseases, most patients with RMDs require regular follow-up visits and routine laboratory monitoring, leading to cumulative out-of-pocket costs over time [14]. Supportive services essential to disease management, such as physiotherapy and occupational therapy, represent an additional societal burden, as these services are often not fully covered by health insurance, even when available. The October 7, 2023, war in Gaza resulted in significant fatalities and long-term disabilities, further increasing pressure on the healthcare system and complicating healthcare service delivery [18, 19]. Together, these barriers undermine continuity of care and long-term disease management for patients with chronic rheumatic conditions.

28.2.1.4 Psychosocial Impact and Mental Health

The ramifications of the long conflict on health are profound. In addition to the rising toll of deaths, injuries, and long-term disabilities, many patients suffer from significant psychological distress, mental health-related problems, and chronic pain syndrome associated with chronic exposure to violence, insecurity, and social adversity [9]. In a study conducted in 2013, Palestine was reported to have the highest burden of mental disorders in the Eastern Mediterranean Region [20]. Such psychosocial stressors may exacerbate disease activity, amplify pain perception, and worsen functional impairment in patients with chronic RMDs.

Healthcare professionals also face considerable mental, emotional, and professional strain. During the COVID-19 pandemic, health system pressures, workforce shortages, and scarcity of antirheumatic medications, including biologic therapies, further intensified these difficulties [12, 21]. Prolonged exposure to such conditions contributes to burnout, moral distress, and workforce attrition, ultimately compromising the delivery of specialized rheumatology care.

28.2.1.5 Vaccination

Prior to the escalation of conflict, Palestine maintained high coverage of routine childhood immunization, including polio and measles-containing vaccines, with several antigens reaching coverage levels close to 99% in 2019, according to WHO/

UNICEF estimates. The subsequent decline in vaccination coverage reflects broader disruption of preventive health services and increases the risk of vaccine-preventable disease outbreaks, particularly among patients with RMDs receiving immunosuppressive therapies [22].

Simultaneously, extensive damage to water and sewage systems, contamination of water sources, waste accumulation, overcrowding, and malnutrition have further heightened the transmission of communicable diseases. As a result, outbreaks of scabies, chickenpox, hepatitis A, respiratory, and enteric infections have been reported, alongside the re-emergence of polio [23]. These risks are especially pronounced among vulnerable groups, including children and immunocompromised individuals, such as patients with RMDs, who are more susceptible to infection-related complications.

28.2.1.6 Research

Research addressing RMDs worldwide focuses on countries with high resources, with limited representation from conflict-affected regions [24]. Research in Palestine faces many obstacles, including funding, time, and incentives. Movement restrictions and administrative barriers further complicate data collection and multi-center collaboration. As a result, the true burden and long-term outcomes of patients with RMDs remain under-documented, limiting evidence-based planning and policy development.

28.2.2 Lebanon and Syria

Lebanon and Syria, like Palestine, have been greatly affected by the surrounding conflict in the MENA region. Both countries have endured years of civil war. Current challenges include political instability, hyperinflation, workforce issues, and limited access to healthcare services. The economic crisis and the COVID-19 era have strongly affected medical supplies and storage, as well as access to hospitals and clinics, due to electricity shortages and fuel scarcity [25].

In Lebanon, the management of RMDs has traditionally relied on a broad range of conventional and biologic disease-modifying antirheumatic drugs (DMARDs), with access supported through a combination of public coverage, private insurance, and pharmaceutical assistance programs. However, during periods of political instability, economic collapse, and conflict, the availability of essential medications has been intermittently disrupted [26]. In recent years, there were shortages of commonly used medications, including methotrexate, leflunomide, sulfasalazine, and hydroxychloroquine, resulting in treatment delays, forced substitutions, or interruptions for some patients. These disruptions reflect supply chain instability and financial constraints rather than the absence of therapeutic infrastructure, highlighting the vulnerability of chronic disease management during crises.

Similarly, obstacles to effective rheumatology care include emigration of rheumatologists, a limited number of pediatric rheumatologists in Lebanon and Syria, and constrained financial resources for continuing medical education and research excellence.

In 2013, the Lebanese government estimated that more than 1.5 million Syrian refugees were residing in Lebanon, representing an increase of over 25% in the country's population. However, the healthcare response has remained insufficient, further straining an already overburdened system marked by staffing shortages, limited access to essential medications, and inadequate medical infrastructure [27, 28]. A nearly two-fold increase in services related to vaccination, management of communicable diseases, and NCDs, including hypertension, cardiovascular diseases, diabetes mellitus, chronic respiratory diseases, and arthritis, was documented at the primary healthcare level [29]. According to a study conducted in 2016, the prevalence of NCDs among Syrian refugees in Lebanon was 7.4% for hypertension, 3.8% for chronic lung diseases, 3.3% for diabetes, and 7.9% for arthritis [30]. Additionally, mental health disorders, including post-traumatic stress disorder (PTSD) and depression, as well as infectious diseases like cutaneous leishmaniasis, have been widely reported among the Syrian refugee population [31–33].

The explosion at Beirut port in August 2020, caused by ammonium nitrate, was considered one of the most devastating blasts in recent history. This tragic incident resulted in the loss of over 204 lives, with more than 6500 people injured and approximately 300,000 individuals displaced from their homes. Many of the affected victims continue to experience conditions such as complex regional pain syndrome, post-traumatic stress disorder, depression, and chronic pain syndrome to this day [34].

In Syria, the challenges extend beyond what was previously mentioned. During the height of the Syrian conflict in 2017, there was a significant increase in gunshot and blast-related injuries. More civilians were killed or injured by aircraft than by any other weapon [8, 35]. Numerous factors contribute to the delay in timely surgical care in humanitarian settings, such as security concerns, geographical distances, limited transportation options, restricted access due to checkpoints, and inadequate prehospital stabilization for critical injuries [36]. Consequently, rheumatology colleagues in Syria have observed an increase in patients with complex regional pain syndrome.

Following political developments in late 2024 and 2025, the repatriation of displaced Syrians increased. The United Nations High Commissioner for Refugees (UNHCR) estimated that more than 1.16 million Syrians returned from neighboring countries since December 2024, including over 383,000 from or via Lebanon, contributing to a gradual reduction in registered refugee numbers in host countries [37].

28.2.3 Iraq

During the 1970s and 1980s, Iraq was considered one of the leading Arab countries in providing free universal healthcare services and education. However, decades of armed conflict, economic sanctions, and political instability have resulted in substantial deterioration of the health system. The Iran–Iraq War, the 1991 Gulf War, prolonged international embargoes, and recurrent internal conflicts severely undermined healthcare infrastructure, staffing, and supply chains, leading to chronic shortages of medical personnel and essential medicines [38]. Access to healthcare services became increasingly restricted, with widening geographic disparities in service availability [38].

The public sector remains the principal provider of healthcare services through a nationwide network of primary healthcare centers (PHCCs) and public hospitals, where services are offered at minimal cost. PHCCs deliver primary curative and preventive care and constitute the first point of contact for most patients. Smaller health centers serve rural communities, whereas more advanced and better-equipped centers are concentrated in urban areas. Nevertheless, PHCC performance is significantly constrained by inadequate organizational practices, workforce shortages, and limited pharmaceutical supplies.

Post-2003 recovery efforts resulted in a modest expansion in the number of PHCCs nationally; however, remarkable regional disparities persist. The Kurdistan Region has demonstrated comparatively faster improvements in infrastructure and service delivery than central and southern Iraq [39]. Despite systemic limitations, PHCCs remain a critical healthcare resource, particularly for underprivileged and rural populations.

Patients requiring secondary and tertiary care are referred from PHCCs to public hospitals. However, referral access remains limited due to the inadequate number and uneven distribution of hospitals across governorates. It has been estimated that only approximately 40% of Iraqis have reliable access to referral services [39]. Hospital services are heavily concentrated in major urban centers, and the density of hospital beds remains low, with Iraq ranking among the lowest in hospital bed ratios compared with neighboring countries [40]. These structural constraints restrict timely access to advanced diagnostic and specialized care.

In response to limitations within the public sector, the private healthcare sector has expanded and now provides a growing share of secondary and tertiary services [39]. However, Iraq does not have a formal health insurance system, and private healthcare is predominantly financed through out-of-pocket payments [39, 40]. Although public healthcare services are officially provided free of charge, prolonged conflict and the impact of sanctions significantly reduced service availability and quality. As a result, many patients increasingly turned to private providers, thereby incurring substantial financial burdens [40].

The conflict against the Islamic State of Iraq and the Levant (ISIL) further exacerbated existing vulnerabilities. Widespread destruction and disruption of health facilities left numerous hospitals and clinics unable to provide even basic services, and reconstruction efforts remain incomplete years after liberation [41]. The conflict also triggered massive internal displacement, generating protracted humanitarian and protection needs. Millions of Iraqis were displaced and required life-saving assistance in internally displaced persons (IDP) camps [42]. Conditions in temporary shelters were frequently inadequate, characterized by shortages of safe water, shelter, medicines, and essential services, thereby increasing health risks among displaced populations [43].

The COVID-19 pandemic placed additional strain on an already strained health system. Chronic shortages of medical supplies, insufficient human resources, and prolonged waiting times in public hospitals were further intensified during the pandemic, prompting many patients to seek care in the private sector despite high out-of-pocket costs [44]. In some rheumatology centers, virtual clinics were rapidly implemented to ensure continuity of care for patients with chronic autoimmune and inflammatory diseases, reflecting adaptive strategies in response to system constraints.

Efforts to restore damaged infrastructure and strengthen service delivery are ongoing. The government has formally adopted universal health coverage as a national policy objective, affirming health as a constitutional right and guaranteeing access to healthcare services with minimal financial contribution from citizens [45]. Within rheumatology services, these policy directions have been accompanied by gradual improvements in access to various DMARDs, although disparities in availability persist. In parallel, initial policy measures were introduced to facilitate the reintegration of returning physicians and improve workforce retention through enhanced employment opportunities and financial incentives. Nevertheless, further workforce planning strategies are required to ensure adequate employment opportunities for recent medical graduates and to address persistent staffing gaps across governorates.

28.2.4 Yemen

The prolonged armed conflict in Yemen has severely damaged the country's health infrastructure and drastically reduced the functionality of health facilities [46]. According to the WHO, nearly half of all health facilities in Yemen are only partially functioning or completely out of service due to shortages of staff, medicines, equipment, electricity, and fuel, reflecting the near collapse of the health system and widespread disruption of services [47]. Conflict-related destruction of hospitals, clinics, and support services, along with ongoing economic decline and access barriers, has left millions without adequate medical care and increased the burden of both acute and chronic diseases [48].

The humanitarian crisis has also triggered massive internal displacement, with millions of Yemenis forced to flee their homes into informal settlements and camps where basic services are scarce and access to healthcare is severely limited. Displaced families face compounded vulnerabilities due to damaged infrastructure, inadequate sanitation and hygiene services, and barriers to reaching functioning health facilities [49]. These conditions have significantly increased health risks and further weakened the capacity of the health system to deliver essential services.

Recurrent outbreaks of diarrheal diseases, largely attributed to contaminated water supplies and the collapse of sanitation systems, have been widely reported during the conflict [50]. Enteric infections are established triggers of reactive arthritis, a form of acute infectious-related inflammatory arthritis, and may therefore contribute to additional musculoskeletal morbidity in this population. Yemen has also experienced endemic circulation of viral infections such as dengue fever and chikungunya [51], further increasing the infectious disease burden. Overall, nearly 80% of the country's population, approximately 30 million people, require humanitarian assistance [52].

Primary healthcare services are not adequately equipped to support these patients, necessitating referral to secondary or tertiary healthcare facilities in major cities where rheumatologists are based. The ongoing conflict continues to disrupt medical services and create additional barriers for patients with RMDs seeking care. The closure of healthcare facilities, checkpoints, and fuel shortages significantly affects patients' ability to access necessary medical care. In rural areas, ambulance services for referral patients are often unavailable or ineffective due to chronic fuel shortages [53].

The quality of medicine storage and the availability of essential medicines in both public and private pharmacies have been substantially affected by the ongoing conflict and weakened health infrastructure [54]. Essential medicines were available in only about half of public health outlets, and poorly maintained supply chains, infrastructure damage, and frequent power outages have disrupted cold-chain storage and compromised pharmaceutical services [54]. These deficiencies may contribute to reduced clinical effectiveness of treatments and limit the functionality of care facilities, including those providing services for patients with RMDs. As a result, many patients must pay out of pocket for medications, while access to synthetic DMARDs remains limited, and the high cost of biological therapies makes them largely unaffordable. Some patients who can afford it travel abroad to obtain treatment, while others rely on special requests through private pharmacies.

Healthcare workers, including rheumatologists, have experienced a considerable amount of psychological stress and faced numerous challenges in providing services in such harsh conditions, contributing to internal displacement of qualified staff and voluntary migration outside Yemen [53]. Refugees from conflict-affected areas have reported experiencing PTSD, fibromyalgia, insomnia, and anxiety, highlighting the urgent need for mental health support [55].

Yemen is also experiencing significant setbacks in education, research, and medical training. The current political instability, economic decline, and ongoing conflict pose major obstacles to establishing and sustaining specialty training programs, including rheumatology. In addition, access to medical textbooks, scientific journals, and online academic resources remains limited, further constraining medical education and research development [56].

28.2.5 Sudan

Sudan's prolonged armed conflicts have had a profound impact on population health and economic stability. The Second Sudanese Civil War (1983–2005) resulted in an estimated one to two million deaths and the displacement of millions of civilians across southern Sudan [57, 58]. The prolonged conflict severely damaged infrastructure, disrupted livelihoods, and contributed to recurrent famine crises.

In response to widespread famine and civilian suffering, Operation Lifeline Sudan (OLS) was established in 1989 under United Nations auspices as a coordinated humanitarian mechanism [58, 59]. OLS functioned as a UN "umbrella" structure bringing together the United Nations Children's Fund (UNICEF), the World Food Programme (WFP), and numerous international and local non-governmental organizations to deliver humanitarian assistance to populations in both government-held and rebel-held areas [60]. This arrangement was considered unprecedented in a civil war context, as it permitted cross-line humanitarian access under negotiated agreements.

Over the years, OLS coordinated emergency airlifts, food distribution, vaccination campaigns, and basic health services delivery in remote and conflict-affected areas where road access was limited or unsafe [60]. Despite these efforts, repeated cycles of armed conflict continued to disrupt health services, agricultural production, and economic stability.

More recently, the 2023 armed conflict has again severely affected Sudan's health system and economy. The ongoing conflict has resulted in contraction of economic activity, widespread displacement, food insecurity, destruction of health facilities, shortages of medical supplies, and disruption of essential public services [61]. The humanitarian crisis has further strained an already fragile healthcare infrastructure, limiting access to treatment for chronic and acute diseases alike.

These developments have occurred in a system already challenged by long-standing weaknesses in financing, workforce retention, and equitable service distribution. As a result, patients with chronic diseases, including RMDs, face additional barriers to diagnosis, follow-up, and access to essential therapies. Reduced public investment in health and interruptions in supply chains have further compromised continuity of care [61]. Moreover, disruptions in medical education and postgraduate training have contributed to a persistent shortage of skilled healthcare professionals, further limiting service capacity [62].

28.2.5.1 Rheumatology Care During Conflict

Patients with RMDs have been disproportionately affected during periods of conflict, as outpatient clinics were intermittently closed and access to essential medications and follow-up investigations was compromised. The absence of comprehensive health insurance further exacerbated the situation, given the relatively high cost of disease-modifying therapies and biologic agents.

Both patients and healthcare professionals in Sudan continue to face significant logistical and financial challenges. The ongoing economic crisis, compounded by political instability and supply chain disruptions, has limited timely diagnosis and continuity of care, thereby increasing the risk of disease progression, irreversible joint damage, long-term comorbidities, and avoidable complications.

28.2.5.2 Infections

Chikungunya has emerged as an important public health challenge in Sudan in recent years. On 31 May 2018, the state ministry of health in the Red Sea State reported the first four suspected cases of chikungunya fever. The outbreak expanded rapidly over the following months and became the largest chikungunya outbreak ever documented in the country. Between May 2018 and March 2019, a total of 48,763 cases were reported nationwide, with almost all cases occurring in Kassala and Red Sea States in eastern Sudan, while smaller outbreaks and sporadic cases were documented in several other states [63]. WHO also reported the rapid geographic spread of the outbreak in 2018 and highlighted its public health significance [64].

Chikungunya virus infection is transmitted by Aedes mosquitoes, particularly *Aedes aegypti*. Clinically, it presents with an acute onset of fever and severe arthralgia. Although the acute illness is often self-limiting, musculoskeletal symptoms may persist in a substantial proportion of patients. Chronic manifestations most commonly include persistent polyarthralgia, and in some cases, chronic inflammatory arthritis, tenosynovitis, and enthesopathy have been described, creating diagnostic and management challenges for rheumatologists [65].

In addition to chikungunya, rheumatologists practicing in Sudan face further diagnostic complexity because several endemic infectious diseases can mimic RMDs. Tuberculosis, malaria, dengue, and other viral infections may present with fever, arthralgia, or inflammatory features, often requiring extensive evaluation to distinguish infectious from autoimmune etiologies [63, 65].

The COVID-19 pandemic placed an additional burden on Sudan's already weakened health system. SARS-CoV-2 was first confirmed in Sudan in March 2020, and response measures diverted limited resources toward emergency care, reducing access to routine health services [66]. Across low-resource settings, the pandemic disrupted outpatient clinics, limited laboratory capacity, and created barriers to the diagnosis and follow-up of chronic conditions [67]. Rheumatology services across Africa were similarly affected, with reduced specialist access and delays in treatment continuity [68]. In Sudan, these pressures further restricted care for non-COVID conditions, particularly among vulnerable and chronically ill patients [69]. Although post-COVID inflammatory manifestations, including reactive and inflammatory arthritis, were increasingly reported [70], the more pressing challenge during the pandemic was preserving continuity of care amid severe resource constraints.

28.2.6 Somalia

Decades of protracted conflict, political instability, and recurrent humanitarian crises have profoundly affected Somalia's health system, limiting its ability to deliver consistent care for chronic NCDs, including RMDs. Health service delivery in

Somalia remains fragmented and heavily dependent on external donor support, rendering essential services vulnerable to insecurity, funding interruptions, and workforce shortages. According to the WHO, sustaining even basic health services in Somalia is challenging under these conditions, with chronic disease care often deprioritized during acute emergencies [71, 72].

Similar to other conflict-affected settings in the Arab region, Somalia's prolonged instability has delayed diagnosis and disrupted continuity of care for patients with chronic RMDs. Humanitarian assessments in Somalia consistently report that such barriers disproportionately affect individuals requiring long-term treatment rather than episodic care, increasing the risk of disease flares, irreversible damage, and disability [73].

Effective RMD management depends on access to diagnostic laboratories, imaging, rehabilitation services, and structured referral pathways. These components are often absent, unaffordable, or concentrated in urban centers [74]. To our knowledge, there are currently no formally trained rheumatologists practicing in Somalia. Consequently, patients with RMDs are likely managed within general medical services, frequently at primary or secondary care levels with limited resources. The absence of specialist-led services restricts access to advanced diagnostics, structured follow-up, and multidisciplinary care. In such settings, chronic inflammatory diseases are typically managed according to the capacity of general medical services and the availability of essential medicines rather than through dedicated rheumatology pathways. This situation reflects broader challenges in addressing NCDs in Somalia, where health systems have historically focused on infectious diseases and emergency care [75].

Emerging analyses suggest that pragmatic, context-adapted strategies may help mitigate these gaps. Integrating basic musculoskeletal and inflammatory arthritis care into primary healthcare and humanitarian clinics, task-sharing with trained general clinicians, ensuring availability of a core list of essential medicines, and using simplified monitoring protocols are among the most feasible approaches in Somalia's current context. Long-term improvement, however, depends on health system recovery efforts that strengthen governance, workforce capacity, and service integration, which are critical prerequisites for sustainable rheumatology care in post-conflict and fragile settings [72, 76].

Across the reviewed countries, several recurring structural challenges emerged that collectively undermine the delivery of rheumatic care; these cross-cutting themes are summarized in Table 28.1.

Table 28.1 Common challenges affecting rheumatic care in conflict-affected Arab countries

Domain	Observed pattern across countries	Key implications for rheumatic care
Health System Barriers		
Infrastructure	Damage to hospitals and clinics, electricity interruptions, limited internet connectivity, and reduced rehabilitation capacity.	Limits the ability to deliver consistent outpatient and inpatient rheumatology services.
Diagnostics	Restricted access to laboratory testing, imaging services, and structured referral pathways.	Delays diagnosis and disease monitoring, increasing the risk of irreversible joint damage.
Medicines	Disrupted pharmaceutical supply chains resulting in recurrent shortages of rheumatic medications and very limited access to biologic agents and targeted synthetic therapies.	Patients unable to maintain disease-modifying therapy, leading to disease flares and disability.
Human Capital Barriers		
Workforce	Migration of specialists, workforce attrition, and unsafe working conditions.	Severe shortage of rheumatologists in conflict-affected regions, reducing access to specialist care.
Training & Education	Interrupted medical education and limited continuing professional development opportunities.	Weakens long-term capacity to train and retain rheumatology specialists.
Economic and Policy Barriers		
Financial Barriers	Limited insurance coverage, high out-of-pocket costs, and donor-dependent service provision.	Catastrophic health expenditure for patients; fragile, unsustainable service models.
Chronic Disease Care	Deprioritization of non-communicable diseases during acute emergencies and humanitarian crises.	Rheumatic diseases overlooked in emergency health responses, worsening long-term outcomes.

28.3 Strategies to Strengthen Rheumatic Care in Conflict-Affected Areas of the Arab World

Despite the contextual differences between countries, shared structural challenges are evident. Across all reviewed countries, common themes emerged: workforce attrition, medicine shortages, inequitable access to specialist care, and disrupted training. These recurring patterns highlight the need for coordinated regional strategies tailored to fragile and conflict-affected settings.

Strengthening rheumatic care in conflict-affected settings requires coordinated policy, infrastructure, workforce, and research initiatives. A central priority is the development of regionally adapted, standardized guidelines for the management of RMDs, alongside guaranteed access to essential medications such as methotrexate, colchicine, leflunomide, sulfasalazine, and hydroxychloroquine. Ensuring consistent availability of these core therapies is fundamental to preventing irreversible disease damage and disability.

Although biologic therapies are indicated for selected RMDs, their high cost presents a substantial barrier in fragile and resource-limited settings. Promoting the regulated use of biosimilars, supported by clear national prescribing policies, may enhance affordability while maintaining safety and efficacy.

In areas affected by active conflict, innovative service delivery models may be necessary. Establishing specialized care hubs in relatively stable neighboring regions, protected humanitarian zones, or cross-border referral centers may allow patients continued access to advanced diagnostics and specialist expertise [77]. Comparable approaches have been implemented in oncology, where cross-border and regional cancer care initiatives have provided continuity of treatment for patients displaced by conflict [78]. Adapting similar models to rheumatology could help mitigate service disruptions during periods of instability.

While sustainable improvement in rheumatic care ultimately depends on political stability and the resolution of armed conflict, health system recovery efforts must also include strategic investment in data and service evaluation. Once basic security and infrastructure are restored, the establishment of rheumatology registries and real-world studies can support objective assessment of disease burden, treatment gaps, and outcomes. Such data are essential for guiding continuous quality improvement and informing long-term regional policy decisions during post-conflict rebuilding.

Workforce sustainability remains a cornerstone of long-term reform. Competitive remuneration, improved working conditions, and structured opportunities for continuing medical education are necessary to reduce outward migration and workforce attrition among rheumatologists. Strategic efforts to train and retain specialists, particularly in underserved areas, are essential for ensuring service continuity. Notably, the marked shortage of trained pediatric rheumatologists across the Arab region warrants urgent strategic investment.

Ultimately, strengthening rheumatic care in conflict settings requires coordinated, system-level approaches that align broader health system recovery with specialty-specific needs. Figure 28.1 summarizes the key strategies to improve rheumatic care in conflict-affected Arab countries.

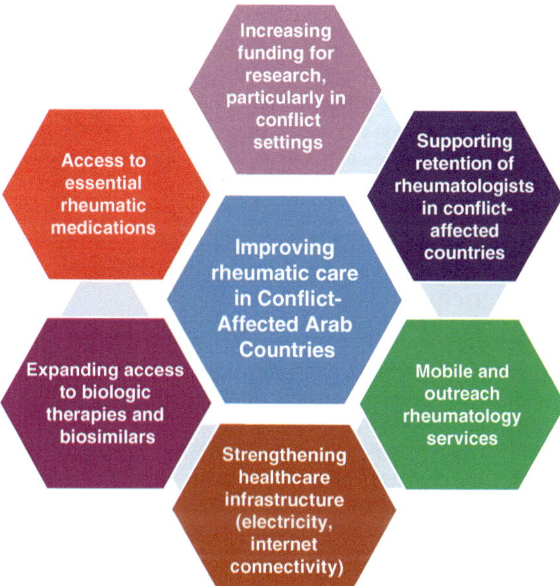

Fig. 28.1 Key strategies to improve rheumatic care in conflict-affected Arab countries

28.4 Conclusion

Across all reviewed countries, recurring patterns of workforce attrition, medicine shortages, and disrupted continuity of care highlight the fragility of chronic rheumatic disease management in conflict-affected settings. Armed conflict and prolonged instability have weakened health systems and disproportionately affected patients with rheumatic and musculoskeletal diseases (RMDs), compromising infrastructure, workforce capacity, training, and access to essential therapies.

Beyond immediate traumatic injuries, conflict environments are associated with rising burdens of non-communicable diseases (NCDs), infectious triggers of inflammatory arthritis, psychological distress, and long-term disability. Treatment interruptions, supply chain instability, healthcare worker migration, and financial hardship further undermine outcomes for patients with chronic RMDs.

Strengthening rheumatic care in fragile contexts requires pragmatic short-term strategies to preserve access to essential medications and maintain service delivery, alongside sustained long-term health system recovery focused on workforce development, equitable financing, and integration of rheumatology within broader NCD frameworks. Durable progress ultimately depends on stability, effective governance, and sustained efforts toward peace. Although this chapter centers on Arab countries, the lessons outlined are applicable to fragile and conflict-affected settings globally.

Conflict of Interest All the authors declare no conflict of interest.

Disclaimer The views and opinions expressed in this chapter are those of the authors and do not necessarily reflect the official policy or position of their affiliated institutions or organizations.

ChatGPT (version 5.2, OpenAI) was used solely for language editing and structural refinement. All scientific content, interpretations, and conclusions are entirely the responsibility of the authors.

References

1. Kuncic A. How similar are Arab countries and what are their Characteristics. 2016 [cited 2026 May 15]. Available from: https://archive.unescwa.org/sites/www.unescwa.org/files/page_attachments/l1600151.pdf.
2. World Bank. Population, total – Arab World [Internet]. Washington, DC: World Bank [cited 2026 May 15]. Available from: https://data.worldbank.org/indicator/SP.POP.TOTL?locations=1A.
3. United Nations, Department of Economic and Social Affairs, Population Division. World population prospects 2024: summary of results [Internet]. New York: United Nations; 2024 [cited 2026 May 15]. Available from: https://population.un.org/wpp/assets/Files/WPP2024_Summary-of-Results.pdf.
4. United Nations Economic and Social Commission for Western Asia (ESCWA). Real sizes of Arab economies between 2017 and 2023 [Internet]. Beirut: ESCWA; 2025 Mar 3 [cited 2026 May 15]. Available from: https://www.unescwa.org/news/escwa-releases-new-report-real-sizes-arab-economies-between-2017-and-2023.
5. Tiliouine H, Meziane M. The history of well-being in the Middle East and North Africa (MENA). In: Estes RJ, Sirgy MJ, editors. The pursuit of human well-being: the untold global history (international handbooks of quality-of-life). 1st ed. Cham: Springer International Publishing; 2017. p. 287–312.
6. Rahim HFA, Sibai A, Khader Y, Hwalla N, Fadhil I, Alsiyabi H, et al. Non-communicable diseases in the Arab world. Lancet. 2014;383(9914):356–67.
7. Coutts A, Stuckler D, Batniji R, Ismail S, Maziak W, McKee M. The Arab Spring and health: two years on. Int J Health Serv. 2013;43(1):49–60. https://doi.org/10.2190/HS.43.1.d.
8. Fares JKHH, Fares MY, Salhab HA, Fares Y. Conflict medicine in the Arab world. In: Laher I, editor. Handbook of healthcare in the Arab world. Cham: Springer; 2020. p. 2503–18.
9. Giacaman R, Rabaia Y, Nguyen-Gillham V, Batniji R, Punamaki RL, Summerfield D. Mental health, social distress and political oppression: the case of the Occupied Palestinian Territory. Glob Public Health. 2011;6(5):547–59. https://doi.org/10.1080/17441692.2010.528443.
10. World Health Organization, Regional Office for the Eastern Mediterranean (WHO-EMRO). Right to health in the Occupied Palestinian Territory. Cairo: WHO-EMRO; 2018 [cited 2026 May 15]. Available from: https://www.emro.who.int/images/stories/palestine/documents/who_right_to_health_2018_web-final.pdf.
11. Beiraghdar F, Momeni J, Hosseini E, Panahi Y, Negah SS. Health crisis in Gaza: the urgent need for international action. Iran J Public Health. 2023;52(12):2478–83. https://doi.org/10.18502/ijph.v52i12.14309.
12. World Health Assembly, 72. Health conditions in the Occupied Palestinian Territory, including East Jerusalem, and the occupied Syrian Golan: report by the Director-General. World Health Organization [Internet]. 2019 [cited 2026 May 15]. Available from: https://iris.who.int/items/565eb8c9-5e7e-40a9-93a2-4426b1cd8fa8.
13. World Health Organisation. Monthly report on Health Access. Barriers for patients in the occupied Palestinian territory [Internet] [cited 2026 May 15]. Available from: https://www.un.org/unispal/wp-content/uploads/2022/05/WHOAPRILMONTHLYRPT_260522.pdf.

14. Mataria A, Khatib R, Donaldson C, Bossert T, Hunter DJ, Alsayed F, et al. The health-care system: an assessment and reform agenda. Lancet. 2009;373(9670):1207–17. https://doi.org/10.1016/S0140-6736(09)60111-2.
15. Aljadba G, Elkhatib Z, Hamad K, Shah S, Zeidan W, Albeik S, et al. UNRWA's health service in Gaza: challenges and response to the October 2023 crisis. East Mediterr Health J. 2025;31(2):73–6. https://doi.org/10.26719/2025.31.2.73.
16. Palestinian Central Bureau of Statistics (PCBS) [Internet] [cited 2026 Feb 1]. Available from: https://www.pcbs.gov.ps/site/881/default.aspx.
17. Marie M, Hannigan B, Jones A. Resilience of nurses who work in community mental health workplaces in Palestine. Int J Ment Health Nurs. 2017;26(4):344–54. https://doi.org/10.1111/inm.12229.
18. World Health Organization. Conflict in Israel and the occupied Palestinian territory and region [Internet]. 2026 [cited 2026 May 15]. Available from: https://www.who.int/emergencies/situations/conflict-in-Israel-and-oPt.
19. Crawford NC. The human toll of the Gaza war: direct and indirect death from 7 October 2023 to 3 October 2025. Watson Institute, Brown University. 2025 [cited 2026 May 15]. Available from: https://costsofwar.watson.brown.edu/sites/default/files/2025-10/Human-Toll-in-Gaza_Costs-of-War_Crawford_7-October-2025.pdf.
20. Charara R, Forouzanfar M, Naghavi M, Moradi-Lakeh M, Afshin A, Vos T, et al. The burden of mental disorders in the Eastern Mediterranean region, 1990-2013. PLoS One. 2017;12(1):e0169575. https://doi.org/10.1371/journal.pone.0169575.
21. Hammoudeh W, Kienzler H, Meagher K, Giacaman R. Social and political determinants of health in the occupied Palestine territory (oPt) during the COVID-19 pandemic: who is responsible? BMJ Glob Health. 2020;5(9) https://doi.org/10.1136/bmjgh-2020-003683.
22. UNICEF. Immunization country profiles. United Nations Children's Fund. State of Palestine, July 2025 [cited 2026 May 15]. Available from: https://data.unicef.org/resources/immunization-country-profiles/.
23. Boussaa S, Dardona Z, Amane M. Challenges and risk factors for infectious diseases in Gaza due to the current conflict. East Mediterr Health J. 2025;31(2):127–33. https://doi.org/10.26719/2025.31.2.127.
24. Kumar B. Global health inequities in rheumatology. Rheumatology (Oxford). 2017;56(1):4–5. https://doi.org/10.1093/rheumatology/kew064.
25. Bizri AR, Khachfe HH, Fares MY, Musharrafieh U. COVID-19 pandemic: an insult over injury for Lebanon. J Community Health. 2021;46(3):487–93.
26. Bizri AR, Khalil PB. A Lebanese physician's dilemma: not how, but with what? Lancet. 2021;398(10303):841.
27. Refaat MM, Mohanna K. Syrian refugees in Lebanon: facts and solutions. Lancet. 2013;382(9894):763–4.
28. Holmes D. Chronic disease care crisis for Lebanon's Syrian refugees. Lancet Diabetes Endocrinol. 2015;3(2):102.
29. El Arnaout N, Rutherford S, Zreik T, Nabulsi D, Yassin N, Saleh S. Assessment of the health needs of Syrian refugees in Lebanon and Syria's neighboring countries. Confl Heal. 2019;13(1):1–14.
30. Doocy S, Lyles E, Hanquart B, Woodman M. Prevalence, care-seeking, and health service utilization for non-communicable diseases among Syrian refugees and host communities in Lebanon. Confl Heal. 2016;10(1):1–17.
31. Doocy S, Lyles E, Roberton T, Akhu-Zaheya L, Oweis A, Burnham G. Prevalence and care-seeking for chronic diseases among Syrian refugees in Jordan. BMC Public Health. 2015;15(1):1–10.
32. Bizri NA, Alam W, Khoury M, Musharrafieh U, Ghosn N, Berri A, et al. The association between the Syrian crisis and cutaneous Leishmaniasis in Lebanon. Acta Parasitol. 2021;66(4):1240–5.

33. Kazour F, Zahreddine NR, Maragel MG, Almustafa MA, Soufia M, Haddad R, et al. Post-traumatic stress disorder in a sample of Syrian refugees in Lebanon. Compr Psychiatry. 2017;72:41–7.
34. Al-Hajj S, Dhaini HR, Mondello S, Kaafarani H, Kobeissy F, DePalma RG. Beirut ammonium nitrate blast: analysis, review, and recommendations. Front Public Health. 2021;9:657996. https://doi.org/10.3389/fpubh.2021.657996.
35. OKeeffe J, Vernier L, Cramond V, Majeed S, Carrion Martin AI, Hoetjes M, et al. The blast wounded of Raqqa, Syria: observational results from an MSF-supported district hospital. Confl Health. 2019;13(1):1–9.
36. Wong EG, Dominguez L, Trelles M, Ayobi S, Hazraty KR, Kasonga C, et al. Operative trauma in low-resource settings: the experience of Medecins Sans Frontieres in environments of conflict, postconflict, and disaster. Surgery. 2015;157(5):850–6. https://doi.org/10.1016/j.surg.2014.12.021.
37. UNHCR. Lebanon – Syrian Returns & Movements Snapshot (30 November 2025). United Nations High Commissioner for Refugees. 2025 [cited 2026 May 15]. Available from: https://data.unhcr.org/en/documents/details/120035.
38. Al Hilfi TK, Lafta R, Burnham G. Health services in Iraq. Lancet. 2013;381(9870):939–48. https://doi.org/10.1016/S0140-6736(13)60320-7.
39. Cetorelli V, Shabila NP. Expansion of health facilities in Iraq a decade after the US-led invasion, 2003-2012. Confl Health. 2014;8:16. https://doi.org/10.1186/1752-1505-8-16.
40. Mohsin K, Mula-Hussain L, Gilson R. HealthCare Access Barrier (HCAB) framework for the barriers to cancer care during conflicts: perspective from Iraq. BMJ Oncol. 2024;3(1):e000252. https://doi.org/10.1136/bmjonc-2023-000252.
41. Ibrahim S, Al-Dahir S, Al Mulla T, Lami F, Hossain SMM, Baqui A, et al. Resilience of health systems in conflict affected governorates of Iraq, 2014-2018. Confl Health. 2021;15(1):76. https://doi.org/10.1186/s13031-021-00412-2.
42. United Nations High Commissioner for Refugees (UNHCR). Iraq Situation. UNHCR; 2025 [cited 2026 May 15]. Available from: https://www.unhcr.org/emergencies/iraq-situation.
43. Euro-Mediterranean Human Rights Monitor. Exiled at home: internal displacement resulted from the armed conflict in Iraq and its humanitarian consequences. Euro-Med Monitor; 2021 [cited 2026 May 15]. Available from: https://euromedmonitor.org/en/article/4464/Exiled-At-Home:-Internal-displacement-resulted-from-the-armed-conflict-in-Iraq-and-its-humanitarian-consequences.
44. Physicians for Human Rights. Challenges faced by the Iraqi health sector in responding to COVID-19. PHR; 2021 [cited 2026 May 15]. Available from: https://phr.org/our-work/resources/challenges-faced-by-the-iraqi-health-sector-in-responding-to-covid-19/.
45. Republic of Iraq, Ministry of Health. National Health Policy 2014–2023. Baghdad: Ministry of Health. 2014 [cited 2026 May 15]. Available from: https://faolex.fao.org/docs/pdf/irq208883E.pdf.
46. El Bcheraoui C, Jumaan AO, Collison ML, Daoud F, Mokdad AH. Health in Yemen: losing ground in war time. Glob Health. 2018;14(1):1–12.
47. World Health Organization. Yemen crisis: health infrastructure and services update. WHO; 2024 [cited 2026 May 15]. Available from: https://www.who.int/emergencies/situations/yemen-crisis.
48. Wikipedia contributors. Health in Yemen. Wikipedia, The Free Encyclopedia. 2026 [cited 2026 May 15]. Available from: https://en.wikipedia.org/wiki/Health_in_Yemen.
49. Internal Displacement Monitoring Centre (IDMC). Impacts on health in Yemen (internal displacement and health access). IDMC 2020 [cited 2026 May 15]. Available from: https://api.internal-displacement.org/sites/default/files/publications/documents/IDMC_ImpactsonHealthinYemen.pdf.
50. Dureab F, Shibib K, Yé Y, Jahn A, Müller O. Cholera epidemic in Yemen. Lancet Glob Health. 2018;6(12):e1283.

51. Furuya-Kanamori L, Liang S, Milinovich G, Soares Magalhaes RJ, Clements AC, Hu W, et al. Co-distribution and co-infection of chikungunya and dengue viruses. BMC Infect Dis. 2016;16(1):1–11.
52. Devi S. Yemen's health system has "collapsed", warns UN. Lancet. 2021;397(10289):2036.
53. Elnakib S, Elaraby S, Othman F, BaSaleem H, AlShawafi NAA, Al-Gawfi IAS, et al. Providing care under extreme adversity: the impact of the Yemen conflict on the personal and professional lives of health workers. Soc Sci Med. 2021;272:113751.
54. Mohamed Ibrahim MI, Alshakka M, Al-Abd N, Bahattab A, Badulla W. Availability of essential medicines in a country in conflict: a quantitative insight from Yemen. Int J Environ Res Public Health. 2020;18(1) https://doi.org/10.3390/ijerph18010175.
55. Al-Smadi AM, Tawalbeh LI, Gammoh OS, Ashour AF, Shajrawi A, Attarian H. Relationship between anxiety, post-traumatic stress, insomnia and fibromyalgia among female refugees in Jordan: a cross-sectional study. J Psychiatr Ment Health Nurs. 2021;28(4):738–47.
56. Muthanna A, Sang G. State of university library: challenges and solutions for Yemen. J Acad Librariansh. 2019;45(2):119–25.
57. Council on Foreign Relations. Global conflict tracker: power struggle in Sudan. CFR; 2025 [cited 2026 May 15]. Available from: https://www.cfr.org/global-conflict-tracker/conflict/power-struggle-sudan.
58. International Development Committee (UK Parliament). Report on OLS establishment, negotiations, sectors, and NGO involvement. 1998 [cited 2026 May 15]. Available from: https://publications.parliament.uk/pa/cm199798/cmselect/cmintdev/872/87205.htm.
59. Operation Lifeline Sudan. Wikipedia, The Free Encyclopedia [cited 2026 May 15]. Available from: https://en.wikipedia.org/wiki/Operation_Lifeline_Sudan.
60. Taylor-Robinson SD. Operation Lifeline Sudan. J Med Ethics. 2002;28(1):49–51. https://doi.org/10.1136/jme.28.1.49.
61. Mohamed EMA, Lucero-Prisno DE. The effects of Sudan's armed conflict on economy and health: a perspective. Health Sci Rep. 2025;8(2):e70424. https://doi.org/10.1002/hsr2.70424.
62. Wharton G, Ali OE, Khalil S, Yagoub H, Mossialos E. Rebuilding Sudan's health system: opportunities and challenges. Lancet. 2020;395(10219):171–3.
63. El Bushra HE, Habtewold BW, Al Gasseer N, Mohamed RE, Mohamednour SA, Abshar M, et al. Outbreak of chikungunya fever in Sudan, 2018–2019. Juniper Online J Public Health. 2019;4(4):555644. https://doi.org/10.19080/JOJPH.2019.04.555644.
64. World Health Organization. Chikungunya—Sudan. Disease Outbreak News. 15 Oct 2018 [cited 2026 May 15]. Available from: https://www.who.int/emergencies/disease-outbreak-news/item/15-october-2018-chikungunya-sudan-en.
65. Staples JE, Breiman RF, Powers AM. Chikungunya fever: an epidemiological review of a re-emerging infectious disease. Clin Infect Dis. 2009;49(6):942–8. https://doi.org/10.1086/605496.
66. COVID-19 pandemic in Sudan. Wikipedia [cited 2026 May 15]. Available from: https://en.wikipedia.org/wiki/COVID-19_pandemic_in_Sudan.
67. Fekadu G, Bekele F, Tolossa T, Fetensa G, Turi E, Getachew M, et al. Impact of COVID-19 pandemic on chronic diseases care follow-up and current perspectives in low resource settings: a narrative review. Int J Physiol Pathophysiol Pharmacol. 2021;13(3):86–93.
68. Akintayo RO, Akpabio AA, Kalla AA, Dey D, Migowa AN, Olaosebikan H, et al. The impact of COVID-19 on rheumatology practice across Africa. Rheumatology (Oxford). 2021;60(1):392–8. https://doi.org/10.1093/rheumatology/keaa600.
69. Babiker MA. COVID-19 and Sudan: the impact on economic and social rights in the context of a fragile democratic transition and suspended constitutionalism. J Afr Law. 2021;65(S2):311–31. https://doi.org/10.1017/S0021855321000383.
70. Ciaffi J, Vanni E, Mancarella L, Brusi V, Lisi L, Pignatti F, et al. Post-acute COVID-19 joint pain and new onset of rheumatic musculoskeletal diseases: a systematic review. Diagnostics (Basel). 2023;13(11) https://doi.org/10.3390/diagnostics13111850.

71. World Health Organization. Sustaining health services in Somalia amid unprecedented funding challenges [Internet]. Geneva: WHO. 2025 [cited 2026 May 15]. Available from: https://www.who.int/news-room/feature-stories/detail/who-sustaining-health-services-in-somalia-amid-unprecedented-funding-challenges.
72. United Nations. Somalia Humanitarian Needs and Response Plan (HNRP) 2026. Mogadishu: United Nations; 2026 [cited 2026 May 15]. Available from: https://somalia.un.org/sites/default/files/2026-01/Somalia_HNRP_2026.pdf.
73. Médecins Sans Frontières (MSF). Somalia: Deadly consequences of obstacles to health care. 2024 Aug 9 [cited 2026 May 15]. Available from: https://www.doctorswithoutborders.org/latest/somalia-deadly-consequences-obstacles-health-care.
74. Abdi YH, Abdi MS, Bashir SG, Ahmed NI, Abdullahi YB. The state of public health in Somalia: top 5 challenges and strategies for improvement. Public Health Challeng. 2025;4(4):e70138. https://doi.org/10.1002/puh2.70138.
75. Mohamud KM. Equity in health funding: an analysis of the essential package of health services (EPHS) in Somalia (2021–2026). Discov Health Sys. 2025;4(1):132. https://doi.org/10.1007/s44250-025-00302-x.
76. European Basic Health Services Agency (EBA). Rebuilding a health system—experiences from Somalia. Stockholm: EBA. 2024 [cited 2026 May 15]. Available from: https://eba.se/app/uploads/2024/12/Rebuilding-a-health-system-%E2%80%93-experiences-from-Somalia.pdf.
77. Sirohi B, Chalkidou K, Pramesh CS, Anderson BO, Loeher P, El Dewachi O, et al. Developing institutions for cancer care in low-income and middle-income countries: from cancer units to comprehensive cancer centres. Lancet Oncol. 2018;19(8):e395–406. https://doi.org/10.1016/S1470-2045(18)30342-5.
78. Skelton M, Alameddine R, Saifi O, Hammoud M, Zorkot M, Daher M, et al. High-cost cancer treatment across borders in conflict zones: experience of Iraqi patients in Lebanon. JCO Glob Oncol. 2020;6:59–66. https://doi.org/10.1200/JGO.19.00281.

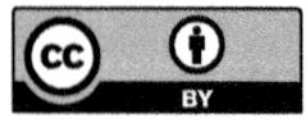

Chapter 29
COVID-19 Crisis and Rheumatology Care in the Arab World

Nelly Ziadé, Wafa Hamdi, Martin Lee, Krystel Aouad, and Manal El Rakawi

Abstract The coronavirus pandemic 2019 (COVID-19) is the most significant public health concern in current times. In addition to its massive morbidity and mortality toll, the pandemic significantly impacted social interactions and global economies.

As a group, the Arab countries ranked 12th in the list of most affected countries in terms of the total number of cases (31,304 cases/1,000,000 population) and ninth in the list of deaths worldwide (383 deaths per 1,000,000 population as of March 2023). Many disparities in epidemiology, infection rate, and clinical outcomes were observed within the Arab countries, which may be attributed to differences in the population's age, ethnicity, vaccination rates, and healthcare systems.

N. Ziadé (✉)
Rheumatology Department, Faculty of Medicine, Saint Joseph University, University Medical Center Hôtel-Dieu de France, Beirut, Lebanon
e-mail: nelly.zoghbi@usj.edu.lb

W. Hamdi
Rheumatology Department, Kassab Institute, Tunis, Tunisia

Tunis Faculty of Medicine, University of Tunis, El Manar, Tunisia
e-mail: wafa.hamdi@fmt.utm.tn

M. Lee
Northumbria Healthcare Trust, North Shields, UK
e-mail: martinlee@doctors.org.uk

K. Aouad
Saint George Hospital University Medical Center, Saint George University of Beirut, Beirut, Lebanon
e-mail: krystel.aouad@hotmail.com

M. El Rakawi
Rheumatology Department, Douera Hospital, Faculty of Medicine Saad Dahlab, Blida, Algeria
e-mail: m.elrakawi@gmail.com

K. A. Alnaqbi, G. Aldabie (eds.), *Rheumatic Diseases in the Arab World*,
https://doi.org/10.1007/978-981-92-0967-5_29

Patients with chronic rheumatic and musculoskeletal diseases (RMDs) were particularly affected, as many of them are generally immunocompromised and vulnerable to infection. Data from the Arab League of Associations for Rheumatology (ArLAR) highlighted the deleterious consequences of the COVID-19 pandemic on the continuity of rheumatology care, the persistence of chronic medication (particularly hydroxychloroquine), the patient's mental health, and the overall income, which are all key predictors of disease prognosis. Studies also highlighted the negative impact on rheumatologists, with a significant reduction in outpatient and inpatient activities and an important effect on physicians' mental health.

In addition to the risk of infection, the main challenges in managing patients with RMDs during the pandemic included the difficulty of access to rheumatology care, lack of proper access to telehealth, shortage of essential anti-rheumatic drugs, and a negative impact on mental health and economic levels. All these factors were associated with a low persistence of chronic anti-rheumatic drugs and poor disease control.

These challenges were addressed through a series of strategies, including the development and dissemination of the best practice guidelines for the use of telehealth in rheumatology by the ArLAR, the conduct of studies investigating the acceptability of the COVID-19 vaccination in patients with RMDs and healthcare providers, and the promotion of awareness campaigns targeting patients with RMDs and the general population.

Rheumatologists were compelled to leave their comfort zone, adopt new technologies, promote public health, and fulfill their duties as role models to patients. These are crucial practice lessons that will remain in the future.

Keywords COVID-19 · Rheumatology · Arab countries · Public health · Telemedicine · Vaccination · Rheumatic diseases · Rheumatology · Pandemics · COVID-19 Vaccines · SARS-CoV-2

29.1 Introduction

The coronavirus disease 2019 (COVID-19) is caused by a novel coronavirus, the severe acute respiratory syndrome coronavirus (SARS-CoV-2), that can cause illnesses ranging from a common cold to a fatal SARS [1]. COVID-19 emerged in December 2019 in Wuhan, China, quickly becoming a global outbreak [1, 2]. It was first declared a public health emergency of international concern by the World Health Organization (WHO) in January 2020 [3], then a pandemic in March 2020 [4]. In addition to the massive morbidity and mortality toll making COVID-19 the most significant public health concern in current times, the pandemic also significantly impacted social interactions and global economies due to lockdowns and social distancing measures [5].

Patients with chronic rheumatic and musculoskeletal diseases (RMDs) were particularly affected, as many of them are generally immunocompromised and vulnerable to infection. At the beginning of the pandemic, recommendations based on firm levels of evidence were lacking concerning guiding anti-rheumatic treatment decisions, and patients who could not access their rheumatologists were compelled to self-modify their treatment [6, 7]. Furthermore, these patients suffered from significant drug shortages as many of their cornerstone therapies were diverted for COVID-19 treatment.

This chapter will discuss the impact of the pandemic on the Arab countries as a whole first, mainly Arab patients with rheumatic diseases, challenges in managing patients with RMDs, strategies to mitigate the pandemic toll, and lessons learned for future pandemics.

29.2 COVID-19 Pandemic in the Arab Countries in General

29.2.1 Epidemiology

COVID-19 has spread worldwide since the first outbreak in December 2019 in China. As of March 19, 2023, more than 682,454,253 confirmed cases of COVID-19 and 6,227,291 deaths have been reported, including 655,312,322 recovered cases [8, 9]. Facing the increasing number of cumulative cases and deaths, many countries implemented strict measures to limit the spread of the infection [10]. Therefore, monitoring and evaluating the morbidity and mortality related to COVID-19 was of obvious interest.

Here, we used data from the WHO and Worldometer websites [8, 9] to present a global overview of COVID-19 epidemiology in the Arab world since the beginning of the pandemic.

The Arab world includes 22 countries with a total population of 453,437,120 as of March 19, 2023. The United Arab Emirates (UAE), followed by Egypt, was the first to report COVID-19 cases on January 29, 2020, and February 14, 2020, respectively [11, 12]. A total of 14,194,238 confirmed COVID-19 cases per million population were reported in the Arab countries; Bahrain, Lebanon, Jordan, Qatar, and Kuwait recorded the highest infection rates (Table 29.1). Compared to the countries most affected by COVID-19 with the highest total number of cases, the Arab countries ranked 12th; the USA, India, and France were at the top of the list (Table 29.2). Furthermore, the Arab countries recorded a high number of tests (10,475,973 tests per million population).

Table 29.1 Description of COVID-19 cases in the Arab countries as of March 19, 2023 (ranked by total cases per million)

Arab countries	Total population	Cumulative COVID-19 cases	Total cases per millions	Total tests per million population	Total recovered	% recovered
Bahrain	1,783,983	713,856	400,147	6,034,319	709,460	99.38
Lebanon	6,684,849	1,233,535	184,527	717,380	1,087,587	88.17
Jordan	10,300,869	1,746,997	169,597	1,669,945	1,731,007	99.08
Qatar	2,979,915	495,856	166,399	1,364,257	494,555	99.74
Kuwait	4,380,326	664,402	151,679	1,930,391	660,237	99.37
Palestine	5,345,541	621,008	116,173	575,907	615,445	99.10
UAE	10,081,785	1,054,873	104,632	199,569,240	1,036,819	98.29
Tunisia	12,046,656	1,151,333	95,573	415,381	NA	NA
Oman	5,323,993	399,449	75,028	4,695,724	384,669	96.30
Libya	7,040,745	507,201	72,038	352,777	500,750	98.73
Iraq	42,164,965	2,465,545	58,474	463,523	2,439,497	98.94
Morocco	37,772,756	1,272,526	33,689	344,038	1,256,151	98.71
Saudi Arabia	35,844,909	831,311	23,192	1,261,389	817,862	98.38
Djibouti	1,016,097	15,690	15,441	301,094	15,427	98.32
Mauritania	4,901,981	63,668	12,988	206,030	62,441	98.07
Comoros	907,419	9048	9971	N/A	8838	97.68
Algeria	45,350,148	271,548	5988	5091	182,893	67.35
Egypt	106,156,692	515,792	4859	34,792	442,182	85.73
Syria	19,364,809	57,478	2968	7553	54,314	94.50
Somalia	16,841,795	27,324	1622	23,778	13,182	48.24
Sudan	45,992,020	63,853	1388	12,240	58,538	91.68
Yemen	31,154,867	11,945	383	10,579	9124	76.38
Total/mean	**453,437,120**	**14,194,238**	**31,304**	**10,475,973**	**12,580,978**	**88.63**

Data extracted as of 19 March 2023 from WHO [8] and Worldometer [9]
UAE United Arab Emirates

As for the mortality rates, the cumulative number of deaths in all Arab countries was 173,794, with the highest total numbers in Tunisia, Iraq, Egypt, Morocco, and Jordan. However, considering the difference in population size, the highest deaths per 100,000 were reported in Tunisia, Lebanon, Jordan, Palestine, and Libya (Table 29.3).

These results showed some discrepancies between the Arab countries (Tables 29.1 and 29.3). For instance, Tunisia reported the highest mortality rate in the Arab world, but it did not report the highest infection rate. On the contrary, Bahrain recorded the highest number of confirmed cases per million population without being at the top of the list of countries with the highest mortality rate. Lebanon was among the top 3 countries with the highest number of confirmed and recovered

Table 29.2 Top 20 affected countries with COVID-19, including the Arab countries as a group (ranked by total cases of COVID-19)

Countries	Total population	Cumulative COVID-19 cases	Total cases per million	Total tests per million	Total recovered	% recovered
World		682,454,253	87,553		655,312,322	
USA	334,805,269	105,920,573	316,365	3,494,614	103,493,314	97.71
India	1,406,631,776	44,695,420	31,775	654,124	44,158,703	98.80
France	65,584,518	39,697,820	605,293	4,139,547	39,450,425	99.38
Germany	83,883,596	38,297,037	456,550	1,458,359	37,936,100	99.06
Brazil	215,353,593	37,145,514	172,486	296,146	36,249,161	97.59
Japan	125,584,838	33,374,303	265,751	770,798	21,709,584	65.05
South Korea	51,329,899	30,690,223	597,901	307,892	30,491,853	99.35
Italy	60,262,770	25,651,205	425,656	4,465,893	25,320,467	98.71
United Kingdom	68,497,907	24,423,396	356,557	7,628,357	24,153,182	98.89
Russia	145,805,947	22,506,199	154,357	1,875,095	21,851,580	97.09
Turkey	85,561,976	17,042,722	199,186	1,902,052	NA	
Arab countries	453,437,120	14,194,238	31,304	10,475,973	12,580,978	88.63
Spain	46,719,142	13,783,163	295,022	10,082,298	13,632,061	98.90
Vietnam	98,953,541	11,527,139	116,490	867,342	10,614,857	92.09
Australia	26,068,792	11,277,613	432,610	3,024,116	11,237,319	99.64
Taiwan	23,888,595	10,231,343	428,294	1,286,903	10,014,375	97.88
Argentina	46,010,234	10,044,957	218,320	776,264	9,912,836	98.68
Netherlands	17,211,447	8,605,996	500,016	1,509,718	8,566,167	99.54
Iran	86,022,837	7,575,927	88,069	643,478	7,340,279	96.89
Mexico	131,562,772	7,507,743	57,066	149,809	6,740,445	89.78

Data extracted as of 19 March 2023 from WHO [8] and Worldometer [9]
USA United States of America, *UK* United Kingdom

cases and among the top 2 countries with the highest mortality rate compared to other Arab countries. These differences observed between countries may be related to many factors such as the population age, the number of tests, vaccination rates, the political stability of the country, healthcare systems, as well as general public health measures and precautions in handling the pandemic.

Compared to the top 20 most affected countries by COVID-19, the Arab countries had a relatively low mortality rate (383 deaths per 1,000,000 population). This finding may be related to the younger age of the Arab population (median age 18–33 years) compared to other countries, leading to less disease severity and a lower mortality rate [12]. Nevertheless, it is important to note that only 45.54% of the Arab population was reported to be fully vaccinated, and the percentage of recovered cases (88.63%) was not among the highest recovery rates compared to the rest of the world (Tables 29.2 and 29.4).

Table 29.3 Description of the COVID-19 deaths in the Arab countries (ranked by deaths per 1,000,000)

Arab countries	Total population	Total COVID deaths	Deaths/ 1,000,000	Vaccinated (%)[a]
Tunisia	12,046,656	29,345	2436	54.14
Lebanon	6,684,849	10,851	1623	35.37
Jordan	10,300,869	14,122	1371	44.68
Palestine	5,345,541	5404	1011	35.67
Libya	7,040,745	6437	914	17.99
Bahrain	1,783,983	1557	873	72.10
Oman	5,323,993	4628	869	59.70
Iraq	42,164,965	25,375	602	19.75
Kuwait	4,380,326	2570	587	78.33
Morocco	37,772,756	16,296	431	63.72
Saudi Arabia	35,844,909	9624	268	73.00
Qatar	2,979,915	688	231	98.99
Egypt	106,156,692	24,613	232	40.16
UAE	10,081,785	2349	233	99.01
Mauritania	4,901,981	997	203	33.07
Djibouti	1,016,097	189	186	35.17
Comoros	907,419	161	177	45.66
Syria	19,364,809	3164	163	12.9
Algeria	45,350,148	6881	152	14.78
Sudan	45,992,020	5023	109	24.12
Somalia	16,841,795	1361	81	41.09
Yemen	31,154,867	2159	69	2.59
Total/mean	**453,437,120**	**173,794**	**383**	**45.54**

Data extracted as of 19 March 2023 from WHO [8] and Worldometer [9]
UAE United Arab Emirates
[a]Persons fully vaccinated, including the last dose of primary series

29.2.2 Prognosis of COVID-19 Infection in the Arab Population

The relationship between ethnicity and clinical outcomes from COVID-19 is unclear. However, studies have suggested associations between ethnicity and morbidity and mortality [13–16]. Some of these studies showed that individuals of some ethnicities, such as Black and Asian ethnicities, were at increased risk of COVID-19 and poorer clinical outcomes (i.e., Intensive Therapy Unit (ITU) admission, mechanical ventilation, and death) compared to White individuals. However, other studies have not confirmed these associations. They have suggested that those racial disparities in COVID-19 outcomes may be partially attributed to higher

Table 29.4 Description of the COVID-19 deaths in the top ten affected countries including the Arab countries as a group (ranked by total number of deaths)

Countries	Total population	Total COVID deaths	Deaths per 1,000,000	Vaccinated (%)[a]
World		6,819,383	874.9	65.13
USA	334,805,269	1,151,279	3439	68.62
Brazil	215,353,593	699,634	3249	51.29
India	1,406,631,776	530,802	377	16.49
Russia	145,805,947	396,834	2722	NA
Mexico	131,562,772	333,310	2533	44.23
Peru	33,684,208	219,648	6521	NA
United Kingdom	68,497,907	208,458	3043	74.59
Italy	60,262,770	188,750	3132	82.96
Arab countries	453,437,120	173,794	383	45.54
Germany	83,883,596	169,661	2023	76.42
France	65,584,518	165,314	2521	78.96

Data extracted as of 19 March 2023 from WHO [8] and Worldometer [9]
[a]Persons fully vaccinated, including the last dose of primary series

comorbidity rates, such as rates of cardiometabolic diseases and/or socioeconomic differences.

To add complexity to research into the effects of ethnicity on the clinical outcomes of COVID-19, different strains of the COVID-19 virus have become more predominant as the global pandemic has progressed since the first cases were reported in 2019. These various strains of COVID-19 may affect the clinical outcomes in different ethnic populations in different ways.

Data specifically looking at clinical outcomes of COVID-19 in the Arab population is sparse. Many systematic reviews and meta-analyses investigating clinical outcomes and ethnicity stratify populations into White, Black, Hispanic, Asian, and Mixed/Other but do not specifically report populations of Arab descent.

A single-center retrospective, observational study by Deeb et al. published in 2021 aimed to identify comorbidities associated with in-hospital death among patients hospitalized for COVID-19 in Abu Dhabi, UAE [17]. It also aimed to assess if ethnicity was correlated with an increased risk of death. This study stratified patients into Arabic, South Asian, African, Filipino, and other subsets. Comorbidities such as diabetes mellitus, hypertension, cardiovascular disease, chronic renal disease, liver disease, and malignancy were associated with a higher risk of morbidity. Higher death rates were seen in the Arab Levant population, although differences between ethnicities did not reach statistical significance.

A recent single-center, retrospective study [18] examined ethnicity-specific features of 560 hospitalized patients with confirmed COVID-19 in Dubai, UAE. Compared to other ethnic groups, Caucasian or East Asian patients had the more severe disease; however, they had a lower comorbidity risk profile. On the other hand, patients from the Middle East had a high-risk factor profile despite a similar disease severity.

Another retrospective analysis of COVID-19 investigated the role of ethnicity on the clinical outcomes of COVID-19 in Kuwait [19]. This study, which included 290 Arabs and 115 South Asians, found statistically higher COVID-19 ITU admission rates and death rates in the South Asian group compared to the Arab group. The results of this study suggested a possible role of ethnicity in COVID-19 clinical outcomes and prognosis. Although the results of this study did not show a meaningful difference in the prevalence of comorbidities between the two ethnic groups, this data could have been influenced by a number of factors other than the genetics of ethnicities, such as living in highly populated accommodation, manual occupation, and lower socioeconomic status.

Also, a cross-sectional socio-demographic study of Jewish and Arab communities looking at morbidity in the first wave of COVID-19 in Israel found that morbidity rates in Jewish communities were consistently higher than in Arab communities [20]. Arab communities in Israel during the first wave of COVID-19 were relatively less affected by the COVID-19 pandemic than Jewish communities, despite their relative poverty, minority status, and prevalent multi-generational households. However, analysis of the second wave of COVID-19 in Israel demonstrated a rise in morbidity in Arab communities and the disappearance of the previously reported negative association of morbidity with Arab ethnicity [21]. These findings were further supported by subsequent data analysis comparing the first to the second wave of COVID-19 infection in Israel [22]. This analysis confirmed a lower incidence, hospitalization, and mortality from COVID-19 in the Arab population compared to Jewish communities during the first wave of COVID-19 in Israel. However, during the second and third waves, these trends reversed, with the incidence and mortality in Arab communities reaching and surpassing rates in Jewish communities. These observations highlight the hypothesis that distinct waves and strains of COVID-19 may affect clinical outcomes in ethnic populations in different ways.

Finally, data from the COVID-19 Vaccination in Auto-Immune Diseases (COVAD) international study [23, 24], a self-reported e-survey, included 19,199 participants (patients with RMDs and controls) from 110 countries and found a similar hospitalization rate (1.9%) in participants from the Arab countries and others. Compared to non-Arab countries, participants from Arab countries reported higher COVID-19 rates. The disease profile was similar, except for a higher proportion of fever and cough and a lower proportion of anosmia/ageusia and skin rashes in participants from the Arab countries.

In summary, the role of ethnicity in COVID-19 outcome disparities is likely to be multifactorial in nature. Genetic factors may account for some ethnic disparities, although the variation in genes within ethnic groups, such as Arabs who are unified by the Arab language rather than a common origin, may be very high. Socioeconomic factors may also contribute to ethnic and racial disparities in COVID-19 clinical outcomes.

29.2.3 General Management Guidelines per Country

Early in the pandemic, the WHO declared that governments should apply strict preventive measures to limit the spread of the virus [25]. Thus, most Arab countries developed specific strategies for that purpose [26–28].

Strict containment measures established at the pandemic's start helped limit the first wave in many countries. However, the situation has diverged with the gradual lifting of these measures. While some countries in the Arab region managed to flatten the curve of infections at some point, the health situation appeared much more fragile in other regions, thus deepening the gap and aggravating the situation of particularly vulnerable patients [27].

Epidemiologic data showed that certain countries managed to control the pandemic through a combination of mitigation, suppression, and elimination strategies. Mitigation strategies focused on protecting the most vulnerable while flattening the peak (e.g., as in the Swedish model). Suppression strategies were aimed at lowering case numbers and outbreaks (e.g., in the UK, Jordan, and Morocco), while elimination strategies tried to exclude the disease and prevent community transmission (Australia, New Zealand, Bahrain, and the UAE).

Notably, healthcare systems in the Arab countries were not sufficiently equipped to handle all healthcare needs related to COVID-19, particularly issues relating to administration, equity, finance, the supply side of healthcare, and the usage of information technology [26].

Specific guidelines for the treatment of COVID-19 were elaborated by health authorities in Arab countries, aiming to standardize the patient's care by adapting it to the country's financial, infrastructural, and human resources and capacities. These guidelines are summarized in Table 29.5. Most guidelines were published by the national Ministry of Health (MOH) in collaboration with specialized scientific societies or dedicated COVID-19 committees in early 2020 [29–37]. Most addressed the issues of case identification, diagnosis, isolation measures, and management guidelines. However, very few handled specific cases of immunocompromised individuals.

Table 29.5 COVID-19 general management guidelines in the Arab countries

Country	Date	Author	Guidance for diagnosis	Guidance for isolation	Prevention guidelines	Treatment guidelines	Chapter for immunosuppressed patients	Reference
Bahrain	July 2020	The National Taskforce for Combating the Coronavirus (COVID-19)	√	√	√	√		[29]
Egypt	2020	Ministry of Health and Population	√		√	√		[30]
Kuwait	January 2020	Infection Control Directorate—MOH	√	√	√			[31]
Lebanon	March 2020	The Lebanese Society of Infectious Diseases and Clinical Microbiology—MOH	√	√	√	√	√	[32]
Morocco	April 2020	National Guidelines on Management of COVID-19 in Morocco	√	√	√	√		[33]
Oman	June 2020	Directorate General of Specialized Medical Care, MOH	√		√			[34]
Qatar	2020	MOH	√	√	√			[33]
Saudi Arabia	April 2022	MOH	√	√	√	√	√	[35]
Tunisia	August 2020	INEAS—MOH	√	√	√	√		[36]
UAE	2020	MOH	√	√	√	√		[37]

INEAS National Instance for Health Evaluation and Accreditation, *MOH* Ministry of Health, *UAE* United Arab Emirates

29.3 COVID-19 Pandemic and Rheumatic Diseases in the Arab Countries

Patients with chronic RMDs are a particularly susceptible group affected by the COVID-19 pandemic [38]. Although the risk of infection was found to be similar or mildly increased between patients with RMDs and the normal population [39, 40], large international population studies had conflicting results. Some studies showed an increased risk of severe COVID-19 infections and higher mortality among some patients with RMDs [41, 42], due to the use of immunosuppressive medications as well as to some RMDs manifestations [43, 44].

29.3.1 Epidemiology

For patients with RMDs, the incidence rate of COVID-19 did not differ from the general population [45, 46]; however, data regarding RMDs patients in Arab countries were scarce. Data from the COVAD study showed a slightly higher reported rate of COVID-19 in patients with RMDs from Arab countries (20%) compared to non-Arab countries (12%) [23]. However, the infectious disease duration was shorter in Arab patients (16 versus 19 days).

29.3.2 Prognosis of COVID-19 Infection in Arab Patients with Rheumatic Diseases

A systematic review published in 2021 aimed to quantify the risk of COVID-19 and disease severity among people with RMDs compared to those without these conditions [47]. This review included little or no data from patients with RMDs living in Arab countries and identified an increased prevalence of COVID-19 in these patients compared to the general population (RR 1.53; 95% CI 1.16–2.01). The odds of hospitalization, ICU admission, and mechanical ventilation were similar in patients with and those without RMDs, although the mortality rate was increased in patients with RMDs (OR 1.74; 95% CI 1.08–2.80). The increased risk of COVID-19 and poor clinical outcomes may be due to several factors, such as underlying disease, associated comorbidities, or treatments used to control the symptoms of these diseases. For example, some studies have suggested an association between using B-cell-depleting therapies such as rituximab and worse COVID-19 outcomes [48].

A review studying the association between ethnicity and COVID-19 clinical outcomes in patients with RMDs was published in 2021 [49]. This study examined patients from the United States (US) with RMDs and COVID-19 who were included in the COVID-19 Global Rheumatology Alliance physician registry. In this review, ethnicity was defined as White, African American, Latin American, Asian, or Other/

Mixed Race. Similar to the general US population findings, racial/ethnic minorities with rheumatic disease and COVID-19 had increased odds of hospitalization and ventilatory support.

Data from Qatar highlighted potential risks regarding COVID-19 in patients with RMDs in the Arab world. One retrospective case-control study compared the viral load of SARS-CoV-2 between patients with and without RMDs [50]. The viral load of SARS-CoV-2 in patients with RMDs was significantly higher at baseline testing and remained higher until day 24. This data may indicate that patients with RMDs were at a higher risk of infection and prolonged potential transmission than those without. A further retrospective single-center, matched case-control cohort study from the same group aimed to evaluate whether there was clinical evidence that patients with RMD infected with SARS-CoV-2 were at a higher risk of poorer outcomes than those without RMDs [51]. The study found that severe SARS-CoV-2 infection (defined by the requirement for oxygen therapy support, need for invasive or non-invasive mechanical ventilation, or use of glucocorticoids) was more common in the RMD group than in the control group (14.9% vs. 5.8%; $p < 0.001$).

Moreover, according to the COVAD study [23], patients from Arab countries reported more COVID-19 symptoms, particularly a higher proportion of fever, fatigue, muscle aches, headache, cough, and diarrhea, compared to non-Arab countries. However, both groups required the same hospitalization rate in this study (2.1%).

Furthermore, some epidemiological studies based on e-surveys evaluated the impact of COVID-19 on patients with RMDs. The Arab Adult Arthritis Awareness (AAAA) group, a special interest group working under the umbrella of the Arab League of Associations for Rheumatology (ArLAR), conducted two studies in 2020 to evaluate the impact of the COVID-19 pandemic on patients with chronic RMDs in the Arab countries (HANDLING study) [6] and on the rheumatology practice (HARMONIC study) [7].

The first survey, named "HANDLING" (How are the rheumatology patients dealing with the COVID-19 pandemic?), was disseminated online through social media and patients' association channels in May 2020, and a total of 2163 patients were included in the analysis. The study highlighted the deleterious consequences of the COVID-19 pandemic on the continuity of rheumatology care, the persistence of chronic medication, and patients' mental health, all key predictors of disease prognosis. In summary, 82% reported a negative impact on access to rheumatology care. Access to chronic anti-rheumatic drugs was compromised in 31% of patients, particularly hydroxychloroquine (47%). In addition, the pandemic had a negative impact on mental health (66%) and income (62%). Factors associated with a negative mental impact of the COVID-19 pandemic were identified: positive personal infection with SARS-CoV-2 (OR: 4.93; 95% CI: 1.38–17.61, p:0.014), isolation due to COVID-19 (OR: 2.45; 95% CI: 1.86–3.25, $p < 0.001$), fewer visits to the rheumatologist (OR: 1.97, 95% CI: 1.29–2.99, p 0.017), difficulty of access to hydroxychloroquine (OR: 1.86; 95% CI: 1.34–2.59, $p < 0.001$), negative impact on income (OR: 1.28, 95% CI: 0.90–1.80, p 0.014), and persistence of medications (OR: 0.36; 95% CI: 0.16–0.84 $p < 0.001$). The mental health impact needed to be specifically addressed, as it may be a significant trigger for rheumatic disease flares and its direct effect on patients' overall well-being. The study also identified marked disparities in the negative impact of the pandemic among different regions in the Arab world.

On the other hand, data from the HARMONIC (How are the Arab rheumatologists dealing with the COVID-19 pandemic?) study included 858 rheumatologists (27% of all registered rheumatologists in the Arab countries). The study identified a 65% reduction in outpatient activity, 69% in hospitalization, and 71% in drug shortages. The impact on the physicians' mental health was reported at 77% and on income at 43%.

The relative scarcity of data on clinical outcomes from COVID-19 infection in patients with RMDs in the Arab population highlights the need for future research in this chronically understudied ethnicity.

29.3.3 *Specific Management Recommendations for Patients with RMDs in the Arab Countries*

The European Alliance of Associations for Rheumatology (EULAR) and the American College of Rheumatology (ACR) developed specific recommendations that addressed several aspects of SARS-CoV-2 and were meant for patients with RMDs and their caregivers. These recommendations covered the general measures and prevention of SARS-CoV-2 infection, the management of RMDs when local social measures were in effect, the management of COVID-19 in the context of RMDs, and the prevention of infections other than SARS-CoV-2 [46, 52, 53].

The AAAA—ArLAR special interest group translated those recommendations to make them widely available to patients and physicians in Arab countries [54].

Some scientific rheumatology societies in Arab countries developed specific local guidelines, recommendations, and points to consider for patients with RMDs and for physicians adapted to each country's epidemiological specificity and capacities (Table 29.6) [35, 55–57]. These recommendations tried to answer several relevant and hot questions in times of crisis, particularly on how to manage patients treated by immunosuppressants and biologics, how physicians can avoid COVID-19 themselves, how to raise patient awareness and provide education and advice on preventive measures, how to organize the consultations (classic consultation/teleconsultation), how to manage a patient suspected to have COVID-19 in the office, what prophylactic treatment against COVID-19 to consider, and finally, the prescription and dispensing of chloroquine and hydroxychloroquine to rheumatic patients. Those recommendations were communicated via documents made available to doctors and patients through websites and social networks.

Table 29.6 Arab countries' guidelines for the treatment of COVID-19 in patients with rheumatic disease list

Country	Date	Author	Publication	Key Topics	Reference
Algeria	November 2021		El-Hakim journal	Management of patients with no sign of COVID-19 Management of suspected cases Management of confirmed cases (SARS-Cov +) and management of newly diagnosed patients with RMDs Recommendations for specific situations (pregnant women)	[55]
Kuwait	October 2021	Kuwait Association of Rheumatology	Current Rheumatology Reviews	Management of patients with RMDs in various clinical scenarios: screening protocols in an infusion clinic, medication protocols for stable patients, care for patients with suspected or confirmed COVID-19 infections, and whether they are stable, in a disease flare, or newly diagnosed conditions for the hospital admission	[56]
Morocco	April 2020	Moroccan Society of Rheumatology	SMR website And Revue Marocaine de Rhumatologie	How can doctors avoid bringing the coronavirus home? Awareness and education of the patient on the preventive measures Organization of consultations (classic consultation and teleconsultation) Management of patients on immunosuppressant treatment in the hospital Management of a patient with RMD treated with Biologics How to manage a patient suspected of COVID-19 in the office? Prophylactic treatment against COVID-19 Spondyloarthritis and nonsteroidal anti-inflammatory drugs	[57]

SMR Moroccan Society of Rheumatology, *SSRSA* Saudi Society for Rheumatology

29.4 Challenges in the Proper Management of the COVID-19 Pandemic in the Arab Countries

Identifying the barriers and obstacles to optimal health care during the COVID-19 crisis was a vital step in overcoming the crisis and a golden opportunity to learn how to improve overall patient care by adopting new approaches such as telehealth.

Emerging evidence on biological and non-biological factors implicated in worse outcomes in people with RMDs affected by the COVID-19 pandemic, whether infected with the virus or not, calls for the need to use more novel frameworks and holistic ways of studying disease [58]. In fact, considering COVID-19 in a pandemic framework was particularly relevant in this context because it emphasizes the synergistic condition that interacts with and exacerbates pre-existing conditions such as RMDs and social conditions [59]. Thus, identifying barriers and facilitators to optimal management of RMDs in this context was fundamental to addressing the pandemic and its health inequalities, particularly in developing countries (Fig. 29.1).

Barriers to online consultations included poor access to the Internet for some patients, low-quality Internet connections on either side, a lack of user-friendly medical files, and psychological reluctance from patients regarding online consultations (most patients prefer face-to-face consultations) [60]. According to the HARMONIC study [52], the top unmet needs in COVID-19 management were the availability of a telehealth platform, access to anti-rheumatic drugs (biologics and hydroxychloroquine), access to personal protective equipment, and patient and physician education.

The continuity of health care was very challenging during waves of virus transmission. Telehealth represented an additional solution for some situations, such as social distancing or mobility restrictions due to the pandemic. Besides, it proved also to be a sustainable solution for patients with chronic diseases. Therefore, implementing a telehealth platform was an essential pillar in overcoming barriers and obstacles to better health care for patients with rheumatic diseases. Thus, discussing the modalities of telehealth and its legal implementation framework in the Arab region was an important step. This unmet need led to the development of Best Practice Guidelines (BPG) for the use of telehealth in rheumatology in the Arab region (TIROL study) to identify the main barriers and facilitators of telehealth and to provide rheumatologists with a practical toolkit for the implementation of telehealth [61]. The barriers to telehealth in the Arab countries were identified in Table 29.7 and included concerns about the quality of care and technical difficulties as priorities.

Drug shortage was a major challenge that was laid by the pandemic [62]. Thus, medication persistence was strongly recommended by raising awareness among patients and other stakeholders, such as governments, which needed to ensure the availability of medications [27].

Dispensing Personal Protective Equipment (PPE) was sometimes a difficult challenge during the COVID-19 pandemic. Thus, working with health authorities to guarantee the availability of PPE for healthcare professionals (HCPs) is a crucial step to improving safety at work and in patient care.

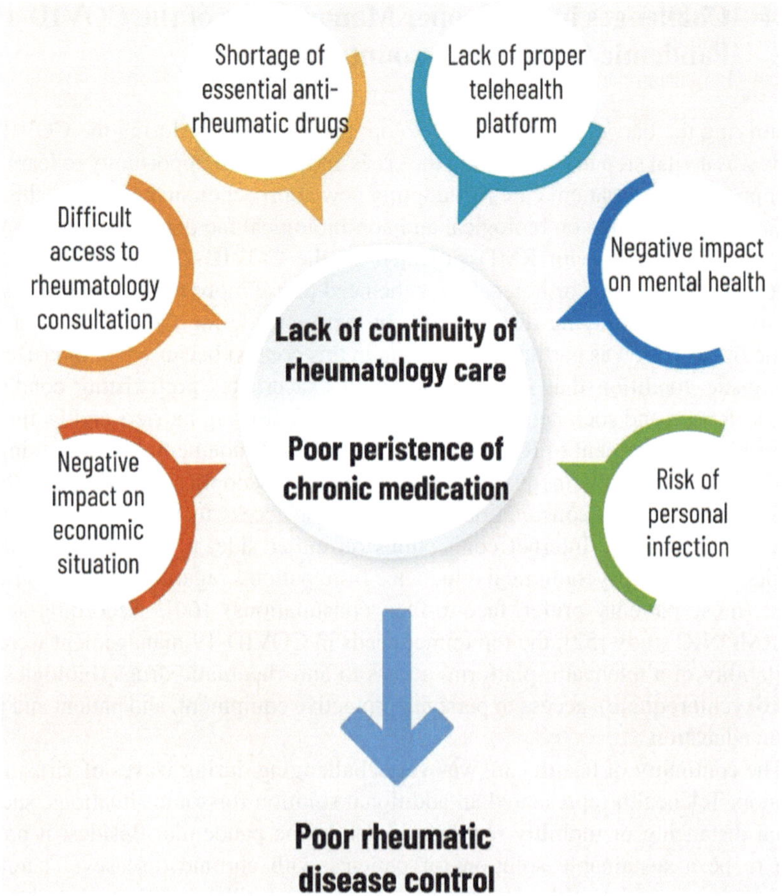

Fig. 29.1 Impact of the COVID-19 pandemic on patients with rheumatic and musculoskeletal diseases

Patient education was an essential aspect of patient care that needs to be developed by establishing unified guidance for rheumatology patients during the pandemic and the transitional deconfinement period and by promoting channels of patient education and advocacy for rheumatology. Besides, continuous medical education for physicians is also vital for promoting healthcare by developing unified practice guidelines for rheumatologists in the Arab region.

The HARMONIC and HANDLING study findings were confirmed by a British qualitative study including 1543 patients and 111 clinicians. This study demonstrated that the pandemic exposed and exacerbated existing healthcare system weaknesses. Moreover, it highlighted increasing barriers to rheumatology patients accessing care. Furthermore, without concerted action such as rebuilding trust, improving administrative systems, and providing more support for clinicians,

Table 29.7 Physician and patient-related barriers to telehealth in the Arab countries, ranked by order of priority

Rank	Physician-related barriers	Patient-related barriers
1	Concern about the quality of care (impossible to do a complete clinical exam, lack of non-verbal communication, patient distraction during the visit)	Concern about the quality of care or proper communication
2	External technical difficulties such as poor Internet connection or suitable equipment	Internal technical difficulties such as lack of familiarity with technology
3	Internal technical difficulties such as lack of familiarity with e-Health and lack of trained staff	External technical difficulties such as poor Internet connection or unsuitable equipment
4	Lack of motivation (lack of reimbursement)	Resistance to change
5	Absence of legal framework: inter-country licensure laws need for credentialing at multiple sites, and liability concerns	Lack of motivation or unclear benefit (patient lives near the healthcare facility, elderly patients with more spare time)

barriers to care and negative impacts of the pandemic on trust, medical relationships, medical security, and patients may persist in the longer term [63].

29.5 Strategies to Control the Pandemic and Improve Rheumatology Care

Early in the pandemic, governments and international bodies used strategies to control the pandemic, including social distancing, lockdown measures, and awareness campaigns. In addition, vaccination campaigns were implemented later when vaccines became available for public use.

Based on the HANDLING and HARMONIC surveys [52, 53], several domains for an action plan to improve the care of patients with chronic rheumatic diseases in Arab countries were proposed:

- Telehealth: Establish a reliable telehealth platform to maintain the continuity of care for patients with rheumatic diseases.
- Drug persistence: Increase patient awareness about the need to maintain chronic treatment unless advised otherwise by the rheumatologist.
- Drug availability: Increase government awareness about maintaining chronic treatment and avoiding drug shortages.
- Mental health: Acknowledge and address the significant mental impact and possible association with disease flares.
- Communication: Use social media to disseminate general guidance to reach the maximum number of patients and encourage establishing and registering patients' associations and groups.

In the following section, telehealth and vaccination will be discussed.

29.5.1 Telehealth

Many studies have highlighted the harmful effect of the COVID-19 pandemic on the continuity of rheumatology care due to confinement, service closure, and postponed consultations, with consequent repercussions on patient adherence, monitoring, and management of their chronic diseases and delay in diagnosis and management for new patients [64, 65]. During this period, many face-to-face appointments were replaced by consultations via telephone or video consultation [64].

Telehealth is an alternative to face-to-face visits in situations of confinement or difficult access in the event of remoteness and is defined by the WHO as "the offering of health care services, where distance is an essential aspect, by all healthcare practitioners using information and communication technology such as mobile consultation, video calling, written report or protected email, to share valid information for the diagnosis, treatment, and prevention of disease, research, and evaluation, and for the continuing education of health care providers, all in the interest of advancing the health of individuals and their communities" [66]. Telehealth can positively impact disease activity and improve medication adherence and self-efficacy levels in patients with rheumatoid arthritis.

In the Arab countries, the need for telehealth was highlighted both in the patients' HANDLING and the rheumatologists' HARMONIC study [52, 53]. They showed that 99% of Arab patients would accept a teleconsultation in case they were offered one (50% through an Internet consultation and 49% through a traditional phone call). On the other hand, only 54% of rheumatologists agree to use telehealth, and an additional 24% would use it only if it is reimbursed. In fact, telehealth remained insufficiently used for reasons of legislation and technology [67]. The impact of the visit to the rheumatologist was less in the Gulf countries, where there is more of an established infrastructure for remote visits [52].

The suggestion of an action plan to improve the care of patients with chronic rheumatic diseases was to set up a reliable telehealth platform to maintain continuity of care and shorten the time taken to care for new patients.

The ArLAR developed BPG for telehealth in rheumatology (TIROL study) with four general principles and 12 statements to provide rheumatologists with consensus guidelines in compliance with the laws and regulations applicable in each country. Specific issues, such as access to electricity and the safe use of technology in Arab countries, were highlighted [62] (Table 29.8). The definition adopted for rheumatology was "a synchronous exchange of medical information between a patient and a rheumatologist via audio or audiovisual electronic communication to improve the patient's health status." The main concerns were quality of care, good communication, safety, and confidentiality, whereas the main positive element was the increased access to care during periods of confinement. Due to different local regulations in the Arab countries, the ArLAR advised abiding by local jurisdictional regulations of the physician's location and using clinical judgment when deciding to implement telehealth.

Table 29.8 Concepts tackled in the ArLAR best practice guidelines for telehealth in rheumatology

General principles
1. Definition of a rheumatology teleconsultation
2. Access and continuity of care
3. Improving disease outcome
4. Quality of medical care
Best Practice statements
1. Informed consent
2. Confidentiality
3. Documentation
4. Shared decision
5. Physical examination
6. Patient-reported outcomes
7. Safe prescription
8. Fees and reimbursement
9. Ethical considerations
10. Rheumatologist training
11. Technical infrastructure and equity
12. Research

It is essential that remote consultations be adapted and well-targeted [68], which allows for efficiency in diagnosis and patient self-management. However, delays in diagnosis and a decreased likelihood of immunosuppressive treatment switching during the COVID-19 pandemic were reported with telehealth, in contrast to better attendance at appointments [69].

A selection of patients eligible for teleconsultation is necessary, and a triage system to help rheumatologists select patients was proposed in the ArLAR BPG [62]. Patients who were eligible for a teleconsultation visit were follow-up patients who were stable or had minor flares that only needed minor changes in chronic treatments and new patients without a complex diagnosis (i.e., osteoporosis, patient education, and shared decision-making about a management plan). However, many cases were inappropriate for a teleconsultation visit, such as new patients with a complex diagnosis, follow-up patients with a flare that required important changes in chronic treatment, or patients needing procedures.

Implementing telehealth may disadvantage many vulnerable patients with poor access to telehealth [64]; on the other hand, it might promote equity by allowing rheumatology access for patients living in remote areas without physical access to a rheumatologist.

Further studies are needed to determine the best uses of telehealth for primary and subspecialty care management of patients with rheumatic diseases in order to optimize efficacy.

29.5.2 Vaccination Against SARS-Cov2: Acceptability in the Arab Countries

In December 2020, the novel vaccines against COVID-19 were authorized for use [70], leading to a worldwide consensus for mass vaccination, hoping to decrease the COVID-19 pandemic burden and return to normalcy [71]. However, 18 months later, in July 2021, only 28% of the world population had received at least one dose of the COVID-19 vaccine, with only 1.1% of people in low-income countries having received at least one dose [72].

Indeed, the perception of vaccines among the public was still conflicted due to decreased awareness, access to healthcare, and falsified information, resulting in vaccine avoidance and skepticism among patients [73–75].

Due to some reports about a higher risk of COVID-19 complications due to rheumatic diseases or anti-rheumatic treatments, protecting patients with RMDs against COVID-19 infection was highly prioritized from the beginning of the vaccination campaigns. Nevertheless, the vaccines raised even more challenges and concerns regarding safety and efficacy issues in this high-risk group [76, 77]. To address these concerns, international scientific associations advised using vaccines, as they were considered safe for these patients, including those treated with immunosuppressive medications [46, 53, 78]. However, despite these reassuring statements, studies showed that patients with RMDs were reluctant to receive the COVID-19 vaccine due to fear of side effects, disease flare-ups, and the lack of information regarding the novel vaccines, with the willingness to take the vaccine ranging from 54% to 93% [79–81].

According to the international COVAD study, the most used vaccines in the Arab countries by patients and controls were Pfizer, Sinopharm, and AstraZeneca (accounting for over 90% of respondents). Compared to non-Arab countries, patients with RMDs from Arab countries reported fewer vaccine adverse events, namely injection site reactions, fatigue, headache, chills, nausea/vomiting, rash, and diarrhea. Patients withheld anti-rheumatic drugs before vaccination in 17% of cases, similarly in Arab and non-Arab countries, except for biologics, which were less withheld in Arab countries. However, the number of days of drug withholding was lower in the Arab countries (13 vs. 22 days).

To address vaccine acceptability, a study among 3176 participants from 19 Arab countries (ARCOVAX study) was conducted among 1595 patients and 1517 HCPs [82]. It showed that patient acceptability was 63%, within the same range as in international studies [79, 80, 83]. Compared to web-based surveys conducted in the general population in some Arab countries, acceptability in this study was higher than the results reported from Jordan (3100 participants, acceptability of 37%) and Kuwait (2368 participants, acceptability of 53%), suggesting non-specific hesitancy related to RMDs [84–86].

As for HCPs, the acceptability was higher than that of an international study (74%) conducted earlier but was in the same range as a Canadian study, also conducted in December 2020, including 2761 HCPs, which reported an acceptability of 80.9% [87].

Interestingly, the ARCOVAX study confirmed the influence of the physician, especially the rheumatology specialist, to convince the patients to vaccinate. In fact, 57% of the undecided patients and 40% of the unwilling would take the vaccine if the doctor recommended it, and 61% specifically trust their rheumatologist as a source of information about the COVID-19 vaccine. This finding confirms similar results from studies conducted in different cultural backgrounds and should be seriously considered when conducting any vaccine awareness campaign [79, 80, 83, 88].

As for the HCPs, acceptability increased more significantly if the vaccine was mandatory by law, suggesting that different strategies should be used to encourage the HCPs to vaccinate. These strategies should not be neglected, as they will also indirectly impact the population's vaccination. Indeed, even before the COVID-19 era, African experiences showed that one of the pillars of the vaccine's success in the population is its uptake by the HCPs [89].

Vaccine hesitancy stems from multiple factors, including the absence of information on vaccines, the belief that vaccines are unnecessary to protect against diseases, and the lack of access to vaccination [90]. Some of the strongest predictors of acceptability were feeling that it is important to be personally vaccinated and the effects of vaccine uptake on the population in general. Furthermore, a history of previous influenza vaccination predicted acceptability.

In 2019, the WHO named vaccine hesitancy as one of the top ten threats to global health [91], which should be addressed rigorously in any vaccination campaign. The main reasons for vaccine avoidance among patients with RMDs were the lack of information regarding the vaccines, the use of new technology, fear of flare-ups of their disease, and side effects of the vaccine [79, 88].

In the ARCOVAX study, the most significant concerns regarding the vaccine in the patient group were the fear of side effects, the lack of experience, and concerns regarding vaccines in general. In the HCPs group, the greatest concerns were the lack of experience and concerns about government health crisis management [82]. This highlights the need for better communication about the efficacy and, mainly, safety data in a timely and transparent manner to build the much-needed trust in vaccines.

Other factors associated with vaccine acceptability in the literature were older age, male gender, and higher education (Table 29.9).

Table 29.9 Factors associated with vaccination hesitancy in the Arab countries

Healthcare system-related	Patient-related	Disease-related
1. Low country GDP 2. Concerns about health crisis management by governments 3. Suspected link between pharmaceutical companies and governments	1. Fear of side effects 2. Concerns regarding vaccines in general 3. Younger age 4. Female gender 5. Lower level of education	1. Lack of experience 2. Vaccine might be less efficacious 3. Vaccine might induce disease flares

GDP Gross Domestic Product

29.6 Conclusion

In conclusion, the COVID-19 pandemic severely impacted the world population, including those living in the Arab countries, and caused unprecedented economic and mental consequences. In particular, the negative impact affected patients with RMDs more harshly due to drug shortages and lack of access to rheumatology care.

The initial control strategies included lockdowns, social distancing, and early screening. Thereafter, strategies included measures meant to persist in the future, such as campaigns to motivate patients to vaccinate and the development of frameworks for telehealth implementation in rheumatology clinics.

Rheumatologists were compelled to leave their comfort zone, adopt new technologies, promote public health, and fulfill their duties as role models to patients. These are crucial practice lessons that will remain in the future.

Conflict of Interest The authors declare that they have no conflicts of interest.

References

1. Wu Z, McGoogan JM. Characteristics of and important lessons from the coronavirus disease 2019 (COVID-19) outbreak in China: summary of a report of 72 314 cases from the Chinese Center for Disease Control and Prevention. JAMA. 2020;323(13):1239–42. https://doi.org/10.1001/jama.2020.2648.
2. Tang D, Comish P, Kang R. The hallmarks of COVID-19 disease. PLoS Pathog. 2020;16(5):e1008536. https://doi.org/10.1371/journal.ppat.1008536.
3. Eurosurveillance editorial team. Note from the editors: World Health Organization declares novel coronavirus (2019-nCoV) sixth public health emergency of international concern. Euro Surveill. 2020;25(5):200131e. https://doi.org/10.2807/1560-7917.ES.2020.25.5.200131e.
4. World Health Organization. Coronavirus disease (COVID-19) pandemic [Internet]. Available from: https://www.who.int/europe/emergencies/situations/covid-19 [cited 2025 Oct 19].
5. Parmet WE, Sinha MS. Covid-19 – The law and limits of quarantine. N Engl J Med. 2020;382(15):e28. https://doi.org/10.1056/NEJMp2004211.
6. Ziadé N, El Kibbi L, Hmamouchi I, Abdulateef N, Halabi H, Hamdi W, et al. Impact of the COVID-19 pandemic on patients with chronic rheumatic diseases: a study in 15 Arab countries. Int J Rheum Dis. 2020;23(11):1550–7. https://doi.org/10.1111/1756-185X.13960.

7. Ziadé N, Hmamouchi I, El Kibbi L, Abdulateef N, Halabi H, Abutiban F, et al. The impact of COVID-19 pandemic on rheumatology practice: a cross-sectional multinational study. Clin Rheumatol. 2020;39(11):3205–13. https://doi.org/10.1007/s10067-020-05428-2.
8. WHO. WHO Coronavirus (COVID-19) Dashboard. Vol. 35. 2021. Available from: https://covid19.who.int [cited 2025 Oct 19].
9. Worldometer. COVID Live – Coronavirus Statistics – Worldometer [Internet]. 2020. Available from: https://www.worldometers.info/coronavirus/ [cited 2025 Oct 19].
10. Alandijany TA, Faizo AA, Azhar EI. Coronavirus disease of 2019 (COVID-19) in the Gulf Cooperation Council (GCC) countries: current status and management practices. J Infect Public Health. 2020;13(6):839–42. https://doi.org/10.1016/j.jiph.2020.05.020.
11. Alwahaibi N, Al Maskari M, Al Dhahli B, Al Issaei H, Al-Jaaidi S, Al Bahlani S. One-year review of COVID-19 in the Arab world. Qatar Med J. 2021;2021(3):66. https://doi.org/10.5339/qmj.2021.66.
12. Alwahaibi N, Al-Maskari M, Al-Dhahli B, Al-Issaei H, Al-Bahlani S. A review of the prevalence of COVID-19 in the Arab world. J Infect Dev Ctries. 2020;14(11):1238–45. https://doi.org/10.3855/jidc.13270.
13. Pan D, Sze S, Minhas JS, Bangash MN, Pareek N, Divall P, et al. The impact of ethnicity on clinical outcomes in COVID-19: a systematic review. EClinicalMedicine. 2020;23:100404. https://doi.org/10.1016/j.eclinm.2020.100404.
14. Sze S, Pan D, Nevill CR, Gray LJ, Martin CA, Nazareth J, et al. Ethnicity and clinical outcomes in COVID-19: a systematic review and meta-analysis. EClinicalMedicine. 2020;29:100630. https://doi.org/10.1016/j.eclinm.2020.100630.
15. Magesh S, John D, Li WT, Li Y, Mattingly-App A, Jain S, et al. Disparities in COVID-19 outcomes by race, ethnicity, and socioeconomic status: a systematic-review and meta-analysis. JAMA Netw Open. 2021;4(11):e2134147. https://doi.org/10.1001/jamanetworkopen.2021.34147. Erratum in: JAMA Netw Open 2021 Dec 1;4(12):e2144237. https://doi.org/10.1001/jamanetworkopen.2021.44237.
16. Raharja A, Tamara A, Kok LT. Association between ethnicity and severe COVID-19 disease: a systematic review and meta-analysis. J Racial Ethn Disparities. 2021;8(6):1563–72. https://doi.org/10.1007/s40615-020-00921-5.
17. Deeb A, Khawaja K, Sakrani N, AlAkhras A, Al Mesabi A, Trehan R, et al. Impact of ethnicity and underlying comorbidity on COVID-19 in-hospital mortality: an observational study in Abu Dhabi, UAE. Biomed Res Int. 2021;2021:6695707. https://doi.org/10.1155/2021/6695707.
18. Al Zahmi F, Habuza T, Awawdeh R, Elshekhali H, Lee M, Salamin N, et al. Ethnicity-specific features of COVID-19 among Arabs, Africans, South Asians, East Asians, and Caucasians in The United Arab Emirates. Front Cell Infect Microbiol. 2022;11:773141. https://doi.org/10.3389/fcimb.2021.773141.
19. Ali H, Alshukry A, Marafie SK, AlRukhayes M, Ali Y, Abbas MB, et al. Outcomes of COVID-19: disparities by ethnicity. Infect Genet Evol. 2021;87:104639. https://doi.org/10.1016/j.meegid.2020.104639.
20. Birenbaum-Carmeli D, Chassida J. Covid-19 in Israel: socio-demographic characteristics of first wave morbidity in Jewish and Arab communities. Int J Equity Health. 2020;19(1):153. https://doi.org/10.1186/s12939-020-01269-2.
21. Birenbaum-Carmeli D, Chassida J. Health and socio-demographic implications of the COVID-19 second pandemic wave in Israel, compared with the first wave. Int J Equity Health. 2021;20(1):1–12. https://doi.org/10.1186/s12939-021-01445-y.
22. Saban M, Myers V, Peretz G, Avni S, Wilf-Miron R. COVID-19 morbidity in an ethnic minority: changes during the first year of the pandemic. Public Health. 2021;198:238–44. https://doi.org/10.1016/j.puhe.2021.07.018.
23. Sen P, Gupta L, Lilleker JB, Aggarwal V, Kardes S, Milchert M, et al. COVID-19 vaccination in autoimmune disease (COVAD) survey protocol. Rheumatol Int. 2022;42(1):23–9. https://doi.org/10.1007/s00296-021-05046-4.

24. Sen P, Ravichandran N, Nune A, Lilleker JB, Agarwal V, Kardes S, et al. COVID-19 vaccination-related adverse events among autoimmune disease patients: results from the COVAD study. Rheumatology (Oxford). 2022;62(1):65–76. https://doi.org/10.1093/rheumatology/keac305.
25. Anderson RM, Heesterbeek H, Klinkenberg D, Hollingsworth TD. How will country-based mitigation measures influence the course of the COVID-19 epidemic? Lancet. 2020;395(10228):931–4. https://doi.org/10.1016/S0140-6736(20)30567-5.
26. Falah HH. Legal and health response to COVID-19 in the Arab countries. Risk Manag Healthc Policy. 2021;(14):1141–54. https://doi.org/10.2147/RMHP.S297565.
27. OECD. Covid-19 crisis response in MENA countries. Organisation for Economic Co-operation and Development; 2020. p. 1–32. [cited 2026 May 17]. Available from: https://www.oecd.org/en/publications/2020/11/covid-19-crisis-response-in-mena-countries_1dd1478d.html.
28. AlFattani A, AlMeharish A, Nasim M, AlQahtani K, AlMudraa S. Ten public health strategies to control the Covid-19 pandemic: the Saudi experience. IJID Reg. 2021 Dec;1:12–9. https://doi.org/10.1016/j.ijregi.2021.09.003.
29. National Health Regulatory Authority. Bahrain COVID-19 National Protocols [Internet]. [cited 2026 May 17]. Available from: https://www.nhra.bh/Media/Announcement/MediaHandler/GenericHandler/documents/Announcements/NHRA_News_MOH%20ALERT_Bahrain%20COVID-19%20National%20Protocols_20200701.pdf.
30. General Authority for Healthcare Accreditation and Regulation (GAHAR). Guidelines for COVID-19 disease hospital readiness: structural & operational checklist [Internet]. Cairo: GAHAR; [cited 2026 May 17]. Available from: https://admin.gahar.gov.eg/uploads/media/guidelines-for-covid-19-disease-hospital-readiness.pdf.
31. Kim SB, Huh K, Heo JY, Joo EJ, Kim YJ, Choi WS, Kim YJ, Seo YB, Yoon YK, Ku NS, Jeong SJ, Kim SH, Peck KR, Yeom JS. Interim Guidelines on Antiviral Therapy for COVID-19. Infect Chemother. 2020;52(2):281–304. https://doi.org/10.3947/ic.2020.52.2.281.
32. Moghnieh R, Yared Sakr N, Kanj SS, Musharrafieh U, Husni R, Jradeh M, et al. The Lebanese Society for Infectious Diseases and Clinical Microbiology (LSIDCM) guidelines for adult community-acquired pneumonia (CAP) in Lebanon. J Med Liban. 2014;62(1):40–7. https://doi.org/10.12816/0002626.
33. Naciri A, Sine H, Baba MA, Bouchriti Y, Kharbach A, Achbani A. National guidelines on management of coronavirus disease COVID-19 in Morocco. Eur J Med Ed Teach. 2020;13(1):em2003. https://doi.org/10.30935/ejmets/8014.
34. Ministry of Health, Directorate General of Health Services and Programmes. Guideline of management of the SARS-CoV-2 (COVID-19) coronavirus epidemic. MoH/DGSMC/GUD/029/Vers.01. Effective Date: Nov 2020. [cited 2026 May 17]. Available from: https://moh.gov.om/en/approved-documents/dg-of-health-services-and-programmes/guideline-of-management-of-the-sars-cov-2-covid-19-coronavirus-epidemic-in-hemodialysis/.
35. Saudi Arabia Ministry of Health. Saudi MoH protocol for adults patients suspected of/confirmed with COVID-19: supportive care and antiviral treatment of suspected or confirmed COVID-19 infection [Internet]. [cited 2026 May 17]. Available from: https://www.moh.gov.sa/en/Ministry/MediaCenter/Publications/Documents/MOH-therapeutic-protocol-for-COVID-19.pdf.
36. INEAS. Les guides de l'INEAS direction qualité des soins et sécurité des patients: recommandations de prise en charge des patients âgés suspects ou confirmés de la COVID-19 [Internet]. 2020. p. 1–310. [cited 2026 May 17]. Available from: https://aturea.org/pdf_ppt_docs/blog/63.pdf.
37. Abbas Zaher W, Ahamed F, Ganesan S, Warren K, Koshy A. COVID-19 crisis management: lessons from The United Arab Emirates leaders. Front Public Health. 2021;9:724494. https://doi.org/10.3389/fpubh.2021.724494.
38. Furer V, Rondaan C, Agmon-Levin N, van Assen S, Bijl M, Kapetanovic MC, et al. Point of view on the vaccination against COVID-19 in patients with autoimmune inflammatory rheumatic diseases. RMD Open. 2021;7(1):e001594. https://doi.org/10.1136/rmdopen-2021-001594.

39. Monti S, Balduzzi S, Delvino P, Bellis E, Quadrelli VS, Montecucco C. Clinical course of COVID-19 in a series of patients with chronic arthritis treated with immunosuppressive targeted therapies. Ann Rheum Dis. 2020;79(5):667–8. https://doi.org/10.1136/annrheumdis-2020-217424.
40. Tomelleri A, Sartorelli S, Campochiaro C, Baldissera EM, Dagna L. Impact of COVID-19 pandemic on patients with large-vessel vasculitis in Italy: a monocentric survey. Ann Rheum Dis. 2020;79(9):1252–3. https://doi.org/10.1136/annrheumdis-2020-217600.
41. Serling-Boyd N, D'Silva KM, Hsu TY, Wallwork R, Fu X, Gravallese EM, et al. Coronavirus disease 2019 outcomes among patients with rheumatic diseases 6 months into the pandemic. Ann Rheum Dis. 2021;80(5):660–6. https://doi.org/10.1136/annrheumdis-2020-219279.
42. Williamson EJ, Walker AJ, Bhaskaran K, Bacon S, Bates C, Morton CE, et al. Factors associated with COVID-19-related death using OpenSAFELY. Nature. 2020;584(7821):430–6. https://doi.org/10.1038/s41586-020-2521-4.
43. FAI2R /SFR/SNFMI/SOFREMIP/CRI/IMIDIATE consortium and contributors. Severity of COVID-19 and survival in patients with rheumatic and inflammatory diseases: data from the French RMD COVID-19 cohort of 694 patients. Ann Rheum Dis. 2021;80(4):527–38. https://doi.org/10.1136/annrheumdis-2020-218310.
44. Strangfeld A, Schäfer M, Gianfrancesco MA, Lawson-Tovey S, Liew JW, Ljung L, et al. Factors associated with COVID-19-related death in people with rheumatic diseases: results from the COVID-19 Global Rheumatology Alliance physician-reported registry. Ann Rheum Dis. 2021;80(7):930–42. https://doi.org/10.1136/annrheumdis-2020-219498.
45. Favalli EG, Monti S, Ingegnoli F, Balduzzi S, Caporali R, Montecucco C. Incidence of COVID-19 in patients with rheumatic diseases treated with targeted immunosuppressive drugs: what can we learn from observational data? Arthritis Rheumatol. 2020;72(10):1600–6. https://doi.org/10.1002/art.41388.
46. Mikuls TR, Johnson SR, Fraenkel L, Arasaratnam RJ, Baden LR, Bermas BL, et al. American college of rheumatology guidance for the management of rheumatic disease in adult patients during the COVID-19 pandemic: version 3. Arthritis Rheumatol. 2021;73(2):e1–e12. https://doi.org/10.1002/art.41596.
47. Conway R, Grimshaw AA, Konig MF, Putman M, Duarte-García A, Tseng LY, et al. SARS-CoV-2 infection and COVID-19 outcomes in rheumatic diseases: a systematic literature review and meta-analysis. Arthritis Rheumatol. 2022;74(5):766–75. https://doi.org/10.1002/art.42030.
48. Sparks JA, Wallace ZS, Seet AM, Gianfrancesco MA, Izadi Z, Hyrich KL, et al. Associations of baseline use of biologic or targeted synthetic DMARDs with COVID-19 severity in rheumatoid arthritis: results from the COVID-19 Global Rheumatology Alliance physician registry. Ann Rheum Dis. 2021;80(9):1137–46. https://doi.org/10.1136/annrheumdis-2021-220418.
49. Gianfrancesco MA, Hyrich KL, Gossec L, Strangfeld A, Carmona L, Mateus EF, et al. Rheumatic disease and COVID-19: initial data from the COVID-19 Global Rheumatology Alliance provider registries. Lancet Rheumatol. 2020;2(5):e250–3. https://doi.org/10.1016/S2665-9913(20)30095-3.
50. Alsaed O, Chaponda M, Elsayed E, Ashour H, Almaslamani M, Al Emadi S. Durability of the humoral response to mRNA-based anti-SARS-CoV-2 vaccines in patients with autoimmune rheumatic disease, a comparative study. Ann Rheum Dis. 2022;81:961. https://doi.org/10.1136/annrheumdis-2022-eular.3593.
51. Alsaed O, Alemadi S, Satti E, Becetti K, Saleh R, Ashour H, et al. Risk of severe SARS-CoV-2 infection in patients with autoimmune rheumatic diseases in Qatar: a cohort matched study. Qatar Med J. 2022;2022(3):24. https://doi.org/10.5339/qmj.2022.24.
52. Landewé RB, Machado PM, Kroon F, Bijlsma HW, Burmester GR, Carmona L, et al. EULAR provisional recommendations for the management of rheumatic and musculoskeletal diseases in the context of SARS-CoV-2. Ann Rheum Dis. 2020;79(7):851–8. https://doi.org/10.1136/annrheumdis-2020-217877.

53. Bijlsma JW, EULAR COVID-19 Task Force. EULAR 2021 updated viewpoints on SARS-CoV-2 vaccination in patients with RMDs: a guidance to answer patients' questions. Ann Rheum Dis. 2022;81(6):786–8. https://doi.org/10.1136/annrheumdis-2021-221965.
54. ArLAR Arab League of Associations for Rheumatology [Internet]. [cited 2026 Jun 17]. Available from: https://www.arabrheumatology.org.
55. Haouichat C, Rahal F, Djennane M, Khaled T, Dahou B, Ladjouze A, Djoudi H. Rhumatismes inflammatoires chroniques et COVID-19: recommandations nationales [Internet]. Algiers: Revue Médicale Algérienne; 2020 [cited 2026 May 17]. Available from: https://el-hakim.net/wp-content/uploads/2021/02/AL_5._Rhumatismes_inflammatoires_chroniques_et_COVID-19.pdf.
56. Baron F, Alhajeri H, Abutiban F, Almutairi M, Alawadhi A, Aldei A, et al. Rheumatologic aspects of the COVID-19 pandemic: a practical resource for physicians in Kuwait and the Gulf region as recommended by the Kuwait Association of Rheumatology. Curr Rheumatol Rev. 2022;18(2):108–16. https://doi.org/10.2174/1573397117666211007091256.
57. Societe Marocaine de Rhumatologie. Guide Pratique COVID-19 [Internet]. [cited 2026 May 17]. https://rmr.smr.ma/archives/articles/guide-pratique-de-la-societe-marocaine-de-rhumatologie-covid-19.
58. Nikiphorou E, Alpizar-Rodriguez D, Gastelum-Strozzi A, Buch M, Peláez-Ballestas I. Syndemics & syndemogenesis in COVID-19 and rheumatic and musculoskeletal diseases: old challenges, new era. Rheumatology (Oxford). 2021;60(5):2040–5. https://doi.org/10.1093/rheumatology/keaa840.
59. Horton R. Offline: COVID-19 is not a pandemic. Lancet. 2020;396(10255):874. https://doi.org/10.1016/S0140-6736(20)32000-6.
60. Bonfá E, Gossec L, Isenberg DA, Li Z, Raychaudhuri S. How COVID-19 is changing rheumatology clinical practice. Nat Rev Rheumatol. 2021;17(1):11–5. https://doi.org/10.1038/s41584-020-00527-5.
61. Ziade N, Hmamouchi I, El Kibbi L, Daou M, Abdulateef N, Abutiban F, et al. Telehealth in rheumatology: the 2021 Arab League of Rheumatology best practice guidelines. Rheumatol Int. 2022;42(3):379–90. https://doi.org/10.1007/s00296-021-05078-w.
62. Abualfadl E, Ismail F, Shereef RRE, Hassan E, Tharwat S, Mohamed EF, et al. Impact of COVID-19 pandemic on rheumatoid arthritis from a multi-centre patient-reported questionnaire survey: influence of gender, rural-urban gap and north-south gradient. Rheumatol Int. 2021;41(2):345–53. https://doi.org/10.1007/s00296-020-04736-9.
63. Sloan M, Harwood R, Gordon C, Bosley M, Lever E, Modi R, et al. Will 'the feeling of abandonment' remain? Persisting impacts of the COVID-19 pandemic on rheumatology patients and clinicians. Rheumatology (Oxford). 2022;61(9):3723–36. https://doi.org/10.1093/rheumatology/keab937.
64. Mehta B, Jannat-Khah D, Fontana MA, Moezinia CJ, Mancuso CA, Bass AR, et al. Impact of COVID-19 on vulnerable patients with rheumatic disease: results of a worldwide survey. RMD Open. 2020 Oct;6(3):e001378. https://doi.org/10.1136/rmdopen-2020-001378.
65. Dejaco C, Alunno A, Bijlsma JW, Boonen A, Combe B, Finckh A, et al. Influence of COVID-19 pandemic on decisions for the management of people with inflammatory rheumatic and musculoskeletal diseases: a survey among EULAR countries. Ann Rheum Dis. 2021;80(4):518–26. https://doi.org/10.1136/annrheumdis-2020-218697.
66. World Health Organization. Digital Health [Internet]. [cited 2026 May 17]. Available from: https://www.who.int/health-topics/digital-health#tab=tab_1.
67. Al-Samarraie H, Ghazal S, Alzahrani AI, Moody L. Telemedicine in middle eastern countries: progress, barriers, and policy recommendations. Int J Med Inform. 2020;141:104232. https://doi.org/10.1016/j.ijmedinf.2020.104232.
68. Zhu W, De Silva T, Eades L, Morton S, Ayoub S, Morand E, et al. The impact of telerheumatology and COVID-19 on outcomes in a tertiary rheumatology service: a retrospective audit. Rheumatology (Oxford). 2021;60(7):3478–80. https://doi.org/10.1093/rheumatology/keab201.

69. McDougall J. Leveraging telemedicine as an approach to address rheumatic disease health disparities. Rheum Dis Clin N Am. 2021;47(1):97–107. https://doi.org/10.1016/j.rdc.2020.09.008.
70. World Health Organization. COVID-19 vaccine tracker and landscape [Internet]. [cited 2026 May 17]. Available from: https://www.who.int/publications/m/item/draft-landscape-of-covid-19-candidate-vaccines.
71. Hasan T, Beardsley J, Marais BJ, Nguyen TA, Fox GJ. The implementation of mass-vaccination against SARS-CoV-2: a systematic review of existing strategies and guidelines. Vaccines (Basel). 2021;9(4):326. https://doi.org/10.3390/vaccines9040326.
72. Mathieu E, Ritchie H, Rodés-Guirao L, Appel C, Gavrilov D, Giattino C, et al. Our World in Data. Coronavirus (COVID-19) vaccinations [Internet]. Oxford: Global Change Data Lab; [cited 2026 May 17]. Available from: https://ourworldindata.org/covid-vaccinations.
73. Principi N, Esposito S. Early vaccination: a provisional measure to prevent measles in infants. Lancet Infect Dis. 2019;19(11):1157–8. https://doi.org/10.1016/S1473-3099(19)30520-1.
74. Patel MK, Orenstein WA. Classification of global measles cases in 2013–17 as due to policy or vaccination failure: a retrospective review of global surveillance data. Lancet Glob Health. 2019;7(3):e313–20. https://doi.org/10.1016/S2214-109X(18)30492-3.
75. Lazarus JV, Ratzan SC, Palayew A, Gostin LO, Larson HJ, Rabin K, et al. A global survey of potential acceptance of a COVID-19 vaccine. Nat Med. 2021;27(2):225–8. https://doi.org/10.1038/s41591-020-1124-9. Erratum in: Nat Med 2021 Feb;27(2):354. https://doi.org/10.1038/s41591-020-01226-0.
76. Sonani B, Aslam F, Goyal A, Patel J, Bansal P. COVID-19 vaccination in immunocompromised patients. Clin Rheumatol. 2021;40(2):797–8. https://doi.org/10.1007/s10067-020-05547-w.
77. Velikova T, Georgiev T. SARS-CoV-2 vaccines and autoimmune diseases amidst the COVID-19 crisis. Rheumatol Int. 2021;41(3):509–18. https://doi.org/10.1007/s00296-021-04792-9.
78. Tam LS, Tanaka Y, Handa R, Li Z, Lorenzo JP, Louthrenoo W, et al. Updated APLAR consensus statements on care for patients with rheumatic diseases during the COVID-19 pandemic. Int J Rheum Dis. 2021;24(6):733–45. https://doi.org/10.1111/1756-185X.14124.
79. Felten R, Dubois M, Ugarte-Gil MF, Chaudier A, Kawka L, Bergier H, et al. Vaccination against COVID-19: expectations and concerns of patients with autoimmune and rheumatic diseases. Lancet Rheumatol. 2021;3(4):e243–5. https://doi.org/10.1016/S2665-9913(21)00039-4.
80. Boekel L, Hooijberg F, van Kempen ZLE, Vogelzang EH, Tas SW, Killestein J, et al. Perspective of patients with autoimmune diseases on COVID-19 vaccination. Lancet Rheumatol. 2021;3(4):e241–3. https://doi.org/10.1016/S2665-9913(21)00037-0.
81. Ammitzbøll C, Thomsen MK, Erikstrup C, Hauge EM, Troldborg A. National differences in vaccine hesitancy: a concern for the external validity of vaccine studies. Lancet Rheumatol. 2021;3(5):e324. https://doi.org/10.1016/S2665-9913(21)00083-7.
82. El Kibbi L, Metawee M, Hmamouchi I, Abdulateef N, Halabi H, Eissa M, et al. Acceptability of the COVID-19 vaccine among patients with chronic rheumatic diseases and health-care professionals: a cross-sectional study in 19 Arab countries. Lancet Rheumatol. 2022;4(3):e160–3. https://doi.org/10.1016/S2665-9913(21)00368-4.
83. Gaur P, Agrawat H, Shukla A. COVID-19 vaccine hesitancy in patients with systemic autoimmune rheumatic disease: an interview-based survey. Rheumatol Int. 2021;41(9):1601–5. https://doi.org/10.1007/s00296-021-04938-9.
84. El-Elimat T, AbuAlSamen MM, Almomani BA, Al-Sawalha NA, Alali FQ. Acceptance and attitudes toward COVID-19 vaccines: a cross-sectional study from Jordan. PLoS One. 2021;16(4):e0250555. https://doi.org/10.1371/journal.pone.0250555.
85. Alqudeimat Y, Alenezi D, AlHajri B, Alfouzan H, Almokhaizeem Z, Altamimi S, et al. Acceptance of a COVID-19 vaccine and its related determinants among the general adult population in Kuwait. Med Princ Pract. 2021;30(3):262–71. https://doi.org/10.1159/000514636.
86. Qattan AMN, Alshareef N, Alsharqi O, Al Rahahleh N, Chirwa GC, Al-Hanawi MK. Acceptability of a COVID-19 vaccine among healthcare workers in the Kingdom of Saudi Arabia. Front Med (Lausanne). 2021;8:644300. https://doi.org/10.3389/fmed.2021.644300.

87. Dzieciolowska S, Hamel D, Gadio S, Dionne M, Gagnon D, Robitaille L, et al. Covid-19 vaccine acceptance, hesitancy, and refusal among Canadian healthcare workers: a multicenter survey. Am J Infect Control. 2021 Sep;49(9):1152–7. https://doi.org/10.1016/j.ajic.2021.04.079.
88. Yurttas B, Poyraz BC, Sut N, Ozdede A, Oztas M, Uğurlu S, et al. Willingness to get the COVID-19 vaccine among patients with rheumatic diseases, healthcare workers and general population in Turkey: a web-based survey. Rheumatol Int. 2021;41(6):1105–14. https://doi.org/10.1007/s00296-021-04841-3.
89. Wirsiy FS, Nkfusai CN, Ako-Arrey DE, Dongmo EK, Manjong FT, Cumber SN. Acceptability of COVID-19 vaccine in Africa. Int J MCH AIDS. 2021;10(1):134–8. https://doi.org/10.21106/ijma.482.
90. Troiano G, Nardi A. Vaccine hesitancy in the era of COVID-19. Public Health. 2021;194:245–51. https://doi.org/10.1016/j.puhe.2021.02.025.
91. World Health Organization. Ten threats to global health in 2019 [Internet]. [cited 2026 May 17]. Available from: https://www.who.int/news-room/spotlight/ten-threats-to-global-health-in-2019.

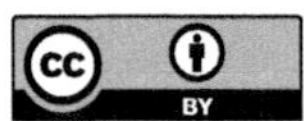

Chapter 30
Future Directions of Rheumatology Care in the Arab World

Khalid A. Alnaqbi

Abstract Rheumatic and musculoskeletal diseases represent a growing health burden across the Arab world, necessitating strategic reforms in workforce development, clinical services, education, research infrastructure, and patient engagement. Building on the region's historical legacy of medical scholarship, this chapter presents a forward-looking framework for strengthening rheumatology care systems across the 22 Arab countries. Key domains addressed include workforce expansion and distribution, modernization of clinical services, personalized medicine, biosimilars and innovative therapies, telemedicine integration, accreditation of rheumatology centers, fellowship and nursing program development, procedural skill enhancement, and regional research collaboration. Emerging digital innovations, including artificial intelligence, wearable devices generating digital biomarkers, and computational disease models such as digital twins, are also discussed as potential tools to support earlier diagnosis, continuous disease monitoring, and personalized treatment strategies. Structural barriers to research growth are analyzed, and a multilevel roadmap is proposed to transition from identifying systemic gaps to implementing sustainable solutions. This approach can enhance care quality, reduce disparities, and position the Arab world as a meaningful contributor to global rheumatology science.

Keywords Arab countries · Rheumatic diseases · Health workforce · Health services accessibility · Patient-centered care · Accreditation · Research capacity building · Precision medicine · Artificial intelligence · Digital health

---

K. A. Alnaqbi (✉)
Rheumatology Division, Sheikh Tahnoon bin Mohammed Medical City, SEHA/PureHealth, Al Ain, UAE

Internal Medicine Department, College of Medicine and Health Sciences, UAE University, Al Ain, UAE

College of Medicine, RAK Medical and Health Sciences, Ras Al Khaimah, UAE
e-mail: kalnaqbi@gmail.com; kalnaqbi@seha.ae

K. A. Alnaqbi, G. Aldabie (eds.), *Rheumatic Diseases in the Arab World*,
https://doi.org/10.1007/978-981-92-0967-5_30

30.1 Introduction

Long before the scientific flourishing of the Islamic Golden Age, ancient Egyptian civilization (3300 BCE to 525 BCE) made important contributions to medical knowledge. Medical papyri such as the Edwin Smith and Ebers texts describe systematic approaches to diagnosis, anatomy, and treatment, representing some of the earliest recorded clinical observations [1]. Although separated by centuries, these early developments in medical organization and documentation took place in a region that would later become part of the Arab world.

The scientific renaissance of early Islamic civilization represents one of the most remarkable knowledge movements in human history. Between the eighth and fourteenth centuries, major urban centers such as Baghdad, Damascus, Cairo, and Cordoba became hubs of translation, scholarship, experimentation, and clinical practice. This created a unified scholarly language and enabled cultural exchange and cumulative intellectual development [2, 3]. Scholars not only preserved earlier knowledge but expanded it, laying foundations in medicine, optics, mathematics, pharmacology, and hospital organization that later influenced medical scholarship in Europe during the renaissance [3–5].

The term 'Arab world' does not imply ethnic or religious homogeneity. The scientific vitality of the classical Islamic Golden Age was not confined to Arab Muslims alone. It included Persian, Syriac, Andalusian, Central Asian, and other scholars, as well as Muslim, Christian, and Jewish physicians and scientists working within a shared intellectual framework. This intellectual diversity was particularly evident in regions such as Al-Andalus (Islamic Spain), where scholars from different religious and cultural backgrounds interacted within vibrant centers of learning for several centuries [6]. For example, Hunayn ibn Ishaq (c. 809–873 CE), a Christian physician, led major translation efforts of Galenic medicine, while Ibn Sina (Avicenna, 980–1037 CE), a Persian Muslim polymath, authored *The Canon of Medicine*, a medical encyclopedia that shaped teaching and clinical practice in both the Islamic world and medieval Europe for centuries [2, 4]. This diversity is also reflected in the work of Maimonides (1138–1204 CE), a Jewish physician and philosopher who lived within the Islamic world and integrated Greek, Islamic, and Jewish medical traditions into a coherent clinical and ethical framework [7].

A well-known story about the physician Al-Razi (Rhazes, c. 865–925 CE) illustrates the observational approach of the time. When asked to choose the best site for a hospital in Baghdad, he reportedly placed pieces of meat in different districts and selected the location where decomposition occurred most slowly, reasoning that it indicated healthier environmental conditions [8]. The story reflects broader principles of environmental awareness, observation, and rational decision-making that characterized hospital development. Importantly, the bimaristan was not merely a place of care but also a foundational site of medical training, clinical documentation, and an early public health organization [9].

Building on the historical legacy of scientific vitality in the Arab world, the future of rheumatology care must now be shaped by deliberate and coordinated action across the region. This chapter outlines a forward-looking framework to strengthen rheumatology care across the Arab world. It proposes actionable strategies across key domains: workforce development, modernization of clinical services, accreditation and quality reform, education and training redesign, research infrastructure, and digital transformation. Rather than presenting fragmented recommendations, the chapter introduces an integrated roadmap that aligns short-term achievable steps with medium- and long-term system-building goals.

30.2 Manpower

The combined population of the 22 Arab League countries is estimated to be approximately 480 million in 2024 [10]. In this book, the term "Arab world" refers to these countries, a regional grouping defined primarily by membership in the League of Arab States, where Arabic is the official language and an important component of shared cultural and political identity [11]. Across this large and diverse population, many remote and underserved areas face limited access to specialized care, including rheumatology services. Epidemiological and workforce studies indicate that the rheumatology workforce in Arab countries remains suboptimal relative to population needs. A recent survey by the Arab League of Associations for Rheumatology (*A*rLAR) *R*esear*ch* Group (ARCH) reported a mean density of 0.84 practicing rheumatologists per 100,000 population across 16 Arab countries [12]. However, substantial variation exists between countries, ranging from 0.06 per 100,000 in Sudan to 1.86 per 100,000 in Tunisia, and projected workforce expansion may not keep pace with expected population growth of approximately 20% by 2032. Moreover, waiting times for rheumatology consultations remain prolonged (averaging 20 days), reflecting the imbalance between demand and supply of specialists.

Reliable data on the number of pediatric rheumatologists are even scarcer, but available evidence and regional clinical experience suggest that the majority of pediatric cases across the region are diagnosed and managed by adult rheumatologists or general pediatricians rather than by specialists trained in pediatric rheumatology. This underscores the need to expand both adult and pediatric rheumatology training pathways to improve access to care, reduce diagnostic delays, and meet population health needs.

In addition to increasing overall workforce numbers, coordinated system-level policies are required to address geographic maldistribution. Evidence from the region demonstrates significant disparities in physician distribution across health regions [13]. International experience further indicates that financial incentives alone may have a limited impact unless combined with broader retention strategies [14]. The World Health Organization (WHO) recommends multifaceted approaches, including financial incentives, professional support, improved working conditions, and career development pathways, to enhance recruitment and retention in rural and remote settings [15]. In the Arab context, incentive-based models, such as commuting allowances, protected outreach clinics, housing benefits, and academic recognition, may therefore help improve access to specialist services, including rheumatology, in underserved regions.

Women constitute a substantial and growing proportion of the rheumatology workforce in Arab countries, with female rheumatologists comprising more than half of practitioners in several countries. However, despite this strong representation, women remain under-represented in senior leadership roles at many national rheumatology societies, highlighting the need to support and promote female leaders in rheumatology [16]. Encouragingly, the Gulf region demonstrates notable progress in this regard. As of March 2026, women serve as presidents of five national rheumatology societies or associations in the six Gulf countries, reflecting a more favorable trajectory toward gender balance in professional leadership within this subregion.

Collectively, these findings underscore the need for coordinated workforce reform across training, distribution, and leadership domains, as summarized in Table 30.1.

Table 30.1 Strategic priorities for strengthening the rheumatology workforce in the Arab world

Strategic area	Priority action	Rationale	Implementation horizon
Workforce planning	Establish regional workforce mapping and forecasting systems	Align training capacity with demographic trends and disease burden	*Short term*
Rural distribution	Introduce retention incentives for underserved and remote areas	Reduce geographic disparities in access to care	*Short–medium term*
Fellowship expansion	Increase accredited adult and pediatric rheumatology fellowship positions	Address specialist shortage and improve rheumatologist-to-population ratio	*Short–medium term*
Integrated training	Develop joint adult–pediatric rheumatology training pathways	Strengthen continuity of care and address pediatric workforce gaps	*Medium term*
Allied health capacity	Establish rheumatology nurse specialist certification programs Integrate clinical pharmacists into multidisciplinary rheumatology teams	Support multidisciplinary care and improve service efficiency Optimize medication safety, adherence, and biologic therapy monitoring	*Medium term*
Leadership development	Promote equitable female leadership within national rheumatology societies	Ensure equitable representation and sustainable institutional growth	*Medium–long term*

Implementation horizons: Short term = 0–2 years; Medium term = 3–5 years; Long term = 6+ years

30.3 Advancing Clinical Services

This section outlines key priority domains that will shape the evolution of rheumatology services across the Arab world.

30.3.1 Early Diagnosis and Screening

Training non-specialist clinicians in musculoskeletal (MSK) history-taking and physical examination improves early detection and referral of inflammatory arthritis. In the Kingdom of Saudi Arabia (KSA), primary care physicians trained by rheumatologists in MSK examination techniques showed fair-to-moderate agreement with rheumatologists in detecting synovitis and other signs of inflammatory arthritis, supporting the feasibility of such educational interventions in general medical settings [17]. Additionally, programs that combine training with structured referral guidelines and decision-support tools have been shown to reduce referral delays and increase confidence among primary care clinicians [18].

Additionally, with appropriate training in focused MSK examination and recognition of inflammatory arthritis, physiotherapists can accurately identify inflammatory presentations [19, 20]. In remote or underserved settings, they may help to detect suspected cases and facilitate timely referral when specialist evaluation is limited or unavailable. Examples of such training include extended-practice models such as the Advanced Clinician Practitioner in Arthritis Care (ACPAC) program offered by the University of Toronto in Canada, which equips physiotherapists with advanced skills in assessment, diagnosis, triage, and management of arthritis and other MSK disorders [21].

A structured framework for enhancing early detection and screening capacity across the Arab region is presented in Table 30.2.

30.3.2 Innovative Therapies

Globally, the use of biological therapies has transformed rheumatology care over the past three decades by enabling targeted management of inflammatory diseases. In the Arab world, there is growing interest in expanding the availability and affordability of these treatments by facilitating biosimilar adoption, which can reduce costs and potentially increase patient access to effective biologic-level therapies [22].

Consensus-based expert recommendations from the Gulf Cooperation Council (GCC) region highlight that biosimilars can reduce financial barriers and prevent underutilization of necessary treatments while maintaining comparable quality, safety, and efficacy to reference biologics [23]. The first Arab consensus-based

Table 30.2 Strategic priorities to enhance early diagnosis and screening of rheumatic diseases in the Arab world

Strategic domain	Key action	Expected impact	Implementation level
Standardized referral pathways	Develop and implement clear early arthritis referral criteria for primary care physicians.	Reduced diagnostic delay and faster access to rheumatology services.	*National* *Institutional*
AI-supported triage systems	Develop digital symptom-checker tools and decision-support algorithms to facilitate referrals.	Improved triage efficiency and optimized specialist utilization.	*National* *Institutional*
Primary care training	Provide structured musculoskeletal examination training workshops led by rheumatologists.	Improved recognition of synovitis and inflammatory presentations.	*National* *Institutional*
Decision-support tools	Introduce standardized electronic referral templates and screening checklists.	Reduced inappropriate referrals and improved diagnostic accuracy.	*Institutional*
Physiotherapist integration	Train physiotherapists in inflammatory arthritis screening and structured referral models.	Enhanced case detection in remote and underserved areas.	*National* *Institutional*
Undergraduate curriculum reform	Integrate focused musculoskeletal screening and inflammatory arthritis modules into medical and physiotherapy schools.	Long-term improvement in early disease recognition.	*Academic* *National* *Regional*
Public awareness campaigns	Launch campaigns highlighting early symptoms of inflammatory arthritis.	Earlier self-referral and reduced patient delay.	*National* *Community*

Implementation levels: Institutional = single facility; National = country-wide policy; Regional = multi-country Arab region; Community = public/community level; Academic = universities and training institutions
AI Artificial Intelligence

biosimilars value framework was recently published for GCC countries [24]. The expert panel proposed a value framework based on trust, cost savings, and contextual considerations and emphasized educational initiatives to increase stakeholder awareness, improve biosimilar knowledge, and support policymakers and decision-makers in promoting biosimilar adoption across high-income and low- to middle-income settings in the region.

Beyond biosimilars, Janus kinase (JAK) inhibitors and other targeted synthetic therapies have emerged as important treatments for inflammatory RMDs [25]. However, access to these agents remains uneven across the Arab world, particularly in countries affected by conflict or political instability. Fragile health systems, disrupted supply chains, and limited funding restrict access to modern therapies. Strengthening health infrastructure and political stability will be essential to improve equitable access to essential and innovative therapies and enhance patient outcomes.

30.3.3 Precision Medicine

Medicine rarely creates a unique therapy for each person. Instead, patients are grouped into biologically defined categories. Because of this, many experts prefer the term "precision medicine," which reflects stratified treatment rather than completely individualized care. Precision medicine, sometimes referred to as personalized medicine, aims to integrate biomarkers, genomic data, and immune profiling to guide treatment, improve efficacy, monitor disease activity, and minimize adverse effects. Advancements in genetics, molecular biology, transcriptomics, and systems biology are paving the way for precision medicine in rheumatology [26].

Available routine biomarkers that are widely used in clinical practice for the diagnosis and monitoring of rheumatic diseases include autoantibody panels such as anti-citrullinated protein antibodies (ACPA), rheumatoid factor, antinuclear antibodies (ANA), anti-dsDNA, and extractable nuclear antigen antibodies (ENA). In addition, inflammatory markers such as C-reactive protein (CRP), erythrocyte sedimentation rate (ESR), and calprotectin are commonly used to assess disease activity. Commercially available genetic biomarkers are HLA-B27 and HLA-B51. Beyond these established biomarkers, numerous molecular markers are currently being investigated in research settings. These include serum cytokine profiles (e.g., IL-6, TNF-α, IL-17, IL-37), synovial tissue molecular signatures such as B-cell, macrophage, and fibroblast subsets, and pharmacogenetic markers (e.g., MTHFR and HLA variants) that may help predict therapeutic response or adverse drug reactions in the future [27].

Several initiatives across the Arab world support the development of personalized medicine. Regional genomic resources, such as the Catalogue for Transmission Genetics in Arabs (CTGA) and other variant databases, facilitate the translation of genetic research into clinical practice by cataloguing disease-associated variants in Arab populations [28, 29]. National genomic programs have also been launched in KSA, the UAE, Qatar, and Egypt, aiming to map population-specific genetic variation and establish reference datasets to support precision healthcare [30].

Building on these genomic initiatives, translational genomic research is emerging in rheumatology, with studies beginning to identify genetic loci, biomarkers, and potential therapeutic targets relevant to clinical care. For example, a multinational genome-wide association study in Arab populations (Jordan, Lebanon, KSA, Qatar, and the UAE) identified both established and novel genetic loci associated with rheumatoid arthritis (RA), including two Arab-specific associations at 5q13 and 17p13 [31]. In addition, a multi-omics study from the UAE, combining different molecular data layers (e.g., genes and proteins), has shown how integrated molecular profiling can identify candidate biomarkers and therapeutic targets that may inform individualized treatment strategies in RA [32]. In pediatric rheumatology, genomic investigations from the UAE have demonstrated the clinical utility of next-generation sequencing and whole-exome sequencing for diagnosis and management, with genetic findings directly informing therapeutic decisions in most cases [33].

Despite its significant potential, the implementation of precision medicine in rheumatology across the Arab region still faces several challenges. These include limited biobanking infrastructure and governance frameworks, financial and sustainability constraints affecting genomic and biobanking research, difficulties in sharing data across institutions, and the need for stronger ethical and regulatory oversight to ensure the responsible management of genomic and clinical data [30, 34].

30.3.4 Telemedicine and Digital Health

Telemedicine and digital health technologies expanded rapidly during the COVID-19 pandemic and have become increasingly relevant in rheumatology practice [35]. These tools can improve access to specialist care, particularly in remote or underserved areas, through virtual consultations, remote disease monitoring, and mobile health applications for patient self-management. The ArLAR has recently published best practice guidelines for telehealth that can be adapted across Arab countries [36]. Tele-rheumatology is particularly suitable for follow-up care, disease monitoring, and medication counseling, whereas initial assessments, active or complex disease, and visits requiring procedures or detailed physical examination are generally better conducted in person. Despite these advances, tele-rheumatology remains underutilized in parts of the region due to infrastructural limitations, including inconsistent internet connectivity, limited digital platforms, and socioeconomic barriers.

30.3.5 Artificial Intelligence in Rheumatology

Artificial intelligence (AI) is expected to transform diagnosis, imaging interpretation, treatment selection, and disease monitoring [37]. Machine-learning algorithms can analyze complex datasets such as electronic medical records (EMRs), laboratory data, imaging studies, and genomic information [38]. In MSK imaging, AI tools are being explored to detect inflammatory lesions on magnetic resonance imaging (MRI) and assist in disease classification in conditions such as RA and axial spondyloarthritis (axSpA) [37].

Although peer-reviewed publications from Arab countries remain limited, regional interest in AI-based rheumatology research is increasing. A multicenter study from the UAE, Jordan, KSA, and Spain developed an AI system capable of automatically detecting sacroiliitis lesions on MRI in patients with axSpA [39]. Another study from Qatar introduced a hybrid deep-learning model for MRI-based classification of ankylosing spondylitis with high diagnostic accuracy [40]. AI may also support clinical triage and early diagnostic assessment. A study from the UAE evaluating a proprietary rule-based engine and GPT-4 for the initial assessment of rheumatology referrals demonstrated strong agreement between AI-generated differential diagnoses and rheumatologist evaluations [41].

30.3.6 Wearable Devices and Digital Biomarkers

Wearable devices increasingly monitor physical activity, sleep, and physiological parameters in patients with RMDs. Accelerometer-based sensors quantify physical activity, sedentary behavior, heart rate, and other physiological signals, enabling continuous real-world monitoring of patient health status. For example, wearable trackers have been used in patients with axSpA to measure physical activity and sedentary behavior and explore their relationship with disease activity and functional outcomes [42].

These technologies can generate digital biomarkers, defined as objective physiological or behavioral measurements collected through digital devices, including step count, physical activity levels, heart rate variability, and sleep metrics. A recent systematic review reported that digital biomarkers derived from wearable devices correlate with fatigue and activity levels across several chronic diseases, including RA and systemic lupus erythematosus (SLE), suggesting their potential to complement traditional patient-reported outcomes [43]. Studies using wearable devices and ecological momentary assessment in RA also demonstrate the feasibility of remote monitoring of symptoms, physical activity, and sleep [44]. However, published research specifically evaluating wearable-derived digital biomarkers in RMDs from Arab countries remains very limited, highlighting an important research gap.

30.3.7 Digital Twins and Computational Disease Models

Alongside advances in AI and precision medicine, another emerging technological concept is the development of digital or virtual twins. A digital twin can be defined as a computational replica of a patient, organ, or biological system that integrates multidimensional data and simulates its behavior to inform clinical decisions. These models continuously integrate clinical, molecular, imaging, and real-world data to predict disease progression and evaluate potential therapeutic interventions [45].

In rheumatology, digital twins represent an emerging technological concept with significant potential to transform disease understanding and treatment. For example, researchers have constructed large computational maps of immune and cellular pathways in the arthritic joint and converted them into executable models capable of reproducing disease mechanisms and identifying potential therapeutic targets [46].

In the future, integrating EMRs, imaging data, disease registries, and multi-omics datasets could enable the creation of patient-specific digital twins capable of predicting disease trajectories and optimizing individualized treatment strategies.

Although digital twin technologies are rapidly expanding in biomedical research, applications in RMDs remain limited, and no well-documented digital twin studies in rheumatology originating from Arab countries have yet been reported, highlighting an important opportunity for future regional research.

30.3.8 Patient-Centered Care

Patient-centered care is a core principle of modern rheumatology and includes clear communication, attention to patient goals and values, and shared decision-making when more than one reasonable treatment option exists. Incorporating patient preferences can improve engagement with care plans and align treatment choices with patients' daily lives [47]. Studies from the region suggest that many Arabic-speaking patients value involvement in decisions, but a substantial proportion (nearly 75%) still prefer a more physician-led approach, particularly in chronic disease care [48]. In rheumatology settings, regional studies on treatment preferences in RA also highlight the importance of discussing options with patients and incorporating preferences into therapy selection [49, 50].

Non-profit and charitable associations for patients with RMDs represent an important yet underdeveloped component of care in several Arab countries. These organizations can provide patient education, psychosocial support, advocacy for access to treatment, and participation in research and health policy dialogue. The Rheumatism Association and the Fibro Association in KSA are examples of structured charitable initiatives that support patients with RMDs through medical services, disease awareness, education, and community engagement programs serving both local and expatriate communities [51, 52]. Expanding similar models across the Arab world could complement clinical services and strengthen patient-centered rheumatology care systems.

The priority actions required to advance personalized medicine, innovative therapies, digital integration, and patient-centered care across the Arab region are summarized in Table 30.3.

30.4 Accreditation of Rheumatology Centers

Conceptual frameworks for centers of excellence emphasize specialized expertise, high-impact research, quality service delivery, leadership, and external accreditation as essential components to ensure standardized processes and alignment with recognized quality indicators and performance standards [53]. Formal evaluation frameworks (e.g., patient-centered standards of care and multidisciplinary quality indicators) have been developed in other regions and demonstrate how structured quality standards can enhance clinical outcomes and patient engagement [54].

Table 30.3 Strategic priorities to advance clinical innovation and patient-centered rheumatology care in the Arab world

Strategic domain	Key actions	Expected impact	Implementation level
Innovative therapies	Promote cost-effective biosimilar implementation aligned with regional value frameworks	Expanded access to biologic therapies and reduced financial barriers	*National Policy*
	Develop equitable reimbursement and insurance models for advanced biologics and targeted synthetic therapies	Reduced treatment disparities across socioeconomic groups	*National*
	Establish real-world pharmacovigilance and effectiveness registries for innovative medications	Improved safety monitoring and context-specific evidence generation	*Institutional Regional*
Personalized medicine	Develop precision-based treatment protocols integrating genomic, transcriptomic, and biomarker data into clinical decision-making	Improved therapeutic targeting, optimized treatment response, and reduced adverse events	*Institutional National*
	Establish regional biobanks and multi-omics research platforms linked to rheumatology registries	Generation of population-specific data to guide regional precision medicine	*National Regional*
	Integrate national genomics initiatives into rheumatology research frameworks and strengthen genomic infrastructure, data-sharing frameworks, and research capacity	Translation of genomic discoveries into clinical practice and equitable implementation of personalized medicine across the region	*National*
Telemedicine and digital health	Expand tele-rheumatology services across primary and secondary care networks	Improved access to specialist consultation in remote and underserved regions	*Institutional Regional*
	Implement secure digital platforms for remote monitoring and patient self-management	Enhanced continuity of care and reduced travel burden	*Institutional*
	Strengthen digital infrastructure and internet access in rural areas	Reduced geographic inequities in specialist care	*National*
Artificial intelligence in rheumatology	Integrate AI-based clinical decision-support and imaging analysis within EMR systems	Earlier diagnosis, improved imaging interpretation, and enhanced clinical decision-making	*Institutional National*

(continued)

Table 30.3 (continued)

Strategic domain	Key actions	Expected impact	Implementation level
Wearable devices and digital biomarkers	Promote the use of wearable technologies to monitor physical activity, sleep patterns, and physiological signals in patients with RMDs	Continuous real-world monitoring of disease activity and functional status. Generation of region-specific evidence and improved adoption of digital health technologies	*Institutional National*
	Develop digital biomarker frameworks integrating wearable data with patient-reported outcomes and clinical registries	Earlier detection of disease flares and improved longitudinal disease monitoring	*Institutional Regional*
Digital twins and computational disease models	Develop computational models of RMDs integrating clinical, imaging, and molecular data	Improved understanding of disease mechanisms and identification of novel therapeutic targets	*Research Institutional*
	Integrate EMRs, registries, imaging databases, and multi-omics datasets to build patient-specific disease models	Prediction of disease progression and individualized treatment strategies	*National Regional*
	Establish interdisciplinary collaborations between rheumatologists, data scientists, and computational biologists	Acceleration of digital twin research and innovation in rheumatology	*Institutional Regional*
Patient-centered care	Integrate shared decision-making approaches into routine rheumatology consultations	Improved treatment adherence and patient engagement in care planning	*Institutional*
	Integrate patient-reported outcome measures (PROMs) into routine clinical practice	Improved disease monitoring and alignment with patient priorities	*Institutional*
	Support the development of non-profit patient associations and charitable organizations for patients with RMDs	Improved patient education, psychosocial support, advocacy for treatment access, and participation in research and policy dialogue	*National*

Implementation levels: Institutional = single facility; National = country-wide policy; Regional = multi-country Arab region; Policy = legislative or regulatory action
AI Artificial Intelligence, *EMR* Electronic Medical Record, *RMDs* Rheumatic and Musculoskeletal Diseases

In the Arab world, accreditation of rheumatology-specific patient-centered programs remains extremely rare. Unlike several medical specialties, there are no widely adopted regional accreditation systems for rheumatology programs to ensure consistent delivery of care across centers. International rheumatology bodies such as the European Alliance of Associations for Rheumatology (EULAR) and the Asia Pacific League of Associations for Rheumatology (APLAR) function as accrediting authorities by formally designating centers of excellence through structured application processes, defined evaluation criteria, and fixed-term certification periods with mandatory renewal [55, 56].

Beyond specialty-specific accreditation frameworks, broader hospital and clinical program accreditation models, such as those offered by Joint Commission International (JCI), are available globally [57]. JCI's Clinical Care Program Certification (CCPC) provides accreditation for disease-specific clinical programs that demonstrate integrated, evidence-based, and multidisciplinary care pathways. However, their application to rheumatology programs in Arab countries remains limited. In 2019, four rheumatology clinical care programs at Al Ain Hospital in the UAE received JCI accreditation for juvenile idiopathic arthritis, ankylosing spondylitis, SLE, and RA [58]. The accreditation was not renewed following disruptions related to the COVID-19 pandemic. As of March 2026, no rheumatology CCPC has been reported in any Arab country [59].

Sharing experiences across Arab countries in developing structured rheumatology programs highlights the importance of standardized frameworks. This supports the potential establishment of a regional rheumatology accreditation body tailored to the Arab context. For additional details on standards and accreditation concepts, refer to the Chap. 23.

30.5 Rheumatology Education and Training Programs

Continuous professional development through continuing medical education (CME), workshops, and conferences is essential to keep rheumatologists and allied health professionals updated on evolving diagnostic tools and therapies. Most Arab countries actively participate in national and regional scientific meetings and continuing medical education activities, such as conferences and workshops. However, systematic integration of CME within structured career development frameworks, including formal accreditation and requirements tied to licensure or professional advancement, remains highly variable across the region, with some countries having mature systems and others lacking formal structures or mandatory requirements [60].

To help address these disparities in access to structured educational resources, the ArLAR offers an educational library that serves as a centralized, freely accessible repository of webinars and tailored educational content (in English and French), including recordings of past scientific sessions and expert-led discussions on current topics in rheumatology [61].

30.5.1 Rheumatology Fellowship Training Programs

The sustainability of rheumatology services in Arab countries depends on structured fellowship training programs. Health authorities in each country should regularly assess the national workforce needs for both adult and pediatric rheumatologists and align fellowship intake with projected population demands for RMDs. Workforce planning is influenced by multiple determinants, including demographic growth, epidemiologic burden of RMDs, political stability, healthcare financing, and national prioritization of specialized care [62].

Several Arab countries have successfully established national rheumatology fellowship programs. However, there is heterogeneity in accreditation standards, curriculum structure, research exposure, and exit examinations. In 2023, the Arab Board of Health Specializations established the Arab Board of Rheumatology, providing a unified regional framework for specialist certification. The program lasts two years [63].

The integration of fellows within rheumatology departments provides multiple academic and system-level benefits:

1. Academic enrichment: Trainees stimulate critical appraisal of evidence and encourage case-based literature review, fostering an academic culture within clinical practice [64].
2. Research productivity: Fellows often contribute to clinical research, registry development, quality improvement initiatives, and manuscript preparation [65].
3. Multidisciplinary development: Fellowship training promotes interdisciplinary collaboration with radiology, rehabilitation, immunology, and primary care, strengthening integrated models of RMD care.
4. Practice productivity: The presence of trainees can support service delivery and contribute to clinical productivity. In supervised settings, fellows may enhance productivity metrics and complement the attending workforce while maintaining quality of care [66]. This benefit is relevant in both government and private practice environments.
5. Service expansion: Structured supervision allows optimization of patient throughput and facilitates expansion of specialized clinics or service lines while maintaining quality standards [67].
6. Succession planning: Training programs contribute to long-term workforce sustainability and ensure continuity of rheumatology services [67].

As of March 2026, based on the author's personal communication and the information presented in the country-specific chapters of this book, several Arab countries have established local rheumatology specialization or fellowship programs, including Kuwait, KSA, Qatar, the UAE, Jordan, Syria, Lebanon, Palestine, Iraq, Egypt, Sudan, Algeria, Tunisia, and Morocco. However, the availability, accreditation structure, duration, and recognition of these programs vary considerably across the region. In some countries, rheumatology training is delivered through nationally accredited subspecialty programs, while in others it remains integrated within broader internal medicine training frameworks or relies on overseas certification pathways. In contrast, a number of Arab countries currently lack formally structured national rheumatology specialization programs and depend on international training systems.

Enhanced collaboration among rheumatology fellowship programs across Arab countries could standardize curricula, promote trainee exchange, and harmonize competency-based assessments. Academic partnerships, joint virtual teaching sessions, regional grand rounds, and collaborative research networks may help reduce disparities in training quality and improve patient outcomes across the region.

30.5.2 Rheumatology Nursing Programs

Across the Arab region, there is a recognized shortage of nurses with specialized training in rheumatology. Although general nursing education exists throughout the Arab world, there are no formal postgraduate or specialist training pathways specifically for rheumatology nursing [68]. This gap presents a challenge to the delivery of comprehensive multidisciplinary rheumatology care and may contribute to unmet needs in chronic disease management.

Internationally, the role of rheumatology nurses has been clearly defined. The 2018 update of the EULAR recommendations emphasizes that rheumatology nurses are integral members of the healthcare team and should provide needs-based patient education, support shared decision-making, participate in comprehensive disease management, and contribute to improved access to care and patient satisfaction [69]. The recommendations also highlight the importance of continuous specialty education and the development of extended nursing roles following appropriate training.

In high-income countries, rheumatology nurse-led care models have demonstrated improved patient perceptions of care, equivalent or superior clinical outcomes, and potential cost-effectiveness for conditions such as RA [68, 70]. Specialist nurses also contribute to improved patient education, medication management, monitoring for adverse drug reactions, and coordination of care within multidisciplinary teams [71].

30.5.3 Enhancing Procedural Skills

30.5.3.1 Musculoskeletal Ultrasonography Programs

MSK ultrasonography has become an increasingly important tool in modern rheumatology practice. It improves diagnostic accuracy in inflammatory arthritis, enhances early detection of synovitis, and supports treatment monitoring and treat-to-target strategies [72]. International guidelines, including EULAR recommendations, recognize MSK ultrasound as a valuable adjunct in the assessment and management of RA and other inflammatory RMDs [73].

Despite its growing importance, structured ultrasound training is not uniformly embedded within all rheumatology fellowship curricula worldwide. As a result, many rheumatologists pursue additional certification through international courses such as those offered by the EULAR and the American College of Rheumatology (ACR) [74, 75]. EULAR has developed a standardized multilevel training framework for rheumatologic ultrasonography [75], and EULAR-endorsed courses have been conducted in several Arab countries, including the UAE and Qatar, supporting regional capacity building [76, 77]. The ArLAR Musculoskeletal Sonography Group (regional initiative) supports training and collaboration with international bodies to enhance MSK ultrasonography education in the Arab region [78].

30.5.3.2 Nailfold Capillaroscopy

Nailfold video capillaroscopy (NVC) is an essential diagnostic and prognostic tool in systemic sclerosis and other connective tissue diseases. It is incorporated into the 2013 ACR/EULAR classification criteria for systemic sclerosis and is recommended for the evaluation of Raynaud's phenomenon and microvascular involvement [79]. Given its recognized clinical value, appropriate training in capillaroscopy is increasingly important for rheumatology practice.

However, structured training in capillaroscopy varies across fellowship programs and is not yet universally integrated into rheumatology training curricula. A dedicated curriculum has been shown to increase fellows' confidence and ability to perform and interpret nailfold capillaroscopy, supporting its inclusion in educational programs [80]. Research from the Arab region remains limited. However, emerging data from Qatar reported that severe NVC patterns in systemic sclerosis were associated with Raynaud's phenomenon and digital ulcers, supporting the clinical value of NVC in regional cohorts [81].

Table 30.4 summarizes a strategic framework to enhance rheumatology education and training programs in the Arab world.

30.6 Research in Rheumatology

Collaborative research initiatives across Arab countries can accelerate progress through shared data platforms, multicenter trials, and coordinated resources, improving understanding and management of RMDs across diverse healthcare systems. Over the past decade, multinational collaborative efforts across the Arab region have generated important publications [36, 82–86].

To further strengthen regional collaboration, the ARCH group of ArLAR was established in June 2021 [87]. The group has since published several studies addressing diverse aspects of RMDs and patient care [12, 88, 89]. In addition to research

Table 30.4 Strategic framework for enhancing rheumatology education and training programs in the Arab world

Strategic domain	Key actions	Expected impact	Implementation level
1. Digital Learning Platforms	Develop centralized online portals hosting recorded lectures, case discussions, procedural demonstrations, guideline updates, and regional consensus documents	Equitable access regardless of geography; continuous knowledge updating; cost-effective expansion	*Institutional/ National*
2. Regional Exchange Fellowship Programs	Establish formal inter-country exchange rotations among accredited Arab rheumatology training centers to expose fellows to diverse case-mix, subspecialty clinics, procedural training, and research environments	Harmonized competencies, reduced training disparities, strengthened regional collaboration, and capacity building in under-resourced settings	*National/ Regional*
3. Mentorship Networks	Establish structured mentorship programs linking trainees and early career rheumatologists with regional and international experts for case discussions, research supervision, and career guidance	Improved clinical decision-making, enhanced academic productivity, strengthened leadership, and regional talent retention	*Institutional/ National*
4. Protected Research Time During Training	Allocate dedicated research blocks within fellowship curricula, supported by institutional policies and funding mechanisms	Increased research output, registry development, multinational study participation, and cultivation of clinician-scientists	*Institutional*
5. Multidisciplinary Team Training Models	Develop joint training activities involving rheumatologists alongside radiologists (e.g., MRI for axSpA), rehabilitation specialists, nurses, pharmacists, immunologists, and primary care physicians	Strengthened team-based care, improved service coordination, enhanced patient-centered outcomes, and readiness for complex chronic disease management	*Institutional*

(continued)

Table 30.4 (continued)

Strategic domain	Key actions	Expected impact	Implementation level
6. Development of Rheumatology Nursing Curricula	Advocate for structured rheumatology nursing curricula within nursing colleges and universities, supported by regional professional bodies and workforce planning initiatives	Strengthened multidisciplinary care, improved chronic disease management, and enhanced workforce capacity	*National / Policy*
7. Integration of Structured Procedural Training (Musculoskeletal Ultrasound and Capillaroscopy)	Integrate musculoskeletal ultrasonography and nailfold video capillaroscopy training within Arab rheumatology fellowship curricula	Enhanced procedural competency, improved diagnostic precision, early diagnosis, improved risk stratification, and reduced reliance on external imaging	*Institutional/ National*

Implementation levels: Institutional = single facility; National = country-wide policy; Regional = multi-country Arab region; Policy = legislative or regulatory action
axSpA Axial SpondyloArthritis, *MRI* Magnetic Resonance Imaging

output, ARCH has organized online seminars and workshops focused on research methodology, outcome measures, and cohort development, often involving regional and international experts.

A major milestone in advancing regional academic collaboration was the establishment of the *Arab Journal of Rheumatology* in 2021 under the umbrella of ArLAR [90]. Published in English, this journal represents a unified academic platform for disseminating research from across the Arab region, with an editorial board composed primarily of expert rheumatologists and researchers from Arab countries. Although the journal remains relatively new and faces financial and logistical challenges, it reflects a collective commitment to strengthening regional scientific output.

30.6.1 Challenges of Conducting Rheumatology Research in the Arab World

Despite progress in regional collaboration, several structural and systemic barriers continue to limit the growth and global impact of rheumatology research, particularly in Arab countries [91, 92]. Addressing these challenges is important for improving patient outcomes, informing healthcare policies, and advancing the field globally. Below are key obstacles limiting research progress in rheumatology within the region.

30.6.1.1 Under-Representation in Global Research Initiatives

Patients from Arab countries remain under-represented in international multicenter clinical trials and high-impact rheumatology publications, with regional research output accounting for a small proportion of global rheumatology literature [93]. This under-representation limits the availability of region-specific data and reduces the visibility of Arab populations in global evidence generation and policy development.

For example, rheumatology research from the region includes relatively few randomized controlled trials (RCTs), and several countries report limited or no locally conducted RCTs [94]. Consequently, many trials evaluating biologic therapies for RMDs have recruited predominantly from North America and Europe, with minimal participation from Middle Eastern or North African populations. As a result, evidence on treatment outcomes in Arab populations remains limited, despite potential genetic and environmental factors that may influence disease expression and therapeutic response.

30.6.1.2 Limited Research Infrastructure

In many Arab countries, research infrastructure remains insufficiently developed [93]. Key challenges include limited protected research time, lack of research coordinators, absence of registries, and limited digital research infrastructure [92, 95]. Furthermore, access to biostatisticians and clinical epidemiologists is often limited, constraining methodological rigor and large-scale data analysis. Without expert guidance in study design, statistical analysis, and data interpretation, researchers often struggle to produce robust and publishable results—a gap that is particularly problematic for complex studies requiring advanced statistical modeling.

30.6.1.3 Funding Constraints and Competing Priorities

Research funding for RMDs remains limited in many regions, particularly in low- and middle-income countries. Compared with fields such as infectious diseases and oncology, which benefit from more established global funding mechanisms, rheumatology research often receives less dedicated support [96]. Furthermore, many funding agencies restrict awards to domestic investigators or prioritize nationally focused projects, limiting opportunities for multinational collaboration [91, 92]. Securing financial support for multicenter regional studies, therefore, remains challenging, especially in resource-constrained settings.

30.6.1.4 Mentorship, Research Culture, and Workforce Engagement

Limited availability of structured mentorship programs for early career investigators represents a significant barrier to research sustainability. Heavy clinical demands may further constrain protected time for scholarly activity, particularly in private or semi-private healthcare environments [91, 96]. This pattern may be influenced by limited exposure to research methodologies during training, modest institutional incentives, and the perception that research is not consistently associated with clear professional advancement. These factors may contribute to gaps in regional data on disease patterns and treatment outcomes. Similar challenges have been described in other resource-constrained regions, including sub-Saharan Africa [92].

Collaborative research culture varies across institutions. A common challenge is the substantial reliance on principal investigators to drive all aspects of the research process—from study design and data collection to analysis and manuscript preparation. This imbalance may contribute to inefficiencies and delays and may affect overall research quality. The limited development of multidisciplinary research teams—ideally including senior and junior rheumatologists, biostatisticians, and methodologists—together with an underdeveloped patient support group infrastructure, may further restrict the capacity to conduct comprehensive, high-quality studies [91, 96].

30.6.1.5 Administrative and System-Level Barriers

At the system level, governance and health research structures strongly influence research sustainability in the Arab region. In the Eastern Mediterranean Region, key weaknesses include limited national health research policies, weak stewardship frameworks, inadequate monitoring systems, and insufficient sustained investment in research capacity [97]. These structural gaps limit long-term systematic planning and hinder the effective translation of research findings into policy and practice.

In many Arab countries, research production is not consistently aligned with national health priorities. This reflects fragmented institutional coordination and limited integration between research institutions and policymaking bodies [98, 99]. In addition, the absence of structured knowledge transfer mechanisms reduces the use of locally generated evidence in health decision-making.

Operationally, regional situational analyses of health research systems identify weaknesses in research governance processes, including complex and fragmented regulatory and ethical approval procedures, limited institutional research management capacity, and insufficient coordination to ensure efficient oversight and implementation of research activities [97, 100]. These governance and administrative constraints extend beyond individual investigators and shape the broader research environment across many Arab countries.

These recurring barriers are summarized in Table 30.5, which outlines the principal challenges affecting rheumatology research across the Arab world.

Table 30.5 Key challenges to rheumatology research in the Arab world

Challenge	Key contributing factors	Impact
1. Under-representation in global research	Exclusion from multicenter trials and registries; insufficient region-specific data; under-representation in high-impact journals	Limited integration of Arab data into global evidence base; reduced influence on global guidelines and policy
2. Limited research infrastructure	No protected research time; lack of coordinators, registries, and biostatisticians	Poor methodological rigor; limited publishable output
3. Funding constraints and competing priorities	Prioritization of high-mortality diseases; scarce multicenter grants	Few RMD-focused studies; restricted research scope
4. Mentorship, culture, and workforce gaps	No mentorship programs; heavy clinical load; low motivation; substantial reliance on PI	Unsustainable research pipelines; low productivity
5. Administrative and system-level barriers	Weak national research policies; fragmented governance and institutional coordination; limited knowledge translation mechanisms; complex regulatory and ethical approval processes; limited research management systems	Limited policy translation; inefficient oversight; poor long-term planning

RMD Rheumatic and Musculoskeletal Disease, *PI* Principal Investigator

30.6.2 Transforming Rheumatology Research in the Arab World: From Gaps to Action

Research systems do not improve by chance; they improve through deliberate design, sustained effort, and institutional commitment [101]. In the Arab world, rheumatology research faces structural, institutional, and cultural challenges that have been outlined throughout this book. Addressing these challenges requires coordinated action at multiple levels—from individual clinicians and trainees, through institutional systems and governance structures, to regional collaboration and patient engagement.

Table 30.6 proposes a practical and adaptable roadmap for strengthening rheumatology research capacity and impact across Arab countries, recognizing that implementation strategies may vary depending on national context and available resources.

At the institutional level, maintaining continuous dialogue with hospital leadership is essential. Research should not be viewed as secondary to clinical service but as an integral component of high-quality healthcare. Conducting research enhances patient engagement, fosters innovation, strengthens institutional reputation, and may ultimately translate into increased patient trust, physician productivity, and sustainable revenue models [102, 103].

Bridging the gap between academic and hospital-based rheumatologists is equally important. University-based clinicians should actively collaborate with full-time hospital rheumatologists, while hospital-based clinicians with research

Table 30.6 Strategic actions to strengthen rheumatology research capacity in Arab countries across multiple levels

Level	Key barriers addressed	Strategic actions	Expected outcomes
Individual (Clinicians and Researchers)	Limited methodological skills Low research motivation	Engage with experienced researchers Attend research methodology courses Seek mentorship Collaborate in ongoing research projects	Improved research competence Increased research productivity
Training (Undergraduate and Postgraduate)	Limited early exposure to research	Attract students/residents through structured rotations Integrate research training into curricula Require trainee research projects for graduation Involve trainees in consensus initiatives Offer research methodology courses Develop structured mentorship programs Establish clinical epidemiology programs	Stronger research culture in early career development
Institutional/ Organizational	Limited research infrastructure Lack of protected research time Weak institutional coordination	Establish research infrastructure (protected time, offices, biostatistics support, digital platforms) Recognize and incentivize research contributions Form multidisciplinary research teams Maintain engagement with hospital leadership Support internal and external grant applications Encourage publication in national/regional journals	Sustainable research infrastructure Higher-quality research outputs Stronger institutional research culture

(continued)

Table 30.6 (continued)

Level	Key barriers addressed	Strategic actions	Expected outcomes
Regional Collaboration	Fragmented research networks Limited multicenter studies	Strengthen regional research networks Develop shared data platforms Harmonize research protocols Establish sustainable disease registries Share best practices in registry development Facilitate cross-country collaboration Support national/regional rheumatology journals Develop online networking platforms for researchers	Increased research visibility Greater region-specific evidence generation Enhanced multicenter collaboration
Patient Engagement and Dissemination	Limited patient involvement in research	Educate patients about research participation Involve patients in surveys and consensus processes Disseminate research findings publicly Engage policymakers to translate evidence into practice	More patient-centered research Greater societal and policy impact

questions should seek academic partnerships to design and implement methodologically sound studies. Such bidirectional collaboration strengthens both clinical relevance and scientific rigor.

Capacity building should also include training in scientific writing and research dissemination skills. Structured educational sessions on manuscript preparation, responding to peer-review comments, and managing rejection constructively can empower researchers across the region [104]. Given that English is not the first language in all Arab countries, some investigators face challenges in translating complex scientific ideas into clear academic writing. Mentorship and the responsible use of language-support tools—including artificial intelligence-based applications used strictly for grammar and stylistic refinement—may help reduce this barrier while preserving scientific integrity.

At the regional level, collaborative research between Arab countries requires support at governmental, institutional, and professional society levels. Recognition of RMDs as a health priority by ministries of health is fundamental. Regional collaboration allows diverse perspectives and expertise to converge, facilitating the generation of region-specific evidence and consensus-based guidance. Although consensus-based recommendations remain limited in the Arab region, meaningful progress has emerged in recent years, including the ArLAR telehealth recommendations and Gulf-based consensus initiatives on biosimilars and axSpA [23, 24, 36, 105].

Patient engagement represents another cornerstone of sustainable healthcare and research development. Involving patients in shared decision-making, awareness initiatives, and quality improvement processes enhances transparency, relevance, and societal trust, consistent with international best practices in collaborative health systems [106]. In the Arab region, structured initiatives such as the Arab Adult Arthritis Awareness campaigns demonstrate how culturally tailored engagement strategies can strengthen patient education, outreach, and community trust [88].

Promoting transparency and fairness within research culture is essential. Clear authorship criteria [107], equitable access to research opportunities, and transparent processes in collaboration strengthen trust within the scientific community and encourage broader participation.

Finally, research impact does not end with publication. Effective dissemination through regional and international conferences, endorsement by ministries of health and professional societies, responsible use of social media, and support from regional journals are important to translating research findings into practice and policy. Supporting emerging regional journals, such as the *Annals of Rheumatology and Autoimmunity* [108] and the *Arab Journal of Rheumatology* [90], can strengthen the regional research ecosystem. In addition, expanding publication opportunities for researchers from countries affected by economic hardship or conflict may promote broader participation in regional research.

Together, these actions reflect a shift from identifying gaps to building solutions. The future of rheumatology research in Arab countries will depend not only on resources but also on collective vision, collaboration, and sustained commitment.

30.7 Conclusion

The future of rheumatology care in the Arab world will depend on translating vision into structured systems that improve equitable patient outcomes. Although progress has been made in clinical innovation, workforce development, research collaboration, and education, significant disparities remain across the region. The Arab world includes 22 countries with substantial variation in resources, conflict burden, digital maturity, academic capacity, insurance systems, and regulatory environments. Addressing these differences will require coordinated efforts to expand the rheumatology workforce, strengthen training and accreditation pathways, develop research infrastructure, and promote patient engagement and digital transformation.

Strengthening rheumatology care is not only a clinical priority but also a health system responsibility. Investment in research capacity, equitable access to innovative therapies, multidisciplinary care models, and patient support networks will be essential for building sustainable services. The region's long tradition of scientific scholarship illustrates that transformative progress is possible when institutions prioritize knowledge, collaboration, and inclusive research.

Emerging technologies such as digital health platforms, artificial intelligence, wearable monitoring, and computational disease modeling may further support more personalized and data-driven care. With sustained collaboration and system-level reform, the Arab world has the opportunity to improve outcomes for patients with rheumatic diseases and contribute more actively to global advances in rheumatology.

Acknowledgments The author thanks Prof. Robert D. Inman (Professor of Medicine and Immunology, University of Toronto, Canada), Dr. Suad Hannawi (Consultant Rheumatologist, Emirates Health Services, UAE), and Dr. Ghaydaa Aldabie (Consultant Rheumatologist, Farwaniya Hospital, Kuwait) for reviewing earlier drafts of this chapter and for their valuable comments and suggestions.

Disclaimer The views and opinions expressed in this chapter are those of the author and do not necessarily reflect the official policy or position of their affiliated institutions or organizations. In addition, ChatGPT (version 5.2, OpenAI) was used solely for language editing. All scientific content, interpretations, and conclusions are the author's own.

Conflict of Interest None.

References

1. Metwaly AM, Ghoneim MM, Eissa IH, Elsehemy IA, Mostafa AE, Hegazy MM, et al. Traditional ancient Egyptian medicine: a review. Saudi J Biol Sci. 2021;28(10):5823–32. https://doi.org/10.1016/j.sjbs.2021.06.044.
2. Gutas D. Greek thought, Arabic culture: the Graeco-Arabic translation movement in Baghdad and early Abbasid society. 1st ed. London: Routledge; 1998.
3. Saliba G. Islamic science and the making of the European renaissance. Cambridge: MIT Press; 2011.
4. Pormann PE, Savage-Smith E. Medieval Islamic medicine. Edinburgh: Edinburgh University Press; 2007.
5. Arraez-Aybar LA, Bueno-Lopez JL, Raio N. Toledo School of Translators and their influence on anatomical terminology. Ann Anat. 2015;198:21–33. https://doi.org/10.1016/j.aanat.2014.12.003.
6. Menocal MR. The ornament of the world: how Muslims, Jews, and Christians created a culture of tolerance in medieval Spain. Boston: Little, Brown and Company; 2002. 315 p.
7. Gesundheit B. Maimonides' appreciation for medicine. Rambam Maimonides Med J. 2011;2(1):e0018. https://doi.org/10.5041/RMMJ.10018.
8. Hajar R. The air of history (part IV): great Muslim physicians Al Rhazes. Heart Views. 2013;14(2):93–5. https://doi.org/10.4103/1995-705X.115499.
9. Asad MR, Almansour M, Kazmi SY, Alzahrani RE, Ahmed MM, Nazeer M. Educational paradigms in Islamic medical history: a review. J Pharm Bioallied Sci. 2024;16(Suppl 1):S56–S9. https://doi.org/10.4103/jpbs.jpbs_969_23.
10. United Nations Economic and Social Commission for Western Asia (UNESCWA). Demographic trends in the Arab region. 2025 Mar 13. [cited 2026 May 16]. Available from: https://www.unescwa.org/news/demographic-trends-arab-region-rapid-population-growth-and-impactful-changes.
11. Al-Wer E. Variation in Arabic languages. In: Brown K, editor. Encyclopedia of Language & Linguistics. Oxford: Elsevier; 2006. p. 341–4. https://doi.org/10.1016/B0-08-044854-2/01527-3.
12. Ziade N, Hmamouchi I, Haouichat C, Baron F, Al Mayouf S, Abdulateef N, et al. The rheumatology workforce in the Arab countries: current status, challenges, opportunities, and future needs from an ArLAR cross-sectional survey. Rheumatol Int. 2023;43(12):2281–92. https://doi.org/10.1007/s00296-023-05427-x.

13. Kattan W, Alshahrani A. Navigating the 2022 physician workforce dynamics in Saudi Arabia: a study of regional distribution. Open Public Health J. 2025;18:e18749445418574. https://doi.org/10.2174/0118749445418574251007111758.
14. Jobalayeva B, Khismetova Z, Glushkova N, Kozhekenova Z, Abzaliyeva A, Berikuly D, et al. The impact of incentive scheme on rural healthcare workforce availability: a case study of Kazakhstan. Hum Resour Health. 2024;22(1):23. https://doi.org/10.1186/s12960-024-00905-0.
15. Ajuebor O, Boniol M, McIsaac M, Onyedike C, Akl EA. Increasing access to health workers in rural and remote areas: what do stakeholders' value and find feasible and acceptable? Hum Resour Health. 2020;18(1):77. https://doi.org/10.1186/s12960-020-00519-2.
16. Ziade N, Hmamouchi I, El Kibbi L. Women in rheumatology in the Arab league of associations for rheumatology countries: a rising workforce. Front Med (Lausanne). 2022;9:880285. https://doi.org/10.3389/fmed.2022.880285.
17. Magliah R, Hafiz W, Alahmadi ZA, Siddiqui MI, Ahmed HM, Attar SM, et al. Early diagnosis of inflammatory arthritis by primary care physicians following training by a rheumatologist. Open Access Rheumatol. 2019;11:315–21. https://doi.org/10.2147/OARRR.S222630.
18. Bourgeois C, Sanchez-Lucas M, Olmedo-Galindo J, Schiaffino MT, Del Rio T, Molina-Collada J, et al. Improving early referrals for inflammatory arthritis through primary care engagement: a quality improvement initiative. Rheumatol Adv Pract. 2025;9(4):rkaf129. https://doi.org/10.1093/rap/rkaf129.
19. Passalent L, Hawke C, Lawson DO, Omar A, Alnaqbi KA, Wallis D, et al. Advancing early identification of axial Spondyloarthritis: an interobserver comparison of extended role practitioners and rheumatologists. J Rheumatol. 2020;47(4):524–30. https://doi.org/10.3899/jrheum.180787.
20. Ehrmann Feldman D, Bernatsky S, Orozco T, El-Khoury J, Desmeules F, Laliberte M, et al. Physical therapists' ability to distinguish between inflammatory and noninflammatory arthritis and to appropriately refer patients to a rheumatologist. Arthritis Care Res (Hoboken). 2020;72(12):1747–54. https://doi.org/10.1002/acr.24081.
21. Ahluwalia V, Inrig T, Larsen T, Shupak R, Papneja T, Karasik A, et al. An advanced clinician practitioner in arthritis care (ACPAC) maintains a positive patient experience while increasing capacity in rheumatology community care. J Multidiscip Healthc. 2021;14:1299–310. https://doi.org/10.2147/JMDH.S304206.
22. El Zorkany B, Al Ani N, Al Emadi S, Al Saleh J, Uthman I, El Dershaby Y, et al. Biosimilars in rheumatology: recommendations for regulation and use in middle eastern countries. Clin Rheumatol. 2018;37(5):1143–52. https://doi.org/10.1007/s10067-018-3982-9.
23. Alnaqbi KA, Al Adhoubi N, Aldallal S, Al Emadi S, Al-Herz A, El Shamy AM, et al. Consensus-based overarching principles and recommendations on the use of Biosimilars in the treatment of inflammatory arthritis in the Gulf region. BioDrugs. 2024;38(3):449–63. https://doi.org/10.1007/s40259-023-00642-1.
24. Alnaqbi KA, Al-Jedai A, Farghaly M, Omair MA, Hamad A, Abutiban FMA, et al. Expert consensus recommendations on a Biosimilars value framework for the Gulf cooperation council countries. Ther Innov Regul Sci. 2025;59(1):153–63. https://doi.org/10.1007/s43441-024-00716-4.
25. Huston KK. Recent advances in rheumatology. Mo Med. 2025;122(5):433–9.
26. Guthridge JM, Wagner CA, James JA. The promise of precision medicine in rheumatology. Nat Med. 2022;28(7):1363–71. https://doi.org/10.1038/s41591-022-01880-6.
27. Colina M, Campana G. Precision medicine in rheumatology: the role of biomarkers in diagnosis and treatment optimization. J Clin Med. 2025;14(5) https://doi.org/10.3390/jcm14051735.
28. Centre for Arab Genomic Studies (CAGS). Home page [Internet]. Dubai (UAE): CAGS. [cited 2026 May 16]. Available from: http://www.cags.org.ae/.
29. Vatsyayan A, Sharma P, Gupta S, Sandhu S, Venu SL, Sharma V, et al. DALIA- a comprehensive resource of disease alleles in Arab population. PLoS One. 2021;16(1):e0244567. https://doi.org/10.1371/journal.pone.0244567.

30. Abdelhafiz AS, Ahram M, Ibrahim ME, Elgamri A, Gamel E, Labib R, et al. Biobanks in the low- and middle-income countries of the Arab Middle East region: challenges, ethical issues, and governance arrangements-a qualitative study involving biobank managers. BMC Med Ethics. 2022;23(1):83. https://doi.org/10.1186/s12910-022-00822-8.
31. Saxena R, Plenge RM, Bjonnes AC, Dashti HS, Okada Y, Gad El Haq W, et al. A multinational Arab genome-wide association study identifies new genetic associations for rheumatoid arthritis. Arthritis Rheumatol. 2017;69(5):976–85. https://doi.org/10.1002/art.40051.
32. Tariq MH, Advani D, Almansoori BM, AlSamahi ME, Aldhaheri MF, Alkaabi SE, et al. The identification of novel therapeutic biomarkers in rheumatoid arthritis: a combined bioinformatics and integrated multi-omics approach. Int J Mol Sci. 2025;26(6) https://doi.org/10.3390/ijms26062757.
33. Fathalla BM, Alsarhan A, Afzal S, El Naofal M, Abou Tayoun A. The genomic landscape of pediatric rheumatology disorders in the Middle East. Hum Mutat. 2021;42(4):e1–e14. https://doi.org/10.1002/humu.24165.
34. Elhussein A, Baymuradov U, Consortium NA, Elhadad N, Natarajan K, Gursoy G. A framework for sharing of clinical and genetic data for precision medicine applications. Nat Med. 2024;30(12):3578–89. https://doi.org/10.1038/s41591-024-03239-5.
35. Avouac J, Marotte H, Balsa A, Chebbah M, Clanche SL, Verhagen LAW, et al. Teleconsultation in rheumatology: a literature review and opinion paper. Semin Arthritis Rheum. 2023;63:152271. https://doi.org/10.1016/j.semarthrit.2023.152271.
36. Ziade N, Hmamouchi I, El Kibbi L, Daou M, Abdulateef N, Abutiban F, et al. Telehealth in rheumatology: the 2021 Arab league of rheumatology best practice guidelines. Rheumatol Int. 2022;42(3):379–90. https://doi.org/10.1007/s00296-021-05078-w.
37. Xu L, Bressem K, Adams L, Poddubnyy D, Proft F. AI for imaging evaluation in rheumatology: applications of radiomics and computer vision-current status, future prospects and potential challenges. Rheumatol Adv Pract. 2025;9(2):rkae147. https://doi.org/10.1093/rap/rkae147.
38. Stoel BC, Staring M, Reijnierse M, van der Helm-van Mil AHM. Deep learning in rheumatological image interpretation. Nat Rev Rheumatol. 2024;20(3):182–95. https://doi.org/10.1038/s41584-023-01074-5.
39. Alnaqbi KA, Fragío-Gil JJ, K H, Statache G, Abouelnadar A, Almarzooqi A, et al. Deep learning tool for lesion detection in axial spondyloarthritis patients with active sacroiliitis on magnetic resonance imaging [abstract]. Arthritis Rheumatol. 2025;77(Suppl 9)
40. Gharib M, Khandakar A, Ayari M, Al emadi S. ASembleNet: a hybrid AI model for MRI-based classification of ankylosing spondylitis [abstract]. Arthritis Rheumatol. 2025;77(Suppl 9)
41. Badsha H, Khan B, Harifi G, Raman AJS. Artificial intelligence in rheumatology: evaluation of a proprietary rule engine and GPT-4 for the initial assessment of rheumatology cases [abstract]. Ann Rheum Dis. 2024;83(Suppl 1):2112. https://doi.org/10.1136/annrheumdis-2024-eular.1942.
42. Soulard J, Carlin T, Knitza J, Vuillerme N. Wearables for measuring the physical activity and sedentary behavior of patients with axial Spondyloarthritis: systematic review. JMIR Mhealth Uhealth. 2022;10(8):e34734. https://doi.org/10.2196/34734.
43. Aboagye NY, Hinchliffe C, Del Din S, Ng WF, Baker KF, Baker MR. Systematic review: digital biomarkers of fatigue in chronic diseases. NPJ Digit Med. 2025;8(1):602. https://doi.org/10.1038/s41746-025-01939-x.
44. Tung HY, Galloway J, Matcham F, Boalch A, Shand G, Norton S. Feasibility of remote measurement in intensive longitudinal data collection for rheumatoid arthritis patients commencing a new treatment. Rheumatol Adv Pract. 2025;9(3):rkaf078. https://doi.org/10.1093/rap/rkaf078.
45. Drummond D, Gonsard A. Definitions and characteristics of patient digital twins being developed for clinical use: scoping review. J Med Internet Res. 2024;26:e58504. https://doi.org/10.2196/58504.
46. Zerrouk N, Auge F, Niarakis A. Building a modular and multi-cellular virtual twin of the synovial joint in rheumatoid arthritis. NPJ Digit Med. 2024;7(1):379. https://doi.org/10.1038/s41746-024-01396-y.

47. Morrison T, Foster E, Dougherty J, Barton J. Shared decision making in rheumatology: a scoping review. Semin Arthritis Rheum. 2022;56:152041. https://doi.org/10.1016/j.semarthrit.2022.152041.
48. Alzubaidi H, Samorinha C, Saidawi W, Hussein A, Saddik B, Scholl I. Preference for shared decision-making among Arabic-speaking people with chronic diseases: a cross-sectional study. BMJ Open. 2022;12(4):e058084. https://doi.org/10.1136/bmjopen-2021-058084.
49. Fayad F, Ziade NR, Merheb G, Attoui S, Aiko A, Mroue K, et al. Patient preferences for rheumatoid arthritis treatments: results from the national cross-sectional LERACS study. Patient Prefer Adherence. 2018;12:1619–25. https://doi.org/10.2147/PPA.S168738.
50. Bukhari RI, Alamr R, Alsindi RA, Hafiz BF, Gadah AA, Awad NA, et al. Preferred mode of therapy among patients in rheumatoid arthritis Saudi database: a cross-sectional study. Cureus. 2023;15(6):e41014. https://doi.org/10.7759/cureus.41014.
51. Rheumatism Association [Internet]. Arabic. Saudi Arabia. [cited 2026 May 16]. Available from: https://rheumatism.org.sa.
52. Fibro Association. Saudi Fibromyalgia Care Association [Internet]. Arabic. Saudi Arabia. [cited 2026 May 16]. Available from: https://fibro.sa/.
53. Manyazewal T, Woldeamanuel Y, Oppenheim C, Hailu A, Giday M, Medhin G, et al. Conceptualising centres of excellence: a scoping review of global evidence. BMJ Open. 2022;12(2):e050419. https://doi.org/10.1136/bmjopen-2021-050419.
54. Frank JR, Taber S, van Zanten M, Scheele F, Blouin D, International Health Professions Accreditation Outcomes C. The role of accreditation in 21st century health professions education: report of an international consensus group. BMC Med Educ. 2020;20(Suppl 1):305. https://doi.org/10.1186/s12909-020-02121-5.
55. European Alliance of Associations for Rheumatology (EULAR). EULAR Centres of Excellence. [cited 2026 May 16]. Available from: https://www.eular.org/eular-centres-of-excellence.
56. Asia-Pacific League of Associations for Rheumatology (APLAR). APLAR Centre of Excellence Collaboration. [cited 2026 May 16]. Available from: https://aplar.org/collaboration/center-of-excellence/.
57. The Joint Commission. Clinical Care Program Certification. [cited 2026 May 16]. Available from: https://www.jointcommission.org/en/certification/clinical-care-program.
58. Alnaqbi KA, Fazal F, Namas R. From sand to excellence: a deep dive into Abu Dhabi's rheumatology landscape. Mediterr J Rheumatol. 2024;35(1):73–82. https://doi.org/10.31138/mjr.011123.fst.
59. Joint Commission International: Who We Are – JCI-Accredited Organizations [Internet]. 2026. [cited 2026 May 16]. Available from: https://www.jointcommission.org/en/about-us/recognizing-excellence/find-accredited-international-organizations.
60. Sherman L, Aboulsoud S, Chappell K. An overview of continuing medical education/continuing professional development Systems in the Middle East and North Africa: a mixed methods assessment. J CME. 2024;13(1):2435737. https://doi.org/10.1080/28338073.2024.2435737.
61. Arab League of Associations for Rheumatology (ArLAR). Educational Library [Internet]. [cited 2026 Mar 8]. Available from: https://www.arabrheumatology.org/educational-library.
62. Dejaco C, Putrik P, Unger J, Aletaha D, Bianchi G, Bijlsma JW, et al. EULAR 'points to consider' for the conduction of workforce requirement studies in rheumatology. RMD Open. 2018;4(2):e000780. https://doi.org/10.1136/rmdopen-2018-000780.
63. Alnaqbi KA, Al Cheikh SA. Shaping the future: the transformative path of the Arab Board of Rheumatology. Cureus. 2023;15(9):e45624. https://doi.org/10.7759/cureus.45624.
64. Karpinski J, Ajjawi R, Moreau K. Fellowship training: a qualitative study of scope and purpose across one department of medicine. BMC Med Educ. 2017;17(1):223. https://doi.org/10.1186/s12909-017-1062-5.
65. Zimmerman R, Alweis R, Short A, Wasser T, Donato A. Interventions to increase research publications in graduate medical education trainees: a systematic review. Arch Med Sci. 2019;15(1):1–11. https://doi.org/10.5114/aoms.2018.81033.

66. Valentine J, Poulson J, Tamayo J, Valentine A, Levesque J, Jenks S. Impact of medical trainees on efficiency and productivity in the emergency department: systematic review and narrative synthesis. West J Emerg Med. 2024;25(5):767–76. https://doi.org/10.5811/westjem.18574.
67. Alweis R, Donato A, Terry R, Goodermote C, Qadri F, Mayo R. Benefits of developing graduate medical education programs in community health systems. J Community Hosp Intern Med Perspect. 2021;11(5):569–75. https://doi.org/10.1080/20009666.2021.1961381.
68. Uthman I, Almoallim H, Buckley CD, Masri B, Dahou-Makhloufi C, El Dershaby Y, et al. Nurse-led care for the management of rheumatoid arthritis: a review of the global literature and proposed strategies for implementation in Africa and the Middle East. Rheumatol Int. 2021;41(3):529–42. https://doi.org/10.1007/s00296-020-04682-6.
69. Bech B, Primdahl J, van Tubergen A, Voshaar M, Zangi HA, Barbosa L, et al. 2018 update of the EULAR recommendations for the role of the nurse in the management of chronic inflammatory arthritis. Ann Rheum Dis. 2020;79(1):61–8. https://doi.org/10.1136/annrheumdis-2019-215458.
70. Yang L, Xiang P, Pi G, Wen T, Liu L, Liu D. Effectiveness of nurse-led care in patients with rheumatoid arthritis: a systematic review and meta-analysis. BMJ Open Qual. 2025;14(1) https://doi.org/10.1136/bmjoq-2024-003037.
71. Stoilova S, Popova-Belova S, Geneva-Popova M. Nurses' role in patient education for managing inflammatory joint diseases: insights from a cross-sectional survey in Bulgarian rheumatology clinics. Healthcare (Basel). 2025;13(19) https://doi.org/10.3390/healthcare13192516.
72. Di Matteo A, Mankia K, Azukizawa M, Wakefield RJ. The role of musculoskeletal ultrasound in the rheumatoid arthritis continuum. Curr Rheumatol Rep. 2020;22(8):41. https://doi.org/10.1007/s11926-020-00911-w.
73. Costantino F, Carmona L, Boers M, Backhaus M, Balint PV, Bruyn GA, et al. EULAR recommendations for the reporting of ultrasound studies in rheumatic and musculoskeletal diseases (RMDs). Ann Rheum Dis. 2021;80(7):840–7. https://doi.org/10.1136/annrheumdis-2020-219816.
74. American College of Rheumatology (ACR). Rheumatology Musculoskeletal Ultrasound (RHMSUS) Certification [Internet]. [cited 2026 May 16]. Available from: https://rheumatology.org/rhmsus-certification.
75. European Alliance of Associations for Rheumatology (EULAR). Musculoskeletal Ultrasound Courses. EULAR Education Platform [Internet]. [cited 2026 May 16]. Available from: https://edu.eular.org/totara/catalog/index.php?catalog_cat_browse=75&orderbykey=time&itemstyle=narrow.
76. MENA Conference. Musculoskeletal sonography course, basic level, 14–17 December 2012 [Internet]. MENA Conference Archive [Internet]. 2012. [cited 2026 May 16]. Available from: https://archive.menaconference.com/mena_archives/Musculoskeletal%20Sonography%20Course%20,%20Basic%20Level%20-%2014th%20to%2017th%20December%202012.pdf.
77. Qatar Rheumatology Society. Qatar rheumatology society home page [internet]. Doha (Qatar): 2026. [cited 2026 May 16]. Available from: https://qrheumsoc.org/.
78. Arab League of Associations for Rheumatology (ArLAR). Musculoskeletal Sonography Group (MSSG) [Internet]. [cited 2026 Mar 8]. Available from: https://www.arabrheumatology.org/arlar-mssg.
79. Cutolo M, Herrick AL, Distler O, Becker MO, Beltran E, Carpentier P, et al. Nailfold Videocapillaroscopic features and other clinical risk factors for digital ulcers in systemic sclerosis: a multicenter, Prospective Cohort Study. Arthritis Rheumatol. 2016;68(10):2527–39. https://doi.org/10.1002/art.39718.
80. Hatzis C, Lerner D, Paget S, Cutolo M, Smith V, Spiera R, et al. Integration of capillary microscopy and dermoscopy into the rheumatology fellow curriculum. Clin Exp Rheumatol. 2017;35(5):850–2.
81. Kunjumon NM, Alam F, Al Emadi S, Becetti K. The 9th annual Saudi Society for Rheumatology Conference Abstracts Presented at the 9th SSRC 2023. Nailfold Videocapillaroscopy patterns and associated clinical features in systemic sclerosis in Qatar. Ann Rheumatol Autoimmun. 2023;3(1):14–21. https://doi.org/10.4103/ara.ara_3_23.

82. Darzi A, Harfouche M, Arayssi T, Alemadi S, Alnaqbi KA, Badsha H, et al. Adaptation of the 2015 American College of Rheumatology treatment guideline for rheumatoid arthritis for the eastern Mediterranean region: an exemplar of the GRADE Adolopment. Health Qual Life Outcomes. 2017;15(1):183. https://doi.org/10.1186/s12955-017-0754-1.
83. Arayssi T, Harfouche M, Darzi A, Al Emadi S, Alnaqbi KA, Badsha H, et al. Recommendations for the management of rheumatoid arthritis in the eastern Mediterranean region: an adolopment of the 2015 American College of Rheumatology guidelines. Clin Rheumatol. 2018;37(11):2947–59. https://doi.org/10.1007/s10067-018-4245-5.
84. Ziade N, El Kibbi L, Hmamouchi I, Abdulateef N, Halabi H, Hamdi W, et al. Impact of the COVID-19 pandemic on patients with chronic rheumatic diseases: a study in 15 Arab countries. Int J Rheum Dis. 2020;23(11):1550–7. https://doi.org/10.1111/1756-185X.13960.
85. El Kibbi L, Metawee M, Hmamouchi I, Abdulateef N, Halabi H, Eissa M, et al. Acceptability of the COVID-19 vaccine among patients with chronic rheumatic diseases and health-care professionals: a cross-sectional study in 19 Arab countries. Lancet Rheumatol. 2022;4(3):e160–e3. https://doi.org/10.1016/S2665-9913(21)00368-4.
86. Hmamouchi I, Abi Najm A, El Kibbi L, Metawee M, Halabi H, Abdulateef N, et al. How to optimize recruitment strategies of patients with rheumatic and musculoskeletal diseases for online surveys: experience from an international study. Rheumatol Int. 2023;43(4):705–12. https://doi.org/10.1007/s00296-022-05195-0.
87. Arab League of Associations for Rheumatology (ArLAR). ArLAR Research Group (ARCH) [Internet]. [cited 2026 Mar 8]. Available from: https://www.arabrheumatology.org/arch.
88. El Kibbi L, Halabi H, Masri B, Hmamouchi I, Metawee M, Alnaqbi K, et al. Shaping awareness about rheumatic and musculoskeletal diseases in the Arab region: the Arab adult arthritis awareness group initiative. Arab J Rheumatol. 2024;2(1):1–6. https://doi.org/10.4103/ajr.ajr_3_24.
89. Ziade N, Abbas N, Hmamouchi I, El Kibbi L, Maroof A, Elzorkany B, et al. Is the patient-perceived impact of psoriatic arthritis a global concept? An international study in 13 Arab countries (TACTIC study). Rheumatol Int. 2024;44(5):885–99. https://doi.org/10.1007/s00296-024-05552-1.
90. Arab Journal of Rheumatology [Internet]. [cited 2026 May 16]. Available from: https://journals.lww.com/ajrh/pages/default.aspx.
91. Al Maini M, Adelowo F, Al Saleh J, Al Weshahi Y, Burmester GR, Cutolo M, et al. The global challenges and opportunities in the practice of rheumatology: white paper by the world forum on rheumatic and musculoskeletal diseases. Clin Rheumatol. 2015;34(5):819–29. https://doi.org/10.1007/s10067-014-2841-6.
92. Tikly M, McGill P. Epidemiology: the challenge of practicing rheumatology in Africa. Nat Rev Rheumatol. 2016;12(11):630–1. https://doi.org/10.1038/nrrheum.2016.170.
93. Bayoumy K, MacDonald R, Dargham SR, Arayssi T. Bibliometric analysis of rheumatology research in the Arab countries. BMC Res Notes. 2016;9:393. https://doi.org/10.1186/s13104-016-2197-x.
94. Jawad ASM, Hasbani GE, Uthman I. Rheumatology research in Arab countries. Saudi Med J. 2024;45(5):542. https://doi.org/10.15537/smj.2024.45.5.20240362.
95. Alnaimat F, Sweis NJ, Sweis JJG, Ascoli C, Korsten P, Rubinstein I, et al. Reproducibility and rigor in rheumatology research. Front Med (Lausanne). 2022;9:1073551. https://doi.org/10.3389/fmed.2022.1073551.
96. Bilsborrow JB, Pelaez-Ballestas I, Pons-Estel B, Scott C, Tian X, Alarcon GS, et al. Global rheumatology research: frontiers, challenges, and opportunities. Arthritis Rheumatol. 2022;74(1):1–4. https://doi.org/10.1002/art.41980.
97. Ismail SA, McDonald A, Dubois E, Aljohani FG, Coutts AP, Majeed A, et al. Assessing the state of health research in the eastern Mediterranean region. J R Soc Med. 2013;106(6):224–33. https://doi.org/10.1258/jrsm.2012.120240.
98. El-Jardali F, Lavis JN, Ataya N, Jamal D. Use of health systems and policy research evidence in the health policymaking in eastern Mediterranean countries: views and practices of researchers. Implement Sci. 2012;7:2. https://doi.org/10.1186/1748-5908-7-2.

99. AlKhaldi M, Al-Surimi K, Meghari H. Health policy and systems research in the Arab world: concepts, evolution, challenges, and application necessity for COVID-19 pandemic and beyond. In: Laher I, editor. Health policy and systems research in the Arab world. Cham: Springer Nature Switzerland AG; 2020. https://doi.org/10.1007/978-3-319-74365-3_62-1.
100. Sheblaq N, Al Najjar A. The challenges in conducting research studies in Arabic countries. Open Access J Clin Trials 2019;11:57–66. doi:https://doi.org/10.2147/OAJCT.S215738.
101. Sitthi-Amorn C, Somrongthong R. Strengthening health research capacity in developing countries: a critical element for achieving health equity. BMJ. 2000;321(7264):813–7. https://doi.org/10.1136/bmj.321.7264.813.
102. Yoong SL, Bolsewicz K, Reilly K, Williams C, Wolfenden L, Grady A, et al. Describing the evidence-base for research engagement by health care providers and health care organisations: a scoping review. BMC Health Serv Res. 2023;23(1):75. https://doi.org/10.1186/s12913-022-08887-2.
103. Marzban S, Najafi M, Agolli A, Ashrafi E. Impact of patient engagement on healthcare quality: a scoping review. J Patient Exp. 2022;9:23743735221125439. https://doi.org/10.1177/23743735221125439.
104. Ngutete Mukundwa P, Alayande BT, Iradukunda D, Fenta B, Bucyibaruta G, Ojomo O, et al. Building research capacity in the global south: insights from a scientific writing workshop. BMC Med Educ. 2026; https://doi.org/10.1186/s12909-026-08811-w.
105. Alnaqbi KA, Aldabie G, Enizi AA, Abdulkarim S, Satti E, Lawati TA, et al. 2025 consensus-based recommendations for the referral, diagnosis, monitoring, and management of axial spondyloarthritis in the Arabian gulf countries. Semin Arthritis Rheum. 2025;75:152828. https://doi.org/10.1016/j.semarthrit.2025.152828.
106. Nabil Y, Eldaw A, El-Shourbagy D, Ibrahim D, Alturkistani H, Alshahrani M, et al. Unmet needs and strategies to promote patient engagement in the Arab world: experts' opinion. Cureus. 2024;16(3):e56804. https://doi.org/10.7759/cureus.56804.
107. International Committee of Medical Journal Editors. Defining the role of authors and contributors. In: Recommendations for the Conduct, Reporting, Editing, and Publication of Scholarly Work in Medical Journals [Internet]. ICMJE. [cited 2026 May 16]. Available from: https://www.icmje.org/recommendations/browse/roles-and-responsibilities/defining-the-role-of-authors-and-contributors.html.
108. Annals of Rheumatology and Autoimmunity [Internet]. [cited 2026 May 16]. Available from: https://journals.lww.com/aora/pages/default.aspx.

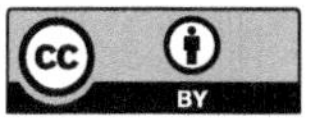

GPSR Compliance

The European Union's (EU) General Product Safety Regulation (GPSR) is a set of rules that requires consumer products to be safe and our obligations to ensure this.

If you have any concerns about our products, you can contact us on ProductSafety@springernature.com

In case Publisher is established outside the EU, the EU authorized representative is:

Springer Nature Customer Service Center GmbH
Europaplatz 3
69115 Heidelberg, Germany

Batch number: 10406357

Printed by Printforce, the Netherlands

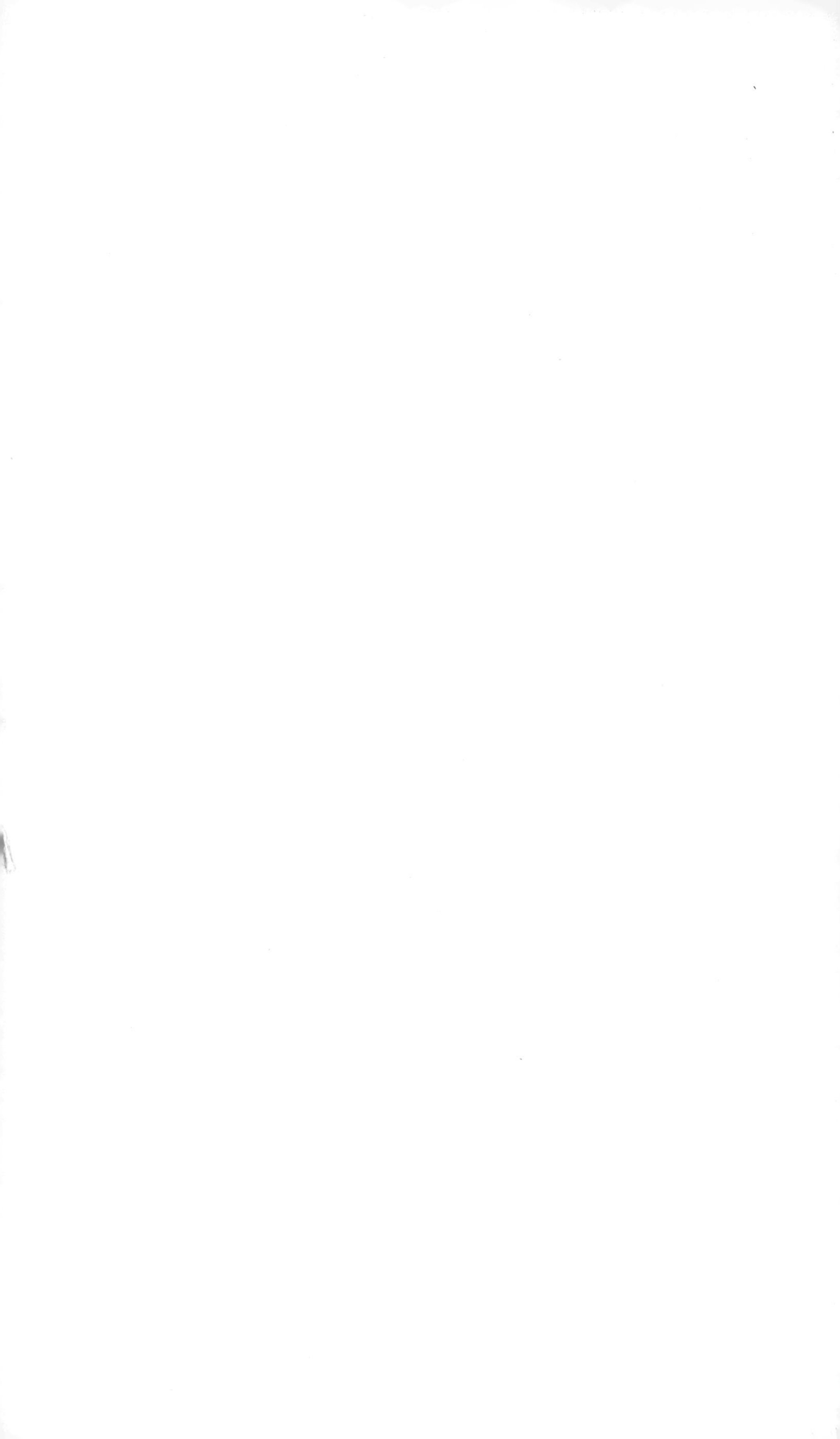